ANNALS OF
THE NEW YORK ACADEMY
OF SCIENCES

Volume 830

EDITORIAL STAFF

Executive Editor
BILL BOLAND

Managing Editor
JUSTINE CULLINAN

Associate Editor
TRUMBULL ROGERS

The New York Academy of Sciences
2 East 63rd Street
New York, New York 10021

IMMUNOLOGIC DISEASES
OF THE EAR

ANNALS OF THE NEW YORK ACADEMY OF SCIENCES
Volume 830

IMMUNOLOGIC DISEASES OF THE EAR

Edited by Joel M. Bernstein, Howard S. Faden, Donald Henderson, Allen F. Ryan, Maurizio Barbara, and Antonio Quaranta

The New York Academy of Sciences
New York, New York
1997

Library of Congress Cataloging-in-Publication Data

Immunologic diseases of the ear / edited by Joel M. Bernstein . . . [et al.].
    p.   cm. — (Annals of the New York Academy of Sciences, ISSN 0077-8923 ; v. 830)
    Includes bibliographical references and index.
    ISBN 1-57331-100-6 (cloth : alk. paper). — ISBN 1-57331-101-4 (paper : alk. paper)
    1. Ear—Diseases—Immunological aspects—Congresses.
I. Bernstein, Joel M.   II. New York Academy of Sciences.
III. Series.
    [DNLM: 1. Ear Diseases—immunology—congresses.   W1 AN626YL v.830 1997]
Q11.N5   vol. 830
[RF122]
500 s—dc21
[617.8'079]
DNLM/DLC
for Library of Congress   97-42727
                                           CIP

&/PCP
Printed in the United States of America
ISBN 1-57331-100-6 (cloth)
ISBN 1-57331-101-4 (paper)
ISSN 0077-8923

ANNALS OF THE NEW YORK ACADEMY OF SCIENCES

Volume 830
December 29, 1997

IMMUNOLOGIC DISEASES OF THE EAR[a]

Editors
JOEL M. BERNSTEIN, HOWARD S. FADEN, DONALD HENDERSON, ALLEN F. RYAN,
MAURIZIO BARBARA, AND ANTONIO QUARANTA

Conference Organizers
JOEL M. BERNSTEIN, HOWARD S. FADEN, DONALD HENDERSON, MAURIZIO BARBARA,
ANTONIO QUARANTA, ALLEN F. RYAN, SALVATORE IURATO, AND E. CASSANDRO

CONTENTS

[a]This volume contains the papers from a conference entitled *Immunological Diseases of the Ear*, which was held in Positano, Italy, on October 24–26, 1996.

Part 3. Immunologic and Inflammatory Mechanisms Causing Complications in Otitis Media

Part 4. Immunology of the Inner Ear

Part 5. Animal Models of Autoimmune Disease of the Inner Ear

Part 6. Human Immunological and Viral Diseases of the Inner Ear

Part 7. New Horizons in the Immunology of the Ear

Financial assistance was received from:

Contributors

- AMPLIFON S.p.A.—MILAN, ITALY
- ASTA MEDICA—MILAN
- AUDIOMEDICAL -POMPEI
- BRISTOL-MYERS SQUIBB COMPANY
- CENTER FOR HEARING AND DEAFNESS, STATE UNIVERSITY OF NEW YORK AT BUFFALO
- CONNAUGHT LABORATORIES, INC.
- ELI LILLY COMPANY
- PFIZER INC.
- SMITHKLINE BEECHAM
- THE UPJOHN COMPANY
- WYETH-AYERST LABORATORIES

Preface

JOEL M. BERNSTEIN,[a] HOWARD FADEN,[b] DONALD HENDERSON,[c]
ALLEN F. RYAN,[d] MAURIZIO BARBARA,[e] AND ANTONIO QUARANTA[f]

*[a]4949 Harlem Road
Amherst, New York 14226*

*[b]Department of Pediatrics
Children's Hospital of Buffalo
219 Bryant Street
Buffalo, New York 14222*

*[c]State University of New York at Buffalo
Center for Hearing and Deafness
Hearing Research Laboratory
215 Parker Hall
Buffalo, New York 14214*

*[d]ENT Department
University of California at San Diego
9500 Gilman Drive
La Jolla, California 92093-0666*

*[e]Department of Otolaryngology
University "La Sapienza"
Rome, 00185 Italy*

*[f]Department of Audiology and Otology
University of Bari
Bari, 70124 Italy*

The immunology of the middle and inner ear is a relatively new field of study. Until recently, the ear and its disorders were not part of mainstream immunology because the prevailing view was that both structures were immunoincompetent. In 1987, Bernstein and Ogra published *Immunology of the Ear*, summarizing and integrating clinical and basic research. The book quickly became a standard reference. In the last ten years there has been an enormous volume of literature dealing with cellular and immune mechanisms in the nasopharynx, middle ear, and inner ear. In addition, the new field of molecular biology created a similarly broad fund of knowledge relevant to understanding otitis media (OM) and various types of sensorineural hearing impairments. The importance and prevalence of the problems addressed, as well as the solid advances already made, prompted the organization of a second conference to integrate and analyze data with the ultimate goal of publishing this volume.

The first topic of the symposium, *Immunology of Mucosal Surfaces*, updates our knowledge of secretory IgA and its role in the nasopharynx and middle ear. Recent evidence suggests that children who are colonized by potential pathogens earlier in life and who have a poor local immune response, develop OM earlier in life and tend to become otitis prone. A critical understanding of immune mechanisms involved in the nasopharynx may lead to a better approach to treatment of the disease. This would be an extremely important outcome in light of the failure of antibiotics to eradicate OM and the emergence of antibiotic-resistant bacteria that has occurred over the last forty years.

The middle ear has been considered an immunoincompetent space because the middle-ear mucosa possesses very few lymphocytes, very few capillaries, and no organized lymphoid tissue of its own. However, during infection or allergic diatheses, the inflammatory response leads to the movement of immunologic cells into the middle-ear space. The second topic of the symposium is *Specific Immunologic Mechanisms in the Development of Otitis Media*. Information is presented on the homing of lymphocytes into the middle ear and the sources of those lymphocytes, including areas such as the tonsils and adenoids, the bronchopulmonary lymphoid tissue, Peyer's patches, and other organized mucosal lymphoid tissues. Knowledge gained from discussion of this topic is critical for our understanding of immunological processes and for the development of vaccines for the prevention of OM.

The third topic, *Molecular Basis of Bone Resorption in Chronic Otitis Media with and without Cholesteatoma*, was chosen because the resolution of OM may take weeks or months. The same mechanisms involved in clearing the disease may also be responsible for some complications. Bone resorption has now been documented to occur as a result of nonimmune mechanisms as well as by specific immune mechanisms. The molecular biology of bone resorption is elegantly reviewed by Chole.

Interactions Between the Middle Ear and the Inner Ear is the fourth topic. It has been a topic of several international symposia conducted over the last three years. The pathways of these interactions may be through lymphatics, through the round window, and oval window, or, perhaps, by retrograde extension via nerve fibers. A review of the interactions between middle ear and inner ear is discussed, particularly with regard to bacterial products, viral infection, antibiotics, and inflammatory mediators. These substances may not only cause middle-ear pathology, but may also be responsible for temporary or permanent dysfunction of the inner ear.

The fifth topic addresses *Immunology of the Inner Ear* and includes a review of clinical and experimental animal studies. Since 1987, advances in our understanding of cellular immunology, molecular biology, and genetics have strongly supported the possibility of autoimmunity of the inner ear as one cause of progressive sensorineural hearing loss. Advances in molecular biology using new techniques have suggested that some patients with progressive sensorineural hearing disorders may have a specific antibody directed against heat shock protein 70 (HSP 70). It is interesting to note that this protein in genetically coded on the short arm of chromosome 6, an area that is extremely close to the coding site for HLA antigens. Work from several laboratories suggests that specific HLA antigen haplotypes may be associated with an increased risk of developing inner-ear diseases such as Ménière's disease, strial presbycusis and otosclerosis. Because several inflammatory mediators, such as HSP 70, tumor necrosis factor alpha (TNF-α), and lymphotoxin tumor necrosis factor beta (TNF-β) are coded on chromosome 6, it is interesting to speculate that the HLA antigens may be associated with various inflammatory mediators that are responsible for the development of autoimmune disease of the inner ear. Autoantibodies against these inflammatory mediators may be important markers for the study of disease and for the clinical identification of patients who may respond to immunosuppressive therapy.

The inner ear may be a target for both autoimmunity and systemic immunological diseases. Several papers provide an update of the auditory findings and laboratory tests that are available and could provide the opportunity to specifically diagnose immune-mediated inner-ear disease.

Finally, because antibiotics fail to cure every case of OM, and because children still die of complications associated with this disease, it is obvious that other strategies for the treatment of OM are required. Several papers provide an update on our understanding of prevention of OM with immunization against bacteria and viruses. In addition, viral infections of the inner ear as a cause of otosclerosis and other sensorineural hearing disorders are thoroughly discussed. The volume includes focused reviews of the proceedings by Ogra and Ryan.

The organization of an international symposium with representatives from thirteen countries presents a formidable logistical challenge. Ms. Olimpia Cassano handled arrangements in Italy that were flawless and led to a memorable experience for everyone in attendance. Ms. Carol Altman handled all the presymposium arrangements for speakers and attendees, as well as service as the conference treasurer. Her intelligence and professionalism made a complicated task run smoothly. While every author presents a "perfect" manuscript, Mrs. Judith Maurino helped to organize all the papers into an integrated volume. We also thank Bill Boland and his editorial staff for the fine job they did in producing this volume. Finally, we want to thank the pharmaceutical industry, whose financial support allowed us to bring the speakers together from countries throughout the world.

Mucosal Immunology of the Upper Airways: An Overview[a]

P. BRANDTZAEG,[b] F. L. JAHNSEN, I. N. FARSTAD, AND G. HARALDSEN

Laboratory for Immunohistochemistry and Immunopathology (LIIPAT)
Institute of Pathology
University of Oslo
The National Hospital, Rikshospitalet
N-0027 Oslo, Norway

INTRODUCTION

This review focuses on the role of mucosal immunity in the defense of the upper airways and putative mechanisms of importance for tolerance induction as part of normal mucosal homeostasis. Alterations of the local immune system associated with chronic inflammation are also discussed in the context of aberrant immune regulation and modified leukocyte extravasation. In respiratory mucosae these changes are reflected in a shift of local immunoglobulin (Ig) -producing cells from IgA to an increasing contribution of IgG and often IgD, enhanced or induced expression of endothelial adhesion molecules, and in certain conditions a striking accumulation of eosinophilic granulocytes.

MUCOSAL ANTIBODY DEFENSE

The mucosae of the upper airways are primarily protected by a secretory immune system that is under complex immunoregulatory control.[1] This specific defense system depends on B cells with a remarkable potential for expression of J-chain, an essential component of polymeric immunoglobulins (pIg). The initial induction or priming of these B cells is believed to take place mainly in organized mucosa-associated lymphoid tissue (MALT) that consists of lymphoepithelial structures such as those constituting Waldeyer's pharyngeal ring.[2,3] The primed B cells (and also primed T cells) migrate through lymph and blood to secretory tissues including the airway mucosae where they go through terminal differentiation to Ig-producing plasma cells (see below).

Most Ig produced at such mucosal effector sites normally consists of dimers and larger polymers of IgA, collectively called polymeric IgA (pIgA). A selective transport mechanism exists to "pump" J-chain-containing pIgA through secretory epithelial cells by means of a basolaterally expressed receptor protein called transmem-

[a]Studies in the authors' laboratory were supported by the Norwegian Cancer Society, the Research Council of Norway, the Research Fund for Asthma and Allergy, and the Red Cross Research Fund for Children with Asthma and Allergy.

[b]Author to whom correspondence should be addressed. Phone: +47/22 86 86 34/35/27; fax: +47/22 86 86 40/22 11 22 61; e-mail: per.brandtzag@rh.uio.no

brane secretory component (SC) or the pIg receptor (FIG. 1). Pentameric IgM also contains J-chain, and is therefore subjected to active epithelial transport in a manner similar to pIgA.[1]

The generated secretory antibodies (SIgA and SIgM) perform immune exclusion by inhibiting uptake of soluble antigens and by blocking epithelial colonization of microorganisms (FIG. 1). However, this reinforcement of the mucosal barrier function is highly dependent on intact natural defense mechanisms with which the secretory antibodies normally cooperate in various ways.[2] These innate protective factors include antimicrobial substances such as lactoferrin produced by the mucosal glands

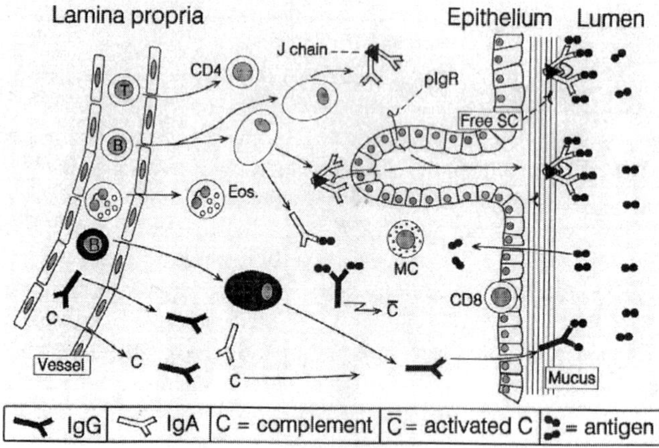

FIGURE 1. Putative balance between normal and altered mucosal homeostasis is determined by the "gatekeeper" function of the microvascular endothelium **(to the left)**. Extravasation is normally restricted largely to MALT-derived primed B and T cells (CD4 and CD8 phenotypes). Such B cells terminate their differentiation in the mucosa mainly as J-chain-expressing plasma cells that produce dimeric IgA. These polymers are readily picked up by the transmembrane secretory component (SC), also called pIg receptor (pIgR), which is expressed basolaterally on glandular epithelial cells **(at the top)**. The resulting secretory IgA antibodies contribute to normal homeostasis in a first line of defense by performing immune exclusion of antigens in the mucus layer on the epithelial surface together with smaller amounts of passively transferred IgG antibodies **(to the right)**. Free SC is generated when unoccupied pIgR is cleaved at the apical face of the epithelial cell. Altered homeostasis **(at the bottom)** is reflected by distorted mucosal B-cell accumulation giving rise to excessive local IgG production combined with increased endothelial and epithelial permeability. The profile of endothelial adhesion molecules is modulated by cytokines to facilitate emigration of B and T cells belonging to the systemic immune system as well as mast cells (MC) armed with IgE and eosinophils (Eos). Serum-derived or locally produced IgG contributes to a second line of defense in the lamina propria by performing immune elimination in an attempt to limit dissemination of foreign antigens. Due to the proinflammatory properties of IgG antibodies, a vicious circle may develop with further increase of endothelial and epithelial penetrability, intensified complement activation, massive attraction of phagocytes, and release of a variety of inflammatory mediators. Such a development may result in aggravation and perpetuation of inflammation as a basis for chronic mucosal disease, but it is counteracted by noninflammatory IgA antibodies in the lamina propria competing for penetrating antigens as schematically depicted.

as well as physical mechanisms such as mucin and the ciliary function in the airways.

It is difficult to evaluate the clinical role of SIgA antibodies, as the possibility of a superimposed protective effect of concurrently elicited systemic immune responses has to be considered. Live mucosal immunogens usually stimulate considerable levels of serum IgG, IgA, and IgM antibodies in addition to a local SIgA response; and the effect of mucosal inflammation on leakage of serum-derived or locally produced IgG antibodies into exocrine secretions during natural infections or after topical application of live virus vaccines is well documented.[2] Such passively transferred IgG would likely be protective according to the principle of "pathotopic potentiation" of local respiratory immunity as described in experimental animals.[2]

In patients with selective IgA deficiency, SIgA is lacking, but it may be satisfactorily replaced by protective "compensatory" SIgM antibodies in addition to mucosal IgG responses in the airways. In other IgA-deficient patients, however, the disordered immune regulation gives rise to a large number of IgD-producing immunocytes in the upper aerodigestive tract.[4] IgD cannot act as a secretory antibody but may, instead, block antibody-mediated defense functions (see below); patients with local overproduction of IgD are in fact prone to have recurrent airway infections.[4] Such observations show that there are large individual variations in the mucosal immune system.

IgA exists as two subclasses, IgA1 being preferentially produced in nasal and bronchial mucosae.[5] This is intriguing in view of the frequent synthesis of IgA1-specific proteases by *Haemophilus influenzae, Streptococcus pneumoniae,* and *Neisseria meningitidis*—three bacteria that tend to produce invasive diseases of the upper respiratory tract. A relationship of this proneness to an enzymatically induced deterioration of regional SIgA-dependent immunity has been proposed.[6] Interestingly, children with atopic allergy have increased amounts of IgA1 split products in their nasopharyngeal secretions,[7] and their nasopharynx may be colonized by IgA1-specific protease-producing bacteria in an early vulnerable period.[8]

RECRUITMENT OF LEUKOCYTES TO MUCOSAL TISSUES

Extravascular recruitment of immune cells and inflammatory cells is controlled by dynamically regulated complementary adhesion molecules expressed on the surface of circulating leukocytes and on the endothelium of venules. Such molecules regulate the trafficking (recirculation) of naive lymphocytes through organized lymphoid tissue and particularly the dissemination (homing) of primed B and T cells to immunological effector sites such as the mucosae, as well as the extravasation of different leukocytes in inflammation.[9,10]

All kinds of cells express various families of adhesion molecules, and some appear more important than others in direction certain leukocytes to selected tissue sites. Receptors on the luminal face of the endothelial cells communicate via corresponding ligands or counterreceptors expressed by circulating leukocytes to initiate their extravasation.[9] This multistep process involves not only several integral surface molecules but also a variety of chemokines (chemoattractant cytokines) derived from extravascular or endothelial cells.[11] The first step is independent of leukocyte activation, being mediated mainly by adhesion molecules (selectins) that react with mucinlike ligands (FIG. 2). The initial attachment (tethering) of the free-flowing leukocytes is relatively loose and allows "rolling" on the endothelium (high "on-off" rate). The leukocytes are then subjected to activation signals provided by various chemoattractants. This leads to cellular polarization and participation of secondary receptor–ligand pairs providing firm adhesion by means of activated leukocyte integrins that bind to endothelial receptors belonging to the Ig gene superfamily.[12] Finally, chemoattractants direct the extravasation of the arrested leukocytes, involving crawling along the endothelium where chemokines are deposited in a solid phase, active diapedesis, and migration into the tissue site, presumably along a gradient of signals.[11]

The endothelial adhesion molecules may be constitutively expressed or are inducible, and they can be modulated by various cytokines, especially in inflammatory lesions (FIG. 3). Animal experiments have suggested an important role for constitutive ICAM-1 (intercellular adhesion molecule-1; member of the Ig superfamily = CD54) in the general influx of leukocytes into the airway mucosa.[9] Still another endothelial receptor, E-selectin (endothelial adhesion molecule-1; previously called ELAM-1 = CD62E) appears to be particularly involved in the extravasation of neutrophils.[9] Tumour necrosis factor-α (TNF-α) and interleukin-1 (IL-1) are important for up-regulation of ICAM-1 on endothelial cells;[13] activated macrophages that secrete these cytokines can therefore enhance the function of ICAM-1. An array of other cytokines and different mediators contribute to the expression of other adhesion molecules on endothelial cells (FIG. 3).

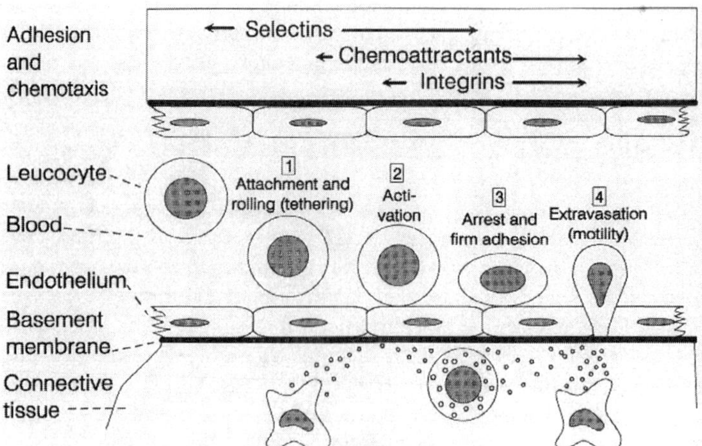

FIGURE 2. Four overlapping sequential steps **(at the top)** in controlled extravasation of leukocytes, involving adhesion molecules as well as chemotactic factors (o) derived from extravascular cells **(at the bottom)**. The free-flowing leukocytes first use activation-independent molecules to interact loosely with endothelial receptors (1). Activation signals (2) lead to participation of secondary receptor–ligand pairs providing firm adhesion (3), and chemoattractants direct the extravasation of the arrested leukocytes (4).

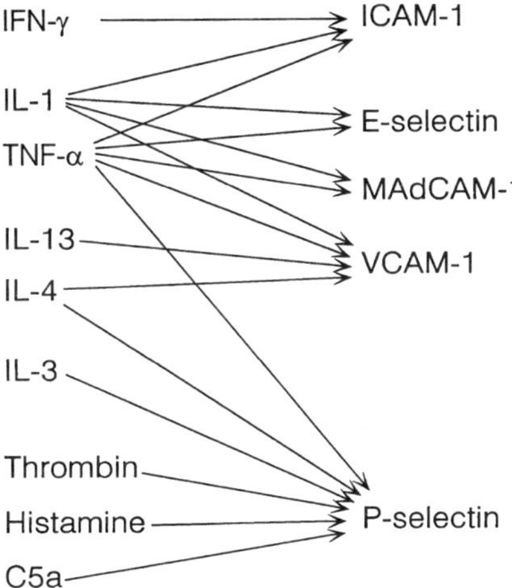

FIGURE 3. Cytokines and other mediators that can induce or upregulate cell-surface expression of various adhesion molecules on endothelial cells.

DISSEMINATION OF IMMUNE CELLS TO MUCOSAL EFFECTOR SITES

Mucosal Homing Mechanisms for Primed B and T Cells

Experimental data have revealed that certain lymphoid adhesion molecules are more strongly expressed by unprimed ("naive") than by primed ("memory") lymphocytes, and vice versa, and some of them are relatively tissue-specific in their function. L-selectin apparently directs naive lymphocytes mainly to peripheral lymph nodes, but also contributes to their recirculation through inductive MALT structures.[10] The integrin α4β7, on the other hand, appears crucial for the homing of primed (memory and effector) lymphocytes, not only to the organized MALT but particularly to mucosal effector sites such as the intestinal lamina propria.[10,11] The endothelial receptor for this integrin is called mucosal addressin cell adhesion molecule-1 (MAdCAM-1), the regulation of which may involve TNF-α and probably other cytokines.[14] Both T and B cells express high levels of α4β7 when they arrive in the intestinal lamina propria and undergo terminal differentiation to effector cells.[15] However, little detailed knowledge is available about lymphocyte homing in the upper airways; the mechanisms may be similar to those operating in the gut, but additional unique features probably exist.[16] The apparent dichotomy between the upper aerodigestive tract and the gut with regard to the isotype pattern (IgA1 versus IgA2) of secretory immunity[5] may depend on different profiles of adhesion molecules expressed by regional B cells and/or by the local microvascular endothelium. Differential immunoregulatory effects of the local microbiota may be involved as well.[5]

A second integrin called αEβ7 is abundantly expressed on intestinal mucosal T lymphocytes, especially on the CD8[+] subset that migrates into the epithelium (FIG. 1), where this integrin binds to E-cadherin.[17] This interaction may explain the retention of intraepithelial lymphocytes (IEL), and αEβ7 is mainly expressed on the predominant CD8[+]IEL subset that bears the ordinary T-cell receptor (TCRα/β) as well as on the minor intraepithelial TCRγ/δ[+] subset. A high level of αEβ7 has recently been shown also on CD8[+]IEL in human airway mucosa.[18]

Induction of Immune Cells in MALT of the Upper Airways

As mentioned earlier, mucosal lymphoid cells are supposed to be primed mainly in various organized MALT structures, which all show principally a similar morphology dominated by secondary (or activated) B-cell follicles with germinal centers covered by a specialized follicle-associated epithelium.[3] Large collections of T cells along with dendritic antigen-presenting cells (APC) are found between the follicles and this epithelium that contains so-called M ("membrane") cells actively transporting foreign antigens inwards from the mucosal surface.[1] These antigens are next presented as immunogenic peptides to T cells after being processed by HLA class II-positive extrafollicular APC, whereas native antigens are presented in immune complexes to B lymphocytes within the germinal centers.[3] In this way memory B cells with high receptor affinity for specific antigen are generated for subsequent distribution through lymph and peripheral blood to various exocrine tissues (FIG. 4).

Experimental animal work on MALT of the upper airways has focused on the paired lymphocytic cell aggregates that occur in rodents at the entrance of the nasopharyngeal duct.[19] The inductive function of this nasal-associated lymphoid tissue (NALT) may be crucial for immunity of the upper aerodigestive tract. In humans, MALT structures of this region are constituted mainly by the palatine tonsils, the nasopharyngeal tonsil (adenoids), and the lingual tonsil that together constitute most of Waldeyer's ring, while the lateral pharyngeal bands are less prominent components.[20] In addition, similar lymphoid structures are often present associated with the larynx (LALT)[21], and also at the entrance of the eustachian tube (TALT), the latter (so-called tubal tonsils) to some extent being inflammation-dependent.[22] Although it remains uncertain whether all these organized lymphoepithelial structures are functionally comparable to NALT in rodents,[19] they are indeed strategically located to orchestrate regional immune functions against both airborne and alimentary antigens (FIG. 4). As discussed below, there is at least circumstantial evidence to suggest that the palatine tonsils and adenoids belong to MALT in addition to giving rise to considerable *in situ* differentiation to plasma cells, the latter feature being unlike the situation in Peyer's patches, which are the best studied parts of gut-associated lymphoid tissue (GALT).[23]

All categories of tonsil contain four lymphoid cell compartments, namely the reticular crypt epithelium, the extrafollicular area, the mantle zones of lymphoid follicles, and the follicular germinal centers.[24,25] Primary follicles are present as early as 16 weeks' gestation, but formation of germinal centers reflecting B-cell activation by exogenous antigens does not take place until shortly after birth; terminal differentiation of B cells to extrafollicular plasma cells can be seen about 2 weeks postnatally.[24] The reticular crypt epithelium is well designed for uptake of antigens both through M cells[24] and by its large content of professional dendritic cells,[25] as well as memory B cells negative for surface (s) IgD (sIgD[-]IgM[+]CD38[+]B7[+])[26,27] with antigen-presenting properties (FIG. 5).

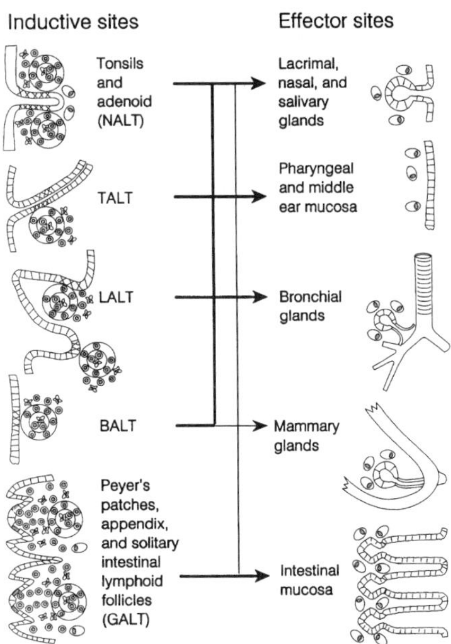

FIGURE 4. Model for putative homing pathways of primed lymphoid cells from inductive sites to effector sites in the integrated mucosal immune system. Presumed compartmentalization is indicated, the *heavier arrows* representing preferential migration routes of primed B and T cells. Homing from gut-associated lymphoid tissue (GALT) appears to be determined mainly by integrin $\alpha4\beta7$ interacting with MAdCAM-1, expressed on the microvascular endothelium in the intestinal lamina propria (see text for details). Other interactions may be more important for immune cells primed in nasal-associated lymphoid tissue (NALT), eusthasian tube-associated lymphoid tissue (TALT), larynx-associated lymphoid tissue (LALT), and bronchus-associated lymphoid tissue (BALT). Among these organized lymphoepithelial structures, NALT has obvious advantages as inductive tissue because of its antigen-retaining crypts (and absence of antigen-degrading digestive enzymes). Lactating mammary glands apparently receive primed immune cells from inductive tissues in both airways and gut.

The germinal centers characteristically arise in T-cell-dependent B-cell responses and are associated with: (1) clonal expansion of B cells; (2) somatic hypermutation in B-cell Ig variable (*Ig V*)-region genes; (3) positive selection of B cells that are able to receive antigen-specific signals by high affinity; (4) subsequent differentiation to memory B cells and plasma cells of various isotypes; and (5) induction of the J-chain gene in a variable subset of B cells.[3] The founder cell for this fascinating B-cell development has recently been tentatively identified within the dark zone of tonsillar germinal centers[27] as a sIgD+IgM+CD38+ proliferative (Ki-67+) lymphocyte subset (FIG. 5).

The tonsillar germinal center reaction normally generates a variable number of intrafollicular Ig-producing immunocytes (plasmablasts and plasma cells (predominated by the IgG (55–72%) and IgA (13–18%) isotypes.[3,24] Both these germinal center immunocyte classes, and those producing IgM or IgD, often express J-chain in normal palatine tonsils and adenoids of children, but in recurrent tonsillitis this expres-

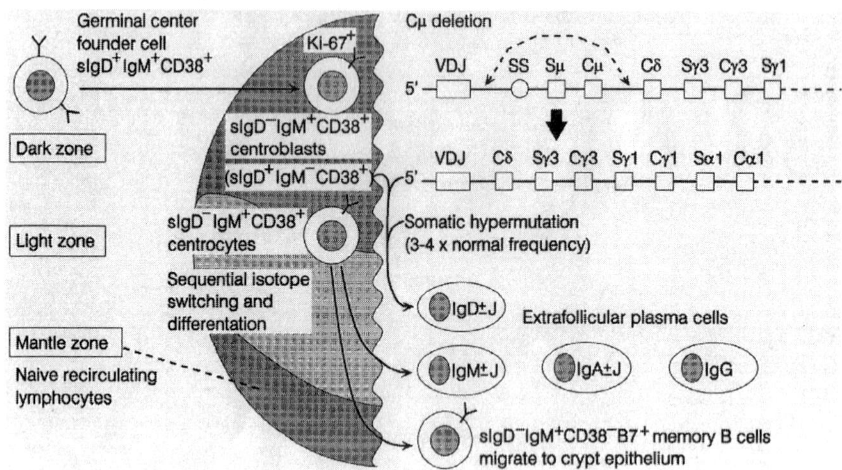

FIGURE 5. B-cell developmental events suggested to take place in the dark and light zones of tonsillar germinal centers, leading to the generation of extrafollicular plasma cells of various isotypes with or without J-chain expression (±J). Precursor cells with activated J-chain gene may also migrate from the germinal centers to regional mucosal effector sites as a basis for secretory IgA immunity (see text for details). In the dark zone there is a subset of B cells with surface IgD (sIgD+IgM−CD38+) that undergo Cμ deletion (*broken curved arrows* at the top) also resulting in loss of the somatic mutation silencer (SS) and the switch region (Sμ) required for further downstream C_H gene switching. These cells moreover undergo a high frequency of somatic mutations and may represent an important precursor subset for IgD-producing plasma cells in the upper airways. (Based partly on Liu *et al.*[59])

sion is considerably reduced.[3,24] The cytokine profiles and other microenvironmental factors determining this B-cell differentiation process remain obscure, but it appears that clonal maturation by massive or repeated antigen stimulation downregulates the J-chain, thus promoting monomer production by the IgA immunocytes.[1,23] Nevertheless, constant heavy chain (C_H) gene switching in tonsillar germinal centers normally gives rise to an even higher percentage of extrafollicular IgA immunocytes with J-chain expression.[3,24] The fact that their isotype is mainly IgA1 (approximately 90%), together with the parallel occurrence of many IgG and some IgD immunocytes, supports the notion that tonsillar B-cell differentiation takes place mainly in a sequential downstream C_H gene-switching fashion.[3,5,24]

Because the J-chain is a key peptide in the formation of pIgA with pIg receptor-binding properties,[1] the tonsillar B-cell differentiation process exhibits features compatible with precursor generation for the SIgA system.[3] It may be visualized that only some of the germinal center-derived pIgA-producing blasts give rise to extrafollicular plasma cells (FIG. 5), whereas an unknown number migrate to regional secretory sites for terminal differentiation there (FIG. 4). The nasopharyngeal tonsil, in addition, has its own secretory immune system, because patches of its surface and crypt epithelium express SC, but this is not true for the palatine tonsils.[24]

Evidence for Homing of Primed Tonsillar B Cells to Regional Mucosal Effector Sites

The finding that nasal and bronchial mucosae, as well as salivary and lacrimal glands, contain an IgA1 and IgD immunocyte distribution similar to that of tonsils,[2,5,24] suggests that these secretory sites are seeded mainly by B-cell blasts generated in tonsillar germinal centers and perhaps in bronchus-associated lymphoid tissue (BALT). Indeed, tonsillar germinal centers contain a subset of B cells (sIgD+IgM−CD38+) in the dark zone that undergo excessive somatic hypermutation (FIG. 5) and probably gives preferentially rise to IgD-producing plasma cells of this region.[27] By contrast, the intestinal lamina propria probably receives most stimulated B cells from GALT (FIG. 4), and IgD-producing plasma cells are virtually absent from the gut, even in selective IgA deficiency.[28] A similar B-cell homing dichotomy within the mucosal immune system has been suggested by studies in the rat, as reviewed elsewhere.[3]

Additional support for an inductive MALT role of the tonsils comes from the preferential appearance of IgA antibodies in parotid sections, recently shown in rabbits after tonsillar antigen exposure.[29] Furthermore, occurrence of IgA-producing plasma in the middle-ear mucosa of guinea pigs has been induced both by BALT and GALT immunization.[30] It is also of great interest that activated human tonsillar B cells transferred to mice with severe combined immunodeficiency, migrated to the lung of these animals but not to their gut mucosa.[31] In keeping with this observation, direct immunization of human palatine tonsils, and particularly nasal vaccination, gave rise to local B-cell responses in tonsils and adenoids as well as specific circulating B cells that apparently did not enter the intestinal mucosa.[32] Moreover, in infants dying of the sudden infant death syndrome, the palatine germinal centers were shown to be overstimulated as revealed by an increased number of IgG and IgA immunocytes; and primed B cells were apparently distributed in excessive numbers to regional secretory sites such as the parotid glands.[3] Together these observations provide indirect evidence for the notion that human tonsils, and perhaps particularly the adenoids, function as NALT and supply secretory sites of the upper aerodigestive tract with stimulated pIgA precursor cells within an integrated mucosal immune system (FIG. 4). The reason for the observed dichotomy in B-cell dissemination between this region and the gut may be differences in homing receptors and vascular addressins as discussed earlier.

To explore the NALT concept in humans, it is important to evaluate the effect of adenotonsillectomy on the regional SIgA levels. The pioneer report by Ogra[33] in 1971 showed that combined tonsillectomy and adenoidectomy in children reduced the level of IgA antibody to poliovirus three- to fourfold in their nasopharyngeal secretions and delayed or abrogated their local immune response to subsequent live poliovaccine. Jeschke and Ströder[34] performed tonsillectomy in children and found that their serum Ig and salivary IgA decreased for up to 3 years. D'Amelio *et al.*,[35] however, observed no salivary IgA reduction (but decreased serum IgA) in previously tonsillectomized adults (16–24 years old). Finally, Cantani *et al.*[36] more recently observed that salivary IgA as well as serum IgA (and less so IgG and IgM) were significantly reduced 4 months after combined tonsillectomy and adenoidectomy in children. More extensive clinical studies are clearly needed to obtain conclusive information.

MAINTENANCE OR ABROGATION OF MUCOSAL HOMEOSTASIS

Antigen presentation to $CD4^+$ T-helper (Th) cells by APC depends on their expression of HLA Class II molecules. Such molecules are also expressed by certain epithelial cells in the tonsils,[24] airway mucosa,[2] and small intestinal villi.[37] It is interesting that Class II-positive epithelial cells can act as APC under *in vitro* experimental conditions. The main effect obtained with gut epithelial cells in such test systems has been activation of $CD8^+$ suppressor cells, as reviewed elsewhere.[38] The epithelium might thus be an important immunoregulatory element for the induction of suppressive mechanisms explaining tolerance or hyporesponsiveness to foreign soluble antigens encountered at mucosal surfaces. This phenomenon is best known in relation to dietary antigens as so-called "oral tolerance" and has been defined particularly by feeding experiments in rodents.[38] The dominating $TCR\alpha/\beta^+CD8^+$ mucosal IEL subset (FIG. 1) could play an important role in this context by downregulating proinflammatory humoral immune responses (IgG and IgE) and T-cell-mediated (Th1-dependent) delayed-type hypersensitivity against harmless environmental antigens.[38] The existence of such a homeostatic control mechanism in humans is strongly suggested by the fact that the normal intestinal mucosa mounts no substantial IgG response[1,37] and contains very few T cells with high levels of recent activation markers such as the IL-2 receptor or CD25.[38]

Immunosuppressive mechanisms similar to oral tolerance apparently operate in the upper airways, particularly against IgE responses to inhalant antigens.[39] Nevertheless, hypersensitivity reactions to allergens and microbial antigens are much more frequent and persistent in the airways than in the gut.[40] It is possible that this disparity to some extent is explained by the relative scarcity of $TCR\alpha/\beta^+CD8^+IEL$ in the airway epithelium. Thus, while only 6–12% $TCR\alpha/\beta^+CD4^+$ IEL are normally present in the jejunum,[37] the latter subset averages 30% in the surface epithelium of normal nasal mucosa.[18] These differences may be explained by local profiles of chemoattractant factors to which $CD8^+$ mucosal T cells are particularly responsive.[41]

There are also other putative immunoregulatory differences between the airways and the gut. Numerous HLA Class II-positive dendritic cells are located within the airway epithelium;[2] they may be involved in antigen uptake and mediate down-regulation or up-regulation of immunity, depending on their state of activation.[39,42] In the normal state, the dendritic cells appear locally inert but transport antigens from the mucosa to the regional lymph nodes, where stimulation of $CD8^+$ regulatory T cells may cause immune deviation with down-regulation of the Th2 cells that are necessary for IgE responses.[40]

Furthermore, ICAM-1 is readily induced basally on airway epithelium in contrast to gut epithelium,[18] and this adhesion molecule may provide a costimulatory signal for T-cell activation by HLA Class II-positive epithelial cells.[38] Therefore, the epithelium of the upper respiratory tract appears to possess properties favoring immunological help instead of suppression. This may contribute to the preferential development of airway allergy through break of immunological tolerance against soluble protein antigens, in addition to a less robust surface barrier function in this region because of the preferential production of IgA1 that is susceptible to bacterial proteases as discussed earlier. Nevertheless, local IgA production will in various ways have a potential for maintaining homeostasis, not only by immune exclusion but also by its anti-inflammatory properties within the lamina propria (FIG. 1). This notion is supported by the effect of local IgA induction on the severity of experimental otitis media in rabbits.[30]

ALTERED MUCOSAL HOMEOSTASIS

Role of IgG and IgE Antibodies, Mast Cells, and Eosinophils

Chronic inflammatory diseases of the airways feature increased numbers of IgG-producing mucosal immunocytes, particularly beneath the surface epithelium.[2] Although IgG may reach the respiratory secretions by passive leakage and thereby enhance immune exclusion (so-called "pathotopic potentiation" or local defense),[2] this antibody class has a proinflammatory and tissue-damaging potential, particularly because of its complement-activating capacity (FIG. 1). A persistent mucosal IgG response may therefore be of immunopathological significance. Local production of IgE is rarely seen in respiratory mucosae; but mast cells "armed" with IgE are common in allergic patients, both in the connective tissue and in the epithelium.[3] Histamine and other inflammatory mediators from activated or degranulated mast cells may cause pathotopic potentiation of local immunity by increasing permeability but may also alter adhesion properties of endothelial cells (FIG. 3) and thereby initiate a vicious immunopathological circle involving IgG antibodies (FIG. 6).

The balance between mucosal protection and hypersensitivity is an intriguing variable that usually is difficult to understand. Environmental factors, such as tobacco smoking, appear to be associated with increased susceptibility to allergic and infectious diseases of the respiratory tract. This may reflect an effect on both immune exclusion and suppression, because IgA and IgG responses are reduced, whereas IgE responses are increased in smokers.[43] In addition, there is likely a genetic impact on the tendency to produce excessive levels of IgE as seen in atopic individuals. Enhanced IgE production and IgE sensitization of mast cells (FIG. 7), as well as other mast cell stimuli such as IgG immune complexes, may in various ways drive the mucosal response toward a chronic inflammatory reaction. Mast cells have been shown to produce an array of cytokines, among these IL-5 and TNF-α, that are important for rapid and prolonged priming of eosinophils and basophils.[44] Activated mast cells also generate IL-4 and the lipid mediator leukotriene B_4, both of which can contribute to the development of a local Th2 response. The cytokine profile of Th2 memory cells is polarized toward IL-4, IL-5, IL-10, and IL-13 secretion;[45] and preferential IgE production as well as extravasation of eosinophils are enhanced by IL-4 and IL-13, while IL-5 appears particularly capable of priming eosinophils for increased mediator release in response to subsequent stimuli.[9,44]

The eosinophil-predominant late-phase allergic reaction may thus have its origin in preferential local activation of Th2-type CD4+ memory cells combined with triggering of mast cells as part of a vicious cycle (FIG. 7). Increasing evidence supports the notion that eosinophils are important proinflammatory cells with the potency to generate several types of lipid and peptide mediators, including a variety of cytokines.[9,44] The mobilization of such cells to mucosal lesions appears to be highly dependent on the vascular cell adhesion molecule-1 (VCAM-1; member of the Ig su-

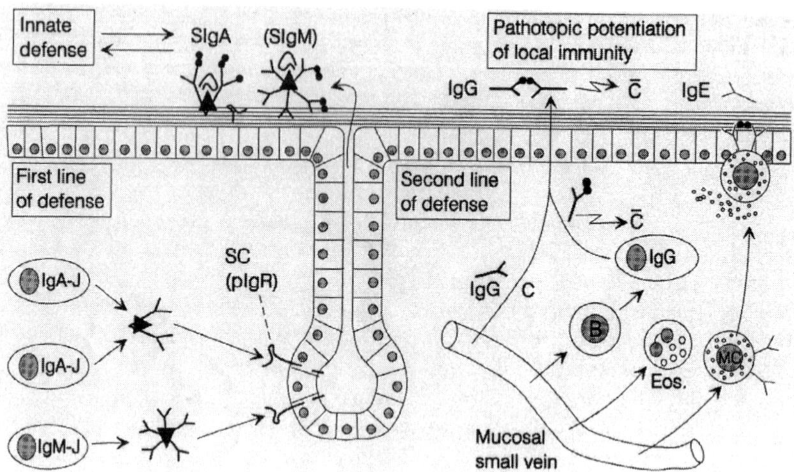

FIGURE 6. Two principles of humoral mucosal defense operative for upper airway protection. The first line of defense is constituted by the antigen (••)-excluding SIgA system (and to a lesser extent SIgM) interacting in a cooperative manner with nonspecific protective factors (innate defense); it originates in J-chain-expressing plasma cells (IgA-J and IgM-J) and depends on SC (pIgR)-mediated epithelial transport of dimeric IgA (and pentameric IgM) antibodies to the mucosal surface **(at the top)**. Paracellular leakage of IgG antibodies through the surface epithelium may also contribute to immune exclusion. The second line of defense depends mainly on IgG and IgE antibodies that can activate inflammatory mechanisms such as the complement (C) cascade and mast cell (MC) degranulation; this type of mucosal protection may result in so-called pathotopic potentiation of local immunity. As it is associated with extravasation of B cells of systemic rather than MALT origin as well as IgE-bearing MC and eosinophils (Eos.), the second defense line may evolve into chronic inflammatory disease. Further details are discussed in the text.

perfamily = CD106) and ICAM-1 that bind the leukocyte integrins β1 (VLA-4) and β2 (LFA-1, Mac-1), respectively.[9] Increased expression of VCAM-1 has been observed on endothelium in nasal mucosa of challenged patients with allergic rhinitis compared with nonatopic controls.[46] *In vitro* experiments have suggested that endothelial VCAM-1 expression is induced selectively by IL-4 and IL-13,[9,47] but other cytokines may also be involved (FIG. 3). Circulating eosinophils from allergic patients are sufficiently primed *in vivo* to adhere and migrate through such stimulated endothelium. Mast cells and activated Th2 lymphocytes are important sources of IL-4 and IL-13 and may therefore be crucial for the recruitment of eosinophils to the allergic mucosa.[44]

We have used nasal polyps to evaluate the expression of E-selectin, ICAM-1, and VCAM-1 *in situ* in relation to the accumulation of eosinophils and neutrophils.[48] The number of eosinophils was well correlated with the percentage of vessels positive for VCAM-1, whereas the two other endothelial adhesion molecules showed no such relationship. This observation supports a central role of VCAM-1 in human eosinophil

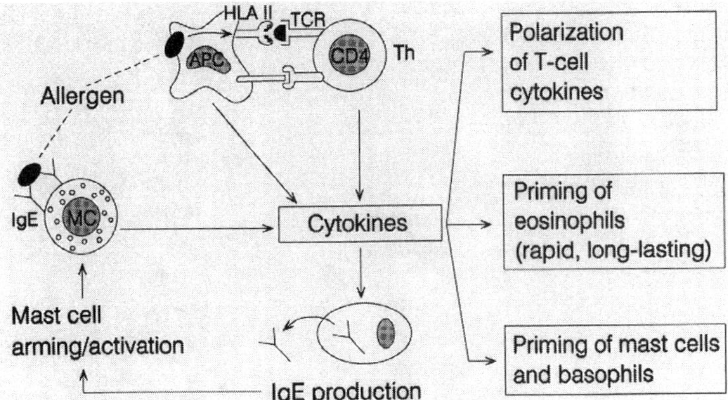

FIGURE 7. Central role played by IgE production and MC arming/activation in the development of a late-phase allergic reaction. Processed allergen is displayed by antigen-presenting cell (APC) in an HLA Class II-restricted manner to CD4[+] T helper (Th) cell, while intact allergen cross-bridges IgE antibodies on the surface of MC, thereby activating it. Cytokines released from activated MC promote polarization of T-cell cytokines to a Th2 pattern as well as priming of eosinophils, mast cells, and basophils. TCR = T-cell receptor.

extravasation. However, experimental evidence suggests a significant contribution to this process of other adhesion molecules such as P-selectin, as well as chemoattractants such as RANTES[44,49] that is produced both by the epithelium[50] and the endothelial cells in human airways (Jahnsen *et al.,* unpublished observations).

The most crucial steps of eosinophil extravasation have to be characterized before rational therapeutic immune intervention can be designed. To this end we have recently established primary cultures of isolated polyp microvascular endothelial cells (PMEC), which respond to cytokines by increased VCAM-1 expression. In particular, IL-4 or IL-13 synergistically enhances the effect of TNF-α and IL-1 in this respect.[51] Our PMEC culture system permits defined functional studies with endothelial cells that may prove more relevant to the airways than human umbilical vein endothelial cells, which traditionally have been used for similar *in vitro* experiments.

Putative Immunopathological Role of IgD Antibodies in Airway Mucosae

The upper airway microbiota may exert a significant impact on human tonsillar B cells that perhaps explains the relatively common occurrence of IgD-producing cells at secretory sites of this region,[5] and particularly the prominent population of such immunocytes seen in many subjects with selective IgA deficiency.[4,28] Most strains of *H. influenzae* and *Moraxella catarrhalis*, frequent colonizers of the upper airways, express an IgD-binding factor (protein D) that likely may trigger the sIgD[+]IgM[-]CD38[+] tonsillar B-cell subset (FIG. 5) by cross-linking sIgD with HLA

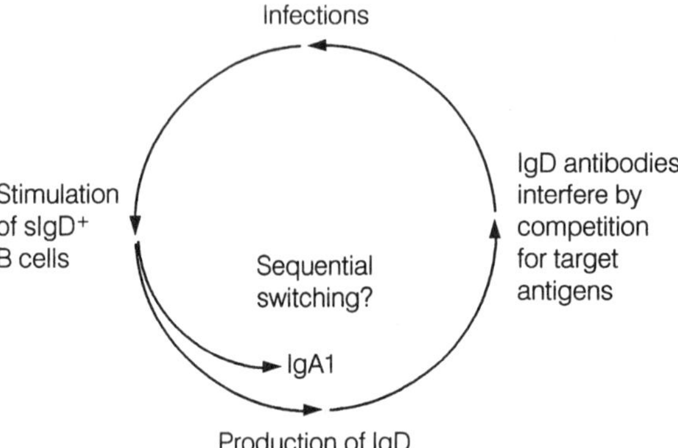

FIGURE 8. Infections of the upper airways may adversely influence the regional development of humoral immunity by bacterial binding to B cells bearing surface IgD (sIgD⁺). Such interaction may enhance production of IgD antibodies that are potentially harmful by interfering with the function of protective antibodies; it may also promote sequential switching of B cells to production of IgA1 antibodies that are susceptible to bacterial proteases.

Class I determinants.[52,53] A similar effect on the sIgD⁺sIgM⁺CD38⁺ germinal center founder cell population (FIG. 5) might in theory favor a sequential differentiation pathway of C_H gene switching and thereby explain the usual predominance of IgA1 production in the upper aerodigestive tract.[5,24]

It is as yet unknown if mucosal IgD production is merely a reflection of such a regional bacterial influence on B-cell differentiation or whether in addition it has immunopathological significance. Recurrent tonsillitis is associated with an increased number of extrafollicular IgD plasma cells,[24,54] and the serum IgD level is increased in some patients with bacterial pneumonia[55] and in cigarette smokers.[56] It is also of interest that IgD is locally produced in secretory otitis media;[57] the mucosal immunocytes may indeed have a tonsillar origin because otitis-prone children often have increased numbers of IgD-producing cells in their adenoids.[58] Further, IgD of local origin appearing in nasopharyngeal secretions of such patients is well correlated with the IgD levels in their middle ear effusions.[58] As mentioned earlier, moreover, infection-prone IgA-deficient patients have remarkably large numbers of IgD-producing immunocytes in their nasal mucosa and paranasal sinus mucosa, and this is reflected in a raised level of IgD in their serum.[4]

Because IgD can neither activate complement nor possesses other known biological amplification properties, it is possible that antibodies of this class may block defense functions of IgG within the mucosae and reduce the immune exclusion efficiency of polymeric antibodies in the secretions. One can hence visualize that pathogenic bacteria of the upper airways in some patients drive a vicious circle involving enhanced production of IgD antibodies with inferior defense properties, and also a sequential B-cell switching pathway leading to preferential production of the more susceptible IgA1 isotype (FIG. 8).

CONCLUSIONS

Immunological defense of the upper airways depends primarily on secretory immunity. The B cells involved are believed to be stimulated in organized mucosa-associated lymphoid tissue (MALT), including the tonsils, the adenoids, and similar regional lymphoepithelial structures. From these inductive sites, the primed cells migrate to secretory effector sites where they differentiate terminally to Ig-producing plasma cells. Locally produced Ig consists mainly of J-chain-containing dimers and larger polymers of IgA (pIgA) that are selectively transported through epithelial cells by a receptor called transmembrane secretory component (SC) or the pIg receptor. Because of the large predominance of the IgA1 subclass in the upper airways, secretory immunity may be inadequate in the face of respiratory bacteria producing IgA1-cleaving proteases. Although IgG can participate in immune exclusion when it reaches the secretions by passive diffusion, its proinflammatory properties render such antibodies of immunopathological importance when elimination of penetrating antigens is unsuccessful. Local overproduction of IgD is also often associated with infections and chronic inflammation in the upper airways. Furthermore, T-helper (Th) cells activated locally may, by a Th2 cytokine profile, promote persistent inflammation with extravasation and priming of inflammatory cells, particularly including eosinophils. This development appears to be part of the late-phase allergic reaction, perhaps initially driven by IL-4 released from mast cells subjected to IgE-mediated or other types of degranulation, and subsequently also by further Th2-cell activation. Eosinophils are potentially tissue-damaging, particularly after priming with IL-5. Various cytokines up-regulate adhesion molecules on endothelial and epithelial cells, thereby enhancing accumulation of eosinophils and perhaps, in addition, causing aberrant immune regulation within the epithelium. Soluble antigens bombarding the mucosal surfaces normally induce various immunosuppressive mechanisms, but such homeostasis appears to be less robust in the airways than oral tolerance to dietary antigens operating in the intestinal immune system.

ACKNOWLEDGMENTS

Hege Eliassen Bryme is thanked for excellent secretarial assistance and Erik Kulø Hagen for the illustrations.

REFERENCES

1. BRANDTZAEG, P. 1995. Molecular and cellular aspects of the secretory immunoglobulin system. APMIS **103:** 1–19.
2. BRANDTZAEG, P. 1984. Immune functions of human nasal mucosa and tonsils in health and disease. *In* Immunology of the Lung and Upper Respiratory Tract, J. Bienenstock, Ed.: 28–95. McGraw-Hill. New York.
3. BRANDTZAEG, P. 1996. The B-cell development in tonsillar lymphoid follicles. Acta Otolaryngol. Suppl. **523:** 55–59.
4. BRANDTZAEG, P., G. KARLSSON, G. HANSSON, B. PETRUSON, J. BJÖRKANDER & L. A. HAN-

SON. 1987. The clinical condition of IgA-deficient patients is related to the proportion of IgD- and IgM-producing cells in their nasal mucosa. Clin. Exp. Immunol. **67:** 626–66.

5. BRANDTZAEG, P. 1992. Humoral immune response patterns of human mucosae: Induction and relation to bacterial respiratory tract infections. J. Infect. Dis. **165**(Suppl 1): S167–S176.

6. KILIAN, M. & M. W. RUSSELL. 1994. Function of mucosal immunoglobulins. *In* Handbook of Mucosal Immunology, P. L. Ogra, J. Mestecky, M. E. Lamm, W. Strober, J. R. McGhee, and J. Bienenstock, Eds.: 127–137. Academic Press. Orlando, Fla.

7. SØRENSEN, C. H. & M. KILIAN. 1984. Bacterium-induced cleavage of IgA in nasopharyngeal secretions from atopic children. Acta Pathol. Microbiol. Immunol. Scand. [C] **92:** 85–87.

8. KILIAN, M., S. HUSBY, A. HØST & S. HALKEN. 1995. Increased proportions of bacteria capable of cleaving IgA1 in the pharynx of infants with atopic disease. Pediatr. Res. **38:** 182–186.

9. MONTEFORT, S., S. T. HOLGATE & P. H. HOWARTH. 1993. Leucocyte-endothelial adhesion molecules and their role in bronchial asthma and allergic rhinitis. Eur. Respir. J. **6:** 1044–1054.

10. BUTCHER, E. C. & L. J. PICKER. 1996. Lymphocyte homing and homeostasis. Science **272:** 60–66.

11. SCHALL, T. J. & K. B. BACON. 1994. Chemokines, leukocyte trafficking, and inflammation. Curr. Opin. Immunol. **6:** 865–873.

12. DEL POZO, M. A., P. SÁNCHEZ-MATEOS & F. SÁNCHEZ-MADRID. 1996. Cellular polarization induced by chemokines: A mechanism for leukocyte recruitment? Immunol. Today **17:** 127–131.

13. REDINGTON, A. E., P. BRADDING & S. T. HOLGATE. 1993. The role of cytokines in the pathogenesis of allergic asthma. Reg. Immunol. **5:** 174–200.

14. SIKORSKI, E. E., R. HALLMANN, E. L. BERG & E. C. BUTCHER. 1993. The Peyer's patch high endothelial receptor for lymphocytes, the mucosal vascular addressin, is induced on a murine endothelial cell line by tumor necrosis factor-α and IL-1. J. Immunol. **151:** 5239–5250.

15. FARSTAD, I. N., T. S. HALSTENSEN, A. I. LAZAROVITS, J. NORSTEIN, O. FAUSA & P. BRANDTZAEG. 1995. Human intestinal B-cell blasts and plasma cells express the mucosal homing receptor integrin $\alpha4\beta7$. Scand. J. Immunol. **42:** 662–672.

16. PICKER, L. J., R. J. MARTIN, A. TRUMBLE, L. S. NEWMAN, P. A. COLLINS, P. R. BERGSTRESSER & D. Y. M. LEUNG. 1994. Differential expression of lymphocyte homing receptors by human memory/effector T cells in pulmonary versus cutaneous immune effector sites. Eur. J. Immunol. **24:** 1269–1277.

17. CEPEK, K. L., S. K. SHAW, C. M. PARKER, G. J. RUSSELL, J. S. MORROW, D. L. RIMM & M. B. BRENNER. 1994 Adhesion between epithelial cells and T lymphocytes mediated by E-cadherin and the $\alpha4\beta7$ integrin. Nature **372:** 190–193.

18. JAHNSEN, F. L., I. N. FARSTAD, J. P. AANESEN & P. BRANDTZAEG. 1997. Phenotypic distribution of T cells in human nasal mucosa differs from that in the gut. Am. J. Respir. Cell Mol. Biol. In press.

19. KUPER, C. F., P. J. KOORNSTRA, D. M. HAMELEERS, J. BIEWENGA, B. J. SPIT, A. M. DUIJVESTIJN, P. J. VAN BREDA VRIESMAN & T. SMINIA. 1992. The role of nasopharyngeal lymphoid tissue. Immunol. Today **13:** 219–224.

20. DOLEN, W. K., B. SPOFFORD & J. C. SELNER. 1990. The hidden tonsils of Waldeyer's ring. Ann. Allergy **65:** 244–250.

21. KRACKE, A., A. S. HILLER, T. TSCHERNIG, M. KASPER, W. J. KLEEMANN, H. D. TRÖGER & R. PABST. 1997. Larynx-associated lymphoid tissue (LALT) in young children. Anat. Rec. **248:** 413–420.

22. MATSUNE, S., H. TAKAHASHI & I. SANDO. 1996. Mucosa-associated lymphoid tissue in middle ear and Eustachian tube in children. Int. J. Pediatr. Otorhinolaryngol. **34:** 229–236.

23. BRANDTZAEG, P. & K. BJERKE. 1990. Immunomorphological characteristics of human Peyer's patches. Digestion **46**(Suppl. 2): 262–273.

24. BRANDTZAEG, P. 1987. Immune functions and immunopathology of palatine and nasopharyngeal tonsils. *In* Immunology of the Ear, J. M. Bernstein and P. L. Ogra, Eds.: 63–106. Raven Press. New York.

25. BRANDTZAEG, P. & T. S. HALSTENSEN. 1992. Immunology and immunopathology of tonsils. Adv. Otorhinolaryngol. **47:** 64–75.

26. LIU, Y.-J., C. BARTHÉLÉMY, O. DE BOUTEILLER, C. ARPIN, I. DURAND & J. BACHEREAU. 1995. Memory B cells from human tonsils colonize mucosal epithelium and directly present antigen to T cells by rapid up-regulation of B7-1 and B7-2. Immunity **2:** 239–248.

27. LIU, Y.-J. & J. BANCHEREAU. 1996. The paths and molecular controls of peripheral B-cell development. Immunologist **4:** 55–66.

28. BRANDTZAEG, P., S. T. GJERULDSEN, F. KORSRUD, K. BAKLIEN, P. BERDAL & J. EK. 1979. The human secretory immune system shows striking heterogeneity with regard to involvment of J chain-positive IgD immunocytes. J. Immunol. **122:** 503–510.

29. FUKUIZUMI, T., H. INOUE, Y. ANZAI, T. TSUJISAWA & C. UCHIYAMA. 1995. Sheep red blood cell instillation of palatine tonsil effectively induces specific IgA class antibody in saliva in rabbits. Microbiol. Immunol. **39:** 351–359.

30. WATANABE, N., H. YOSHIMURA & G. MOGI. 1988. Induction of antigen-specific IgA-forming cells in the middle ear mucosa. Arch Otolaryngol. Head Neck Surg. **114:** 758–762.

31. NADAL, D., B. ALBINI, C. CHEN, E. SCHLÄPFER, J. M. BERNSTEIN & P. L. OGRA. 1991. Distribution and engraftment patterns of human tonsillar mononuclear cells and immunoglobulin secreting cells in mice with severe combined immunodeficiency. Role of the Epstein-Barr virus. Int. Arch. Allergy Appl. Immunol. **95:** 341–351.

32. QUIDING-JÄRBRINK, M. G. GRANSTRÖM, I. NORDSTRÖM, J. HOLMGREN & C. CZERKINSKY. 1995. Induction of compartmentalized B-cell responses in human tonsils. Infect. Immun. **63:** 853–857.

33. OGRA, P. L. 1971. Effect of tonsillectomy and adenoidectomy on nasopharyngeal antibody response to poliovirus. New Eng. J. Med. **284:** 59–64.

34. JESCHKE, R. & J. STRÖDER. 1980. Verlaufsbeobachtung Klinischer und immunologischer Parameter, insbesondere des Speichel-IgA, bei tonsillektomierten Kindern. Klin. Pädiat. **192:** 51–60.

35. D'AMELIO, R., L. PALMISANO, S. LEMOLI, R. SEMINARA & F. AIUTI. 1982. Serum and salivary IgA levels in normal subjects: Comparison between tonsillectomized and non-tonsillectomized subjects. Int. Arch. Allergy Appl. Immunol. **68:** 256–259.

36. CANTANI, A., P. BELLIONI, F. SALVINELLI & L. BUSINCO. 1986. Serum immunoglobulins and secretory IgA deficiency in tonsillectomized children. Ann. Allergy **57:** 413–416.

37. BRANDTZAEG, P., T. S. HALSTENSEN, K. KETT, P. KRAJCI, D. KVALE, T. O. ROGNUM, H. SCOTT & L. M. SOLLID. 1989. Immunobiology and immunopathology of human gut mucosa: Humoral immunity and intraepithelial lymphocytes. Gastroenterology **97:** 1562–1584.

38. BRANDTZAEG, P. 1996. History of oral tolerance and mucosal immunity. Ann. N.Y. Acad. Sci. **778:** 1–27.

39. HOLT, P. G. & C. MCMENAMIN. 1989. Defence against allergic sensitization in the health lung: The role of inhalation tolerance. Clin. Exp. Allergy **19:** 255–262.

40. HOLT, P. G. 1994. Immunoprophylaxis of atopy: Light at the end of the tunnel? Immunol. Today **15:** 484–489.

41. EBERT, E. C. 1995. Human intestinal intraepithelial lymphocytes have potent chemotactic activity. Gastroenterology **109:** 1154–1159.

42. GRABBE, S., S. BEISSERT, T. SCHWARZ & R. D. GRANSTEIN. 1995. Dendritic cells as initia-

tors of tumor immune responses: A possible strategy for tumor immunotherapy? Immunol. Today **16:** 117–121.

43. HOLT, P. 1987. Immune and inflammatory function in cigarette smokers. Thorax **42:** 241–249.

44. DEVRIES, J. E. 1994. Atopic allergy and other hypersensitivities. Editorial overview. Curr. Opin. Immunol. **6:** 835–837.

45. BRANDTZAEG, P., F. L. JAHNSEN & I. N. FARSTAD. 1996. Immune functions and immunopathology of the mucosa of the upper respiratory pathways. Acta Otolaryngol. **116:** 149–159.

46. LEE, B. J., R. M. NACLERIO, B. S. BOCHNER, R. M. TAYLOR, M. C. LIM & F. M. BAROODY. 1994. Nasal challenge with allergen unregulates the local expression of vascular endothelial adhesion molecules. J. Allergy Clin. Immunol. **94:** 1006–1016.

47. BOCHNER, B. S., D. A. KLUNK, S. A. STERBINSKY, R. L. COFFMAN & R. P. SCHLEIMER. 1995. IL-13 selectively induces vascular cell adhesion molecule-1 expression in human endothelial cells. J. Immunol. **154:** 799–803.

48. JAHNSEN, F. L., G. HARALDSEN, J. P. AANESEN, R. HAYE & P. BRANDTZAEG. 1995. Eosinophil infiltration is related to increased expression of vascular cell adhesion molecule-1 in nasal polyps. Am. J. Respir. Cell Mol. Biol. **12:** 624–632.

49. SYMON, F. A., G. M. WALSH, S. R. WATSON & A. J. WARDLAW. 1994. Eosinophil adhesion to nasal polyp endothelium is P-selectin-dependent. J. Exp. Med. **180:** 371–376.

50. BERKMAN, N., A. ROBICHAUD, V. L. KRISHNAN, G. ROESEMS, R. ROBBINS, P. J. JOSE, P. J. BARNES & K. F. CHUNG. 1996. Expression of RANTES in human airway epithelial cells: Effect of corticosteroids and interleukin-4, -10, and -13. Immunology **87:** 599–603.

51. JAHNSEN, F. L., P. BRANDTZAEG, R. HAYE & G. HARALDSEN. 1997. Expression of functional VCAM-1 in cultured nasal polyp-derived microvascular endothelium. Am. J. Pathol. **150:** 2113–2123.

52. RUAN, M., M. AKKOYUNLU, A. GRUBB & A. FORSBERG. 1990. Protein D of *Haemophilus influenzae.* A novel bacterial surface protein with affinity for human IgD. J. Immunol. **145:** 3379–3384.

53. JANSON, H., L. O. HÉDEN, A. GRUBB, M. R. RUAN & A. FORSGREN. 1991. Protein D, an immunoglobulin D-binding protein of *Haemophilus influenzae:* Cloning, nucleotide sequence, and expression in Escherichia coli. Infect. Immun. **59:** 119–125.

54. YAMANAKA, N., H. MATSUYAMA, Y. HARABUCHI & A. KATAURA. 1992. Distribution of lymphoid cells in tonsillar compartments in relation to infection and age. A quantitative study using image analysis. Acta Otolaryngol. **112:** 128–137.

55. NORDBRING, F., C. HÖGMAN & S. G. O. JOHANSSON. 1969. Serum immunoglobulin levels in the course of acute pneumonia. Scand. J. Infect. Dis. **1:** 99–106.

56. BAHNA, S. L., D. C. HEINER & B. A. MYHRE. 1983. Changes in serum IgD in cigarette smokers. Clin. Exp. Immunol. **51:** 624–630.

57. SØRENSEN, C. H. 1983. Quantitative aspects of IgD and secretory immunoglobulins in middle ear effusions. Int. J. Pediatr. Otorhinolaryngol. **6:** 247–253.

58. SØRENSEN, C. H. & P. L. LARSEN. 1988. IgD in nasopharyngeal secretions and tonsils from otitis-prone children. Clin. Exp. Immunol. **73:** 149–154.

59. LIU, Y.-J., C. ARPIN, O. DE BOUTEILLER, C. GURET, J. BANCHEREAU, H. MARTINEZ-VALDEZ & S. LEBECQUE. 1996. Sequential triggering of apoptosis, somatic mutation and isotype switch during germinal center development. Semin. Immunol. **8:** 169–177.

The Microbial Ecology and Immunology of the Adenoid: Implications for Otitis Media

JOEL M. BERNSTEIN,[a,b,d,e] MOLAKALA S. REDDY,[c]
FRANK A. SCANNAPIECO,[c] HOWARD S. FADEN,[b,d]
AND MARK BALLOW[b,d]

[a]*Departments of Otolaryngology and Pediatrics*
School of Medicine and Biomedical Sciences
State University of New York at Buffalo
Buffalo, New York 14222
and
Department of Communicative Disorders and Sciences
State University of New York at Buffalo
Buffalo, New York 14222

[b]*Division of Infectious Diseases*
Children's Hospital of Buffalo
Buffalo, New York 14222

[c]*Department of Oral Biology*
School of Dental Medicine
State University of New York at Buffalo
Buffalo, New York 14222

[d]*Department of Pediatrics*
State University of New York at Buffalo
Buffalo, New York 14222

INTRODUCTION

The nasopharyngeal tonsil (adenoid) is a lymphoepithelial tissue located in a critical position of the upper respiratory tract. It lies adjacent to the eustachian tube orifice and the lateral wall of the nose in close proximity to the ethmoid, frontal, and maxillary sinuses. The adenoid, along with other parts of Waldeyer's ring, are the only lymphoepithelial tissues that protect the lower respiratory tract.

Homeostasis of the bacterial microecology and appropriate local mucosal immune function of this lymphoepithelial organ must be maintained to protect the host

[e]Address for correspondence: Joel M. Bernstein, M.D., Ph.D., 4949 Harlem Rd., Amherst, NY 14226. Phone: 716/839-1600; fax: 716/839-5596; e-mail: jbernste@acsu.Buffalo.edu

from infectious diseases caused by bacteria and viruses as well as from allergic diseases caused by inhalant and food antigens that enter the upper respiratory tract.

The purpose of this communication is to review new concepts of the microecology and immunology of the adenoid as they relate to protection of the upper airway from viral, bacterial, and allergic diseases.

Our laboratory has focused on four areas of research. They include (1) bacterial–mucin interactions in the nasopharynx; (2) the role of viridans streptococci in inhibition of potential pathogens such as nontypeable *Haemophilus influenzae, Moraxella catarrhalis,* and *Streptococcus pneumoniae*; (3) the specific protective role of secretory immunoglobulin A (IgA) against bacteria and viruses; and (4) the cytokine profiles of lymphocytes in the adenoid of both otitis-prone and nonotitis-prone children.

BACTERIAL–NASOPHARYNGEAL MUCIN INTERACTION

Bacterial colonization of epithelial cells usually precedes invasion of tissue and infection. Mucins are purified glycoproteins that are secreted by goblet cells and seromucinous glands of the nose. Mucins may provide receptors for adhesion of bacteria to host surfaces and they may also modulate bacterial colonization by preventing adherence to the epithelial cell wall. We have performed studies to understand the mechanism of nasopharyngeal and middle-ear mucin binding to the three major bacterial agents of otitis media. In our studies, we have purified both human nasopharyngeal and middle-ear mucins and have utilized an overlay binding assay to identify the specific outer membrane proteins (OMPs) that may function as bacterial adhesins. Briefly, middle-ear and nasopharyngeal secretions were fractionated on Sepharose CL-2B in tris-guanidine buffer. Chromatography of nasopharyngeal and middle-ear secretions yielded pools that were then separated on sodium dodecyl sulphate polyacrylamide gels (SDS-PAGE) followed by staining with periodic acid-Schiff reagent to identify the presence of high molecular-weight glycoproteins. OMPs of nontypeable *H. influenzae, M. catarrhalis, Pseudomonas aeruginosa,* and *S. pneumoniae* were isolated according to previously described protocols.[1]

Both human middle-ear (HMEM) and human nasopharyngeal (HNM) mucins were radio-labeled by iodination. Binding of [^{125}] HNM and [^{125}I] HMEM to OMPs of various bacteria were examined by the overlay assay.[2] FIGURES 1–3 summarize the results of our studies. Both [^{125}I] HNM and [^{125}] HMEM bound to two OMPs of nontypeable *H. influenzae* migrating between 45 and 31 kDa. The binding pattern of a representative strain is presented in FIGURE 1. On the basis of electrophoretic mobility and immunoblotting, these two proteins were identified as OMPs P2 and P5. Unequivocal identification of OMPs P2 and P5 was made by employing OMPs of bacterial strains and their respective isogenic mutants lacking the respective OMP in the binding assays. Thus, OMPs of *H. influenzae b* (DL42) and its isogenic mutant lacking OMP P2 and OMPs of nontypeable *H. influenzae* 1128 and its isogenic mutant lacking OMP P5 were employed in this assay to confirm that OMPs P2 and P5 function as adhesins for HNM and HMEM.

In contrast to nontypeable *H. influenzae*, [^{125}I] HNM and [^{125}I] HMEM bound to a single *M. catarrhalis* OMP with a size of approximately 57 kDa (FIG. 1). The 57-kDa component was identified as the CD protein of *M. catarrhalis*.

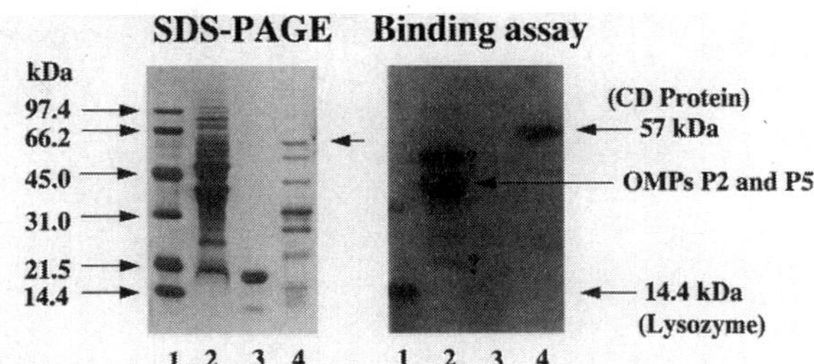

FIGURE 1. Various bacterial OMPs Western transferred to the polyvinylidene difluoride membrane were stained with Coomasie blue. On the **left** SDS-PAGE. **Lane 1:** molecular-weight markers; **Lane 2:** OMPs of NTHi; **Lane 3:** pili subunit of *P. aeruginosa*; **Lane 4:** OMPs of *M. catarrhalis*. On the **right**, autoradiograph demonstrates proteins that bind to [^{125}I] HNM. Proteins involved in binding are marked with *arrowheads* in both panels. The OMPs P2 and P5 of NTHi bind the mucin. The pili subunit of *P. aeruginosa* does not bind to human nasal mucin. The 57-kDa component identified as the CD protein of *M. catarrhalis* is the only protein that binds to purified nasal mucin.

Binding of [^{125}I] HNM and [^{125}I] HMEM to two proteins of *P. aeruginosa*, an adhesin to tracheobronchial mucin, and a subunit of *P. aeruginosa* pili were examined. [^{215}I] HNM and [^{125}I] HMEM bound to a 16-kDa OMP of *P. aeruginosa*, but not to the pilus subunit (FIG. 2). *S. pneumoniae* was bound to human nasal mucin exclusively by 17.5- and 20.5-kDa surface proteins (FIG. 3). HMEM did not bind to the surface proteins of *S. pneumoniae* (FIG. 4). Other surface proteins used in this study bound to both HNM and to HMEM. The significance of the lack of binding of *S. pneumoniae* to purified middle-ear mucin is as yet unknown, but may help to explain the severity of otitis media infection by this organism. Lack of mucin binding may foster colonization and subsequent inflammation. From the observations discussed earlier, it can be concluded that binding involves specific interactions.

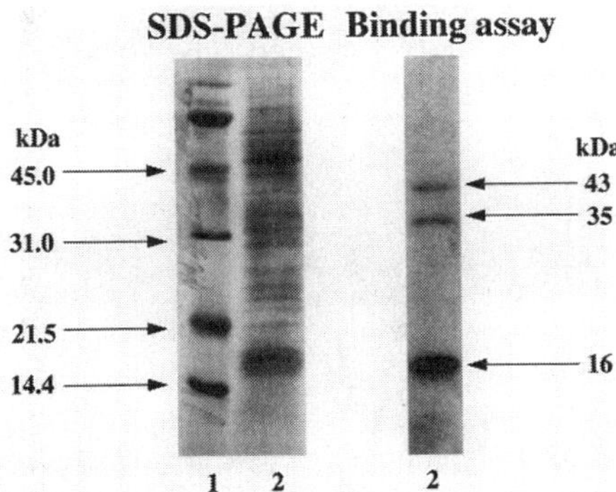

FIGURE 2. 1. SDS-PAGE, and 2. overlay binding assay of *P. aeruginosa* extract. The major protein binding is the 16-kDa protein, which is a nonpilus OMP. Smaller bands at 43 and 35 kDa also bind to the human purified nasal mucin.

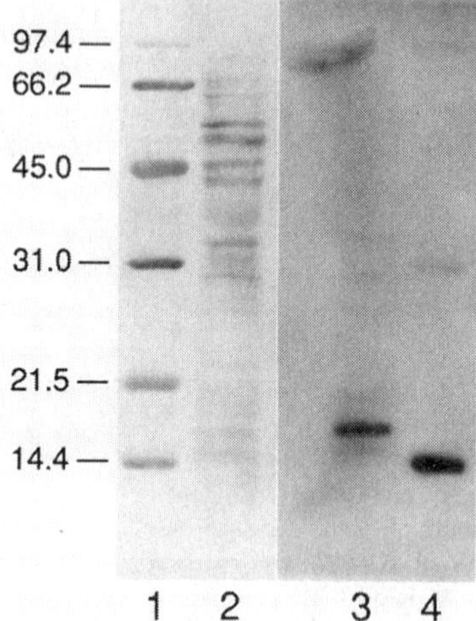

FIGURE 3. *S. pneumoniae* binding to purified human nasal mucin. This overlay binding assay demonstrates the specificity of binding of a major surface protein at 17.5 kDa. **Lane 1:** molecular-weight markers; **Lane 2:** surface proteins of *S. pneumoniae*; **Lane 3:** radio autograph demonstrates binding of 17.5-kDa protein to HNM; **Lane 4:** lysozyme binds to HNM.

Preliminary experiments to identify the HNM or HMEM receptor(s) for OMPs P2 and P5 of nontypeable *H. influenzae* were also conducted. Asialo-[^{125}I] HNM and [^{125}I] HMEM were prepared by mild acid hydrolysis and utilized in the binding studies. Removal of sialic acid resulted in a loss of binding of [^{125}I] HNM and [^{125}I] HMEM to OMPs P2 and P5, indicating a role for sialic-acid-containing oligosaccharides in bacterial binding. This role was confirmed by inhibition studies. Following Western transfer, the polyvinylidene difluoride membrane was incubated with O-glycosidically linked oligosaccharides isolated from fetuin prior to addition of [^{125}I]

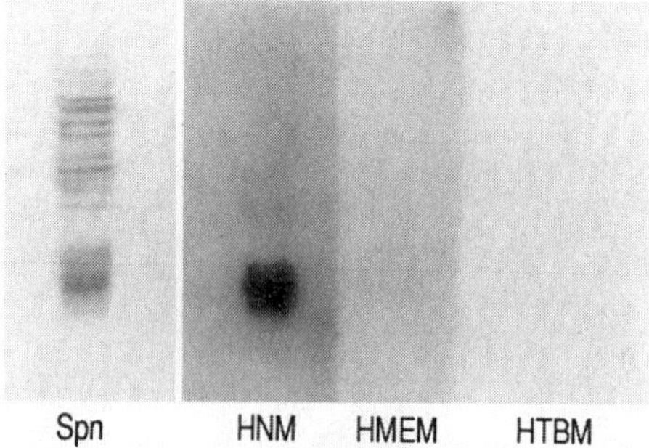

FIGURE 4. Overlay technique demonstrating the presence of a 17.5-kDa OMP of an *S. pneumoniae* lysate to human nasal mucin, but the total absence of binding to both human middle-ear mucin and human tracheobronchial mucin.

HNM or [^{125}I] HMEM. Fetuin O-glycosidically linked oligosaccharides inhibited the binding of [^{125}I] HNM and [^{125}I] HMEM to OMPs P2 and P5. These results are in agreement with those of other studies that found that mucin oligosaccharides function as receptors for bacteria.[3]

In conclusion, isolated nasopharyngeal mucin and middle-ear mucin subunits were utilized in an overlay binding assay to determine the mechanism of binding between mucin and OMPs of nontypeable *H. influenzae, M. catarrhalis, P. aeruginosa,* and *S. pneumoniae.* OMPs P2 and P5 of nontypeable *H. influenzae* appear to function as adhesins for these purified mucins. Sialic-acid-containing oligosaccharides of these purified mucins appear to be the receptors for the bacteria. Further characterization of the mucin receptors and bacterial adhesins is in progress. The demonstration of specific interaction between these bacteria and purified human nasal and middle-ear mucin and the identification of the putative bacterial adhesins provide another potential target for intervention in the colonization process.

BACTERIAL INTERFERENCE AT THE LEVEL OF THE NASOPHARYNX

The orderliness of man's indigenous bacterial flora is impressive. The mucosal surfaces or normal individuals are colonized by well-defined microbial flora. Sites, such as the posterior pharynx, are colonized by a range of species which, within fairly wide limits, maintain their proportions one to another.[4]

The interrelationships among organisms in the nasopharynx provide one of the mechanisms that maintain the bacterial *status quo.* Many organisms in the normal pharynx and nasopharynx are capable of preventing the growth of other bacterial species. The majority of inhibitory species have been identified as alpha hemolytic (viridans) streptococci.[5] Furthermore, previous studies have shown that implantation of viridans streptococci can be established in the pharynx of infants colonized with pathogenic organisms and that successful implantation can result in prompt development of normal pharyngeal flora within 48 h.[6] The interaction of human indigenous microflora and exogenously acquired pathogens has been the subject of sporadic investigation and continuous speculation for many decades; however, only recently has it been demonstrated conclusively that these interactions may enhance man's capacity to resist infection.

We have previously described the microbial ecology of the nasopharyngeal bacterial flora in otitis-prone and non-otitis-prone children[7,8]. Quantitative bacteriology of the adenoid of otitis-prone children demonstrated an inverse relationship between viridans streptococci and nontypeable *H. influenzae.* Factors responsible for this relationship, however, remain to be elucidated. We recently studied two strains of viridans streptococci. One strain (Parker) inhibited all nontypeable *H. influenzae in vitro* so far tested. The second strain, (Booth), did not inhibit any strains of nontypeable *H. influenzae in vitro.* The biochemical profile and antibiotic sensitivity of these two organisms were quite different (TABLE 1).

Utilizing standard taxonomic methods, both the inhibitory and noninhibitory viridans strains were identified as *Streptococcus oralis.* The major difference between

TABLE 1. Comparison of Inhibitor Strain of Viridans Streptococcus (P) and Noninhibitor Viridans Streptococcus (B)

	1[a] Insulin	2[b] NAG	3[c] Gent	4[d] T/S	5[e] PEN	6[f] AMP	7[g] Tet
V.S. (P) (inhibitor strain)	−	+	6	S	S	S	R
V.S. (B) (noninhibitor strain)	+	−	≤1	R	R	R	S

[a]1. Formation of acidic product from carbohydrate utilization.
[b]2. Hydrolysis of p-nitrophyl[B], D-N-acetylglucosamide.
[c]3. Getamicin.
[d]4. Trimethoprin/sulfa.
[e]5. Penicillin.
[f]6. Ampicillin
[g]7. Tetracycline.

the strains was the substantially faster rate of growth of the Parker strain (FIG. 5). Even under anaerobic conditions, the Parker strain grew more rapidly (FIG. 6).

The pH of the broth in which the Parker strain grew was depressed more rapidly (FIG. 7). Hydrogen peroxide was also produced in a shorter period of time by the strain. Many studies were conducted to determine whether a bacteriocin or other soluble product(s) were also produced by this strain that inhibited the growth of nonty-

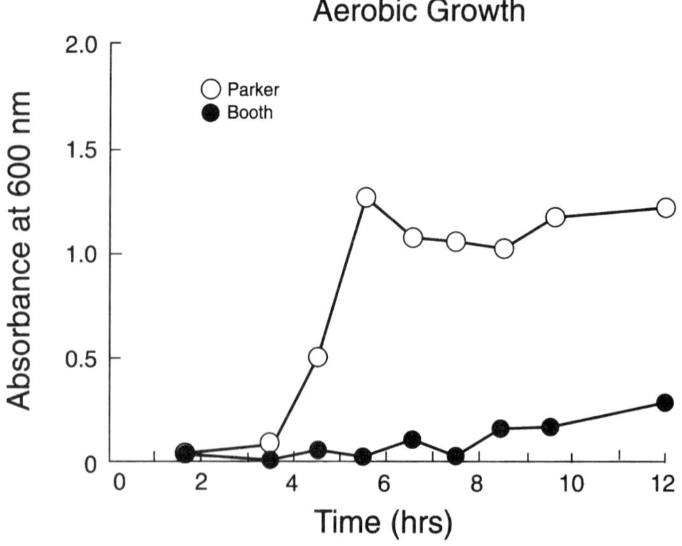

FIGURE 5. Log phase growth of viridans streptococci (Parker) and viridans streptococci (Booth). The kinetics of growth demonstrate rapid growth of the Parker strain compared to the Booth strain.

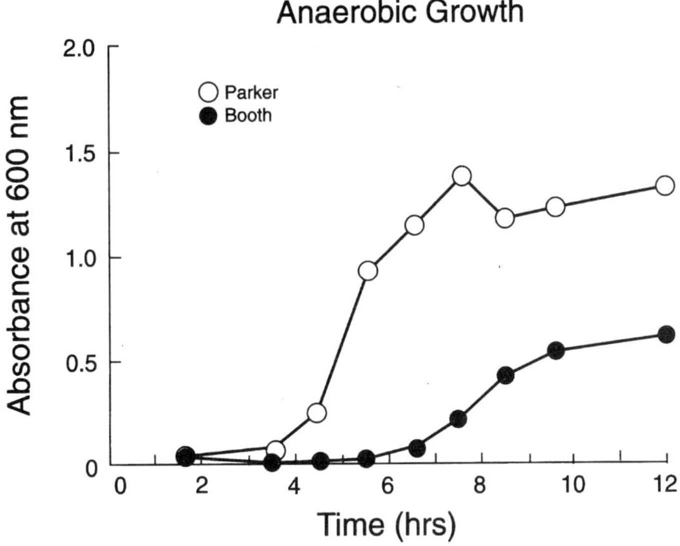

FIGURE 6. Log phase growth in anaerobic environment of viridans streptococci (Parker) and viridans streptococci (Booth). The Parker strain grows more rapidly than the Booth strain.

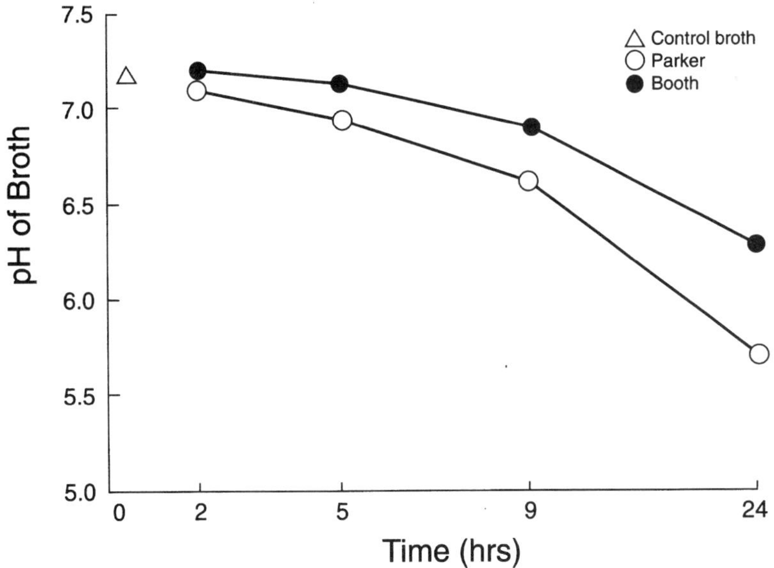

FIGURE 7. The kinetics of pH change between viridans streptococci (Parker) and viridans streptococci (Booth) over a 24-h period. The Parker strain depresses pH of brain–heart infusion (BHI) at a more rapid rate than the Booth strain.

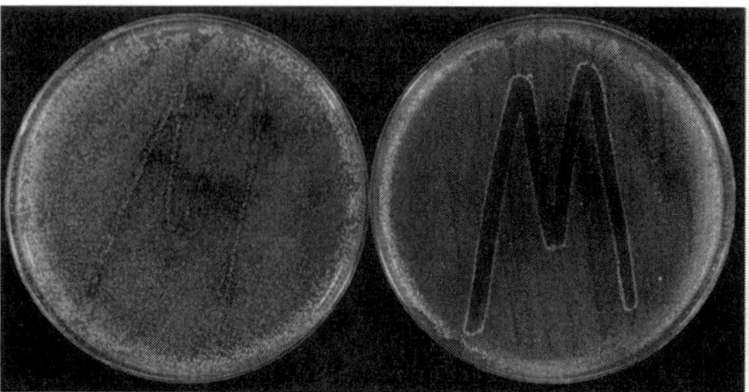

FIGURE 8. Coculture of viridans streptococci (Booth **(left)** and viridans streptococci (Parker) **(right)** with *M. catarrhalis*. The configuration M represents the streaking of the streptococcus over the growth of *M. catarrhalis*. Only the Parker strain causes complete inhibition of growth in the area in which it is streaked. The Booth strain has no inhibitory activity.

peable *H. influenzae*, but none were identified. Our present hypothesis, therefore, is that bacterial interference by *S. oralis* (Parker) may result from a rapid alteration in pH and production of hydrogen peroxide, and possibly by the sequestration of essential nutrients in the nasopharyngeal mucus by this species. That the alteration of pH may be relevant in this ecological niche relates to the average pH of nontypeable *H. influenzae* and that of *S. oralis* at 18 h in broth. The final pH produced by *S. oralis* after 18 h was found to be significantly lower than the pH produced by nontypeable *H. influenzae* in brain–heart infusion broth (TABLE 2).
). It is also well known that oral streptococci are prolific acid procuders and quite tolerant of low pH conditions.[9]

Finally, *S. oralis* (Parker) was also able to inhibit *M. catarrhalis* (FIG. 8) and *S. pneumoniae* (data not shown) when grown side to side on chocolate and blood agar, respectively.

Knowledge of the mechanisms responsible for the alteration of normal flora are extremely important because prevention of colonization with potential pathogens is a major function of the normal flora. Bacterial interference may therefore be a method to protect the nasopharynx from colonization by potential pathogens. The most significant function of the indigenous microflora is its ability to inhibit the implantation of invading organisms (pathogenic or other). Before bacterial pathogens can colonize humans, there must be a break in the activity of the indigenous microflora. It is very possible that the indiscriminate use or inappropriate use of antibiotics can inhibit normal flora and "open the door" to colonization by potential pathogens.

TABLE 2. pH Following 18 h of Incubation with Viridans Streptococci and NTHI in Brain–Heart Infusion Broth

Organism	pH
Viridans streptococci	5.5
NTHI	6.8

There can be no reasonable doubt then that it would be of incalculable benefit to clinical medicine if the composition of the indigenous microflora of man could be manipulated in such a way that bacterial species that are responsible for the beneficial effects of that flora are retained, whereas those that cause detrimental effects are eliminated. This would only be possible, however, if the mechanisms that control the implantation and population size of the microorganisms in the indigenous microflora of the body were better understood.

THE ROLE OF SPECIFIC SECRETORY IgA IN THE NASOPHARYNX AGAINST BACTERIA AND VIRUSES AND ITS IMPLICATION IN OTITIS MEDIA

Adenoidal tissue produces secretory IgA antibody and this antibody serves as the most important specific immunological defense mechanism against colonization of potential pathogens in the upper respiratory tract.[10]

The mechanism whereby secretory IgA acts as a mucosal barrier has been elucidated by investigators studying cell-surface phenomena of phagocytic engulfment and cell adhesiveness.[11] It appears that IgA does not contribute to the hydrophobicity of particles, nor does it enhance phagocytosis. As such, secretory IgA is responsible for at least three biological functions at the level of the mucosal surface.[12] The traditional role of IgA antibodies in mucosal defense has been considered as providing an immune barrier to keep exogenous substances, including microbial pathogens, from penetrating the mucosa. More recently, it has been suggested by *in vitro* and *in vivo* studies that IgA may have additional roles in mucosal defense.[12] For example, during their passage through the lining epithelial cells enroute to the secretion, IgA antibodies may have the opportunity to neutralize intracellular pathogens such as certain bacteria and especially viruses. Also, IgA antibodies in the mucosal lamina propria may complex with antigens and excrete them through the adjacent mucosal epithelium again by the same route to the secretions that is taken by free IgA. These latter functions could aid in recovery from infection. Most clinical studies, have focused on the role of secretory IgA in preventing colonization of bacteria and viruses in the nasopharynx, and subsequently reducing the incidence of inflammatory disease such as otitis media and sinusitis. The nasal mucosa may be the source of protective secretory IgA and the adenoid may serve as the inductive site for development of J-chain-positive IgA B cells that migrate to the nasal mucosa.

The relationship between nasopharyngeal colonization with nonetypeable *H. influenzae* and recurrent otitis media has been assessed in our laboratory by following prospectively children from birth through 12 months of age.[13] Nasopharyngeal secretory IgA reactive to P6 and OMP appears to reduce or eliminate nontypeable *H. influenzae* and is significantly higher in the nasopharyngeal secretions in those children who are colonized less frequently. The results demonstrate a strong relationship between nasopharyngeal colonization patterns and the level of specific secretory IgA against P6 of nontypeable *H. influenzae*. This mucosal immune response appears to be important in the elimination of potential pathogens from the upper respiratory tract, as there is a significant reduction in the incidence of otitis media in these children.

In other studies, human milk secretory IgA antibody to nontypeable *H. influenzae* appears to be protective against nasopharyngeal colonization with this orgranism.[14] The data suggest the protective effects of human milk against otitis media are in part due to inhibition of nasopharyngeal colonization with nontypeable *H. influenzae* by specific secretory IgA antibody. Studies from other laboratories also corroborate the role of secretory IgA as a mucosal defense barrier against respiratory syncytial virus and influenza virus.[15,16] The role of secretory IgA in the nasopharynx in preventing colonization and resultant otitis media with *M. catarrhalis* has yet to be studied.

These studies taken together demonstrate the crucial role of secretory IgA in nasopharyngeal secretions in the defense of the host against bacterial and viral infectious diseases.

Thus far, we have reviewed three different topical strategies to protect the host against colonization of infectious disease particles. They all have in common the basic concept of prevention of colonization of potential pathogens. All three approaches can utilize the topical sprays or suspensions. Specific antibodies directed against bacterial OMPs that function as adhesins, could prevent colonization by directly inhibiting the adherence of bacteria to either nasopharyngeal mucin or nasopharyngeal epithelial cells.

Bacterial interference with the use of a specific strain of viridans streptococcus capable of inhibiting all three bacterial pathogens causing otitis media could be used as a topical spray.

Finally, conserved OMP antigens from the major gram-negative pathogens can induce specific secretory IgA delivered intranasally or orally as a spray.

Th1 AND Th2 CYTOKINE PROFILES IN ADENOIDS: IMPLICATIONS IN OTITIS MEDIA

The development of distinctive subsets of CD4+ T cells during an immune response, distinguished by their ability to produce discrete patterns of cytokines, can determine whether an infectious organism is eradicated or is able to chronically colonize the host. Th1 cells, producing interferon gamma and IL2 mediate immune responses important for the clearance of many infectious organisms, but may be implicated in the immunopathology resulting from organ-specific autoimmune diseases.[17] Th2 cells producing cytokines such as IL4, IL5, IL10, and IL13 were originally defined as helpers of B-cell responses and are now implicated in allergic responses after activation of mast cells and eosinophils. The ability of cytokines such as IL10 and IL4 to inhibit inflammatory as well as Th1-cell-mediated immune responses may explain why cell-mediated and humoral responses are often observed to be mutually exclusive. Th2 subsets are important regulators of cell-mediated immunity.

Our laboratory has been studying the cytokine profiles in the nasopharyngeal tonsil in children with either hypertrophic adenoids without a history of otitis media and in children with recurrent acute otitis media. Data from our laboratory suggest there is a relative decrease in the synthesis of Th1 cytokines, IL2, and IFN-γ, in comparison with the peripheral blood lymphocytes in patients with recurrent otitis media (FIG. 9). In contrast, the Th2 cytokines appear to be synthesized in the same quantities as peripheral blood lymphocytes or, in some cases, greater amounts than the cor-

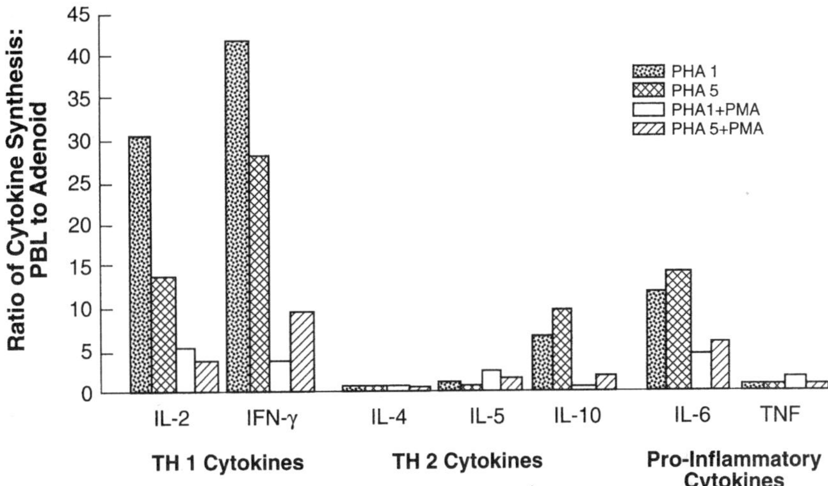

FIGURE 9. Cytokine synthesis: ratio of peripheral blood lymphocytes to adenoids. Summary of findings in the study demonstrate that there is a relative increase in the amount of IL-2 and IFN-γ (Th1 cytokines) in peripheral blood lymphocytes in comparison to adenoidal lymphocytes. In contrast, the production of IL-4, IL-5, and IL-10 (Th2 cytokines) appear to be approximately the same in peripheral blood lymphocytes and adenoidal lymphocytes, suggesting that the adenoidal lymphocytes are capable of producing concentrations of IL-4 and IL-5 that are similar to those of the peripheral blood lymphocytes. IL-6 appears to be produced in greater amounts than the peripheral lymphocytes; TNF-α synthesis appears to be similar in the adenoidal lymphocytes and peripheral blood lymphocytes.

responding peripheral blood mononuclear leukocytes. It should be emphasized that children who were atopic did not appear to have a difference in IL-4 or IL-5 production compared to children who were considered nonatopic. Children with hypertrophic adenoids, or normal-sized adenoids in the absence of otitis media, had higher adenoid levels of IL-2 compared to otitis-prone children, and had lower levels of IFN-γ. Th2 cytokine levels were similar to those of PBL in both groups of children.

Whether or not the apparent imbalance in Th1 production has any clinical significance regarding the development of infectious diseases of the upper respiratory tract is still unclear. Several important concepts may be proposed. The relative ability of the adenoidal lymphocytes to produce IL-4 and IL-5 may be beneficial for the host because the cytokines are important in the production of antibodies that would be directed against potential pathogens. However, a persistence of Th2 cytokines may lead to hyperresponsiveness, which could contribute to a chronic inflammatory state.

Th1 lymphocytes produce IFN-γ, which is important in host defense against viral infection. Viral infections frequently precede most upper respiratory tract maladies in which bacteria invade the middle ear and sinuses. If Th1 cytokines are required for macrophage activation, antigen presentation might be reduced in the early immune response for T-cell-dependent antigens when Th1 cytokines are deficient.

It is apparent that further work in identifying cytokine profiles and their role in modulating the immune response will be advisable in determining the role of the immune response in the nasopharynx and its relationship to the development of inflammation of the eustachian tube and middle ear. Most importantly, defective cytokine production may be responsible for altered IgA synthesis. This could be critical for the homeostasis and defense of the nasopharynx in the prevention of inflammatory disease of the middle ear and sinuses.

SUMMARY

The nasopharyngeal tonsil, or adenoid, is a major inductive site for the synthesis of J-chain-positive B cells that may migrate to other areas of the upper respiratory tract, such as the nasal mucosa, the parotid gland, the lacrimal gland, and the middle ear during inflammation. The production of secretory IgA by both the nasopharyngeal tonsil and the nasal mucosa plays a major role in local immune protection against bacteria and viruses. The release of cytokines from Th1 and Th2 lymphocytes must be appropriate for B cells to produce IgA. The factors or mechanisms responsible for this are not, at present, known, but it appears that there is a difference in the profiles of cytokine secretion by Th1 and Th2 lymphocytes in the adenoids in both otitis-prone, as well as nonotitis-prone children.

We have suggested that if this specific immune system does not protect the host from invasion by potential pathogens, there are other modalities of therapy to protect the nasopharynx from colonization with pathogenic bacteria or viruses. These include the production of specific antibodies against bacterial surface proteins that have been identified as mucin-binding proteins. Alteration of the microbial flora with commensal organisms such as viridans streptococci can be utilized. These α-hemolytic streptococci probably function by producing an acid environment that prevents colonization of organisms such as nontypeable *H. influenzae*. Finally, the induction of specific SIgA by conserved outer membrane protein antigens of potential pathogens may be another strategy in the prevention of colonization of potential bacterial pathogens in the nasopharynx.

REFERENCES

1. MURPHY, T. F. & M. A. APICELLA. 1985. Antigenic heterogeneity of outer membrane proteins of nontypable *Haemophilus influenzae* is a basis for a serotyping system. Infect. Immun. **50:** 15–21.
2. REDDY, R. S., J. M. BERNSTEIN, T. F. MURPHY & H. S. FADEN. 1996. Binding between outer membrane proteins of nontypable *H. influenzae* and human nasopharyngeal mucin. Infect. Immun. **64:** 1477–1479.
3. MURRAY, P. S., M. J. LEVINE, L. A. TABAK & M. S. REDDY. 1982. Specificity of salivary-bacterial interactions. II. Evidence for a lectin on Streptococcus sanguis with specificity for a NeuAcα2,3Galβ1,3GalNAc sequence. Biochem. Biophys. Res. Commun. **106:** 390–396.
4. FRETER, R., H. BRICKNER, M. BOTMEY, D. CLEVEN & A. ARANKI. 1983. Mechanisms that control bacterial population in continuous-flow culture models of mouse large intestinal flora. Infect. Immun. **36:** 676–685.

5. SANDERS, W. E., JR. 1969. Bacterial interference I. Its occurrence among respiratory tract flora and characterization of inhibition of Group A *streptococci* by viridans *streptococci*. Infect. Dis., **120:** 698–707.

6. SPRUNT, K., G. LEIDY & W. REDMAN. 1980. Abnormal colonization of neonates in an ICU: Conversion to normal colonization by pharyngeal implantation of alpha hemolytic streptococcus strain 215. Pediatr. Res. **14:** 308–313.

7. BERNSTEIN, J. M., H. F. FADEN, D. M. DRYJA & J. WACTAWSKI-WENDE. 1993. Microecology of the nasopharyngeal bacterial flora in otitis-prone and non-otitis-prone children. Acta Otolaryngol. (Stockholm) **113:** 88–92.

8. BERNSTEIN, J. M., S. SAGAHTAHERI-ALTAIE, D. M DRYJA & J. WACTAWSKI-WENDE. 1994. Bacterial interference in nasopharyngeal bacterial flora of otitis-prone and non-otitis-prone children. Acta Otolaryngol. (Belg.) **48:** 1–9.

9. VAN HOUTE, J. 1980. Bacterial specificity in the etiology of dental caries. Int. Dent. **301:** 305–326.

10. BRANDTZAEG, P. 1987. Immune functions and immunopathology of palatine and nasopharyngeal tonsils. *In* Immunology of the Ear, J. M. Bernstein and P. L. Ogra, Eds.: 63–106. Raven Press. New York.

11. VAN OSS, C. J. & C. GILLMAN. 1975. Phagocytic engulfment and cell adhesiveness as cell surface phenomena. *In* Micro-organisms and Infectious Diseases, Vol. 2. Decker. New York.

12. LAMM, M. E., J. G. NEDRUD, C. S. KAETZEL & N .B. MAZANEC. 1995. IgA and mucosal defense. APMIS **103:** 241–246.

13. HARABUCHI, Y., H. FADEN, N. YAMANAKA, L. DUFFY, J. WOLF & D. KRYSTOFIK. 1994. Nasopharyngeal colonization with nontypeable Haemophilus influenzae and recurrent otitis media J. Infect. Dis. **170:** 826–866.

14. HARABUCHI, Y., H. FADEN, N. YAMANAKA, L. DUFFY, J. WOLF & D. KRYSTOFIK. 1994. Human milk secretory IgA antibody to nontypeable Haemophilus influenzae: Possible protective effects against nasopharyngeal colonization. J. Pediatr. **124:** 193–198.

15. WELTZIN, R., S. HSU, E. S. MITTLER, K. GEORGAKOPOULIS & T. P. MONATH. 1994. Intranasal monoclonal immunoglobulin A against respiratory syncytial virus protects against upper and lower respiratory tract infections in mice. Antimicrob. Agents Chemother. **38:** 2785–1791.

16. MAZANEC, M., C. S. KAETZEL, M. E. LAMM, D. FLETCHER, J. PETERRA & J. G. NEDRUD. 1995. Intracellular neutralization of Sendai and influenzae viruses by IgA monoclonal antibodies. Adv. Exp. Med. Biol. **371A:** 651–654.

17. O'GARRA, A. & K. MURPHY. 1996. Role of cytokines in development of Th1/Th2 cells. *In* Th1 and Th2 Cells in Health and Disease, S. Romagnani, Ed.:1–13. Karger Press. Basel, Switzerland.

The Immunology of the Host–Parasite Relationship in the Nasopharynx[a]

BRITTA RYNNEL-DAGÖÖ,[b,d] KARIN LINDBERG,[b]
ANDERS SAMULESON,[c] STEN BLOMBERG,[b]
AND JOACHIM FORSGREN[b]

[b]Department of Clinical Sciences
Division of Oto-Rhino-Laryngology
Karolinska Institute
Huddinge Hospital
S-141 86 Huddinge, Sweden

[c]Department of Clinical Sciences
Division of Clinical Bacteriology
Karolinska Institute
Huddinge Hospital
S-141 86 Huddinge, Sweden

INTRODUCTION

The host–parasite relationship in the nasopharynx with bacterial colonization and antigen uptake in the epithelium and lymphatic tissue provides an opportunity for investigating infectious/inflammatory processes and responses in healthy and infection-prone individuals.

The human nasopharynx is a natural reservoir for several bacterial species, including *Streptococcus pneumoniae*, nontypeable *Hemophilus influenzae* (NTHI), and *Moraxella (Branhamella) catarrhalis*.[1] Earlier it was believed that the binding process between the microorganism and the host target cell was a passive event. During the last decade it has become evident that binding initiates a process both in the bacterium and in the host cell with induction of signals and release of mediators.[2]

The microflora is established early in childhood, and longitudinal studies with repeated upper respiratory tract cultures from the same population over several years have contributed to the understanding of the dynamics and turnover of bacteria in these regions. Adherence of pneumococci has been monitored in several epidemiological studies, particularly in the age group 1–2 years,[3] where the colonization rate is about 90%. The epidemiology of NTHI is less well known because of earlier difficulties to classify this species. In one recent study the colonization rate was 35% in preschool children.[4] A decline with increasing age has also been demonstrated.[5]

Recurrent acute otitis media (RAOM) is a common problem in children. Thus, in

[a]This study was supported by grants the Ragnar and Torsten Söderberg Foundation, and from the Swedish Association for Medical Research.

[d]Address for correspondence: Dr. Britta Rynnel-Dagöö, Division of ENT, B53, Huddinge University Hospital, S-141 86 Huddinge, Sweden. Phone: +46858580000; fax: +4687467551.

an epidemiological investigation 5% of children under the age of four were reported to have contracted between 6 and 11 episodes.[6] Carriership is a potential mechanism for pathogenicity since bacteria might invade the eustachian tube and the middle ear and cause disease. In episodes of acute otitis media, the same bacterial strains are found in the nasopharynx and in the middle-ear cavity, as demonstrated with genetic fingerprinting.[7]

The pharyngeal tonsil or adenoid is a part of the mucosa-associated lymphatic tissue, responsible for regional immune functions in the nasopharynx. The epithelium is a site for bacterial attachment and is covered by a viscous secretion, known to bind microorganisms and contain locally produced immunoglobulins.[8] From the surface, deep crypts penetrate into the tissue and are outlined with a specialized epithelium with dendritic cells and macrophages. The adenoid is also highly organized into T- and B-cell areas and possesses the cellular prerequisites for antigen uptake, processing, presentation, and T–B-cell cooperation.[9]

Considerable interest has been focused on the role of cytokines in intercellular interactions.[10] The inflammatory cytokines, interleukin 1β (IL-1β), interleukin 6 (IL-6), and tumor necrosis factor α (TNF-α) are glycoproteins produced by a wide variety of cell types when exposed to bacteria and viruses.[11] These polypeptide hormones mediate a broad spectrum of biological activities, such as triggering of the acute phase response, T- and B-cell proliferation and differentiation.[12] Increased serum cytokine levels have been reported in various bacterial infections with septicemia.

Virtually nothing has been described concerning cytokine production in the nasopharynx. In this compartment, the heavy load of bacteria could imply a stimulus for cytokine production, leading to local cytokine production in the tissue and detectable levels in nasopharyngeal secretions.

By using fluorescent oligonucleotide probes for *in situ* DNA-RNA hybidization, Forsgren *et al.*[13] have obtained evidence that NTHI resides and multiplies intracellularly in human adenoid tissue. The reservoir for these bacterial colonizations seems to be macrophages in the subepithelial layers close to the reticular crypt epithelium. For infection-prone individuals it would probably be of value if this colonization could be diminished or eliminated. This could be achieved by the administration of a drug known to have a good intracellular penetration and an effect against NTHI. Thus azithromycin,[14] a rather new antibiotic, related to macrolides, was given in a randomized study preoperatively to children scheduled for adenoidectomy.

The aim of the present study was to elucidate the production of cytokines in adenoid tissue and as reflected by levels of nasopharyngeal secretions, in healthy and otitis-prone children with and without treatment with antibiotics, in healthy adults, and in individuals with immunodeficiency.

MATERIALS AND METHODS

Patient Group I

The study groups consisted of 46 children, 18 healthy (2–89 months, 8 of which were <18 months, median age 24 months), with 0–1 episodes of acute otitis media;

and 28 children (8–38 months, of which 13 were <18 months, median age 20 months) at risk for development of the otitis-prone condition, with >3 episodes before 1 year of age or 6 episodes before 18 months of age, designated RAOM children. Forty-one of the 46 children were 3 years or younger. Also 21 healthy adults and 19 adults with hypogammaglobulinemia or selective deficiency of IgG3 were included. The healthy adults and the healthy children did not receive prophylactic antibiotics, but 10 of the 28 RAOM children were treated. From 3 RAOM children, no information about antibiotics was available. From 23/28 RAOM and 12/18 healthy children, information about other medical treatment was available; none of them received antihistamins, intranasal corticosteroids, or decongestants. In 4/28 RAOM and 1/18 healthy children, allergy was reported (2 astma, 3 to antibiotics, and 1 to food).

Patient Group II

The study group consisted of healthy children admitted for adenoidectomy because of nasal obstruction due to a large adenoid. Children without a history of middle-ear disease were randomized for treatment with azithromycin (Az group) or for no treatment (control group). To achieve an optimal effect azithromycin treatment was started 10 days before the operation and given in an adequate dose for 5 days. Twenty children were included, 11 in the Az group and 9 in the control group. The mean age distribution was 8.1 years (range 4–12) and 5.8 years (range 3–9) in the Az and control groups, respectively. The male/female ratio was 9/3 for the Az group and 5/4 for the control group. No patient had received antibiotic treatment because of disease during the month prior to adenoidectomy.

Collection and Preparation of Secretions—Patient Groups I and II

Specimens from the nasopharyngeal space were obtained more than 2 h after a meal with a suction device, the Juhn-Tym-Tap via the oral route, and care was taken not to damage the mucosa or to contaminate the sampled material with saliva or blood. In children, the collection had to be done under general anesthesia (in healthy children due to nonotological surgery or adenoidectomy; in RAOM children due to insertion of myringostomy tubes), all given the same type of premedication. All samples were obtained under clinical infection-free conditions, except for those from patients with immunodeficiency.

Because of our current regime with a transmyringeal ventilating tube insertion in young patients at risk for recurrent episodes of middle-ear disease, it was possible to collect nasopharyngeal secretions during the operating procedure. Due to small amounts (30–100 μL) and high viscosity of the nasopharyngeal specimens, the quantity from some individuals was not sufficient for all analyses planned.

The secretions were weighed and diluted 1/10 in PBS. For solubilzation of the secretions, glass beads (2 mm in diameters) were added. The secretions were then centrifuged for 30 min in +4°C at 10,000 rpm. The soluble fractions were immediately frozen at –70°C and stored until analyzed. Sera were obtained from 39 children and from all healthy adults and were centrifuged and stored as previously (patient group I).

Bacterial Culture—Patient Group II

Prior to the operation specimens for nasopharyngeal culture were obtained via the nasal route. A semiquantitative evaluation was performed:++++>100, +++50–99, ++10–49, and +<10 colonies. Excised adenoid tissue was divided asceptically and either frozen and stored in –70°C until further analysis or processed for quantitative bacterial culture, as was described earlier.[13] Briefly, one specimen was weighed and homogenized. After dilution, 0.1 mL samples of tenfold dilution steps were plated onto agar plates in duplicates. *H. influenzae, S. pneumoniae, M. catarrhalis,* and *S. pyogenes* were identified using standard bacteriologic techniques, counted and reported as colony-forming units (CFU)/g adenoid. Statistical evaluation was performed using the Mann–Whithney U-test.

Assays for Detection of Cytokines in Nasopharyngeal Secretions and Serum

Assays for IL-1β, IL-6, and TNF-α were performed with commercially available EASIA kits (Medgenix Diagnostics, Brussels, Belgium—patient group I, and R&D, Minnesota—patient group II). The kits were based on the oligoclonal system in which several Mabs directed against distinct epitopes of IL-1β, IL-6, and TNF-α, respectively, were used. The optical density of the wells was measured at 490 nm by a Microplate Autoreader (Bio Tekinstruments). A standard curve was plotted, and concentrations of the cytokines in the samples were determined by interpolation from the standard curve. The separate EASIA assays have been studied with respect to specificity for IL-1β, IL-6, and TNF-α, respectively. Thus, the IL-1β EASIA does not detect IL-6 and TNF-α, the IL-6 EASIA does not detect IL-1β and TNF-α, and the TNF-α EASIA does not detect IL-1β and IL-6. Minimum detectable concentrations of IL-1β was estimated to be 1–2 pg/mL and for IL-6 and TNF-α, 3 pg/mL. Absorption experiments over night with selected IL-6-containing nasopharyngeal fluids using immobilized antihuman IL-6 antibodies (Genzyme code1618-01) were performed.

Albumin

Albumin was analyzed according to standard laboratory methods (Department of Clinical Chemistry, Huddinge Hospital, Sweden).

Immunohistochemistry of Adenoid Tissue

Specimen of adenoid tissue for fluorescent *in situ* hybridization (FISH) and for immunohistochemistry (IHC) were snap frozen in liquid nitrogen. The frozen tissue

TABLE 1. Mouse Mabs Used for the Detection of Human Cytokines[a]

	Concentration (μg/mL)	Source
IL-1β	10	Genzyme (Cambridge, MA)
IL-2	5	Genzyme (Cambridge, MA)
IL-4	5	Genzyme (Cambridge, MA)
IL-5	25	Genzyme (Cambridge, MA)
IL-6	10	Genzyme (Cambridge, MA)
IL-10	2.5	Serotec (Oxford, UK)
TNF-α	25	R & D Systems (Oxon, UK)
IFN-γ	5	Serotec (Oxford, UK)
IgG$_1$ control (*Aspergillus niger*)	2.5–25	Dakopatts (Glostrup, DK)

[a]Working concentrations and sources.

was cut in sections 6 μm thick and left to air-dry at room temperature overnight. The sections used for IHC were fixed in 4% formaldehyde, permeabilized with 0.1% saponin, and stained with Mabs (TABLE 1) with the modified ABC protocol according to J. Andersson *et al.*[15] Endogenous peroxidase activity was quenched with hydrogen peroxide. Sections were stained in duplicate and subclass-matched irrelevant monoclonal antibodies (*Aspergillus niger*) were used as controls.

The sections stained for the eight different cytokines were studied using ordinary light microscopy. Microscope images were captured with an S-VHS camera and digitized with a RasterOps 24 XLTVs board (RasterOps Corp, Santa Clara, CA) and a personal computer. All cells in the sections were counted, and the respective area positively stained for cytokines was measured and calculated interactively using the IP Lab Spectrum (Signal Analytics Corp., Vienna, Virginia) software for digital image analysis. The result was expressed as area ratio, that is, the mean sum of the surface stained positively for each cytokine divided with the respective section area.

Fluorescent in situ *Hybridization*

The adenoid tissue sections were hybridized *in situ* with a FITC-conjugated oligonucleotide DNA-probe specific for and complementary to *H. influenzae* 16S ribosomal RNA was performed as described earlier.[13]

The result of the FISH was studied using epifluorescence microscopy and the number of *H. influenzae*-containing cells/mm^2 in three consecutive sections was determined for each case. The nonparametric Mann–Whitney U-test was used for statistical comparison.

RESULTS

IL-1β, IL-6, and TNF-α in Nasopharyngeal Secretions

IL-1β: 70 samples of nasopharyngeal secretions were analyzed (FIG. 1). Detectable levels of IL-1β were found in 22 of 40 children (healthy, 11/14; RAOM,

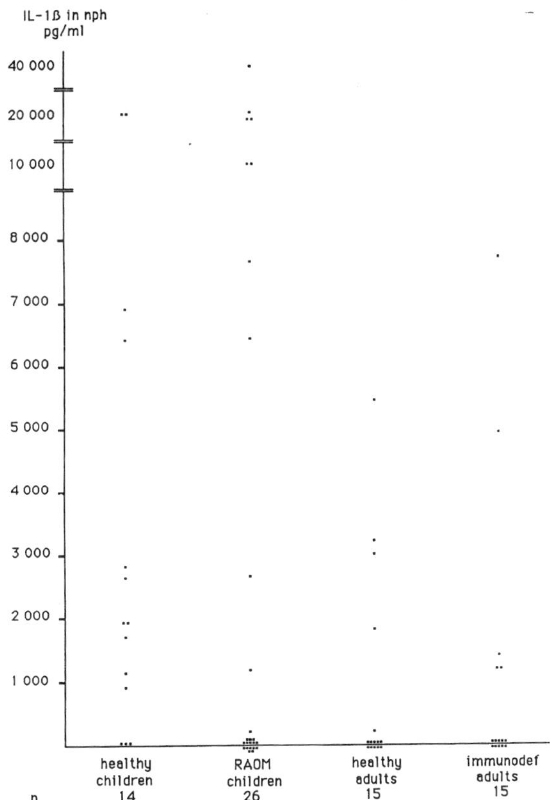

FIGURE 1. The levels of IL-1β in nasopharyngeal secretions from healthy children, children with recurrent episodes of acute otitis media (RAOM), healthy adults, and adults with immunodeficiency syndrome.

11/26), in 5 of 15 healthy adults, and in 5 of 15 adults with immunodeficiency. Healthy children showed significantly ($p < 0.05$) higher levels of IL-β in nasopharyngeal secretions than RAOM children. The levels of IL-1β in healthy were significantly ($p = 0.05$) higher than in healthy adults.

IL-6: 85 samples from nasopharyngeal secretions were analyzed (FIG. 2). Detectable levels of IL-6 were found in 35 of 46 children (healthy, 13/18; RAOM, 22/28), in 4 of 20 healthy adults, and in 6 of 19 adults with hypogammaglobulinemia. Healthy children exhibited higher levels of IL-6 than RAOM children, although the difference was not significant. A significant difference was found when healthy children were compared to healthy adults ($p = 0.05$).

TNF-α: 81 samples of nasopharyngeal secretions were analyzed. In 14 of 42 children (healthy, 7/15; RAOM, 7/27), in 2 of 20 healthy adults, and in 1 of the 19 adults with immunodeficiency detectable levels of TNF-α were seen. The levels of TNF-α in nasopharyngeal secretions were higher in healthy children (not significant) than in RAOM children. Healthy children showed significantly ($p = 0.05$) higher levels than

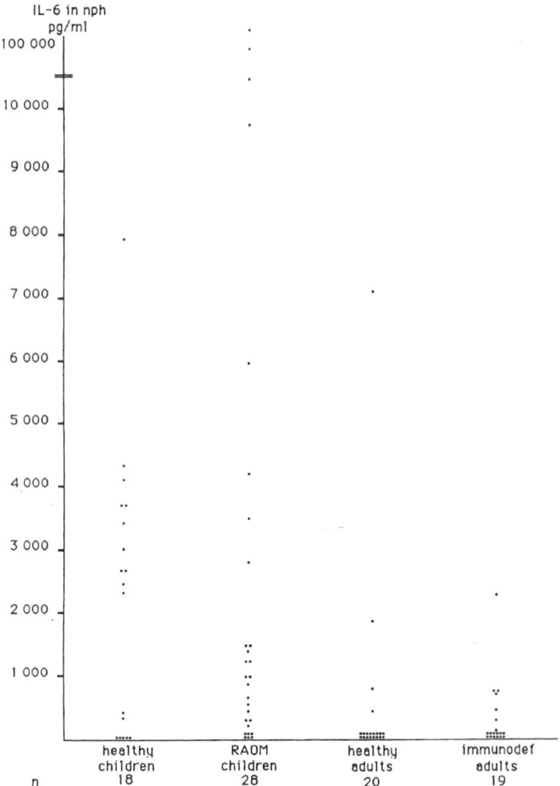

FIGURE 2. IL-6 levels in nasopharyngeal secretions from healthy children, children with recurrent episodes of acute otitis media (RAOM), healthy adults, and adults with immunodeficiency syndrome.

healthy adults. In all but three children with detectable TNF-α, IL-6 was also demonstrated. No differences were found in the levels of IL-1β, IL-6, and TNF-α in nasopharyngeal secretions from healthy adults and adults with hypogammaglobulinemia, respectively.

Possible Effects of Antibiotics on Cytokine Production

Ten of the 26 RAOM children were treated with prophylactic antibiotics, while the remaining 16 children were not. The levels of IL-1β were measured, and there was no significant difference between the groups. Furthermore, cytokine levels were compared in 14 nontreated healthy and 16 nontreated RAOM children (FIG. 3). The 16 nontreated RAOM children exhibited significantly lower levels than the 14 healthy children. This difference was significant ($p = 0.05$). Higher levels of both IL-6 and TNF-α were also seen in the healthy children, but the difference was not significant.

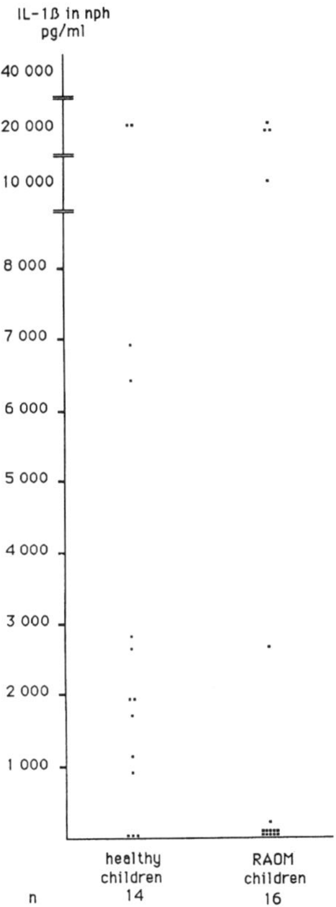

FIGURE 3. The levels of IL-1β in nasopharyngeal secretions in children not treated with antibiotics.

Comparison of IL-1β, IL-6, and TNF-α in Individual Nasopharyngeal Secretions

In all 14 healthy children and in 22 of the 26 RAOM children, one or more of the three cytokines were elevated. Two different patterns were found. Sometimes, high levels of IL-1β were associated with low or undetectable levels of IL-6 and TNF-α, whereas low levels of IL-1β were associated with high levels of IL-6 and TNF-α, especially in RAOM children.

Detectability of Cytokines in Nasopharyngeal Secretions

In order to study the specificity of the detection of cytokines in nasopharyngeal fluid, a number of experiments were undertaken and have been described earlier.[16]

Cytokine Levels in Sera

Selected serum samples, 13 of which were analyzed with respect to IL-1β and 17 with respect to TNF-α showed lower or undetectable levels of these cytokines (IL-1β <112 pg/mL, TNF-α <43 pg/mL). Forty-two sera from the children and healthy adults with IL-6 exceeding 20 pg/mL in nasopharyngeal secretions generally showed negligible levels of IL-6.

Il-1β in Nasopharyngeal Secretions: Patient Group II

Moderately elevated levels of Il-1β were found in samples from all children with no difference between the Az group and the control group (FIG. 4).

Albumin

The albumin concentration was measured both in secretions (mg/L) and in serum (g/L). In secretions, no difference was found between healthy children and RAOM children. The quotient of albumin in secretions (mg/L) and in sera (g/L) was 0.16 in the adult group and 0.38 in the two groups of children ($p = 0.0002$). The higher levels in children indicate a higher degree of leakage from serum.

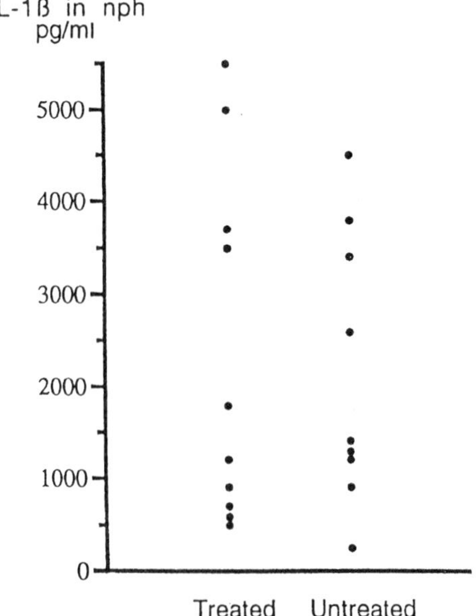

FIGURE 4. The levels of IL-1β in nasopharyngeal secretions in children treated and untreated with azithromycin.

Nasopharyngeal Colonization: Patient Group II

Specimens positive for NTHI or *M. catarrhalis* or from both species (all ++++) were found in 5/9 in the control group. In the Az group positive cultures were found in 3/11 children (all +).

Quantitative Culture from Adenoid Tissue: Patient Group II

The viable counts of the aerobic respiratory tract pathogens *H. influenzae, M. catarrhalis, S. pneumoniae,* and *S. pyogenes* varied from 6.4×10^2 to 7.8×10^6 CFU/g adenoid. Counts of $<10^2$ CFU/g adenoid were not detected in this assay.[13] The presence of the previously listed bacterial species in adenoid cell suspension is summarized (TABLE 1). The concentration of *H. influenzae* in CFU/g adenoid tissue were about 10-fold lower in the group of children treated with azithromycin ($p<0.05$, Mann–Whitney U-test). In brief, in 9/20 children one or more potential pathogens were found in the nasopharyngeal swabs cultures. NTHI were found in five of these children. Ordinary flora only or no growth of bacteria was recorded in the remaining 11 cultures. In the quantitative culture the bacterial load, that is, the sum of colony-forming units (CFUs) of potential pathogens per gram of adenoid tissue ranged from 10^2 cfu/g—the lowest detectable bacterial concentration—to 1.4×10^7 cfu/g. NTHI were found in 12/20 of the quantitative cultures. Seven children had a bacterial load of $<10^5$ cfu/g and 13 children had a bacterial load of $>10^5$ cfu/g.

Fluorescent in situ Hybridization—Patient Group II

In situ hybridization with the AGN-1-FLU probe demonstrated *H. influenzae* in adenoid tissue sections from all 20 patients, including those who were negative for quantitative culture. There was a typical distribution of *H. influenzae* in large mononuclear cells located close to the adenoid cryptepithelium. It has to be pointed out that all specimens were positive. In one case a few bacteria were seen (0.7/section), and in two cases very high numbers (>200/section) were found. All three belonged to the Az group.

Cytokines in Tissue—Patient Group II

Seven children had a bactrial load of $<10^5$ cfu/g, and 13 children had a bacterial load of $>10^5$ cfu/g. In the FISH, the number of *H. influenzae*-containing cells ranged from 0.02 to 40 cells/mm^2, with a mean of 4.4 (median 2.3) cells/mm^2.

All eight cytokines were detected *in situ* in the adenoid tissue. The background staining was low and the negative controls were consistently negative. Positively stained cells were mostly lymphocytes and monocytes/macrophages as judged by morphology and often localized subepithelially (FIG. 5). However, positive epithelial cells were also seen, especially when stained for IL-6 (not shown).

The mean and median area ratios for all cytokines except IL-2 and IFN-γ were

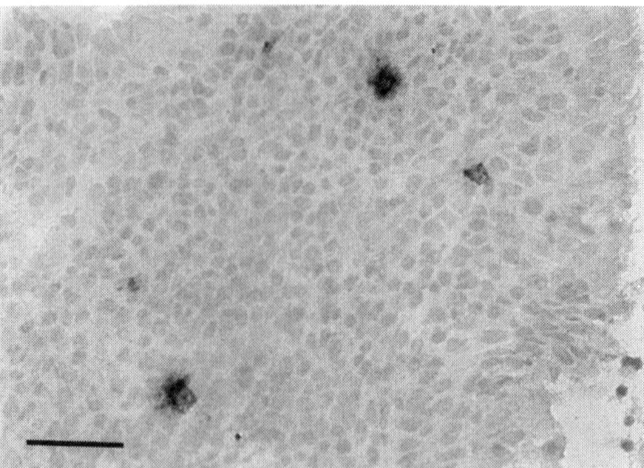

FIGURE 5. Light micrograph showing an adenoid tissue section stained for IL-1β and counterstained with Hematoxylon. Positively stained cells are seen subepithelially. Bar = 50 μm.

higher in the group with one or more potential pathogens as compared to the group with ordinary flora or no growth in the nasopharyngeal swabs cultures (TABLE 2). Statistical significance was reached only for IL-6 ($p = 0.02$). The same tendency to higher area ratio values for all cytokines except IL-2 was also observed in the children with a bacterial load of $> 10^5$ cfu/g as compared to the children with a bacterial load of $> 10^5$ cfu/g in the quantitative culture assay (TABLE 2). Statistical significance was reached for IL-6 and IL-4 ($p < 0.05$).

No correlation was found between the area ratio for any of the detected cytokines and the number of *H. influenzae*-containing cells/mm^2 in the adenoid tissue sections. Nor was any particular cytokine profile found, for example, in terms of quantitative expression of IL-2 and IFN-γ (T$_h$1 cytokines) versus IL-4, IL-5, and IL-10 (T$_h$2 cytokines) in the cases with high numbers as compared to the cases with low numbers of *H. influenzae*-containing cells (data not shown).

DISCUSSION

Although cytokines have been implicated in inflammatory reactions in many diseases, little is known about their role in immune responses to bacteria colonizing mucosal membranes in individuals without clinical signs of infection. The present study provides information about cytokines in nasopharyngeal secretions, cytokine production in the nasopharyngeal mucosa, and adenoid tissue.

Healthy, very young children, one to three years of age, were found to have IL-1β, IL-6, and TNF-α levels in nasopharyngeal secretions, which were significantly higher than in healthy adults. The secretions were found to contain substantial quantities of IL-1β (22 positive of 40), IL-6 (35 positive of 46), and TNF-α (14 positive of 42). In a few cases extremely high levels of IL-1β, IL-6, and TNF-α were detected in the absence of upper respiratory tract infection. Children 3 to 12 years of age all had demonstrable amounts of IL-1β, although lower than in the younger age-group. In

TABLE 2. Mean Area Ratio ($\mu m^2/mm^2 \times 10^6$) in the Adenoid Tissue for the Eight Different Cytokines in the Children with a Bacterial Load of $>10^5$ CFU/g and the Children with a Bacterial Load of $<10^5$ CFU/g in the Quantitative Cultures on Homogenized Adenoid Tissue, Respectively

	N	IL-1β	IL-2	IL-4	IL-5	IL-6	IL-10	TNF-α	INF-γ
$>10^5$ CFU/g	13	12.2	2.6	200	9.4	41	14	30	5.3
$<10^5$ CFU/g	7	4.3	2.8	74	7.6	18	13	35	1.5
p^a		N.S.[b]	N.S.	<0.05	N.S.	<0.05	N.S.	N.S.	N.S.

[a]Mann–Whitney U-test.
[b]N.S. = not significant.

healthy adults and adults with immunodeficiency approximately 30% were found to have detectable levels of IL-1β. It is possible that serum leakage into nasopharynx, a phenomen known to be more prominent in children compared to adults,[8] caused dilution of the nasopharyngeal fluid. Thus, were it not for this dilution it is likely that the levels of cytokines in nasopharyngeal secretions of children, as measured in this study, would have been even more elevated. In contrast, children with recurrent episodes of otitis media exhibited significantly lower nasopharyngeal IL-1β levels than healthy children. IL-6 and TNF-α were also lower, although not significantly. TNF-α was detected less frequently than IL-1β and IL-6, but was correlated to positive IL-6 determinations. The very high IL-β levels in nasopharyngeal fluid was associated with low levels of IL-6 and TNF-α, whereas low levels of IL-1β were found in children with high levels of IL-6 and TNF-α. This pattern was most pronounced in otitis-prone children.

The present observation that children at risk for development of the otitis-prone condition often lacked nasopharyngeal cytokine activity, points to the possibility that they have a local defect in cytokine production. Such a putative defect may be responsible for defective immune reactivity. A defective or immature immune system, mainly demonstrated as low levels of the IgG 2 subclass and of low specific antibody activity against common pneumococcal serotypes or against a highly conserved outer membrane protein from NTHI (P 6) in serum, in a significant number of highly otitis-prone children, has been reported in several prospective controlled studies,[17–19] and may be consistent with the present findings.

The poor cytokine production in RAOM children may be a result of antibiotics. Prophylactic treatment at the time of operation was given to 10 otitis-prone children, and might have reduced bacterial load on mucosa and lymphatic tissue, resulting in lower cytokine levels. However, the fact that the 16 individuals not treated with antibiotics also showed statistically low cytokine production indicate that antibiotics did not supress cytokine induction. In a prospective study of otitis-prone children *H. influenzae* was isolated from the nasopharynx even after antibiotic treatment of AOM in about 70% of the episodes.[20] Despite the fact that it is justified to assume that children requiring antibiotics were more severely affected than those not given any treatment, RAOM children without antibiotic prophylaxis were found to have significantly lower levels of IL-1β. In order to further test the hypothesis of an effect of antibiotics on cytokine production, azithromycin—an antibiotic with documented effect on

NTHI[14] and also other microorganisms in the upper respiratory tract—was given to healthy children in a randomized study. Although quantitative culture from adenoid tissue showed significantly lower amounts of NTHI in specimens from children given antibiotics compared to the control group, nasopharyngeal secretions from both groups of children were found to contain comparable amounts of IL-1β. Azithromycin did not eradicate the bacterial flora and did not supress cytokine production. Thus it might be justified to assume that azithromycin does not hamper an immune response in this region, as reflected by the local production of inflammatory cytokines.

Furthermore, attempts have been made to quantitatively analyze the expression of cytokines in adenoid tissue. Using selected Mabs, permeabilization of the tissue with saponin and a modified ABC protocol for immunohistochemical stainings, it was possible to specifically detect cytokines at the protein level *in situ*. The quantitation of cytokine expression was made feasible and more exact than in traditional semi-quantitative immunomorphometric assays by use of computer assisted image analysis.

The expression of IL-1β, IL-4, IL-5, IL-6, TNF-α and IFN-γ was greater in patients with one or more potential pathogens when compared to patients with normal flora only or no growth of bacteria in the nasopharyngeal swabs cultures. The same tendency was also observed when comparing the group of children with high bacterial load with the group of children with low bacterial load in the quantitative culture on homogenized adenoid tissue. This is in accordance with the finding of higher amounts of IL-1β, in nasopharyngeal secretions from healthy infants with NTHI colonization.[16] The finding of strong expression of IL-4, apparently correlated to the level of bacterial colonization could be interpreted as a sign of activation of the adenoid lymphatic tissue by bacteria—even under clinically infection-free conditions. IL-4 is important in the early differentiation of B cells toward mature antibody-forming plasma cells. We have recently demonstrated the intense proliferative activity in the B-cell areas of the adenoid.[21]

The present results contain several findings that merit consideration and discussion. Accordingly, the high and even extremely high levels of IL-1β, IL-6, and TNF-α in nasopharyngeal secretions in healthy children, and in a minority of adults, and the constant finding of a large number of cytokines in adenoid lymphatic tissue, clearly indicate an activation of the local synthesis in epithelium and/or lymphatic tissue. The high cytokine levels in nasopharyngeal secretions probably depend primarily on the presence of inducing factors such as LPS from gram-negative bacteria. However, it is also possible that the nasopharynx of children contain a relatively large number of potent producer cells in the epithelium, the subepithelial region, or the organized lymphatic tissue.

Epithelial cells in the urinary tract have been found to produce IL-6,[22] and the epithelium in the respiratory tract may also play a role for the cytokine production besides intra- or subepithelial macrophages and T cells. The relatively weak production of cytokines in patients with immunodeficiency diseases, in spite of heavy *H. influenzae* colonization, may reflect that the mucosa of these patients contain few producer cells. Furthermore, the poor cytokine production may constitute a primary reason for defective local immunity.

The lipopolysaccharide (LPS) component of gram-negative bacteria has been shown to induce production of IL-1β, IL-6, TNF-α, and possibly other mediators of inflammation.[11,23] In several models of experimental urinary-tract infections in mice and humans, *E. coli* has been found to be a potent inducer of IL-6.[22,24] *NTHI* is considered the most pathogenic organism associated with chronic secretory otitis media,[25] which is an inflammatory process in the middle-ear cleft. Endotoxin is present in a high percentage of middle-ear effusions,[26] and significant levels of IL-1β, IL-6, and TNF-α have been found in the fluid.[27] Also teichoic acid from gram-positive bacteria can induce cytokine production, and high cytokine levels were demonstrated in serum of sepsis patients with both gram-negative and gram-positive infections.[28,29]

The high nasopharyngeal cytokine levels and the constant finding of cytokines in adenoid tissue may seem reasonable in the light of the fact that the upper respiratory tract is a common site of gram-negative bacterial colonization in children.[4] IL-6 was demonstrable on tissue sections and IL-1β, IL-6, and TNF-α levels were higher in children with demonstrable *H. influenzae* growth in nasopharyngeal cultures than in culture-negative children (data not shown). The capacity of *M. catarrhalis* to induce cytokine production is less well known, but a contribution of LPS from this species to cytokine production cannot be excluded. Also pneumococci may contribute to cytokine induction but only a few children were culture positive in the present study.

Bacterial adherence to epithelial and pharyngeal cells has been extensively studied,[30] but still the mechanisms of colonization are only partly understood. It is a clearly age-dependent phenomenon, and a role of the local immune response in the clearance of bacteria from the mucosa has been postulated.[8] In a recent study of bacterial load on homogenized adenoid lymphatic tissue, *H. influenzae* was found in only 50% of the nasopharyngeal cultures, corresponding to a positive quantitative culture. This suggests that bacteria are harbored in crypts or in the lymphatic tissue.[31] The demonstration of NTHI intracellularly in macrophages, and recently extended using specific anti-LPS monoclonal antibodies,[32] indicates that NTHI may exert a chronic stimulation of local immune activity. However, the lack of correlation between the load of *H. influenzae*-containing cells and the analyzed cytokines may imply that the intracellularly sequestered bacteria go unrecognized by the local immune system. In this preliminary report the exact microenvironment of the *H. influenzae*-containing cells has not been studied, as will be done by simultaneous FISH and IHC for cytokines, as well as for phenotypic cell markers.

One important implication of the present study is that measurements of cytokines in serum do not necessarily reflect a pronounced local synthesis. Thus, the high cytokine levels in nasopharynx were undetectable in serum. These results are consistent with a number of earlier studies demonstrating cytokine production in compartments such as cerebrospinal fluid[11] and urine,[22] but not in serum. Most studies show low or undetectable levels of IL-1, IL-6, or TNF-α in sera of healthy individuals.[22,28,33] Elevated levels of serum cytokines have been found in relation to surgery and trauma,[34] and in patients with sepsis.[28] Elevated levels of cytokines in other serious diseases in infants and children,[35] or in myeloma in adults,[36] have been found. Accumulating data indicate that cytokines involved in both pathological and physiological immune responses are produced predominantly at the site of local antigen stimulation.[15]

In conclusion, this study presents results indicating an activation of cytokine synthesis, especially that of IL-4 and IL-6, in adenoid tissue. This activation is possibly due to the consistent colonization with bacteria, uptake and processing of microorganisms, and the presence of antigens in the lymphatic tissue, and could represent an important aspect of immunological homeostasis at the mucosal site. To our knowledge high cytokine levels have not been reported earlier in healthy individuals, and there is little or no information about defective production in certain individuals. One plausible function of cytokines in nasopharyngeal secretions may be to regulate the local inflammatory response to microrganisms. Elucidation of nasopharyngeal cytokine function requires further studies, and will focus on the differences in local cytokine production with respect to age and the presence of middle-ear disease. The cells responsible for the nasopharyngeal cytokine response remain to be identified.

ACKNOWLEDGMENTS

We particularly thank Dr. Ola Larson, Department of Plastic Surgery, Karolinska Hospital, Stockholm, Sweden, for his assistance in collecting the nasopharyngeal secretions from healthy children.

REFERENCES

1. KAMME, C. & K. LUNDGREN. 1971. Frequency of typeable and nontypeable Haemophilus influenzae strains in children with acute otitis media and results of penicillin V treatment. Scand. J. Infect. Dis. **3:** 225–228.
2. WICK, M., J. MADARA, N. BERNHARD & S. NORMARK. 1991. Molecular crosstalk between epithelial cells and pathogenic microorganisms. Cell **67:** 651–659.
3. GRAY, B., G. CONVERSE & H. DILLON, JR. 1980. Epidemiologic studies of streptococcus pneumoniae in infants: Acquisition, carriage, and infection during the first 24 months of life. J. Infect. Dis. **142(6):** 923–933.
4. TROTTIER, S., K. STENBERG & C. SVANBORG-EDÉN. 1989. Turnover of nontypeable Haemophilus influenzae in the nasopharynx of healthy children. J. Clin. Microbiol. **27:** 2175–2179.
5. KUKLINSKA, D. & M. KILIAN. 1984. Relative proportions of Haemophilus species in the throat of healthy children and adults. Eur. J. Clin. Microbiol. **3:** 249–252.
6. LUNDGREN, K., L. IGVARSSON & B. OLOFSSON. 1984. Epidemic aspects in children with recurrent acute otitis media. *In* Recent Advances in Otitis Media with Effusion: Proceedings of the Third International Symposium, D. Lim, C. Bluestone, J. Klein, and J. Nelson, Eds. Decker. Philadelphia.
7. LOOS, B., J. BERNSTEIN, D. DRYJA, T. MURPHY & D. DICKINSON. 1989. Determination of the epidemiology and transmission of nontypable H. influenzae in children with otitis media by comparison of total genomic DNA restriction fingerprint. Infect. Immun. **57:** 2751–2757.
8. LINDBERG, K., A. FREIJD, B. RYNNEL-DAGÖÖ & L. HAMMARSTRÖM. 1993. Antipneumococcal antibody activity in healthy adults and children. Acta Otolaryngol. (Stockholm). **113:** 673–678.
9. BRANDTZAEG, P. 1987. Immune functions and immunopathology of palatine and nasopharyngeal tonsils. *In* Immunology of the Ear, J. Bernstein and P. Ogra, Eds.: 63–106. Raven Press. New York.
10. DINARELLO, C. 1994. The interleukin-1 family: 10 years of discovery. FASEB. J. **88:** 1314–1325.

11. WAAGE, A., A. HALSTENSEN, R. SHALABY, P. BRANDTZAEG, P. KIERULF & T. ESPEVIK. 1989. Local production of tumor necrosis factor alpha, interleukin 1, and interleukin 6 in meningococcal meningitis. Relation to the inflammatory response. J. Exp. Med. **170:** 1859–1867.

12. BALKWILL, F. & F. BURKE. 1989. The cytokine network. Immunol. Today **10:** 299–304.

13. FORSGREN, J., A. SAMUELSON, A. AHLIN, J. JONASSON, B. RYNNEL-DAGÖÖ & A. LINDBERG. 1994. Heaemophilus influenzae resides and multiplies intracellularly in human adenoid tissue as demonstrated by in situ hybridization and bacterial viability assay. Infect. Immun. **62**(2): 673–679.

14. SCHENTAG, J. & C. BALLOW. 1991. Tissue-directed pharmacokinetics. Am. J. Med. **91**(Suppl. 3A):277–282.

15. ANDERSSON, J., J. ABRAMS, L. BJÖRK, K. FUNA, M. LITTON & K. ÅGREN. 1994. Concomitant in vivo production of 19 different cytokines in human tonsils. Immunology **83:** 16–24.

16. LINDBERG, K., B. RYNNEL-DAGÖÖ & K.-G. SUNDQVIST. 1994 Cytokines in nasopharyngeal secretions; Evidence for defective IL-1b production in children with recurrent episodes of acute otitis media. Clin. Exp. Immunol. **97:** 396–402.

17. PRELLNER, K., O. KALM, G. HARSTEN, J. HELDRUP & V.-A OXELIUS. 1989. Pneumococcal serum antibody concentrations during the first three years of life: A study of otitis-prone and non-otitis-prone children. Int. J. Pediatr. Otorhinolaryngol. **17:** 267–279.

18. FREIJD, A., V.-A OXELIUS & B. RYNNEL-DAGÖÖ. 1985. A prospective study demonstrating an association between plasma IgG2 concentrations and susceptibility to otitis media in children. Scand. J. Infect. Dis. **17:** 115–120.

19. YAMANAKA, N. & H. FADEN. 1993. Low serum IgG antibody levels specific for P6 of nontypeable Haemophilus influenzae in otitis prone children. J. Pediatr. **122:** 212–218.

20. FREIJD, A., S. BYGDEMAN & B. RYNNEL-DAGÖÖ. 1984. The nasopharyngeal microflora of otitis-prone children, with emphasis on H. influenzae. Acta Otolaryngol. (Stockholm) **97:** 117–126.

21. FORSGREN, J. B. RYNNEL-DAGÖÖ & B. CHRISTENSON. 1995. In situ analysis of the immune microenvironment of the adenoid in children with and without secretory otitis media. Ann. Otol. Rhinol. & Laryngol. **104:** 189–196.

22. HEDGES, S., P. ANDERSSON, G. LINDIN-JANSON, P. DE MAN & C. SVANBORG. 1991. Interleukin-6 response to deliberate colonization of the human urinary tract with gram-negative bacteria. Infect. Immun. **59**(1):421–427.

23. VAN SNICK, J. 1990. Interleukin-6: An overview. Ann. Rev. Immunol. **8:** 253–278.

24. DE MAN, P., C. VAN KOOTEN, L. AARDEN, I. ENGBERG, H. LINDER & C. SVANBORG EDÉN. 1989. Interleukin-6 induced at mucosal surface by gram-negative bacterial infection. Infect. Immun. **57**(11): 3383–3388.

25. LIM, D. & T. DEMARIA. 1982. Panel discussion: Pathogenesis of otitis media. Bacteriology and Immunology. Laryngoscope **92:** 278–286.

26. DEMARIA, T., R. PRIOR, B. BRIGGS, D. LIM & H. BRICK. 1984. Endotoxin in middle-ear effusions from patients with chronic otitis media with effusion. J. Clin. Microbiol. **20**(1): 17–17.

27. YELLON, R., G. LEONARD, P. MARUCHA, R. CRAVEN, R. CARPENTER, W. LEHMANN, J. BURLESON & D. KREUTZER. 1991. Characterization of cytokines present in middle ear effusions. Laryngoscope **101:** 165–169.

28. SULLIVAN, J., L. KILPATRICK, A. COSTARINO, S. LEE & M. HARRIES. 1992. Correlation of plasma cytokine elevations with mortality rate in children with sepsis. J. Pediatr. **120:** 510–515.

29. RIESENFELD-ÖRN, I., S. WOLPE, J. GARCIA-BUSTOS, M. HOFFMAN & E. TUOMANEN. 1989. Production of interleukin-1 but not tumor necrosis factor by human monocytes stimulated with pneumococcal cell surface components. Infect. Immun. **57:** 1890–1893.

30. ANDERSSON, B., B. ERIKSSON, E. FALSÉN, A. FOGH, L.-Å. HANSON, O. NYHLÉN, H. PETERSON & C. SVANBORG EDÉN. 1981. Adhesion of streptococcus pneumoniae to human pharyngeal epithelial cells in vitro: Differences in adhesive capacity among strains isolated from subjects with otitis media, septicemia, or meningitis or from healthy carriers. Infect. Immun. **32**(1): 311–317.

31. FORSGREN, J., A. SAMUELSON, A. LINDBERG & B. RYNNEL-DAGÖÖ. 1993. Quantitative bacterial culture from adenoid lymphatic tissue with special references to Haemophilus influenzae age-associated changes. Acta Otolaryngol. (Stockholm) **113:** 668–672.

32. FORSGREN, J., A. SAMUELSON, S. BORELLI, B. CHRISTENSON, J. JONASSON & A. LINDBERG. 1996 Persistence of nontypeable Haemophilus influenzae in adenoid macrophages—A punative colonization mechanism. Acta Otolaryngol. (Stockholm) **166:** 766–773.

33. AKIRA, S. & T. KISHIMOTO. 1992. IL-6 and NF-IL6 in acute-phase response and viral infection. Immunol. Rev. **127:** 25–50.

34. PULLICINO, E., F. CARLI, S. POOLE, B. RAFFERTY & S. MALIK. 1990. The relationship between the circulating concentrations of interleukin 6 (IL-6), tumor necrosis factor (TNF) and the acute phase response to elective surgery and accidental injury. Lymphokine Res. **9**(2): 231–238.

35. HENEY, D., I. LEWIS, S. EVANS, R. BANKS, C. BAILEY & J. WHICHER. 1992. Interleukin-6 and its relationship to C-reactive protein and fever in children with febrile neutropenia. J. Infect. Dis. **165:** 886–890.

36. KAWANO, M., T. HIRANO, T. MATSODA, T. TAGA, Y. HORII, K. IWATO, H. ASAOKU, B. TANG, O. TANABE, H. TANAKA, A. KURAMOTO & T. KISHIMOTO. 1988. Autokrine generation and requirement of BSF-2/IL-6 for human multiple myelomas. Nature **332:** 83–85.

Immunology of the Middle Ear: Role of Local and Systemic Antibodies in Clearance of Viruses and Bacteria

HOWARD S. FADEN[a]

State University of New York at Buffalo
School of Medicine and Biomedical Sciences
Buffalo, New York 14222
and
Division of Infectious Diseases
Children's Hospital of Buffalo
Buffalo, New York 14222

Acute otitis media may be defined as the sudden onset of inflammation in the middle-ear space characterized by ear pain and a bulging, thickened, and immobile tympanic membrane. The middle-ear fluid is typically purulent. A bacterial pathogen is recovered in 75% of the episodes. *Streptococcus pneumoniae* predominates at 35%, followed by nontypeable *Hemophilus influenzae* at 25%, and *Moraxella catarrhalis* at 15%. The remaining 25% of middle-ear fluids are sterile and presumably represent viral infections. Increasing evidence suggests that viruses may participate in more than 50% of all acute otitis media (AOM) episodes; however, pure viral AOM is relatively uncommon.[1]

The natural course of AOM has not been studied in the past decade. A review of articles concerning treatment of AOM demonstrates a spontaneous self-resolution rate between 30 and 80%.[2–6] This rate varies with the specific pathogen from a high rate of 79% with *M. catarrhalis* to a low rate of 11% with *S. pneumoniae*.[7,8] The mechanisms of eradication appear to involve various host defenses, including phagocytosis and destruction within neutrophils, lysis by host products outside of the cell, immunologic destruction by antibody and complement, and drainage of pus from the middle-ear space through the eustachian tube.

Ample evidence has been accumulated that supports the role of serum antibody in protecting the middle-ear space from infection. For example, the incidence of AOM is relatively low during the first six months of life when maternally acquired antibody levels are relatively high in infants. More specifically, antibody concentrations to *S. pneumoniae* in cord blood correlate to susceptibility to the development of pneumococcal otitis media, as does the level of antibody to nontypeable *H. influenzae* in older children.[9–11] Low levels of antibody can be corrected by passive immunization with serum containing high titers of antibody. By passively raising levels of pneumococcal antibody, the frequency of otitis media is reduced.[12] Active immunization with *S. pneumoniae* has also been associated with a reduced frequency of

[a]Address for correspondence: Howard Faden, Children's Hospital of Buffalo, 219 Bryant Street, Buffalo, New York, 14222. Phone: 716/878-7161; fax: 716/888-3804; e-mail: hfaden@ubmede.buffalo.edu

AOM.[13,14] Only pneumococcal types contained in the vaccines were associated with protection, and especially those types that induced a good serologic response.[13,14] These data prove that serum antibody is important in the prevention of AOM in humans.

Animal studies support the same conclusion. Animals passively immunized with antibody to either *S. pneumoniae* or nontypeable *H. influenzae* are protected against the development of AOM.[15,16] The protection is type and strain specific.[16–18] Animals rechallenged in a previously noninfected ear following resolution of an infection in the contralateral ear are protected against reinfection, presumably by serum antibody that diffused into the challenged ear.[17]

In contrast to the plethora of studies conducted on bacterial AOM, little information is available on viral disease. Immunization against influenza virus is associated with a reduction in influenzal disease as well as AOM.[19] It is not known whether or not the reduction in AOM in immunized children reflects decreased viral AOM or protection against secondary bacterial infection.

S. pneumoniae is a gram-positive coccus that most often assumes a diplococcal form. The organism is covered by a large carbohydrate capsule. The capsule is a polymer of repeating oligosaccharides. At present there are more than 84 antigenically different capsular types. Immunity to the pneumococcus is type specific and depends on antibody directed against a short six- or seven-sugar epitope in a particular capsular polysaccharide. Antibody to the capsule is important in opsonophagocytosis. Opsonic activity and IgG and IgM antibody to the capsular polysaccharide highly correlate to protection.[20] Once ingested, *S. pneumoniae* are rapidly destroyed. The specific mechanism of destruction within the neutrophil is unknown. However, it is known that autolysins within *S. pneumoniae* lead to spontaneous death, while host factors such as lysozyme, which function outside of the neutrophil, hasten the destruction.[21,22]

In contrast to capsular polysaccharide, the cell (C) wall polysaccharide is homogeneous throughout all strains. Although the cell wall polysaccharide induces an immune response, the specific antibody does not appear to be protective.[23]

Another antigen that has been shown to be immunogenic and protective is the surface protein A of the pneumococcus.[24] This is an approximately 84-kDa protein. Although this protein is present on all clinically important strains, it is serologically highly variable.[25] The importance of this antigen in human disease is not known.

The natural development of pneumococcal serum antibody is not understood. Gray *et al.*[26] studied a cohort of 82 infants from birth. They were unable to demonstrate consistently the development of serum antibody in response to nasopharyngeal colonization with pneumococci. However, antibody to type 3 pneumococcus was more readily detected after colonization than types 19 or 23. Conversely, serum antibody does not appear to affect colonization. Among children immunized with either an octavalent or 14-valent vaccine, nasopharyngeal colonization remained unaffected regardless of the serum antibody concentration.[27] Parenthetically, the children in this immunization study were less than one year of age at the time of immunization. Immunization of children less than two years of age with pneumococcal vaccine is currently contraindicated because of the poor immune response.[28] In an animal model of otitis media, immunization produced sufficient serum levels of antibody to protect the middle ear against infection; however, nasopharyngeal colonization remained unaffected.[29]

The immune response to *S. pneumoniae* during AOM has been studied in a surprisingly small number of children. In 1974 Sloyer *et al.*[30] used indirect hemagglutination and indirect fluorescence to measure antipneumococcal antibody in acute and convalescent sera as well as middle-ear fluid. Approximately 25% of children developed a systemic immune response that increased with age from 12% for infants less than 1 year of age to 48% for children over 2 years of age. A follow-up study by the same group of investigators demonstrated that middle-ear fluid with pneumococci were cleared more quickly if antibody was present in the middle-ear fluid at the time of diagnosis (75%) than when antibody was absent (18%).[31]

Almost 10 years later, Koskela *et al.*[32] measured the serum antibody response in children with acute pneumococcal otitis media; however, they employed a technique that used exogenous C polysaccharide to remove noncapsular polysaccharide antibodies. The antibody response was clearly related to the capsular type. For example, capsular types 3 and 18 typically induced specific antibodies, while types 6 and 19 rarely did.

Karjalainen *et al.*[33] measured antibody concentrations to all three middle-ear pathogens in middle-ear effusions during AOM, regardless of the inciting agent. They detected antibody to each pathogen in every effusion; however, antibody to the causative agent tended to be more prominent. These data suggest that the antibodies diffuse into the middle-ear space passively due to the acute inflammatory response. Furthermore this study corroborated the findings of Sloyer *et al*;[31] the presence of pneumococcal antibody in middle-ear effusion early in the course of disease was associated with rapid resolution (90%), compared to middle-ear fluid without detectable antibody (57%).

We were fortunate enough to study the systemic and local antibody response in seven children with type-19 pneumococcal otitis media. The children ranged in age from 6 to 29 months with a mean of 15.1 months (TABLE 1). The mean acute serum antibody level of 0.46 µg/mL was not significantly different than the mean convalescent serum antibody level of 0.32 µg/mL. Antibody was concurrently measured in

TABLE 1. IgG-specific Antibody Response (µg/mL) of Children with Acute Otitis Media Due to Type-19 Pneumococcus

		Serum			
Subject	Age (mos.)	Acute	Convalescent	Middle-ear Fluid	Outcome[a]
1	6	0.19	0.20	—	Resolved
2	6	0.19	0.12	< 0.03	Resolved
3	12	0.23	0.21	< 0.03	Persistent
4	15	0.18	0.18	< 0.03	Resolved
5	19	0.16	0.17	< 0.03	Resolved
6	21	0.39	0.28	< 0.03	Resolved
7	29	1.90	1.65	0.15	Persistent

[a]Thirty days post tympanocentesis.

the middle-ear fluids during the acute period. Antibody was detected only in one of six fluids. The one positive middle-ear fluid was recovered from a 29-month-old child who had a relatively high serum antibody concentration. Interestingly, two of the children were unable to resolve their infection despite appropriate antibiotic therapy. Sequential sera and middle-ear fluids demonstrated a failure to develop antibody response in one child and a lack of a local antibody response in the other child (TABLE 2). These data suggest that eradication of pneumococci from the middle-ear space is dependent on the presence of IgG-specific antibody in the middle-ear space. The antibody appears to come from the systemic circulation. Unfortunately young children generate relatively low levels of serum antibody.

Nontypeable *H. influenzae* is a gram-negative pleomorphic coccobacillus. It is not encapsulated like the pneumococcus; rather, it is enclosed by an outer membrane that contains approximately 20 proteins and a lipooligosaccharide (LOS). The heterogeneity of the outer membrane proteins (OMP) provides a basis for typing the various strains.[34] Among the proteins are seven that have been well characterized P1, 2, 4, 5, 6, high molecular weight (HMW) 1, and HMW 2. Most recently, a second family of HMW proteins has been identified.[35] P1, 2, and 5 are heterogeneous, while P4 and 6 are highly conserved. The two HMW proteins are heterogeneous, and unlike the other proteins are detected on only 70–75% of strains.[35] LOS is also fairly heterogeneous.[36]

P2 is the major OMP. It serves as a porin. Recently our laboratory demonstrated a role for P2 in attachment to mucin.[37] P5 and the HMW 1 and 2 proteins have also been shown to play a role in attachment, the former to mucin and the latter to epithelial cells.[37–40]

Antibody to P1, 2, 4, 6, HMW 1 and 2, and LOS are bactericidal. Since P4 and P6 are antigenically stable and highly conserved, an immune response to either antigen should produce an antibody that recognizes all strains of nontypeable *H. influenzae*; in contrast, the antibody responses to P1, 2, HMW1 and 2, and LOS would most likely be strain-specific.

In 1988 we began a series of experiments designed to examine the immune response to nontypeable *H. influenzae* in children with AOM. We first employed an immunodot assay with a prototypic whole bacterial antigen preparation to describe the seroprevalence in the general population. The assay was specific for *H. influenzae*, but did not distinguish homologous from heterologous strains. The initial study

TABLE 2. Serum and Middle-ear Antibody Levels (μg/mL) from Two Children with Persistent Otitis Due to Type-19 Pnemococcus

Subject	Age (mos.)	*S. pneumoniae* × 10^3/mL	Serum	Middle Ear
3	12	1,000	0.23	< 0.3
	13	350	0.21	<0.3
	14	1	0.27	< 0.3
	15	0	0.19	—
7	29	600	1.90	0.15
	30	20	1.65	0.06
	31	0	1.30	—

demonstrated that newborns possessed adult levels of IgG-specific antibody.[41,42] These levels dropped to their lowest point between six months and two years. This time period corresponds to the age when the incidence of AOM is the highest. By four to six years adult levels were reached.

In an effort to utilize a functional antibody test, we next employed a bactericidal assay. Parenthetically, fresh-pooled human serum is able to kill 100% of nontypeable *H. influenzae* strains. Killing of the organism requires both antibody and complement. A total of 21 infants who experienced 29 episodes of otitis media were evaluated.[43] Bactericidal antibody was detected in acute serum of 26% with a mean titer of 0.8 ($\log_2$) and was observed in convalescent serum of 100% subjects at a mean titer of 4.0 ($\log_2$). Unlike the antibody response to *S. pneumoniae*, the bactericidal antibody response to nontypeable *H. influenzae* was not age-dependent. The presence of bactericidal antibody correlated with a reduction in the number of bacteria present in the middle-ear fluid. This suggested that serum antibody entered the middle-ear space.

Examination of the middle-ear fluids was next performed by an immunodot assay with purified homologous outer membrane antigen. This immunodot assay distinguished homologous from heterologous organisms. Strain-specific IgG predominated.[44] It was detected in 91% of the children, compared with IgM in 48%, IgA in 52%, and secretory IgA in 18% (TABLE 3). The titer of specific IgG, 8.2 ($\log_2$) exceeded IgM 3.4 ($\log_2$), IgA 3.7 ($\log_2$), and secretory IgA 1.2 ($\log_2$). Antibody was only detected in middle-ear fluids of individuals who possessed complementary serum antibody.

Further refining of the antibody assay allowed us to examine the response to the highly conserved protein P6.[45] Immunoglobulin G antibody to P6 was detected in 92% of middle-ear fluids compared to 70% for IgM, 78% for IgA, and 45% for secretory IgA. Antibody levels ranged from 249 ng/mL for IgG to a low of 11 ng/mL for IgM. Concentrations of P6-specific IgG in the middle-ear fluid were directly related to the concentration in the serum, $r = 0.89$, and inversely related to the number of bacteria present, $r = -0.62$. These data confirm our earlier studies done with serum bactericidal antibody.

The mechanism of elimination from the middle-ear fluid of nontypeable *H. influenzae* is not known. It is possible that the organisms are killed by the action of specific antibody and complement. It is also possible that the bacteria are opsonized, phagocytosed by neutrophils, and destroyed within the cell.

Nontypeable *H. influenzae* are opsonized by antibody directed against surface

TABLE 3. IgG, IgM, IgA, and sIgA Antibody Responses to Homologous Strains of Nontypeable *H. influenzae* in Middle-ear Fluid

Antibody	Number Positive/Number Tested (%)	P	Antibody Titer ($\log_2$)
IgG	21/23 (91)		8.2 ± 0.1
IgM	11/23 (48)	<0.005	3.4 ± 0.1
IgA	12/13 (52)	<0.005	3.7 ± 0.1
sIgA	3/17 (18)	<0.001	1.2 ± 0.3

From: Faden *et al.*[44]

proteins. At least one report suggests that antibody directed against the P2 protein leads to strain-specific phagocytosis.[46] The necessity for complement in the phagocytic process is somewhat controversial. In our experience, phagocytosis can occur in the presence of antibody alone; however, complement augments the process.[47] In contrast, studies conducted by Troelstra *et al.*[46] and Musher *et al.*[48] attribute greater importance to the role of complement. From our own studies, it is clear that phagocytosis is associated with the release of leukotriene B4, a potent chemoattractant for neutrophils.[47] Thus, the inflammatory response is heightened. We suspect that the inflammatory process permits further influx of serum antibody into the middle-ear space.

In an effort to delineate the roles of inflammation and local immunity on the appearance of antibody in the middle-ear space, we compared antibody levels in the right and left ears of children with bilateral effusions and in whom the organism was present or absent. The IgG-specific antinontypeable *H. influenzae* antibody levels in children with bilaterally infected ears were equivalent, while the levels in the infected side of children with bilateral effusions were higher in the infected side.[44] These findings suggest local production of antibody in the infected side and only passively acquired antibody in the uninfected side. Another interpretation is greater local inflammation in the infected middle-ear mucosa, allowing more serum antibody to cross into the middle-ear space. Supporting this latter interpretation are data from an earlier study in our laboratory that demonstrated higher levels of mediators of inflammation in middle-ear effusions with viable bacteria.[49]

We also obtained sequential tympanocenteses from children with AOM. These studies suggested that as an infection resolved, the level of antibody in the effusion decreased, but serum antibody remained stable or increased (TABLE 4).[41,42] We could not distinguish the effect of inflammation or local antibody production. The majority of data suggest that the antibody present in the middle-ear fluid represents serum antibody that has diffused across an inflamed middle-ear mucosa.

One intriguing observation from our earlier studies suggested that as the number of episodes of otitis media increased and/or the duration of infection persisted, the likelihood of detecting IgM- and IgA-specific antibody middle-ear effusions increased. We examined middle-ear effusions from children with 1–5 episodes, 6–10 episodes, >10 episodes, and those with persistent effusions (TABLE 5).[41] The serum and middle-ear fluid levels of nontypeable *H. influenzae* antibody increased as the number of episodes increased. Although specific IgG, M. and A antibodies were detected in the sera of all children in each group, the same was not true for the middle-ear fluid. IgM- and IgA-specific antibodies were not detected in children with 1–5 episodes. IgA-specific antibodies were absent in the group with 6–10 episodes, while IgM was detected in 25%. In contrast, IgM and IgA antibodies were found in the middle-ear fluids in children with more than 10 episodes, or persistent fluids. Our interpretation of the data is that as the number of episodes increases or the longer the infectious process persists, the more likely a local immune response was responsible for the antibody in the middle-ear fluid.

The third pathogen to be considered is *M. catarrhalis*, formerly called *Neisseria catarrhalis* and *Branhamella catarrhalis*. This organism was once thought to be a nonpathogen. However, in 1965, it was first identified as a cause of AOM.[50] Gradually, the percent of *M. catarrhalis* cases rose to 15% of total episodes. The organism is

TABLE 4. Longitudinal IgG Antibody Response to Nontypeable *H. influenzae* in Serum and Middle-ear Fluid

Subject	Diagnosis	Middle-ear Culture	Time Interval (mos.)	Antibody Titer Serum	MEF
1	ACM	NTHI		25,600	3,200
	PF	NG	4	25,600	400
2	ACM	NTHI		12,800	1,600
	PF	NG	3	12,800	200
3	ACM	NTHI		6,400	100
	PF	NG	2	51,200	<25
4	ACM	NTHI	2	6,400	100
	PF	NG	2	12,800	100
5	ACM	NTHI		1,600	400
	PF	NG	1	25,600	100
	PF	NG	1	6,400	<25
6	ACM	NTHI[a]		1,600	100
	ACM	NTHI[a]	1	12,800	3,200
	PF	NG	2	12,800	800

From: Faden *et al.*[44]

[a]Same strain of NTHI characterized by outer membrane protein distribution.

Abbreviations: ACM—acute otitis media; PF—persistent fluid; NG—no growth.

a gram-negative coccus. It typically assumes a diplococcal form. The organism is readily distinguished from other "Neisserial" organisms by the presence of DNAse and butyryl esterase.

We have learned much about the antigenic makeup of the organism during the past seven years. For instance, eight major proteins, ranging in molecular weight from 21 kDa to 98 kDa, have been identified in the outer membrane.[51] The OMPs have been designated A through H. The OMP patterns are fairly similar between strains. Outer membrane proteins E and G are surface exposed.[52] Outer membrane protein C/D contains a highly conserved epitope.[53] The OMP designated B actually comprises two separate proteins B_1 and B_2. B_1 is important in iron binding and B_2

TABLE 5. Geometric Mean Acute Antibody Titer to Nontypeable *H. influenzae* According to Number of Episodes of Otitis Media in Children with at Least One Episode Due to Nontypeable *H. influenzae*

Episodes	Serum			Middle-ear Effusion		
	G	M	A	G	M	A
1–5	11.7 (7/7)[a]	7.9 (4/4)	5.9 (4/4)	7.8 (8/9)	0.1 (0/5)	0.1 (0/6)
6–10	12.9 (3/3)	5.8 (3/3)	5.6 (3/3)	8.3 (3/3)	4.4 (1/4)	0.1 (0/2)
>10	14.6 (3/3)	9.6 (3/3)	8.3 (3/3)	10.9 (3/3)	4.4 (2/3)	5.3 (3/3)
Persistent	13.1 (4/4)	9.6 (4/4)	5.5 (3/4)	10.5 (5/5)	4.1 (2/4)	6.9 (3/3)

From: Faden *et al.*[41]

[a]Detectable antibody per number tested.

may be important in attachment of the organism. More recently, an HMW proten has been described with a molecular weight between 350 and 720 kDa.[54]

Several studies have measured the immune response to *M. catarrhalis* following respiratory disease.[55–58] At least 50% of the subjects demonstrate a rise in antibody of one of the three immunoglobulin classes.[55–58] Goldblatt *et al.*[59] indicated that IgG 3 antibody recognizes the majority of outer membrane antigens of *M. catarrhalis*. Interestingly, children of less than 4 years of age failed to develop an *M. catarrhalis*-specific IgG 3 antibody response and only manufactured IgG1 and IgG2 antibodies to an 82-kDa protein, protein B_1, or B_2. Antibody to B_2 has been associated with increased clearance of organisms from the airway in an animal model.[60] Most recently, antibody to the HMW protein of *M. catarrhalis* has also been shown to hasten clearance from the airway, and, perhaps equally important, the same authors demonstrated the appearance of antibody to this protein in the convalescent sera from patients with *M. catarrhalis* pneumonia.[61]

Only three studies have examined the immune response to *M. catarrhalis* in children with AOM.[55,62,63] The first was conducted in 1981 by Leinonen *et al.*[55] in Finland. They detected an antibody rise in 50% of the children using a pool of ten strains of *M. catarrhalis* as the antigen in an ELISA assay. We studied the systemic and local antibody response in children by utilizing an ELISA assay with homologous outer membrane antigens.[62] Fifty-seven percent of the children demonstrated a rise in antibody titer in one or more of the immunoglobulin classes. Local antibody consisted of IgG, 100%, IgM, 29%, and IgA, 71%. Both the IgG- and IgA-specific antibody measured in middle-ear fluids appeared to represent local production rather than passive diffusion from the systemic circulation (TABLES 6 and 7).

It is unclear as to how the specific antibodies function to eliminate *M. catarrhalis* from the middle-ear space. Unlike nontypeable *H. influenzae*, which is highly sus-

TABLE 6. Antibody (μg/mL) to Homologous Outer Membrane Antigens of *M. catarrhalis* in Middle-ear Effusions

Patients	IgG	IgM	IgA
14	2.9 ± 2.5	0.2 ± 0.5	1.5 ± 2.0

From: Faden *et al.*[62]

TABLE 7. Comparison of Ratio of IgA and IgG Antibody to Homologous Outer Membrane Antigens of *M. catarrhalis* in Serum and Middle-ear Fluid

	IgA/IgG	
Patients	Serum	Middle-ear Fluid
14	0.2 ± 0.3	1.5 ± 2.1

From: Faden *et al.*[62]

ceptible to killing by fresh-pooled human serum, less than 15% of *M. catarrhalis* strains can be killed by fresh-pooled human serum.[57] It is possible that convalescent sera incubated with homologous organisms demonstrates greater bactericidal activity. We were able to demonstrate increased opsonic activity in convalescent sera of children with AOM compared to acute sera when using homologous outer membrane antigens.[63] It is difficult to hypothesize the mechanism of elimination of *M. catarrhalis* from the middle-ear space until we learn more about the antigenic structure of the organism. However, we currently know that among the three major middle-ear pathogens, *M. catarrhalis* is most readily elimiated from the middle-ear space without antibiotic treatment.[7,8] This implies that the organism must be very susceptible to destruction by one or more of the host's defense mechanisms.

In summary, the majority of evidence suggests that antibody detected in the middle-ear space comes primarily from the systemic circulation, unless the middle-ear process has been persistent. The amount of specific antibody present in the middle-ear space is directly related to the elimination of the organism. Thus, prior exposure to the pathogen through natural means or through immunization should result in prevention of disease.

REFERENCES

1. CHONMAITREE, T., M. J. OWEN, J. A. PATEL, *et al.* 1992. Effect of viral respiratory tract infection on outcome of acute otitis media. J. Pediatr. **120:** 856–862.
2. MYGIND, N., K.-I. MEISTRUP-LARSEN, J. THOMSEN, *et al.* 1981. Penicillin in acute otitis media: A double-blind placebo-controlled trial. Clin. Otolaryngol. **6:** 5–13.
3. VAN BUCHEM, F. L., J. H. M. DUNK & M. A. VAN'T HOF. 1981. Therapy of acute otitis media: Myringotomy, antibiotics, or neither? Lancet **2:** 883–887.
4. BURKE, P., J. BAIN, D. ROBINSON & J. DUNLEAVEY. 1991. Acute red ear in children: Controlled trial of non-antibiotic treatment in general practice. Br. Med. J. **303:** 558–562.
5. KALEIDA, P. H., M. L. CASSELBRANT, H. E. ROCKETTE, *et al.* 1991. Amoxicillin or myringotomy or both for acute otitis media: Results of a randomized clinical trial. Pediatrics **87:** 466–474.
6. VAN BUCHEM, F. L., M. F. PEETERS & M. A. VAN'T HOF. 1985. Acute otitis media: A new treatment strategy. Br. Med. J. **290:** 1033–1037.
7. HOWIE, V. M., R. DILLARD & B. LAWRENCE. 1985. In vivo sensitivity test in otitis media: Efficacy of antibiotics. Pediatrics **75:** 8–13.
8. KLEIN, J. O. 1993. Microbiologic efficacy of antibacterial drugs for acute otitis media. Pediatr. Infect. Dis. J. **12:** 973–975.
9. PRELLNER, K., O. KALM & F. K. PEDERSEN. 1984. Pneumococcal antibodies and complement during and after periods of recurrent otitis. Int. J. Pediatr. Otolaryngol. **7:** 39–49.
10. SALAZAR, J. C., K. A. DALY, M. MUGGLIE, C. LIEBELER, B. LINDGREN & G. S. GIEBINK. 1995. Neonatal type 14 pneumococcal IgG antibody predicts early onset acute otitis media in infancy. Proc. 6th Int. Symp. on Recent Advances in Otitis Media Abstract No. 44, p. 85.
11. SHURIN, P. A., D. I. PELTON, I. B. TAGAR & D. L. KASPER. 1980. Bactericidal antibody and susceptibility to otitis media caused by nontypeable strains of *Haemophilus influenzae*. J. Pediatr. **97:** 364–369.
12. SHURIN, P. A., J. M. REHMUS, C. E. JOHNSON, C. D. MARCHANT, S. A. CARLIN, D. M. SUPER, G. F. VAN HARE, P. K. JONES, D. M. AMBROSINO & G. R. SIBER. 1993. Bacterial polysac-

charide immune globulin for prophylaxis of acute otitis media in high-risk children. J. Pediatr. **123:** 801–810.

13. TEELE, D. W., J. O. KLEIN & THE GREATER BOSTON COLLABORATIVE OTITIS MEDIA STUDY GROUP. 1981. Use of pneumococcal vaccine for prevention of recurrent acute otitis media in infants in Boston. Rev. Infect. Dis. **3:** S113–S118.

14. MAKELA, P. H., M. LEINONEN, J. PUKANDER & P. KARMA. 1981. A study of the pneumococcal vaccine in prevention of clinically acute attacks of recurrent otitis media. Rev. Infect. Dis. **3:** S124–S130.

15. SHURIN, P. A., G. S. GIEBINK, D. L. WEGMAN, D. AMBROSINO, J. RHOLL, M. OVERMAN, T. BAUER & G. R. SIBER. 1988. Prevention of pneumococcal otitis media in chinchillas with human bacterial polysaccharide immune globulin. J. Clin. Microbiol. **26:** 755–759.

16. BARENKAMP, S. J. 1986. Protection by serum antibodies in experimental nontypeable *Haemophilus influenzae* otitis media. Infect. Immun. **52:** 572–578.

17. KARASIC, R. B., C. E. TRUMPP, H. E. GNEHM, *et al.* 1985. Modification of otitis media in chinchillas rechallenged with nontypeable *Haemophilus influenzae* and serological response to outer membrane antigens. J. Infect. Dis. **151:** 273–279.

18. FADEN, H., J., BERNSTEIN, L. BRODSKY, *et al.* 1989. Otitis media in children. I. The systemic immune response to nontypeable *H. influenzae*. J. Infect. Dis. **160:** 999–1004.

19. HEIKKINEN, T., O. RUUSKANEN, M. WARIS, *et al.* 1991. Influenza vaccination in the prevention of acute otitis media in children. Am. J. Dis. Child. **145:** 445–448.

20. ALONSODEVELASCO, E., B. A. T. DEKKER, A. F. M. VERHEUL, R. G. FELDMAN, J. VERHOEF & H. SNIPPE. 1995. Anti-polysaccharide immunoglobulin isotype levels and opsonic activity of antisera: Relationships with protection against *S. pneumoniae* infection in mice. J. Infect. Dis. **172:** 562–565.

21. COONROD, J. D., R. VARBLE & K. YONEDA. 1991. Mechanism of killing of pneumococci by lysozyme. J. Infect. Dis. **164:** 527–532.

22. COTTAGNOUD, P. & A. TOMASZ. 1993. Triggering of pneumococcal autolysis by lysozyme. J. Infect. Dis. **167:** 684–690.

23. MUSHER, D. M., D. A. WATSON & R. E. BAUGHN. 1990. Does naturally acquired IgG antibody to cell wall polysaccharide protect human subjects against pneumococcal infection? J. Infect. Dis. **161:** 736–740.

24. MCDANIEL, L. S., J. S. SHEFFIELD, P. DELUCCHI & D. E. BRILES. 1991. PspA, a surface protein of *Streptococcus pneumoniae*, is capable of eliciting protection against pneumococci of more than one capsular type. Infect. Immun. **59:** 222–228.

25. CRAIN, M. J., W. D. WALTMAN II, J. S. TURNER, J. YOTHER, D. F. TALKINGTON, L. F. MC-DANIEL, B. M. GRAY & D. E BRILES. 1990. Pneumococcal surface protein A is serologically highly variable and is expressed by all clinically important capsular serotypes of *Streptococcus pneumoniae*. Infect. Immun. **58:** 3293–3299.

26. GRAY, B. M., G. M. CONVERSE III, N. HUHTA, R. B. JOHNSTON, JR., M. E. PICHICHERO, G. SCHIFFMAN & H. C. DILLON, JR. 1981. Epidemiologic studies of *Streptococcus pneumoniae* in infants: Antibody response to nasopharyngeal carriage of types 3, 19, and 23. J. Infect. Dis. **144:** 312–318.

27. WRIGHT, P. F., S. H. SELL, W. K. VAUGHN, C. ANDREWS, K. B. MCDONNELL & G. SCHIFFMAN. 1981. Clinical studies of pneumococcal vaccines in infants. II. Efficacy and effect on nasopharyngeal carriage. Rev. Infect. Dis. **3:** S108–S112.

28. IMMUNIZATION PRACTICES ADVISORY COMMITTEE. 1989. Pneumococcal polysaccharide vaccine. MMWR **38:** 64–76.

29. GIEBINK, G. S., I. K. BERZINS, G. SCHIFFMAN & P. G. QUIE. 1979. Experimental otitis media in chinchillas following nasal colonization with type 7F *Streptococcus pneumoniae*: Prevention after vaccination with pneumococcal capsular polysaccharide. J. Infect. Dis. **140:** 716–723.

30. SLOYER, J. L., JR., V. M. HOWIE, J. H. PLOUSSARD, A. J. AMMAN, R. AUSTRIAN & R. B. JOHNSTON, JR. 1974. Immune response to acute otitis media in children. I. Serotypes isolated and serum and middle ear fluid antibody in pneumococcal otitis media. Infect. Immun. **9:** 1028–1032.

31. SLOYER, J. L., V. M. HOWIE, J. H. PLOUSSARD & R. B. JOHNSTON, JR. 1976. Immune response to acute otitis media: Associated between middle ear fluid antibody and the clearing of clinical infection. J. Clin. Microbiol. **4:** 306–308.

32. KOSKELA, M. 1987. Serum antibodies to pneumococcal C polysaccharide in children: Response to acute pneumococcal otitis media or to vaccination. Pediatr. Infect. Dis. J. **6:** 519–526.

33. KARJALAINEN, H., M. KOSKELA, J. LUOTENEN, E. HERVA & P. SIPILA. 1991. Occurrences of antibodies against *Streptococcus pneumoniae, Haemophilus influenzae* and *Branhamella catarrhalis*, in middle ear effusion and serum during the course of acute otitis media. Acta Otolaryngol. (Stockholm) **111:** 112–119.

34. MURPHY, T. F., K. C. DUDAS, J. M. MYLOTTE & M. A. APICELLA. 1983. A subtyping system for nontypeable *Haemophilus influenzae* based on outer-membrane proteins. J. Infect. Dis. **147:** 838–846.

35. BARENKAMP, S. J. & J. W. ST. GEME III. 1996. Identification of a second family of high-molecular-weight adhesion proteins expressed by nontypeable *Haemophilus influenzae*. Molec. Microbiol. **19:** 1215–1223.

36. PATRICK, C. C., A. KIMURA, M. A. JACKSON, L. HERMANSTORFER, A. HOOD, G. H. MCCRACKEN, JR. & E. J. HANSEN. 1987. Antigenic characterization of the oligosaccharide portion of the lipooligosaccharide of nontypeable *Haemophilus influenzae*. Infect. Immun. **55:** 2902–2911.

37. REDDY, M. S., J. M. BERNSTEIN, T. F. MURPHY & H. S. FADEN. 1996. Binding between outer membrane proteins of nontypeable *Haemophilus influenzae* and human nasopharyngeal mucin. Infect. Immun. **64:** 1477–1479.

38. ST. GEME, J. W., III, S. FALKOW & S. J. BARENKAMP. 1993. High-molecular weight proteins of nontypeable *Haemophilus influenzae* mediate attachment to human epithelial cells. Proc. Natl. Acad. Sci. USA **90:** 2875–2879.

39. NOEL, G. J., D. C. LOVE & D. M. MOSSER. 1994. High-molecular weight proteins of nontypeable *Haemophilus influenzae* mediate bacterial adhesion to cellular proteoglycans. Infect. Immun. **62:** 4028–4033.

40. ST. GEME, J. W., III. 1994. The HMW1 adhesion of nontypeable *Haemophilus influenzae* recognizes sialylated glycoprotein receptors on cultured human epithelial cells. Infect. Immun. **62:** 3881–3889.

41. FADEN, H., J. J. HONG, D. A. KRYSTOFIK, J. M. BERNSTEIN, L. BRODSKY, J. STANIEVICH & P. L. OGRA. 1988. Antibody response to nontypeable *Haemophilus influenzae*. *In* Recent Advances in Otitis Media, D. Lim, C. Bluestone, J. Klein, J. Nelson, B. C. Decker, Eds.: 340–343. Toronto/Philadelphia.

42. FADEN, H., D. A. KRYSTOFIK, J. J. HONG, J. M. BERNSTEIN, L. BRODSKY, J. STANIEVICH & P. L. OGRA. 1988. Immune response to nontypeable *Haemophilus influenzae* in the general population and among children with otitis media with effusion. Ann. Otol. Rhinol. Laryngol. **97:** 34–36.

43. FADEN, H., J. M. BERNSTEIN, L. BRODSKY, J. STANIEVICH, D. A. KRYSTOFIK, C. SHUFF, J. J. HONG & P. L. OGRA. 1988. Otitis media in children. I. The systemic immune response to nontypeable *Haemophilus influenzae*. J. Infect. Dis. **160:** 999–1004.

44. FADEN, H., L. BRODSKY, J. M. BERNSTEIN, J. STANIEVICH, D. KRYSTOFIK, C. SHUFF, J. J. HONG & P. L. OGRA. 1989. Otitis media in children: Local immune response to nontypeable *Haemophilus influenzae*. Infect. Immun. **57:** 3555–3559.

45. YAMANAKA, N. & H. FADEN. 1993. Local antibody response to P6 of nontypeable

Haemophilus influenzae in otitis-prone and normal children. Acta Otolaryngol. **113:** 524–529.

46. TROELSTRA, A., L. VOGEL, L. VAN ALPHEN, P. EIJK, H. JANSEN & J. DANKERT. 1994. Opsonic antibodies to outer membrane protein P2 of nonencapsulated *Haemophilus influenzae* are strain specific. Infect. Immun. **62:** 779–784.

47. GAROFALO, R., H. FADEN, S. SHARMA & P. L. OGRA. 1991. Release of leukotriene B$_4$ from human neutrophils after interaction with nontypeable *Haemophilus influenzae*. Infect. Immun. **59:** 4221–4226.

48. MUSHER, D. M., M. HAGUE-PARK, R. E. BAUGHM, R. J. WALLACE & B. COWLEY. 1983. Opsonizing and bactericidal effects of normal human serum on nontypeable *Haemophilus influenzae*. Infect. Immun. **39:** 297–304.

49. BRODSKY, L., H. FADEN, J. M. BERNSTEIN, J. STANIEVICH, G. DECASTRO, B. VOLOVITZ & P. L. OGRA. 1989. Arachidonic acid metabolites in middle ear effusions of children. Ann. Otol. Rhinol. Laryngol. **100:** 589–592.

50. HALSTED, C., M. L. LEPOW, N. BALASSANIAN, *et al.* 1968. Otitis media. Am. J. Dis. Child. **115:** 542–551.

51. BARTOS, L. C. & T. C. MURPHY. 1988. Comparison of the outer membrane proteins of 50 strains of *Branhamella catarrhalis*. J. Infect. Dis. **158:** 761–765.

52. MURPHY, T. F. & L. C. BARTOS. 1989. Surface-exposed and antigenically conserved determinants of outer membrane proteins of *Branhamella catarrhalis*. Infect Immun. **57:** 2938–2941.

53. SARWAR, J., A. A. CAMPAGNARI, C. KIRKHAM & T. F. MURPHY. 1992. Characterization of an antigenically conserved heat-modifiable major outer membrane protein of *Branhamella catarrhalis*. Infect. Immun. **60:** 804–809.

54. KLINGMAN, K. & T. F. MURPHY. 1994. Purification and characterization of a high-molecular-weight outer membrane protein of *Moraxella (Branhamella) catarrhalis*. Infect. Immun. **62:** 1150–1155.

55. LEINONEN, M., J. LUOTENEN, E. HERVA, *et al.* 1981. Preliminary serologic evidence for a pathogenic role of *Branhamella catarrhalis*. J. Infect. Dis. **144:** 570–577.

56. BLACK, A. J. & T. S. WILSON. 1988. Immunoglobulin G. (IgG) serological response to *Branhamella catarrhalis* in patients with acute bronchopulmonary infections. J. Clin. Pathol. **41:** 329–333.

57. CHAPMAN, A. J., D. M. MUSHER, S. JONSSON, *et al.* 1990. Antibody response to P-protein in patients with *Branhamella catarrhalis* infections. Am. J. Med. **88:** S25–S27.

59. GOLDBLATT, D., M. W. TURNER & R. J. LEVINSKY. 1990. *Branhamella catarrhalis*: Antigenic determinants and the development of the IgG subclass response in childhood. J. Infect. Dis. **162:** 1128–1135.

60. HELMINEN, M. E., I. MACIVER, J. L. LATIMER, L. D. COPE, G. H. MCCRACKEN, JR. & E. J. HANSEN. 1993. A major outer membrane protein of *Moraxella catarrhalis* is a target for antibodies that enhance pulmonary clearance of the pathogen in an animal model. Infect. Immun. **61:** 2003–2010.

61. HELMINEN, J. E., I. MACIVER, J. L. LATIMER, J. KLESNEY-TAIT, L. D. COPE, M. PARIS, G. H. MCCRACKEN, JR. & E. J. HANSEN. 1994. A large, antigenically conserved protein on the surface of *Moraxella catarrhalis* is a target for protective antibodies. J. Infect. Dis. **170:** 867–872.

62. FADEN, H., J. HONG & T. MURPHY. 1992. Immune response to outer membrane antigens of *Moraxella catarrhalis* in children with otitis media. Infect. Immun. **60:** 3824–3829.

63. FADEN, H., J. J. HONG & N. PAHADE. 1994. Immune response to *Moraxella catarrhalis* in children with otitis media: Opsonophagocytosis with antigen-coated latex beads. Ann. Otol. Rhinol. Laryngol. **103:** 522–524.

The Role of IgE-mediated Immunity in Otitis Media: Fact or Fiction?

GORO MOGI[a] and MASASHI SUZUKI

Department of Otolaryngology
Oita Medical University
1-1 Idaigaoka, Hazama-machi
Oita-gun, Oita-ken 856-55
Japan

INTRODUCTION

Otitis media with effusion (OME) and allergic rhinitis are common diseases in children. While allergic rhinitis is caused by a typical immunoglobulin-E-mediated (IgE) allergic disorder, the cause and pathogenesis of OME are considered to be multifactorial, involving infection of the tubotympanum, eustachian tube blockage, and allergy. The role of allergy, particularly IgE-mediated immune reactions, in OME has been debated. Recent studies have questioned an allergic etiology of OME on the basis of laboratory findings and experimental data.[1–5] Anatomically, however, there is a continuity of the mucous membrane between the nose and the tympanic cavity via the eustachian tube, and the middle ear mucosa may respond functionally as sensitized tissue in patients with respiratory allergy.

The present communication reviews the evidence for IgE-mediated allergic reactivity in the etiopathogenesis of OME.

IS THERE A HIGH INCIDENCE OF OTITIS MEDIA WITH EFFUSION IN PATIENTS WITH ALLERGY?

The medical literature of the early twentieth century,[6,7] reported a high incidence of OME in allergic patients. In the middle of the century Jordan[8] noted that allergy was associated with OME in 91 (74%) of 123 patients. Lecks[9] evaluated 82 children with OME by scratch skin tests using common environmental, inhalant, pollen, and mold allergens and found a positive reaction in 72 (88%) patients. In a study of 540 children, Draper[10] found OME in 52% of those with allergic rhinitis, but in only 24% of the nonallergic control. These reports, however, appeared before the discovery of IgE. Since 1966, when Ishizaka and Ishizaka[11] identified and purified a reaginic antibody that was recognized as a new class of immunoglobulin called IgE, the mechanism of type I allergic reactions was disclosed, and more precise allergic tests were developed. Using a well-defined, objective definition of OME, Bernstein and Reisman[12] examined 200 consecutive cases presenting to an otolaryngological practice

[a]Author for correspondence. Phone: 0975-86-5910; fax: 0955-49-0762; e-mail: gmogi @oita-med.ac.jp

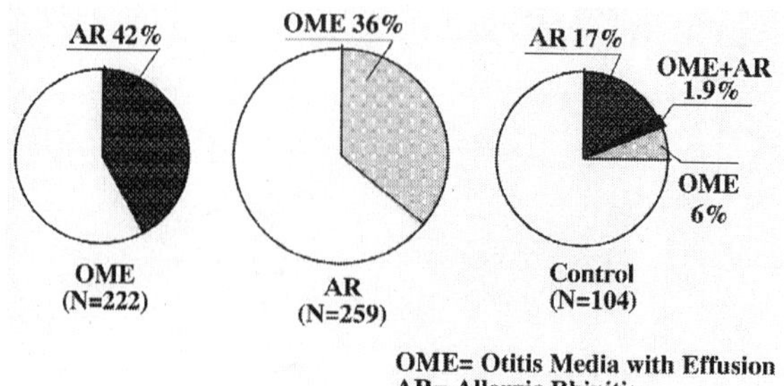

FIGURE 1. Complication ratios of otitis media with effusion and allergic rhinitis.

for evidence of allergy. They reported that 46 of these 200 patients (23%) were allergic. Several authors[13–15] also reported higher frequencies of OME in allergic children compared with age-matched nonallergic children or higher frequencies of allergy in children with OME compared with other diseases. FIGURE 1 shows complication ratios of OME in allergic rhinitis among three age-matched groups (6–8 years of age: mean age 6).[16] OME was confirmed by the presence of fluid in the tympanic cavity using paracentesis, and allergic rhinitis was diagnosed by history, nasal smear, skin test, provocation test, and RIST and RAST. Thus, findings of recent studies indicated that the frequency of allergy in OME patients is significantly higher in comparison with that reported in similarly aged children in the general population.

IS MIDDLE-EAR EFFUSION AN ALLERGIC FLUID?

Since the infiltration of eosinophils is often associated with allergic reactions, cytological study of middle-ear effusion (MEE) and histologic investigation of the middle-ear mucosa obtained from patients with OME have been performed. However, many studies[1,12,17–19] demonstrated that eosinophils were not common in MEE or in the middle ear mucosa. Since the discovery of IgE, many investigators have studied total IgE and specific IgE antibodies in MEE, comparing values in corresponding sera. Mogi *et al.*[20] measured IgE concentration in 96 paired samples of MEE and corresponding serum using a radioactive single radial diffusion technique and found that a majority of the MEE samples had a lower IgE concentration than did the corresponding serum. In only 2 of 96 cases (2.1%) did the IgE concentration in effusion exceed both the 500 ng/mL level and the IgE concentration in the corresponding serum. In a further study by Mogi *et al.*,[21] 179 paired samples of MEE and serum from patients with OME were investigated for the IgE antibody to mites using RAST and 108 paired samples using RIST for estimation of IgE concentration. The study also showed that mean IgE levels of MEE in both serous and mucoid types were significantly lower than those of the sera. Ten of 179 (5.6%) MEE and 8 of 179 (4.5%) serum samples had the IgE antibody to mites. More than half of the patients with this IgE antibody had a nasal allergy. These findings suggested that IgE in MEE is delivered from the serum, and that the allergic state in atopic allergic patients is a predisposing or conditioning factor rather than the cause of the MEE. Bernstein *et al.*[22] evaluated 100 young patients with recurrent OME (allergic and nonallergic) for IgE-mediated hypersensitivity. According to their results, IgE was elevated in 16 of 35 allergic patients (46%) and the IgE/mg protein was higher in MEE than in the corresponding serum of these 16 patients. They hypothesized the local production of IgE in the middle ear of their patients and concluded that IgE-mediated allergic reactions may play a role in the pathogenesis of OME in about 23% of young allergic patients. In contrast with these findings, Phillips *et al.*[23] reported total IgE elevations and increased IgE-bearing cells in all of 26 samples of MEE collected from patients with OME. More recently, Hurst[24] measured eosinophil cationic protein (ECP), which is a histochemical marker of eosinophils in the MEE, of 89 patients with persistent MEE and found that 87.5% of the patients had elevated levels of ECP in the MEE. They also measured 10 biopsy specimens from the middle-ear mucosa and reported that 80% of the mucosal biopsies showed abundant eosinophil infiltration as well as ECP in the subepithelial and intraepithelial tissue. Both of these studies strongly suggested that MEE is an allergic fluid and that the tympanic cavity is a shock organ. However, a number of studies have reported that MEE does not contain total or antigen-specific IgE antibody concentration in excess of that in matched serum.[12,16,20–22,25–27]

If MEE is an allergic fluid, the middle ear could be an allergic shock organ, and IgE-mediated immune reactions would be induced in the tympanic cavity. Miglets[28] provoked OME in passively sensitized monkeys by daily ragweed pollen delivery to the middle-ear mucosa via a eustachian tube catheter and found that the constituents of the provoked MEE were consistent with an allergic origin. However, a verifying study by Doyle *et al.*[29] failed to discover any MEE. The difference between the two experiments was that Doyle *et al.*[29] delivered ragweed pollens to the middle ear via nasopharynx by overpressure, while Miglets delivered ragweed pollens by a eustachian tube catheter. Doyle *et al.*[29] confirmed that the pollen was present in the middle-ear mucosa, but reported that histologic evidence of an allergic reaction was localized to the area of pollen-mucosal contact. Doyle *et al.* suggested that using a catheter may have injured the tubal lumen in the Miglets study, resulting in tubal inflammation that could have led to a middle-ear inflammatory reaction and the production of an effusion. Tomonaga *et al.*[30] made animal models of nasal allergy in guinea pigs by passive sensitization, using the serum of homologous animals containing a specific IgE antibody to antigen (dinitrophenilated(DNP)-ascaris), and injected antigen (DNP-ovalbumin) directly into the tympanic cavity of passively sensitized guinea pigs. Although they found allergic changes in the mucosa lining the tympanic bulla, there was no macroscopic effusion. There are few immunocompetent cells in the middle-ear mucosa in the normal state.[31] However, mast cells are exceptional. There is a significant number of mast cells in the tympanic orifice of the tube and other parts in rats and adults, neonatal, and developing guinea pigs.[32,33] Therefore, the middle ear can be considered to act as an allergic shock organ. However, since the eustachian tube is usually closed, with openings occurring only during swallowing or yawning, and since the eustachian tube offers the only potential pathway for antigen access to the middle ear, inhalant antigens rarely enter the tympanic cavity.[34] Doyle[34] pointed out that there is no established vehicle for introducing antigens in any quantity or with any regularity into the middle-ear space. Because of the difficulty of the antigen delivery, even if the middle ear is a shock organ, IgE-mediated allergic reaction would occur infrequently in the tympanic cavity.

DO ALLERGIC REACTIONS IN THE NASAL MUCOSA INTERFERE WITH EUSTACHIAN TUBE FUNCTION?

The nasal mucosa communicates anatomically with nasopharyngeal and tubal mucosae. Therefore, allergic inflammations in the nasal mucosa may cause edema of the eustachian tube mucosa, resulting in tubal obstruction and dysfunction. A clinical study by Crifo et al.[35] demonstrated that intranasal allergen challenge decreased tubal patency or resulted in complete tubal obstruction in patients with perennial allergic rhinitis. Ackerman et al.[36] observed eustachian tube obstruction after pollen insufflations with different intranasal doses in patients with allergic rhinitis to ragweed or timothy. They compared dose responses and duration of eustachian tube obstruction to patients' serum-IgE antibodies against the causative pollen and found that the induced tubal obstruction was dependent and related to serum-IgE antibody activity. Skoner et al.[37] conducted a similar study of patients with house dust mite nasal allergy and obtained similar results. The findings of these three clinical studies suggest that inflammation in the area of the nasopharynx and tubal orifice can cause tubal obstruction. Although persistent tubal obstruction induces MEE,[38] the tubal obstruction caused by such an allergic inflammatory process does not produce OME.[34]

Tomonaga et al.[30] observed the eustachian tube histologically and functionally after nasal provocation with the antigen in passively sensitized guinea pigs. They found significant allergic reactions in the mucosa of the nose, nasopharynx, and eustachian tube, such as marked infiltration with eosinophils, mast cells, and edema, even though the involvement of histologic changes was limited to as far as the area near the pharyngeal orifice. These changes were noticeable within one hour after the nasal antigen-challenge. Tubal function was evaluated by inflation and deflation tests using tympanometry after the eardrum was perforated. They reported that in comparison to values before the antigen challenge, a significant increase in the opening pressure of the tube was observed at 30 and 60 min after the antigen challenge. FIGURE 2 shows the clearance time of dye from the tympanic cavity to the pharyngeal orifice (unpublished data) in the Tomonaga et al. study.[30] After the induction of nasal allergic reactions, in many cases the exclusion time was significantly delayed. Results of their study indicate that the morphological changes and obstruction of the tube evoked by nasal allergic reactions was transient, culminating in no MEE. These studies suggest that type I allergic reactions of the nose are not an etiologic factor for OME.

In order to investigate the influence of nasal allergic reactions on the clearance of MEE, Mogi et al.[39] made an animal model of allergic rhinitis and OME simultaneously in the same guinea pigs by passive sensitization with IgE antibodies (for allergic rhinitis) and by inoculation of an immunocomplex into the tympanic cavity (for OME). After the inoculation with the immunocomplex, an intranasal antigen challenge was performed. The disappearance of MEE appeared to be delayed in animals in which nasal allergic reactions were induced; however, MEE was not found in those ears that had not been inoculated with the immunocomplex. The results of this study indicate that IgE-mediated allergic reactions of the nose, nasopharynx, and eustachi-

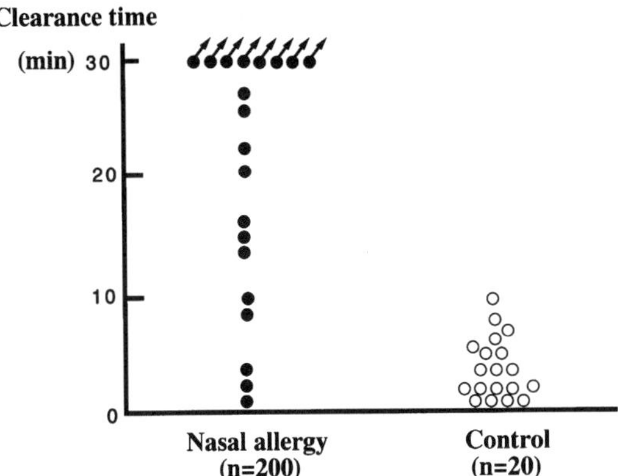

FIGURE 2. The clearance time of dye from the tympanic cavity to the pharyngeal orifice.

an tube constitute a factor indicative of a chronic state of disease, rather than a cause of OME. This finding is consistent with the results of an epidemiological study by Pukander and Karma[40] of 753 infants with acute otitis media; they reported a significantly longer persistence of MEE in infants with a history of allergy as compared with those in a nonallergic control group.

On the basis of their findings, Mogi *et al.*[39] recommended that treatment of allergy be combined with treatment of OME in patients having both allergic rhinitis and OME. In the clinical and experimental studies by Kawauchi *et al.*[41] patients with both OME and allergic rhinitis were divided into two groups. The patients in group A were given azelastine hydrochloride (antiallergic drug) and *s*-carboxymetheylcysteine (S-CMS), while patients in group B were given S-CMC only. S-CMC has been shown to accelerate the clearance of MEE.[42] Kawauchi *et al.* reported a global improvement rate for ear symptoms of 43% in group A and 17% in group B. They induced allergic rhinitis and OME in the same guinea pigs, simultaneously using the method of Mogi *et al.*,[39] and reported that administration of azelastine accelerates the clearance of MEE significantly.

DO ALLERGY AND INFECTION INTERACT WITH EACH OTHER?

It is now generally accepted that infection most often precedes OME. Since bacteria, such as *Streptococcus pneumoniae*, nontypeable *Haemophilus influenzae*, and *Moraxella catarrhalis*, which are the most common pathogens of acute otitis media (AOM), are frequently detected in MEE,[43] and since OME is frequently observed after AOM, persistent MEE is considered a sequela of AOM.[44,45] OME develops subsequent to upper respiratory infection (URI) with respiratory syncytical virus (RSV) and other viruses.[46,47] Acute viral infection leads to profound loss of antibacterial function, such as mucociliary activity, in the host.[48] Doyle *et al.*[49] induced experimental rhinovirus infections in adults with and without allergic rhinitis and demonstrated that rhinovirus infection is associated with significant nasal inflammation, eustachian tube dysfunction, and abnormal middle-ear pressures. More recently, Skoner *et al.*[50] examined cellular immune responses to experimental rhinovirus infection in subjects with allergic rhinitis and in those with nonallergic rhinitis and found a difference in responses between allergic and nonallergic groups.[50] Their data suggest that allergic and nonallergic populations respond differently to upper respiratory virus infection.

Chemical mediators, which are released from mast cells and other inflammatory cells, are the key factor inducing type I allergic reactions. Mast cells are activated by an allergen–IgE antibody complex, resulting in cell degranulation and the release of chemical mediators, such as histamine, heparin, eosinophilic chemotactic factor (ECF), neutrophilic chemotactic factor (NCF), and tryptase (mediators in the acute-phase reactions), as well as arachidonic cascades, such as prostaglandins D_2 (PGD_2) leukotrienes C_4, D_4, E_4, platelet activating factor (PAF), and thromboxian A_2 (mediators in the late-phase reactions). Sugiyama[51] and Ida *et al.*[52] reported the release of histamine from peritoneal mast cells after direct exposure to Sendai virus, and of LTB_4 and LTC_4 by peripheral monocytes upon stimulation by antigen–antibody complexes. Moreover, Welliver *et al.*[53] demonstrated the presence of respiratory syncytical virus-specific IgE (RSV-IgE) and the release of histamine in nasopharyngeal secretions obtained from RSV infected infants. They found RSV-IgE in only one of 19 patients with RSV infection without wheezing, while RSV-IgE was detected in the majority of 60 patients with wheezing. They also correlated the development of RSV-IgE and bronchospasm with the presence and levels of histamine in nasopharyngeal secretions. Virus-specific IgE has also been observed in patients infected with parainfluenza, herpes simplex, and rubella virus.[54] Volovitz *et al.*[55] presented evidence of histamine release and elevation of the level of another chemical mediator, LTC_4, in the respiratory tract of RSV-infected infants manifesting wheezing. These findings suggest that respiratory viral infections may be involved in the activation of mast cells during acute-phase reactions and of other effector cells during late-phase reactions, in a manner similar to type I allergic reactions. Since it was reported that the presence and level of LTC_4 in the nasopharynx were directly related to the degree of eustachian tube obstruction in patients with allergic rhinitis,[56] viral infection may contribute to the pathogenesis of OME in a manner similar to that of respiratory tract allergy.

SUMMARY

As both OME and allergic rhinitis are common among young children, these disorders are occasionally seen in the same patients. Many clinical and experimental studies have denied the allergic etiology of OME, although type I allergic reactions in the nose cause tubal obstruction without inducing MEE because the induced obstruction remains for a short duration. An animal model study demonstrated that allergy-induced tubal obstruction disturbs the clearance of MEE significantly. Since a clinical and an experimental study showed the efficacy of allergic treatment in patients or animals having both diseases, allergy and OME should be treated simultaneously in patients with both diseases. Viral infections of the upper respiratory tract induce viral-specific IgE antibodies, which may cause mucosal inflammatory reactions similar to those seen in type I allergy. Viral infection also triggers bacterial infection. Consequently, viral infection is a critical factor in the etiopathogenesis of OME.

REFERENCES

1. SENTURIA, B. H., C. F. GESSERT, C. D. CARR & E. S. BAUMANN. 1958. Studies concerned with tubotympanitis. Ann. Otol. Rhinol. Laryngol. **67:** 440–467.
2. MOGI, G., S. MAEDA, T. YOSHIDA & N. WATANABE. 1979. Role of atopic allergy in otitis media with effusion. JCE ORL Allergy **41:** 43–49.
3. BERNSTEIN, J. M., E. ELLIS & P. LI. 1981. The fole of IgE-mediated hypersensitivity in otitis media with effusion. Otolaryngol. Head Neck Surg. **89:** 874–878.
4. DOYLE, W. J., T. TAKAHARA & P. FIREMAN. 1985. The role of allergy in with effusion. The pathogenesis of otitis media with effusion. Arch. Otolaryngol. **111:** 502–506.
5. TOMONAGA, K., T. CHAEN, Y. KURONO & G. MOGI. 1990. Type I allergic reactions of the middle ear and eustachian tube: An experimental study. Auris Nasus Larynx. **17:** 121–131.
6. LEWIS, E. R. Otitis media and allergy. Ann. Otol. Rhinol. Laryngol. **38:** 185–188.
7. PROETZ, A. W. 1931. Allergy in the middle and internal ear. Ann. Otol. Rhinol. Laryngol. **40:** 67–76.
8. JORDAN, R. 1949. Chronic secretory otitis media. Laryngoscope **59:** 1002–1015.
9. LECKS, H. I. 1961. Allergic aspects of serious otitis media in children. N.Y. State J. Med. **61:** 2737–2743.
10. DRAPER, W. L. 1967, Secretory otitis media in children: A study of 540 children. Laryngoscope **77:** 636–653.
11. ISHIZAKA, K. & T. ISHIZAKA. 1996. Physicochemical properties of reaginic antibody. 1. Association of reaginic activity with an immunoglobulin other than γA-or γG-globulin. J. Allergy **37:** 169–185.
12. BERNSTEIN, J. M. & R. REISMAN. 1974. The role of acute hypersensitity in secretory otitis media. Trans. Am. Acad. Ophtyalmol. Otolaryngol. **78:** 120–127.
13. SCHUTTE, P. K., D. L. BEALES & R. DALTON. 1981. Secretory otitis media: A retrospective general practice survey. J. Laryngol. Otol. **95:** 17–22.
14. KRAEMER, M. J., M. A. RICHARDSON, N. S. WEISS, C. T. FURUKAWA, G. G. SHAPIRO, W. E. PIERSON & C. W. BIERMAN. 1983. Risk factors for persistent middle ear effusions: Otitis media, catarrh, cigarette smoke exposure, and atopy. JAMA **249:** 1022–1025.
15. TOMONAGA, K., Y. KURONO & G. MOGI. 1988. The role of nasal allergy in otitis media with effusion. A clinical study. Acta Otolaryngol. **458**(Suppl.): 41–47.
16. MOGI, G. 1989. Immunology of the Middle Ear—Etiology and Prophylaxis of Otitis Media with Effusion, Dept. of Otolaryngology, Oita Medical Univ., Oita, Japan.
17. SENTURIA, B. H. 1960. Allergic manifestation in otologic disease. Laryngoscope **70:** 287–297.
18. LIM, D. J. & H. BIRCK. 1971. Ultrastructural pathology of the middle ear mucosa in serious otitis media. Ann. Otol. Rhinol. Laryngol. **80:** 838–853.
19. SPILA, P. & P. KARMA. 1982. Inflammatory cells in mucoid effusion of secretory otitis media. Acta Otolaryngol. **94:** 467–472.
20. MOGI, G., S. HONJO, S. MAEDA, T. YOSHIDA & N. WATANABE. 1974. Immunoglobulin E (IgE) in middle ear effusions. Ann. Otol. Rhinol. Laryngol. **83:** 393–398.
21. MOGI, G., S. MAEDA, T. YOSHIDA & N. WATANABE. 1979. Role of atopic allergy in otitis media with effusion. JCEORL & Allergy **41:** 43–49.
22. BERNSTEIN, J. M., J. LEE, K. CONBOY, E. ELLIS & P. LI. 1985. Further observations on the

role of IgE-mediated hypersensitivity in recurrent otitis media with effusion. Otolaryngol. Head Neck Surg. **93:** 611–615.

23. PHILLIPS, M. J., N. J. KNIGHTS, J. T. MANNING, A. L. ABBOTT & W. G. TRIPP. 1974. IgE and secretory otitis media. Lancet **2:** 1176–1178.

24. HURST, D. S. 1996. Association of otitis media with effusion and allergy as demonstrated by intradermal skin testing and eosinophil cationic protein levels in both middle ear effusions and mucosal biopsies. Laryngoscope **106:** 1128–1137.

25. BOEDTS, D., G. D. GROOTE & J. V. VUCHELEN. 1984. Atopic allergy and otitis media with effusion. Acta Otolaryngol. **414**(Suppl. 108): 108–114.

26. LEWIS, D. M., J. L. SCHRAM, D. J. LIN, H. G. BIRCK & G. GLEICH. 1978. Immunoglobulin E in chronic middle ear effusions: Comparison of RIST, PRIST, RAST, and RIA techniques. Ann. Otol. Rhinol. Laryngol. **87:** 197–201.

27. PALVA, T., T. LEHTINEN & L. HALMEPURO. 1985. Immunoglobulin E in mucoid secretory otitis media. J. Otorhinolaryngol. Relat. Spec. **47:** 220–223.

28. MIGLETS, A. 1973. The experimental production of allergic middle ear effusions. Laryngoscope **83:** 1355–1384.

29. DOYLE, W. J., T. TAKAHARA & P. FIREMAN. 1985. The role of allergy in the pathogenesis of otitis media with effusion. Arch. Otolaryngol. **111:** 502–506.

30. TOMONAGA, K., T. CHAEN, Y. KURONO & G. MOGI. 1990. Type I allergic reactions of the middle ear and eustachian tube: An experimental study. Auris Nasus Larynx **17:** 121–131.

31. ICHIMIYA, I., H. KAWAUCHI & G. MOGI. 1990. Analysis of immunocompetent cells in the middle ear mucosa. Arch. Otolaryngol. Head Neck Surg. **116:** 324–330.

32. WIDEMAR, L., S. HELLSTROM, L.-E. STENFORS & G. D. BLOOM. 1986. An overlooked site of tissue mast cells—The human tympanic membrane. Implications for middle ear affections. Acta Otolaryngol. (Stockholm) **102:** 391–395.

33. WATANABE, T., H. KAWAUCHI, T. FUJIYOSHI & G. MOGI. 1991. Distribution of mast cells in the tubotympanum of guinea pigs. Ann. Otol. Rhinol. Laryngol. **100:** 407–412.

34. DOYLE, W. J. 1994. Etiology of otitis media with effusion: Role of allergy and tubal function. *In* Recent Advances in Otitis Media, G. Mogi, I. Honjo, T. Ishii, and T. Takasaka, Eds.: 53–60. Kugler. Amsterdam/New York.

35. CRIFO, S., S. CITTADINI, E. DESETA & G. ANDRIANI. 1977. Eustachian tube permeability during the nasal provocation test. Rhinology **15:** 81–85.

36. ACKERMAN, M. N., R. A. FRIEDMAN, W. J. DOYLE, J. D. BLUESTONE & P. FIREMAN. 1984. Antigen-induced eustachian tube obstruction: An intranasal provocative challenge test. J. Allergy Clin. Immunol. **73:** 604–609.

37. SKONER, D. P., J. P. DOYLE, A. H. CHAMOVITZ & P. FIREMAN. 1986. Eustachian tube obstruction after intranasal challenge with house dust mite. Arch. Otolaryngol. Head Neck Surg. **112:** 840–842.

38. CASSELBRANT, M. L., E. M. CANTEKIN, D. DIRKMAAT, W. J. DOYLE & C. D. BLUESTONE. 1988. Experimental paralysis of the tensor veli palatini muscle. Acta Otolaryngol. **106:** 178–185.

39. MOGI, G., T. CHAEN & K. TOMONAGA. 1990. Influence of nasal allergic reactions on the clearance of middle ear effusion. Arch. Otolaryngol. Head Neck Surg. **116:** 331–334.

40. PUKANDER, J. & P. H. KARMA. 1988. Persistence of middle ear effusion and its risk factors after an acute attack of otitis media with effusion. *In* Proc. 4th Int. Symp. on Recent Advances in Otitis Media, D. J. Lim, C. D. Bluestone, J. O. Klein, and J. D. Nelson, Eds.:8–11. Decker. Toronto.

41. KAWAUCHI, H., M. SUZUKI, Y. KURONO & G. MOGI. 1995. Clinical and experimental study of azelastine on otitis media with effusion coupled with nasal allergy. *In* Abstracts of the 6th Int. Symp. on Recent Advances in Otitis Media, Fort Lauderdale, Fla., June 4–8, p. 246.

42. Hori, F., H. Kawauchi & G. Mogi. 1994. Effect of S-carboxymethylcysteine on the clearance of middle ear effusion. An experimental study. Ann. Otol. Rhinol. Larayngol. **103:** 567–575.

43. Kurono, Y., K. Tomonaga & G. Mogi. 1988. *Staphylococcus epidermidis* and *Staphylococcus aureus* in otitis media with effusion. Arch. Otolaryngol. Head Neck Surg. **114:** 1262–1265.

44. Shurin, P. A., S. I. Pelton, A. Donner & J. O. Klein. 1979. Persistence of middle ear effusion after acute otitis media in children. New Eng. J. Med. **300:** 1121–1123.

45. Teele, D. W., J. O. Klein & B. A. Rosner. 1989. Epidemiology of otitis media in chidren. Ann. Otol. Rhinol. Laryngol. **89**(Suppl. 68): 5–6.

46. Sarkkinen, H., O. Ruuskanen, O. Meurman, H. Putakka, E. Virolainen & S. Eskola. 1985. Identification of respiratory virus antigen in middle ear fluids of children with acute otitis media. J. Infect. Dis. **151:** 444–448.

47. Giebink, G. S., I. K. Berzins, S. T. Marker & G. Schiffman. 1980. Experimental otitis media after nasal inoculation of *Streptococcus pneumoniae* and influenza A virus in chinchillas. Infect. Immun. **30:** 445–450.

48. Bakaletz, L. O., T. M. Hoepe, T. F. DeMaria & D. J. Lim. 1988. The effect of antecedent influenza A virus infection on the adherence of *Haemophilus influenzae* to chinchilla tracheal epithelium. Am. J. Otolaryngol. **9:** 127–134.

49. Doyle, W. J., D. P. Skoner, P. Fireman, J. T. Seroky, I. Green, F. Ruben, D. R. Kardatzke & J. M. Gwaltney. 1992. Rhinovirus infection in allergic and nonallergic subjects. J. Allergy Clin. Immunol. **89:** 968–978.

50. Skoner, D. P., T. L. Whiteside, J. W. Wilson, W. J. Doyle, R. B. Haberman & P. Fireman. 1993. Effect of rhinovirus 39 infection on cellular immune parameters in allergic and nonallergic subjects. J. Allergy Clin. Immunol. **92:** 732–743.

51. Sugiyama, K. 1977. Histamine release from rat mast cells induced by Sendai virus. Nature **270:** 614–615.

52. Ida, S., J. J. Hooks, R. P. Siraganian & A. L. Notkins. 1977. Enhancement of IgE-mediated histamine release from human basophils by viruses: Role of interferon. J. Exp. Med. **145:** 892–906.

53. Welliver, R. C., D. T. Wong, M. Sun, E. Middleton, R. S. Vaughan & P. L. Ogra. 1981. The development of respiratory syncytical virus-specific IgE and the release of histamine in nasopharyngeal secretions after infection. New Eng. J. Med. **305:** 841–846.

54. Volovitz, B. & P. L. Ogra. 1988. Pathogenesis of viral respiratory tract infection. *In* Proc. 4th Int. Symp. on Recent Advances in Otitis Media, D. J. Lim, C. D. Bluestone, J. O. Klein, and J. D. Nelson, Eds.: 287–290. Decker. Toronto/Philadelphia.

55. Volovitz, B., H. Faden & P. L. Ogra. 1988. Release of leukotrienes in human respiratory tract during viral infection: Implication in virus induced wheezing. J. Pediatr. **112:** 218–222.

56. Volovitz, B., S. L. Osur, J. M. Bernstein & P. L. Ogra. 1988. Leukotriene C4 release in upper respiratory mucosa during natural exposure to ragweed in ragweed-sensitive children. J. Allergy Clin. Immunol. **82:** 414–418.

Immunological Deficiency in "Otitis-prone" Children

NOBORU YAMANAKA,[a] MUNEKI HOTOMI, JUN SHIMADA,
AND AKIHITO TOGAWA

Department of Otolaryngology
Wakayama Medical College
27, 7-Bancho,
Wakayama, 640, Japan

INTRODUCTION

Acute purulent otitis media (AOM) is the type of respiratory tract infection most commonly diagnosed among children. By the end of the third year of life, 50% to 70% of all children have experienced at least one AOM episode. Some children contract frequent, recurrent bouts of AOM. Three or more episodes have been found to occur in 9% to 18% of children during the first year of life and in one-third of all children during their first three years of life.[1] In 1975 Howie *et al.* coined the term "otitis-prone condition" for children with recurrent episodes of AOM.[2] Recent epidemiologic investigations show clearly that recurrent otitis media is a disease of early childhood. Several factors that identify a child at risk for recurrent disease include having the first episode of otitis media early in life, having other family members with recurrent disease, enrollment in day care, and bottle feeding.[1–4] There is, however, increasing evidence for minor immunological deficiencies contributing to proneness to otitis media.

Three bacteria are responsible for the vast majority of ear infections: *Streptococcus pneumoniae* causes between 30 and 50%, nontypeable *Haemophilus influenzae* (NTHI) between 27 and 37%, and *Moraxella catarrhalis* between 11 and 23%.[5–8] The relative distribution of these agents has undergone change over time. For example, NTHI has become a more common cause of otitis media,[6,8] while the incidence of *M. catarrhalis* has increased >20-fold.[7,9] The bacteria causing recurrent episodes of otitis media are the same that cause otitis media, but their relative frequency is different; for reasons not fully understood, NTHI assumes a more prominent role in recurrent disease.[10–14]

IMMUNE RESPONSE TO NONTYPEABLE *H. INFLUENZAE* AND *S. PNEUMONIAE*

H. influenzae occurs with or without a capsule. The encapsulated forms are much more pathogenic than the other types, but the unencapsulated form, that is, nonty-

[a]Phone: 011-81-734-26-8296; fax: 011-81-734-33-6480; e-mail: ynobi@wakayama-med.ac.jp

peable form, is most commonly found in association with upper respiratory tract infection. The NTHI has become the principal cause of both AOM and chronic otitis media with effusion. More than 95% of the strains of *H. influenzae* isolated from nasopharynx and middle ear of children with otitis media represent nontypeable strains.[15] Unlike *S. pneumoniae* NTHI does not possess capsular polysaccharide; rather, it has outer membrane proteins and lipooligosaccharides expressed as surface antigens. Among the approximately 20 outer membrane proteins, at least six are considered major (FIG. 1), and several of them have been shown to be a target for bactericidal antibody.[16,17] More recently, several other less studied ones have been described. Unfortunately, there is a great degree of heterogeneity among outer membrane proteins. Thus, antibody to these proteins may result in strain-specific rather than cross-protective immunity. Both animal and human studies have demonstrated strain-specific protection.[18–21] Among six outer membrane proteins, two outer membrane proteins, P4, molecular weight 30,000 dalton, and P6, molecular weight 16,000 dalton, are antigenically stable and are highly conserved among strains.[22,23] However, Munson and Granoff[24] reported that antiserum directed against P4, when administered to infant rats, was not protective against *H. influenzae*. In contrast, antibody raised to P6 in rabbits was shown to kill a wide spectrum of *H. influenzae* isolates, and was protective.[24,25] For these reasons, P6 has recently been proposed as a potential candidate for vaccine.

The pneumococcal capsular polysaccharide (PCP) is a relevant antigen in the study of protective antibodies. Immunity to pneumococcal infections is closely associated with levels of complement and specific antibodies against PCP.[26] Among different pneumococcal serotypes only a few are clinically important as a cause of otitis media. Type 19 is one of the most common serotypes and is reported to give a poor immune response in spite of showing very high preimmunization antibody levels.[27] On the other hand, serotype 3 is found to evoke increasing levels of naturally occurring antibodies in children up to 5 years of age.[28]

Several immunologic factors were examined previously in children with recurrent otitis media. For example, total immunoglobulin IgG, IgM, and IgA were reportedly

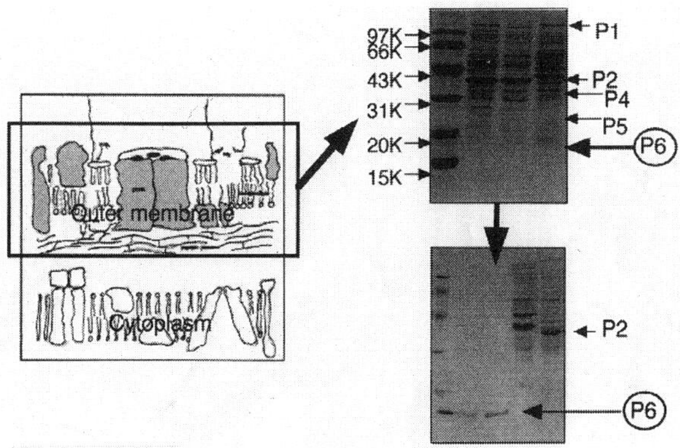

FIGURE 1. Outer membrane proteins and P6 of nontypeable *H. influenzae*.

normal in otitis prone children.[29] However, concentrations of antigen-specific antibody against the common otitis media-associated pneumococcal types 6A and 19F were lower in children with recurrent otitis media.[30,31] Similarly, antibody responses to pneumococcal vaccine were reduced in otitis-prone children.[32]

IgG SUBCLASSES AND THEIR CHANGE WITH AGE

Immunoglobulin G can be separated into distinct subclasses on the basis of antigenic and physiochemical characteristics.[33] Human IgG can be divided into four sublcasses, namely, IgG1 to IgG4. Different trends in the levels of IgG1, IgG2, IgG3, and IgG4 are observed with age. Hayashibara *et al.*[34] reported that the ratio of IgG1 to the total IgG gradually increased until the ages of 2 to 4 years (76.0±6.8%), and decreased thereafter to 60.8±8.6% at 14 to 15 years of age. Conversely, the ratio of IgG2 gradually decreased until the age of 2 to 4 years (17.3±5.6%) and increased thereafter to 32.5±8.2% at the age of 14 to 16 years. The ratio of IgG3 increased rapidly until 4 to 7 months of age (4.8–12.8%), and rapidly decreased thereafter to reach a plateau (about 3.6%) at 4 to 6 years of age. The ratio of IgG4 decreased gradually until 7 to 12 months of age (0.2–1.0%), and increased thereafter until reaching a plateau at 2 to 4 years of age (1.2–1.6%). These subclasses show different biological features, that is, IgG1 and IgG3 are antibodies against protein antigens of such viral particles, and fix complement efficiently. In contrast, IgG2 is an antibody against carbohydrate antigens and polysaccharides, including bacterial capsules such as *S. pneumoniae, H. influenzae* type b, and so forth.[35,36] On the other hand, P6 from NTHI, which doesn't have polysaccharide capsule, elicits IgG1 and IgG3 antibody response.[37]

As a result of catabolism of maternal IgG, the serum levels of IgG in infants decline during the first 6 months of life, showing a period of physiological hypogammaglobulinemia between the ages of 4 to 8 months.[38,39] In addition, the level of IgG2 is the lowest between the ages of 6 months to 2 years. Based on the changes of IgG sublcasses with age described earlier, children of the ages 6 months to 2 years may be most vulnerable to bacterial infections. Hence the significant delay in the onset of production of immunoglobulins in some infants may lead to the recurrent infections in the upper and lower respiratory tract including otitis media.

SPECIFIC IMMUNE RESPONSE TO OUTER MEMBRANE PROTEIN OF NONTYPEABLE *H. INFLUENZAE* IN OTITIS-PRONE CHILDREN

As previously mentioned, P6 of NTHI is highly conserved among strains, and serves as a target for bactericidal antibody. Serum antibody response to P6 has been studied in our laboratory in the general population and both otitis-prone and nonotitis-prone children.[40] Thirty of the subjects were classified as otitis-prone because they had experienced four or more episodes of otitis media in the first year of life or six or more episodes by the second year, or needed placement of tympanostomy tubes.

Anti-P6 antibody levels in the general population are shown in FIGURE 2. At birth,

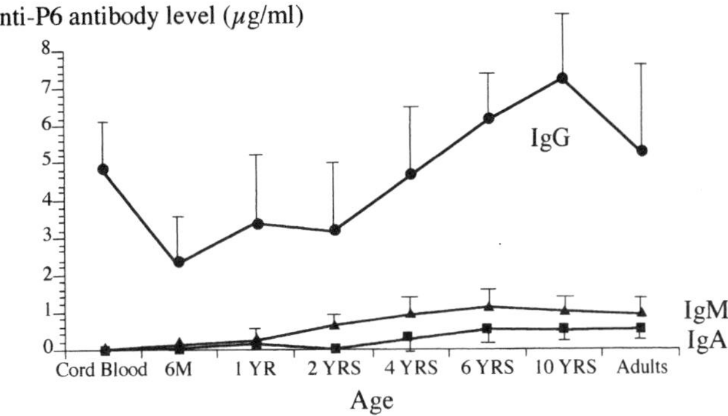

FIGURE 2. Antibody response to P6 of nontypeable *H. influenzae* in the general population.

anti-P6 IgG antibody was found in almost the same level as that of adults, whereas no IgM or IgA antibodies specific for P6 were detected. Anti-P6 antibody levels in the three isotypes studied were lowest at 6 months of age and rose significantly after two years; IgG levels peaked at 10 years, whereas IgM and IgA peaked at 6 years. In every age-group, IgG antibody specific for P6 was in the highest concentration among the three isotypes. Anti-P6 IgG antibody was detected in all individuals in each age group; however, IgM antibody specific for P6 was detected in all individuals older than 6 years of age, and IgA antibody specific for P6 was detected in all individuals only after 10 years of age.

Anti-P6 antibody levels were measured longitudinally in 30 otitis-prone and 13 healthy children on 93 and 32 occasions, respectively. The age at time of sampling varied between one and 92 months. Antibody levels increased 7-fold in the normal group over 36 months compared to less than 3-fold for the otitis-prone group over 48 months (FIG. 3). The levels of antibody in the normal group were significantly higher than those in the otitis-prone group after the age of 18 months. In general, individual antibody levels in otitis-prone individuals did not demonstrate an age-dependent rise.

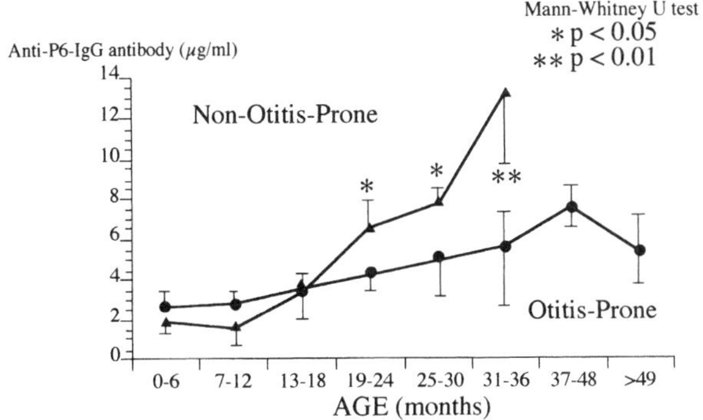

FIGURE 3. IgG antibody response to P6 in otitis-prone and healthy children.

The comparison of anti-P6 IgG antibody between otitis-prone children and healthy children under the age of 6 years are shown in FIGURE 4. It is very interesting to note that 89% of otitis-prone children show the anti-P6 antibody level below 7 μg/mL (mean-2SD of ages 6 months to 6 years in healthy children).[41] Furthermore, children who experienced two or more episodes of otitis media due to NTHI failed to manifest an anamnestic antibody response to P6. Immunoglobulin IgM and IgA antibody responses to P6 in otitis-prone children reached a plateau after 18 months of age, and anti-P6 IgM antibody level remained below the adult serum level even after 4 years of age. Differences in IgM and IgA between otitis-prone and healthy children were not statistically significant.

In our study, otitis-prone children were not unusually vulnerable to infections except otitis media. This fact seems to refute the presence of a broad-based immunologic deficit in the children. However, children who experienced recurrent episodes of otitis media due to NTHI did not mount a normal response to P6 during otitis media, and failed to develop a secondary immune response upon repeated challenge. The failure to recognize P6 as a specific immunogen may account for recurrent infections.

We also examined the local immune response to NTHI in middle-ear fluids and in the nasopharyngeal secretions.[42] The concentration of P6 antibody in the middle ear was inversely related to the number of viable bacteria present in the middle-ear fluids ($r = -0.62$, $p<0.05$), suggesting a direct inhibitory effective antibody on the bacteria. Furthermore, the concentration of P6-specific IgG in the middle ear was directly related to concentration of P6 antibody in the serum ($r = 0.89$, $p<0.001$). These findings again emphasize the importance of specific serum bactericidal antibody of the IgG isotype directed against P6 as being responsible for at least one component in the immune resolution of NTHI in the middle ear. IgA and secretory IgA antibodies to P6 were common (96% and 95%, respectively) and in relatively high concentrations in nasopharyngeal secretions. There was no relationship between nasopharyngeal and serum levels of antibodies, suggesting that antibody in the nasopharynx is predominantly locally produced.

Our data suggest that otitis proneness may be related to specific immunological

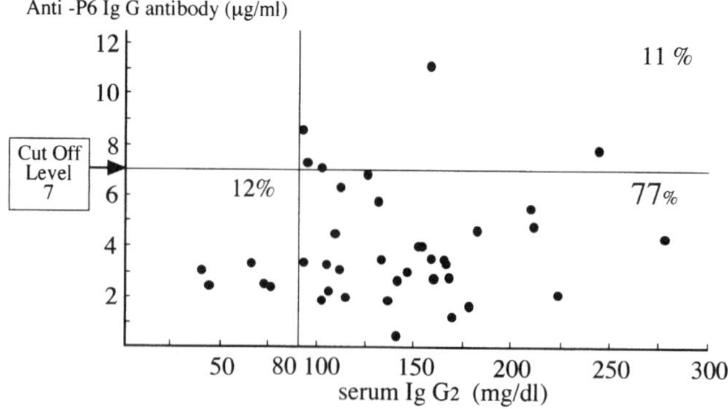

FIGURE 4. P6-antibody response and serum IgG2 level in otitis-prone children.

deficiencies. This defect may be present in both the local and systemic immune systems.

PNEUMOCOCCAL CAPSULAR POLYSACCHARIDE-SPECIFIC IgG SUBCLASS ANTIBODIES

S. pneumoniae is a common pathogenic organism causing respiratory and systemic infections including otitis media in adults and children. In order to assess specific antibody responses to pneumococcal capsular polysaccharide (PCP), polyvalent pneumococcal vaccine has been used as a coating antigen in ELISA.[43] We used a polyvalent pneumococcal vaccine (Pneumovax; Merck Sharp & Dohme, West Point, Pa.) containing 23 serotypes: 1, 2, 3, 4, 5, 6B, 7F, 8, 9N, 9V, 10A, 11A, 12F, 14, 15B, 17F, 18C, 19A, 20, 22F, 23F, and 33F as a coating antigen. Pneumovax-specific IgG subclass antibodies were measured quantitatively by ELISA technique, as described by Kojima *et al.*[44] When measuring Pneumovax-specific IgG1 and IgG2 concentrations in each test serum, the plates were coated with a 1:10 dilution of Pneumovax, and the purified solution containing Pneumovax-specific antibodies was used as a reference standard in the ELISA method.

Evidence from early studies that human antibodies to polysaccharide antigens were largely restricted to IgG2 suggested that susceptibility to pneumococcal infection might be caused by a selective deficiency of IgG2 antibody. In response to reports that IgG2 deficiency is more common than previously appreciated, serum concentration of IgG2 is often used clinically as a marker for susceptibility to infection. In our series of otitis-prone children, only 7% of otitis-prone children showed serum IgG2 levels below 80 mg/mL (2 SD below the mean for age of 1 year) as shown in FIGURE 5. This result brings about skepticism regarding a simple relationship between low serum IgG2 concentrations and susceptibility to infection including otitis media. The study of Pneumovax-specific IgG2 antibody demonstrated that 79% of otitis-prone children had subnormal concentrations of the specific antibody. It is very

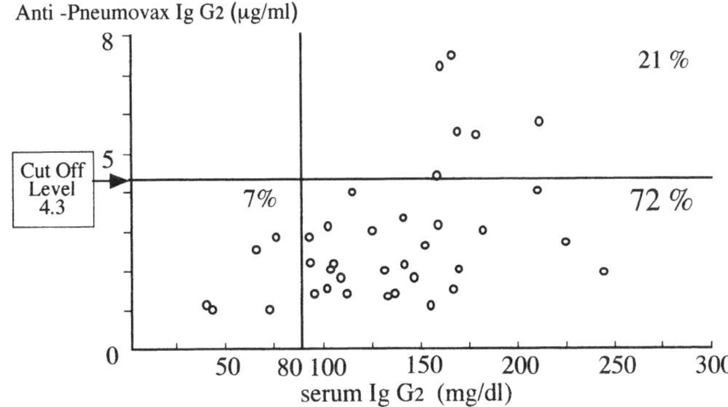

FIGURE 5. Pneumovax-specific IgG2 antibody response and serum IgG2 level in otitis-prone children.

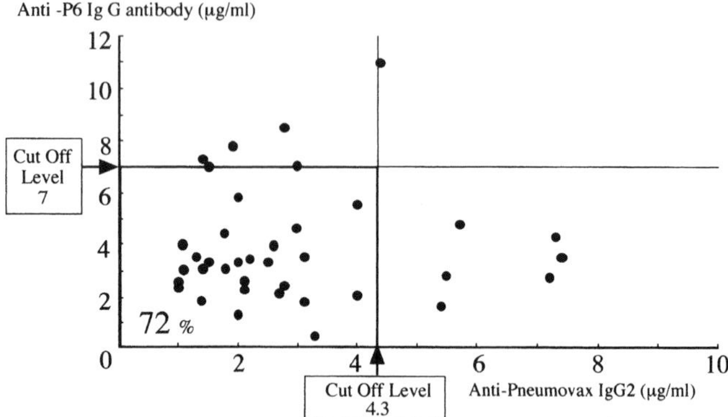

FIGURE 6. P6- and pneumovax-antibody responses in otitis-prone children.

interesting to note that over 90% of the children with subnormal Pneumovax-specific IgG2 antibody level showed normal serum concentrations of IgG2.

Taken together with data of P6-specific antibody in otitis-prone children, this result clearly indicates that pathogen-specific IgG or IgG2 antibodies are highly reliable markers for the otitis-prone condition. Therefore, in a child who is being examined for recurrent otitis media, measurement of the response to pneumococcal capsular polysaccharide and P6 of NTHI should be useful in determining whether immunological deficiency may contribute to the otitis-prone condition.

As shown in FIGURE 6, it is rather striking to note that more than 70% of otitis-prone children showed subnormal serum concentrations in both P6-specific IgG antibody and Pneumovax-specific IgG2 antibody. This result suggests that selective immunological derangement in otitis-prone children may be wider than previously believed.

NEW STRATEGIES FOR THE PREVENTION OF OTITIS MEDIA

The pathogen causing otitis media originates from the adenoid or nasopharyngeal space. Resolution of otitis media by immunological mechanisms within the middle-ear space is most likely the result of pathogen-specific IgG antibodies and complement that reaches the middle ear from the serum. Secretory IgA, on the other hand, may be responsible for coating the bacteria and preventing its attachment to the middle-ear mucosa. Efforts to reduce the otitis-prone condition will include augmenting the production of both systemic-specific IgG antibody and local-specific secretory IgA antibody.

Systemic vaccination with specific outer membrane proteins of NTHI or the use of specific fimbrial proteins, which are conserved in NTHI, may be used to stimulate specific antibodies. Regarding mucosal immunity, an effort to elicit local secretory IgA antibody has just started. Oral immunization may stimulate gut precursors of B cells in Peyer's patches that seed the upper respiratory tract and produce specific IgA in the nasopharyngeal secretion. This has been demonstrated for both NTHI and

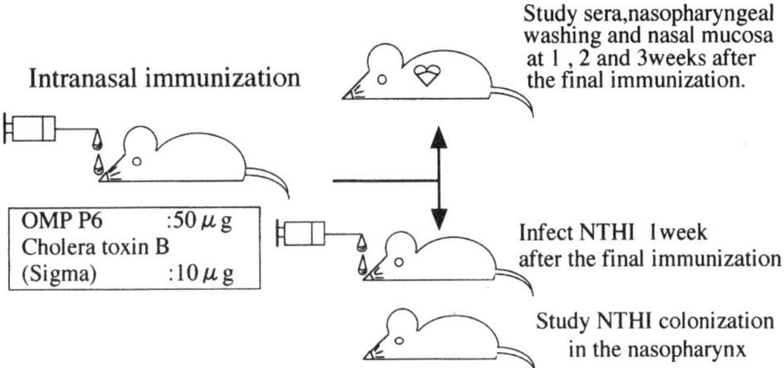

FIGURE 7. Experimental design of intranasal immunization for P6 to mice.

pneumococcus in the experimental animal model.[45,46] Furthermore, there is evidence that oral immunization with bacterial vaccines activate macrophage by stimulating metabolic and functional properties that are characeristic of the activated state and are important for host defense.[47] Recently, evidence has shown that nasal-associated lymphoid tissue (NALT) may play an important role in the immune response in the upper respiratory tract.[48,49] The nasal mucosa may be one of the highly efficient paths for the induction of specific mucosal immunity. Although an equivalent organ or NALT in humans has not been identified yet, nasal immunization may stimulate nasal precursors of B cells in NALT-equivalent organ that may seed immunocompetent cells in the upper respiratory tract and distribute memory cells to the systemic immune organs. These cells will produce immunogen-specific IgA in the nasopharyngeal secretions and IgG in sera.

We designed animal experiments to investigate whether the intranasal immuniza-

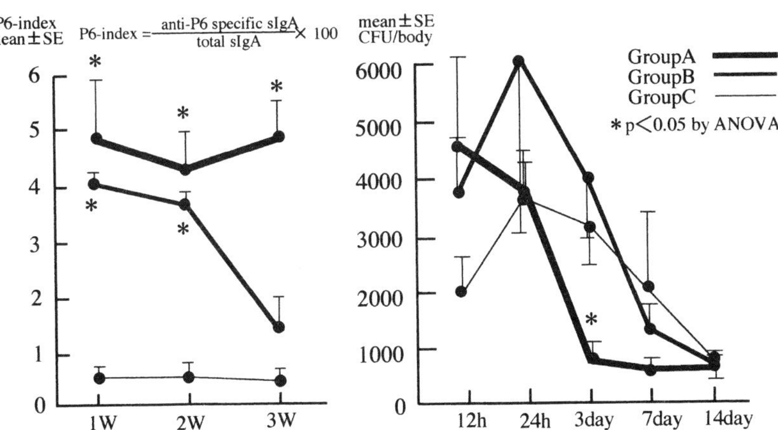

FIGURE 8. P6-specific sIgA in nasopharyngeal secretion and prevention of the colonization of nontypeable *H. influenzae* in the nasopharynx. **Group A:** Immunize P6 for 2 weeks with 2-day interval; **Group B:** immunize P6 with 2-week interval; **Group C:** give PBS for 2 weeks with 2-day interval.

tion of P6 with cholera toxin B subunit (CTB) would induce specific mucosal immunity against NTHI (FIG. 7).[50] As shown in Figure 8a, intranasal immunization of P6 every 2 days for 2 weeks efficiently elicited P6-specific secretory IgA antibody. A good IgG antibody response to P6 was also found by this route of immunization (data are not shown). It is very important to prove that these P6-specific antibodies will protect against infections with *H. influenzae*. Our study showed that the antibodies prevented colonization with NTHI in the nasopharynx of mice (FIG. 8b). Taken together with our results and the fact that P6 is a common antigen among strains of nontypeable and type b *H. influenzae*, intranasal immunization of P6 is one promising strategy for the prevention of infections caused by *H. influenzae* including otitis media.

CONCLUSIONS

1. P6, one of the outer membrane proteins of NTHI is highly conserved among strains.
2. Serum IgG antibody response to P6, and IgG2 antibody response to Pneumovax were studied by the solid-phase ELISA in both otitis-prone and nonotitis-prone children.
3. The failure to recognize P6 and pneumococcal capsular polysaccharide as specific immunogens may account for recurrent otitis media. This result suggests that selective immunological deficiency in otitis-prone children may be wider than previously believed.
4. There is no simple relationship between low serum IgG2 concentrations and susceptibility to otitis media.
5. Intranasal immunization of P6 may be a new strategy for the induction of protective mucosal immunity to *H. influenzae*.

REFERENCES

1. TEELE, D. W., J. O. KLEIN, B. ROSNER & THE GREATER BOSTON OTITIS MEDIA STUDY GROUP. 1989. Epidemiology of otitis media during the first seven years of life in children in greater Boston: A prospective cohort study. J. Infect. Dis. **160:** 83–94.
2. HOWIE, V. M., J. H. PLOUSSARD & J. SLOYER. 1975. The "otitis-prone" condition. Am. J. Dis. Child. **129:** 676–678.
3. HOWIE, V. M. & R. H. SCHWARTZ. 1983. Acute otitis media. Am. J. Dis. Child. **137:** 155–158.
4. SIPILA, M., P. KARMA, J. PUKANDER, M. TIMONEN & M. KATAJA. 1988. The Bayesian approach to the evaluation of risk factors in acute and recurrent otitis media. Acta. Otolaryngol. (Stockholm) **106:** 94–101.
5. VON HARE, G. F., P. A. SHURIN, C. D. MARCHANT, *et al.* 1987. Acute otitis media caused by *Branhamella catarrhalis*: Biology and therapy. Rev. Infect. Dis. **9:** 16–26.
6. FADEN, H., J. BERNSTEIN, J. STANIEVICH, L. BRODSKY & P. L. OGRA. 1992. Effect of prior antibiotic treatment in middle ear disease in children. Ann. Otol. Rhinol. Laryngol. **101:** 87–91.
7. DELBECCARO, M. A., P. M. MENDELMAN, A. F. INGLIS, *et al.* 1992. Bacteriology of acute otitis media. J. Pediatr. **120:** 856–862.

8. OWEN, M. J., R. ANWAR, H. K. NGUYEN, P. R. SWANT, E. R. BANNISTER & V. M. HOWIE. 1993. Efficacy of cefixime in the treatment of acute otitis media in children. Am. J. Dis. Child. **147:** 81–86.

9. MORTINER, E. A., JR. & R. L. WATTERSON, JR. 1956. A bacteriologic investigation in infancy. Pediatrics **17:** 359–366.

10. BJUGGREN, G. & G. TUNEVALL. 1952. Otitis media in children: A clinical and serobacteriological study with special reference to the significance of *Haemophilus influenzae* in relapses. Acta Otolaryngol. (Stockholm) **17:** 311–328.

11. LISTON, T. E., W. S. FOSHEE & C. MCCLASKEY. 1984. The bacteriology of recurrent otitis media and the effect of sulfisoxazole chemoprophylaxis. Pediatr. Infect. Dis. **3:** 20–24.

12. HARRISON, C. J., M. I. MARKS & D. F. WELCH. 1985. Microbiology of recently treated acute otitis media compared with previously untreated acute otitis media. Pediatr. Infect. Dis. **4:** 641–646.

13. CARLIN, S. A., C. D. MARCHANT, P. A. SHURIN, C. E. JOHNSON, D. MURDELL-PANEK & S. J. BARENKAMP. 1987. Early recurrences of otitis media: Reinfection in relapse. J. Pediatr. **110:** 20–25.

14. BLUESTONE, C. D. 1989. Modern management of otitis media. Recent Adv. Pediatr. Otolaryngol. **36:** 1371–1387.

15. BROOK, I. & P. YOCUM. 1989. Quantitative bacterial cultures and beta lactamase activity in chronic suppurative otitis media. Ann. Otol. Rhinol. Laryngol. **98:** 293–297.

16. GNEHM, H. E., S. I. PELTON, S. GULATI & P. A. RICE. 1985. Characterization of antigens from nontypeable *Haemophilus influenzae* recognized by human bactericidal antibodies. J. Clin. Invest. **75:** 1645–1658.

17. MURPHY, T. F., L. C. BARTOS, P. A. RICE, M. B. NELSON, K. C. DUDAS & M. A. APICELLA. 1986. Identification of a 16,600 dalton outer membrane protein on nontypeable *Haemophilus influenzae* as a target for human bactericidal antibody. J. Clin. Invest. **78:** 1020–1027.

18. LOEB, M. R. & D. H. SMITH. 1980. Outer membrane protein composition in disease isolates of *Haemophilus influenzae*: Pathogenic and epidemiological implications. Infect. Immun. **30:** 709–717.

19. BARENKAMP, S. J., D. M. GRANOFF & R. S. J. MUNSON. 1981. Outer membrane protein subtypes of *Haemophilus influenzae* type b and spread of disease in day-care centers. J. Infect. Dis. **144:** 210–217.

20. HANSEN, M. V., D. M. MUSHER & R. E. BAUGHN. Outer membrane proteins of nontypeable *Haemophilus influenzae* and reactivity of paired sera from infected patients with their homologous isolates. Infect. Immun. **47:** 843–846.

21. KARASIC, R. B., C. E. TRUMPP, H. E. GNEHM, *et al.* 1985. Modification of otitis media in chinchillas rechallenged with nontypeable *Haemophilus influenzae* and serological response to outer membrane antigens. J. Infect. Dis. **151:** 273–279.

22. BARENKAMP, S. J., R. S. J. MUNSON & D. M. GRANOFF. 1982. Outer membrane protein and biotype analysis of pathogenic nontypeable *Haemophilus influenzae*. Infect. Immun. **36:** 535–540.

23. MURPHY, T. F., K. C. DUDAS, J. M. MYLOTTE & M. A. APICELLA. 1983. A subtyping system for nontypeable *Haemophilus influenzae* based on outer membrane proteins. J. Infect. Dis. **147:** 838–846.

24. MUNSON, R. S. J., & D. M. GRANOFF. 1985. Purification and partial characterization of outer membrane protein P5 and P6 from *Haemophilus influenzae* type b. Infect. Immun. **49:** 544–549.

25. GREEN, B. A., T. QUINN-DEY, & G. W. ZLOTNICK. 1987. Biologic activities of antibody to a peptidoglycan-associated lipoprotein of *Haemophilus influenzae* against multiple clinical isolates of *H. influenzae* type b. Infect. Immun. **55:** 2878–2883.

26. BROWN, E. J., *et al.* 1982. A quantitative analysis of the interactions of antipneumococcal

antibody and complement in experimental pneumococcal bacteremia. J. Clin. Invest. **69:** 85–98.

27. COWAN, M. J., A. J. AMMAN, D. W. WARA, V. M. HOWIE, L. SCHUTZ, N. DOYLE & M. KAPLAN. 1978. Pneomococcal polysaccharide immunization in infants and children. Pediatrics **62:** 721–727.

28. DOUGLAS, R. M., J. C. PATON, S. J. DUNCAN & D. J. HANSMAN. 1983. Antibody response to pneumococcal vaccination in children younger than five years of age. J. Infect. Dis. **148:** 131–137.

29. BRANFOS-HELANDER, P., T. DAHLBERG & O. NYLEN. 1975. Acute otitis media: A clinical, bacteriological and serological study of children with frequent episodes of acute otitis media. Acta Otolaryngol. (Stockholm) **80:** 399–409.

30. FREIJD, A., L. HAMMAERSTROM, M. A. A. PERSSON & C. I. E. SMITH. 1984. Plasma antipneumococcal antibody activity of the IgG class and subclasses in otitis-prone children. Clin. Exp. Immunol. **56:** 233–238.

31. PRELLNER, K., O. KALM & F. K. PEDERSEN. 1984. Pneumococcal antibodies and complement during and after periods of recurrent otitis. Int. J. Pediatr. Otolaryngol. **7:** 39–49.

32. PELTON, S. I., D. W. TEELE, C. B. REIMER, G. G. DELANGE, G. R. SIBER & THE GREATER BOSTOM OTITIS MEDIA STUDY GROUP. 1988. Immunologic characteristics of children with frequent recurrences of otitis media. *In* Recent Advances in Otitis Media, D. J. Lim, C. D. Bluestone, J. O. Klein, and J. D. Nelson: 143–146. Decker. Toronto/Philadelphia.

33. TERRY, W. & J. FAHEY. 1964. Subclasses of human globulin based on differences in the heavy polypeptide chains. Science **146:** 400–401.

34. HAYASHIBARA, H., K. TANIMOTO, I. NAGATA, Y. HARADA & K. SHIRAKI. 1993. Normal levels of IgG subclasses in childhood determined by a sensitive ELISA. Acta Pediatr. Jpn. **35:** 113–117.

35. SIBER, G. R., P. H. SHUR, A. C. AISENBERG, S. A. WEITZMAN & G. SCHIFFMAN. 1980. Correlations between serum IgG2 concentrations and the antibody response to bacterial polysaccharide antigen. New Eng. J. Med. **303:** 178–182.

36. BARRETT, D. J. & E. M. AYOUB. 1986. IgG2 subclass restriction of antibody to pneumococcal polysaccharides. Clin. Exp. Immunol. **63:** 127–134.

37. YAMANAKA, N. & H. FADEN. 1994. Immune response to P6 of nontypeable *H. influenzae* in otitis-prone children with special reference to IgG subclass. *In* Recent Advances in Otitis Media, G. Mogi, I. Honjo, T. Ishii, and T. Takasaka, Eds.: 489–493. Kugler. Amsterdam/New York.

38. MORELLA, A., F. SKVARIL, W. H. HITZIG & S. BARANDUM. 1972. IgG subclasses: Development of the serum concentrations in "normal" infants and children. Pediatrics **80:** 960–964.

39. OXELIUS, V.-A. 1979. IgG subclass levels in infancy and childhood. Acta Pediatr. Scand. **68:** 23–27.

40. YAMANAKA, N. & H. FADEN. 1993. Antibody response to outer membrane protein of nontypeable *Haemophilus influenzae* in otitis-prone children. J. Pediatr. **122:** 212–218.

41. SHIMADA, J., M. HOTOMI, A. TOGAWA & N. YAMANAKA. 1996. Antibody responses to P6 of nontypeable *H. influenzae* and pneumococcal capsular polysaccharide in otitis-prone children. Submitted for publication.

42. YAMANAKA, N. & H. FADEN. 1993. Local antibody response to P6 of nontypeable *Haemophilus influenzae* in otitis-prone and normal children. Acta Otolaryngol. (Stockholm) **113:** 524–529.

43. WINDEBANK, K. P., J. A. FAUX & H. M. CHAPEL. 1987. ELISA determination of IgG antibodies to pneumococcal capsular polysaccharides in a group of children. J. Immunol. Methods **104:** 143–148.

44. KOJIMA, K., A. ISHIZAKA, E. OSHIKA, *et al.* 1990. Quantitation of IgG subclass antibodies to

pneumococcal capsular polysaccharides by ELISA, using Pneumovax-specific antibodies as reference. Tohoku J. Exp. Med. **161:** 209–215.

45. WATANABE, N., H. KATO & G. MOGI. 1989. Induction of antigen-specific IgA forming cells in the upper respiratory mucosa. Ann. Otol. Rhinol. Laryngol. **98:** 523–529.

46. KURONO, Y., R. SHIMAMURA & G. MOGI. 1992. Inhibition of nasopharyngeal colonization of *Haemophilus influenzae* by oral immunization. Ann. Otol. Rhinol. Laryngol. **101:** 11–15.

47. EMMERICH, B., K. PACHMANN, D. MILATOVIC & H. P. EMSLANDER. 1992. Influence of OM-85BV on different humoral and cellular immune defense mechanisms of the respiratory tract. Respiration **59**(Suppl. 3): 19–23.

49. VAN POPPEL, M. N. M., T. K. VAN DER BERG, E. P. VAN REES, T. SMINIA & J. BIEWENGA. 1993. Reticulum cells in the ontogeny of nasal-associated lymphoid tissue (NALT) in the rat. Cell Tissue Res. **273:** 577–581.

50. HOTOMI, M., J. SHIMADA & N. YAMANAKA. 1997. Induction of specific mucosal immunity to P6 of nontypable *H. influenzae* by intranasal immunization. Submitted for publication.

Are There Immunological or Genetic Markers that can Predict Recurrent Acute Otitis Media?

KARIN PRELLNER[a] AND OLOF KALM

Department of Otorhinolaryngology
University Hospital
S-221 85 Lund
Sweden

RECURRENT ACUTE OTITIS MEDIA

There is no generally accepted definition of otitis proneness. The proposed definitions of this state of multiple recurrent episodes of acute otitis media (rAOM) range from six attacks before the age of 6 years to six episodes within a 12-month period. Approximately 5% of young children suffer from rAOM to such a degree that it causes a clinical problem. Children suffering from rAOM may experience up to 20 attacks before the age of 3 years.[1,2] Early debut of the first AOM attack (before 6 months of age) is a strong risk indicator of rAOM.[2] Viral upper respiratory tract infections often precede AOM, the latter usually regarded as a bacterial infection.

Usually a single AOM episode is not a large problem for the child or its family, in contrast to the stress experienced by families with children contracting frequent recurrent bouts of AOM. For a proper handling of these patients it is of the utmost importance that very early in life, they are identified as children at risk. The importance of heredity is confirmed by ethnic and gender differences in AOM incidence. Also a history of frequent AOM episodes in siblings and/or parents is significantly correlated with rAOM.[2,3]

During the last decade studies have been undertaken, aiming at identifying differences between children with and without rAOM and at predicting which children are at risk. Besides clinical data, the studies have focused on humoral immune factors and genetically determined characteristics. Since humoral immune factors, in contrast to genetically determined characteristics, are influenced by antigenic exposure and the infectious state of the patient, an interpretation of established immunological differences between healthy and rAOM children must be done with great care. Prospective studies initiated before the AOM episodes start are thus of the utmost importance.

MAJOR PATHOGENS

Streptococcus pneumoniae is the bacterium most frequently isolated in AOM, followed by nonencapsulated *Hemophilus influenzae*.[4,5]

[a]Author for correspondence. Phone: +46-46-172162; fax: +46-46-2110968.

On the basis of their various capsular polysaccharides, and according to their antigenic differences or similarities, pneumococci are classified in groups and types, comprising more than 80 known types. Pneumococci of groups 3, 6, 14, 18, 19, and 23 account for 70–80% of pneumococcal AOM episodes, and those of groups 6, 19, and 23 for almost 50%.[6,7] The most commonly isolated types are 6A, 6B, 19F, and 23F.[7] Recurrent AOM is often caused by pneumococci, the same pneumococcal type being almost invariably isolated at recurrence as was isolated at the initial infection.[6] The pneumococcal groups or types vary in their capacity to induce antibody response. The immunogenic capacity of type 3 is good, that of groups 19 and 23 moderate, and that of group 6 poor.[8]

Strains of *H. influenzae* that are nontypeable (NT)—in as much as they do not belong to the known capsular types—are isolated in 90–95% of AOM episodes caused by *H. influenzae*. Which antigens are the most important in eliciting protective antibody response in AOM is still under discussion. Interest has been focused on six outer membrane proteins (P1–P6) and a lipopolysaccharide.

HUMORAL IMMUNE FACTORS RELATED TO HOST DEFENSE AGAINST PNEUMOCOCCI AND *H. INFLUENZAE*

The capsular polysaccharide is proposed to be the most important virulence factor of pneumococci.[9] For normal phagocytosis and killing of pneumococci the bacteria need to be opsonized, that is, coated with specific antibodies and complement (C) cleavage fragments, especially C3b.[10]

H. influenzae is a gram-negative rod and, like most gram-negative bacteria, susceptible to complement-mediated killing. The insertion of the C5b-9 complex onto the outer bacterial membrane results in membrane disorganization and cellular death.

IgG is quantitatively the most important of the serum immunoglobulins.[11] Antibodies to polysaccharide antigens have been supposed to be predominant in the IgG2 subclass. Recent studies on children have, however, shown pneumococcal antibodies to be approximately equally distributed between the IgG1 and IgG2 subclasses.[12,13]

Complement factors are a group of plasma proteins that can be sequentially activated, either through the classic or the alternative pathway. The most important activators of the classic pathway are immune complexes containing IgM or IgG.[14] The first complement factor, C1, is a macromolecule composed of three distinct proteins, C1q, C1r, and C1s. When C1q binds to the Fc portion of IgG or IgM in an appropriate way, this leads to a sequential activation of C1r and C1s, which then splits C4 and later C2, and a complex is formed that converts C3 into the fragments C3a and C3b.[15] C3b is the C cleavage fragment crucial to the opsonization of pneumococci.[10] C3 can also be activated through the alternative pathway (the properdin system). Of utmost importance for the killing of *H. influenzae* is the sequential activation from C3 to C5, of which C5b fuses successively with C6 through C9. Insertion of this complex eventually leads to osmotic rupture of the bacterium.

In pneumococcal otitis media, the alternative pathway can be activated either by intact pneumococci or by pneumococcal cell-wall constituents.[16,17] Furthermore, together with specific antibodies, these pneumococcal antigens can form immune complexes, which then activate the classic pathway. Complexes between C-reactive protein and the common pneumococcal cell-wall polysaccharide (C-polysaccharide) constitute another possible complement activator in otitis media.[17]

Although many immunological studies on capsulated *Hemophilus* strains have been performed, few investigations of NT strains have been reported. In complex with their specific antibodies, their outer membrane proteins—which vary from one NT strain to another[18]—constitute possible activators of the classic pathway of complement in otitis media. The alternative pathway could be activated by the lipopolysaccharide of the cell wall of these bacteria.

Both *in vitro* studies and experimental investigations have shown phagocytosis of pneumococci to be reduced in hypogammaglobulinemic serum and in serum deficient in complement factors.[10,19]

Age-related Physiological Changes

T- and B-lymphocyte function is generally immature during early childhood.[20] Thus, B-lymphocytes of newborns can be triggered to produce IgM at adult levels but not IgG. However, the concentration of total IgG in cord serum is at least as high as that of adults, though it decreases to a minimum by 4½ months of age, followed by a slow increase, adult levels being reached again at 5–7 years of age.[21] The increase of IgG2 and IgG4 subclasses is markedly slower than that of IgG1 and IgG3.[22] The IgM increases during the first three months to 50% of adult levels, the full adult concentration being reached around the age of one year.[21] IgG constitutes about 80% of total serum immunoglobulins, and IgM less than 10%.[11] In contrast to IgM, the IgA concentration increases very slowly and adult levels are not reached until puberty.[21] A switchover from IgM to IgG antibody production against some antigens is known not to occur until the age of 18 to 24 months.[23]

Specific antipneumococcal antibody concentrations are generally lower in healthy children than in adults.[8] With some variation, most of the C components, which are lower in cord serum, increase to adult levels during the first six months of life.[24]

Relations Between Serum Concentrations of Immune Factors and Disease

Individuals with congenital or acquired hypogammaglobulinemia or deficiency of one or two subclasses are known to contract severe acute and chronic bacterial infections,[25,26] and gammaglobulin replacement therapy has been reported to prevent recurrent infections in such categories of patients.[25]

AOM, and especially rAOM, is generally confined to an age group with physiological hypogammaglobulinemia. No differences have been found, however, in the total concentrations of IgG, IgA, or IgM between rAOM children and healthy controls.[27] Increased serum concentrations of specific pneumococcal antibodies, as a result of an AOM attack, have been reported in 25% of the cases studied,[28] as have strain-specific bactericidal antibodies as a result of otitis media caused by NT *H. influenzae*.[29] C activation is noticed in about 50% irrespective of etiologic agent.[30]

Some patients contracting recurrent infections due to pneumococci or *H. influen-*

zae seem to have a low capacity of responding by antibody production to these specific polysaccharides at vaccination, despite having normal total immunoglobulin concentrations. Independent of the total serum IgG concentration, the response to immunization with a vaccine containing several polysaccharide antigens seems to be correlated with the IgG2 subclass concentration.[31] An association between middle-ear effusion antibody concentrations and clearance of the effusion has been demonstrated.[32]

The importance of a functioning C system is demonstrated through the occurrence of serious infections or of immune complex disease in patients with hereditary C component defects.[33] Recurrent severe bacterial infections are particularly seen in patients with C3 deficiency.[33]

In children with single episodes of AOM, the serum concentrations of most C factors were of the same magnitude as those of healthy children without AOM, but a disproportion between C1s and C1q levels, in conjunction with moderate amounts of abnormal complexes of C1r–C1s, was found in those with acute infections[30] (FIG. 1).

Influence of Hereditary Factors

Clinical evidence suggests a hereditary influence on susceptibility to infection by AOM-associated microorganisms. Boys have been reported to show a small but definitely higher incidence of AOM than girls,[34] and children with siblings or one parent with a history of rAOM have been reported to be predisposed to rAOM.[2] Several ethnic differences have also been reported.[3,35] There are also grounds for the idea that the capacity to produce antibodies against several polysaccharide antigens could be genetically determined.[36]

Genetic immunoglobulin markers express immunoglobulin allotypic variants. Markers of the heavy chains of immunoglobulins are designated Gm and markers of the kappa-light-chains are termed Km allotypes.[11] In humans, G2m(n)-positive individuals seem to have higher concentrations of serum IgG2 and IgG4 than people lacking this marker,[37] and G2m(n)-positive individuals were also reported to have higher concentrations of specific antibodies against many polysaccharide antigens and a stronger antibody response on vaccination.[38] The antibody response was found to be better in Km(1)-positive individuals than in Km(1)-negatives.[39]

Associations of varying degrees between the prevalence of hereditary major histocompatibility complex (MHC) class I and II molecules (HLA antigens) and various diseases are well established.[40] Regarding most diseases associated with HLA antigens, the morbidity risk in conjunction with the presence of a given antigen is relatively moderate. A clear exception is the case of ankylosing spondylitis, where the relative risk (RR) of contracting the disease is extremely high (87.4) in a person carrying another MHC class I molecule (HLA-B27).[40] Only few and weak correlations have been found between the occurrence of infectious diseases and HLA antigens.[41]

Blood groups are easily available genetic characters. An association seems to exist between blood-group glycoproteins and antibodies to an otitis-media-associated pathogen (pneumococcus type 14). Glycoproteins with type-14 specificity are likely to be precursors of ABH blood groups and Lewis substances.[42]

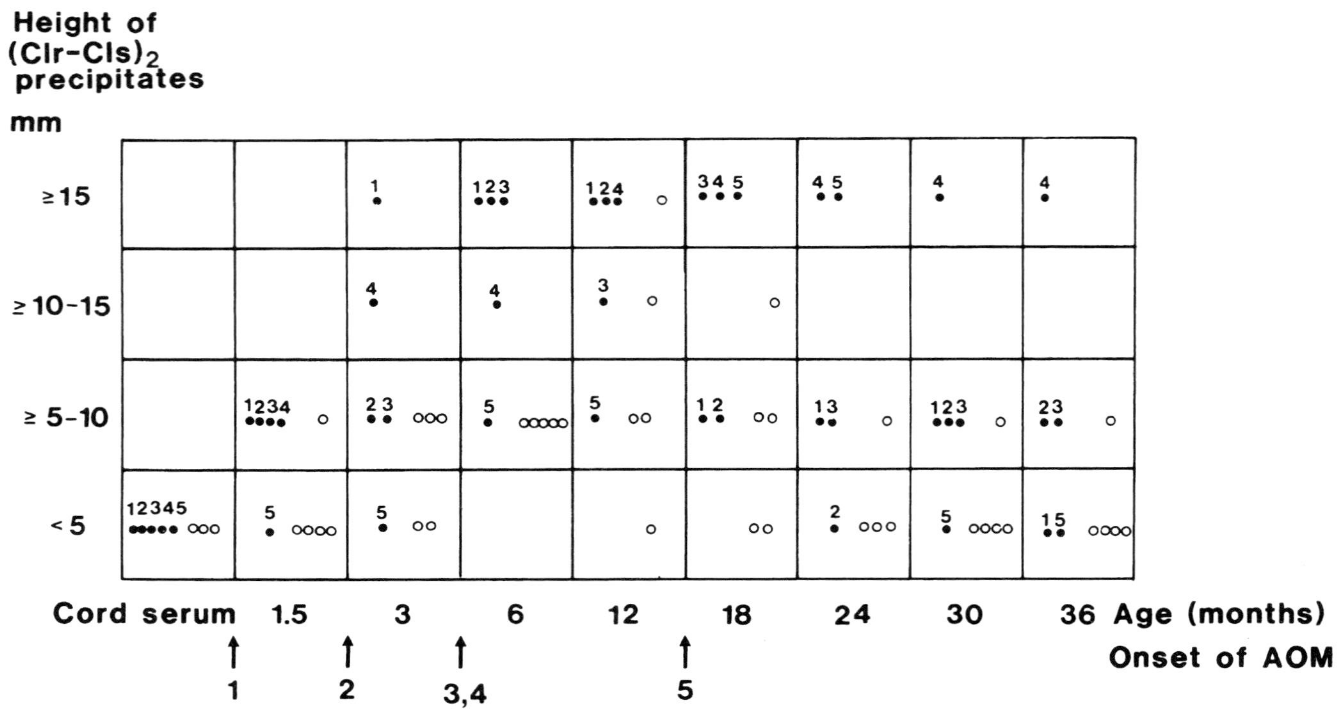

FIGURE 1. Presence and amounts of (Clr-Cls)$_2$ complexes in serum samples obtained at regular intervals from five rAOM children (●) (designated 1–5), and from five healthy children (○). The onset of AOM in each rAOM child is indicated by an arrow. (From Prellner et al.[63] Reprinted with permission.)

WHY ARE CHILDREN MUCH MORE AFFECTED
OF AOM THAN ADULTS?

In children, the eustachian tube is shorter, more horizontal, and the active tubal function is poorer than in adults, and compared with adults the mastoid cell system is considerably smaller in children.[43] Children, unlike adults, often carry potentially pathogenic bacteria in the nasopharynx. The age-related physiological variations, with a relative hypogammaglobulinemia and a relatively poor ability of C activation in young children, probably contribute to why children are more affected than adults.

The younger age groups have a poor ability to synthesize antibodies to polysaccharide antigens, as for example bacterial capsules, in particular the pneumococcal and *H. influenzae* capsules. The antibody production is only weakly stimulated by the pneumococcal types most commonly isolated from children with rAOM. Protein conjugation of the vaccine for *H. influenzae* type b has, however, also dramatically increased its immunogenicity in young children.

WHAT CHARACTERIZES CHILDREN PRONE TO OTITIS MEDIA?

Although the factors previously mentioned can partly explain why most children contract AOM, they do not explain why only a few percent of the children, and not all, suffer from recurrent or prolonged ear problems. Among the humoral immune factors and hereditary characteristics of which otitis-prone children have been reported to differ from nonotitis-prone children are (1) the ABO blood groups, (2) immunoglobulin and subclass concentrations, (3) concentrations of specific serum antibodies and B-cells, (4) HLA antigen prevalences, and (5) complement factors.

ABO Blood Groups

Children with AOM caused by the type-14 pneumococcus have the same distribution of ABO and Lewis blood groups as the normal Swedish population.[6] On the other hand, a significantly lower prevalence of blood group O than in the general population was observed in individuals having been treated for secretory otitis media (SOM).[44] A combination of maternal blood group A and the first attack of middle-ear disease before the first birthday demonstrated a relative risk of 26.77 ($p<0.0001$).[45] Whether these findings reflect a hereditary difference in the immune response to infection or are merely an association between blood groups and anatomical differences is not known.

Immunoglobulin and Subclass Concentrations

The total serum concentrations of IgG, IgA, and IgM are similar in children with and without rAOM.[27] Whether an IgG2 subclass deficiency is present in otitis-prone children is under discussion.[46,47] Children with low IgG2 concentrations were reported to suffer from more infections with *H. influenzae* than those with normal levels.[46]

On the other hand, older age groups of otitis-prone children had similar levels of IgG2 subclasses when compared to controls.[48] Higher levels of total plasma IgG and IgG1 were also noted in this study. Even children with secretory otitis media had raised levels of IgG1. These latter observations were interpreted to be the result of recurrent polyclonal stimulation of the immune apparatus.[48] A deficient SIgA coating observed in rAOM children seems to promote the bacterial attachment to the nasopharyngeal wall.[49]

Concentrations of Specific Serum Antibodies and of B Cells

The serum concentrations of specific antibodies against AOM-associated pneumococcal types (i.e., the poorly immunogenic capsular groups 6 and 19) measured in the main classes IgG and IgA were found to be significantly lower in otitis-prone than in nonotitis-prone children during the first years of life.[47,50] Similar findings were also noted by others.[12] It is of interest that lower concentrations of these antibodies were interestingly seen already in cord serum samples,[47] indicating immunological differences already at birth (FIG. 2). Because cord blood emanates from the mother, it has been speculated that the mothers of some otitis-prone children might

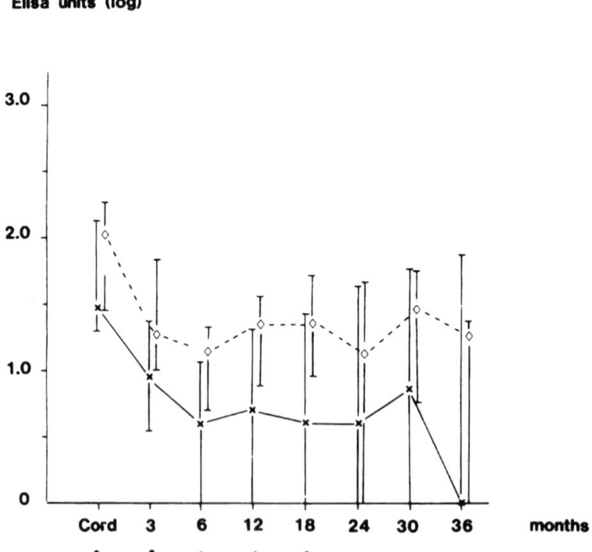

FIGURE 2. Median-specific IgG antibody concentrations (logarithmic values) to pneumococcus type 6A during the first 3 years of life in rAOM children (×) and in healthy children (◇). *Vertical lines* represent one quartile on either side of the median value; (*) denotes statistically significant differences. N.B.: values on the zero-line denote original untransformed values = 0. (From Prellner *et al.*[63] Reprinted with permission.)

be hereditary low-responders to polysaccharide antigens. In spite of probable exposure (infections and colonization) the serum concentrations of specific antibodies remained low in rAOM children aged less than three years.[47] The children thus seem to have a reduced ability to respond immunologically to antigens of otitis-media-associated pneumococci. When analyzing the specific antibody concentrations against the same pneumococcal strains in IgG and IgA subclasses, the otitis-prone children (mean age 1.9 years) were found to have lower concentrations of antibodies to type 6A in the subclasses IgG1, IgG2, IgG3, IgG4, IgA1, and in IgM.[51] At a follow-up at the age of 8 years the antibody concentrations of rAOM children tended to equalize compared to those of controls,[50] and the differences seen had disappeared by adulthood[52] (FIG. 3). The observations discussed, which were found in half the children with rAOM, indicate that rAOM occurs in individuals with a delayed, rather than persisting, inability to mount adequate antibody response against AOM-associated bacteria.

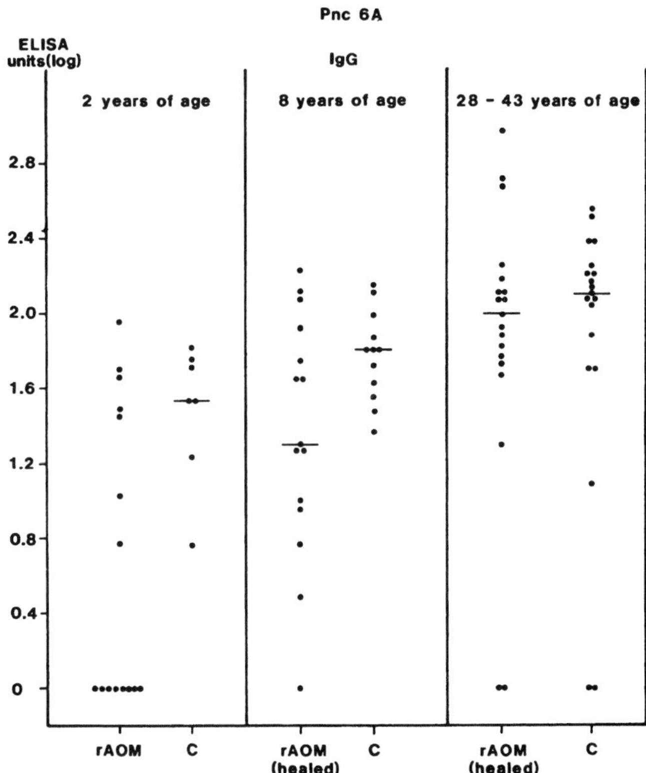

FIGURE 3. Age-related concentrations of IgG antibodies against pneumococcus type 6A in patients with recurrent AOM (rAOM), compared with nonotitis-prone individuals (C). (From Prellner and Kalm.[64] Reprinted with permission.)

Antibodies to nonencapsulated *H. influenzae* have also been reported to be lower in otitis-prone than in nonotitis-prone children[18,53,54] (see Yamanaka *et al.*)[55] Poor antibody response has also been noted at rubella vaccination of rAOM children, indicating that the capacity to mount antibodies to other protein antigens is reduced as well.[56]

At flow cytometry of B-lineage cells, significantly higher concentrations of cells with early B-lineage antigens CD19, CD24, CD20, CD22, and HLA-DR were found in rAOM children (mean age 1.8 years) compared with nonotitis-prone of the same age. After six months the difference had disappeared.[57] The findings mirror a delayed maturation of immunoglobulin-producing cell lines in rAOM children and could in part explain the differences seen between otitis-prone and nonotitis-prone children in IgG subclass concentrations and specific pneumococcal antibodies, and also the poor response to rubella vaccination just described.

Gm and HLA Antigen Prevalences

The distribution of hereditary immunoglobulin allotypes, especially markers of IgG2 (G2m(n)) in rAOM and healthy individuals, did not differ significantly.[58,59] In studies of possible associations between the hereditary HLA antigens and ear disease, HLA-B27—present in 95% of patients with ankylosing spondylitis—has also been found to be associated with chronic ear disease (tympanosclerosis; chronic otitis media).[60] In rAOM the HLA-A2 antigen prevalence was found to be significantly higher in rAOM children (80–90%) than in the general population (55.9%) and the HLA-A3 prevalence lower, but in patients with "chronic SOM" the HLA-A2 and HLA-A3 prevalences were of the same magnitude as in those of controls,[61,62] suggesting divergent influence of heredity on the pathogenesis of rAOM and "chronic SOM." In this context the findings just given are indications of the importance of hereditary factors in rAOM, even if it is not known whether these types of associations are primary or secondary, that is, due to linkage disequilibrium with other HLA factors.[40]

Complement Factors

Disturbances in the activation of complement by the classic pathway have also been observed in rAOM children. Among the aberrations in C activation noted during the acute phase of rAOM are discrepancies between the serum concentrations of the C1 subcomponents C1q and C1s, with C1q below the normal range, and at the same time an excess of C1r–C1s proenzyme complexes is seen (FIG. 1), maybe as a direct consequence of the antibody deficiency just mentioned.[49,63] The disturbances disappear with increasing age. In cord blood from rAOM children, the C1q concentrations were found to be lower than in cord blood from healthy children and even lower in children with early onset of disease.[63] The wide variation of cord blood C1q concentrations within groups and an absence of C1r–C1s complexes, however, speak in favor of the idea that the aberrations are acquired as a result of infection.[63]

CONCLUSION

An increased number of immature blood B-lineage cells, low concentrations of specific IgG serum antibodies to pneumococcal type 6A, being HLA-2 positive, and the first AOM episode before the age of six months, constitute the combination of immunological and hereditary markers that could predict rAOM in a child during its first months of life. For chronic SOM the situation seems much less clear. It must, however, be remembered that factors discussed in this paper probably identify only half of the children at risk. Other factors—e.g., eustachian tube function and external influence (short breast-feeding, type of day care, etc.)—must also be considered.

REFERENCES

1. HOWIE, V. M., J. H. PLOUSSARD & J. SLOYER. 1975. The "otitis-prone" condition. Am. J. Dis. Child. **129:** 676–678.
2. HARSTEN, G., K. PRELLNER, J. HELDRUP, O. KALM & R. KORNFALT. 1989. Recurrent acute otitis media. A prospective study of children during their first three years of life. Acta Otolaryngol. (Stockholm) **107:** 111–119.
3. TEELE, D. W., J. O. KLEIN & B. A. ROSNER. 1980. Epidemiology of otitis media in children. Ann. Otol. Rhinol. Laryngol. **89** (Suppl. 68): 5–6.
4. KLEIN, J. O. 1980. Microbiology of otitis media. Ann. Otol. Rhinol. Laryngol. **89**(Suppl. 68): 98–101.
5. KAMME, C. 1985. Microbiology of acute and secretory otitis media. *In* Treatment of Ear, Nose and Throat Infections: 17–36. National Board of Health and Welfare, Drug Information Committee. Uppsala, Sweden.
6. KAMME, C., M. AGEBERG & K. LUNDGREN. 1970. Distribution of *Diplococcus pneumoniae* types in acute otitis media in children and influence of the types on the clinical course in penicillin V therapy. Scand. J. Infect. Dis. **2:** 183–190.
7. AUSTRIAN, R., V. M. HOWIE & J. H. PLOUSSARD. 1977. The bacteriology of pneumococcal otitis media. Johns Hopkins Med. J. **141:** 104–111.
8. BORGONO, J. M., A. A. McCLEAN, P. P. VELLA, A. F. WOODHOUR, I. CANEPA, W. L. DAVIDSON & M. R. HILLEMAN. 1978. Vaccination and revaccination with polyvalent pneumococcal polysaccharide vaccines in adults and infants. Proc. Soc. Exp. Biol. Med. **157:** 148–154.
9. AUSTRIAN, R. 1981. Some observations on the pneumococcus and on the current status of pneumococcal disease and its prevention. Rev. Infect. Dis. **3**(Suppl.): S1–S17.
10. JOHNSTON, R. B., M. R. KLEMPERER, C. A. ALPER & F. S. ROSEN. 1969. The enhancement of bacterial phagocytosis by serum. The role of complement components and two cofactors. J. Exp. Med. **129:** 1275–1290.
11. GRUBB, R. 1970. The Genetic Markers of Human Immunoglobulins. Springer-Verlg. Berlin.
12. FREIJD, A., L. HAMMARSTROM, M. A. A. PERSSON & C. I. E. SMITH. 1984. Plasma anti-pneumococcal antibody activity of the IgG class and subclasses in otitis prone children. Clin. Exp. Immunol. **56:** 233–238.
13. RYNNEL-DAGOO, B., A. FREIJD & K. PRELLNER. 1985. Antibody activity of IgG subclasses against pneumococcal polysaccharides after vaccination. Am. J. Otolaryngol. **6:** 275–279.
14. AUGENER, W., H. M. GREY, N. R. COOPER & H. J. MULLER-EBERHARD. 1971. The reaction

of monomeric and aggregated immunoglobulins with C1. Immunochemistry **8:** 1011–1020.

15. MULLER-EBERHARD, H. J., M. J. POLLEY & M. A. CALCOTT. 1967. Formation and functional significance of a molecular complex derived from the second and the fourth component of human complement. J. Exp. Med. **125:** 359–380.

16. PRELLNER, K. 1979. Complement activation by pneumococci associated with acute otitis media. Acta Pathol. Microbiol. Scand. C **87:** 213–217.

17. PRELLNER, K. 1981. C1q binding and complement activation by capsular and cell wall components of *S. pneumoniae* type XIX. Acta Pathol. Microbiol. Scand. C **89:** 359–364.

18. SHURIN, P. A., C. D. MARCHANT & V. M. HOWIE. 1984. Bactericidal antibody to antigenically distinct nontypeable strains of *Hemophilus influenzae* isolated from acute otitis media. *In* Recent Advances in Otitis Media with Effusion, D. J. Lim, C. D. Bluestone, J. O. Klein and J. D. Nelson, Eds.: 155–157. Decker. Philadelphia/Toronto.

19. BRACONIER, J. H. & H. ODEBERG. 1982. Granulocyte phagocytosis and killing of virulent and avirulent serotypes of *Streptococcus pneumoniae*. J. Lab. Clin. Med. **100:** 279–287.

20. ANDERSSON, U., G. BIRD & S. BRITTON. 1981. A sequential study of human B lymphocyte function from birth to two years of age. Acta Paediatr. Scand. **70:** 837–842.

21. JOHANSSON, S. G. O. & T. BERG. 1967. Immunoglobulin levels in healthy children. Acta Paediatr. Scand. **56:** 572–579.

22. OXELIUS, V.-A. 1979. IgG subclass levels in infancy and childhood. Acta Paediatr. Scand. **68:** 23–27.

23. PABST, H. F. & H. W. KRETH. 1980. Ontogeny of the immune response as a basis of childhood disease. J. Pediatr. **97:** 519–534.

24. DAVIS, C. A., E. H. VALLOTA & J. FORRISTAL. 1979. Serum complement levels in infancy: Age related changes. Pediatr. Res. **13:** 1043–1046.

25. DWYER, J. M. 1984. Thirty years of supplying the missing link. History of gamma globulin therapy for immunodeficient states. Am. J. Med. **76:** 46–52.

26. OXELIUS, V.-A. 1974. Chronic infections in a family with hereditary deficiency of IgG2 and IgG4. Clin. Exp. Immunol. **17:** 19–27.

27. BRANEFORS-HELANDER, P., T. DAHLBERG & O. NYLEN. 1975. Acute otitis media. A clinical, bacteriological and serological study of children with frequent episodes of acute otitis media. Acta Otolaryngol. (Stockholm) **80:** 399–409.

28. SLOYER, J. L., V. M. HOWIE, J. H. PLOUSSARD, A. J. AMMAN, R. AUSTRIAN & R. B. JOHNSTON. 1974. Immune response to acute otitis media in children. I. Serotypes isolated and serum and middle ear fluid antibody in pneumococcal otitis media. Infect. Immun. **9:** 1028–1032.

29. BERNSTEIN, J. M., H. S. FADEN, B. G. LOOS, T. F. MURPHY & P. L. OGRA. 1992. Recurrent otitis media with nontypeable *Haemophilus influenzae*: The role of serum bactericidal antibody. Int. J. Pediatr. Otorhinolaryngol. **23:** 1–13.

30. PRELLNER, K. & N. I. NILSSON. 1982. Complement aberrations in serum from children with otitis due to *S. pneumoniae* or *H. influenzae*. Acta Otolaryngol. (Stockholm) **94:** 275–282.

31. SIBER, G. R., P. H. SCHUR, A. C. AISENBERG, S. A. WEITZMAN & G. SCHIFFMAN. 1980. Correlation between serum IgG-2 concentrations and the antibody response to bacterial polysaccharide antigens. New Eng. J. Med. **303:** 178–182.

32. SLOYER, J. L., V. M. HOWIE, J. H. PLOUSSARD, G. SCHIFFMAN & R. B. JOHNSTON. 1976. Immune response to acute otitis media: Association between middle ear fluid antibody and the clearing of clinical infection. J. Clin. Microbiol. **4:** 306–308.

33. AGNELLO, V. 1978. Complement deficiency states. Medicine **57:** 1–23.

34. INGVARSSON, L., K. LUNDGREN, B. OLOFSSON & S. WALL. 1982. Epidemiology of acute otitis media in children. A prospective study of acute otitis media in children. 2. Incidence in an urban population. Acta Otolaryngol. (Stockholm) **388**(Suppl.): 29–52.

35. KAPLAN, G. J., J. K. FLESHMAN, T. R. BENDER, C. BAUM & P. S. CLARK. 1973. Long-term effects of otitis media. A ten-year cohort study of Alaskan Eskimo children. Pediatrics **52:** 577–585.

36. NORDEN, C. W., R. H. MICHAELS & M. MELISH. 1975. Effect of previous infection on antibody response of children to vaccination with capsular polysaccharide of *Haemophilus influenzae* type b. J. Infect. Dis. **132:** 69–74.

37. MORELL, A., F. SKVARIL, A. G. STEINBERG, E. VAN LOGHEM & W. D. TERRY. 1972. Correlations between the concentrations of the four subclasses of IgG and Gm allotypes in normal human sera. J. Immunol. **108:** 195–206.

38. AMBROSINO, D. M., G. SCHIFFMAN, E. C. GOTSCHLICH, P. H. SCHUR, G. A. ROSENBERG, G. G. DELANGE, E. VAN LOGHEM & G. R. SIBER. 1985. Correlation between G2m(n) immunoglobulin allotype and human antibody response and susceptibility to polysaccharide encapsulated bacteria. J. Clin. Invest. **75:** 1935–1942.

39. PANDEY, J. P., H. H. FUDENBERG, G. VIRELLA, C. U. KYONG, C. B. LOADHOLT, R. M. GALBRAITH, E. C. GOTSCHLICH & J. C. PARKE. 1979. Association between immunoglobulin allotypes and immune responses to *Haemophilus influenzae* and meningococcus polysaccharides. Lancet **1:** 190–192.

40. SVEJGAARD, A., P. PLATZ & L. P. RYDER. 1983. HLA and disease 1982: A survey. Immunol. Rev. **70:** 193–218.

41. KLEIN, J. O. 1986. Natural History of the Major Histocompatability Complex. Wiley. New York.

42. SCHENKEL-BRUNNER, H. 1973. Incorporation of galactose into blood-groups (ABH) precursor substance by lactose synthetase from human milk. Eur. J. Biochem. **33:** 30–35.

43. LIM, D. J. 1984. Anatomy, morphology, cell biology and pathology of the tubotympanum. *In* Recent Advances in Otitis Media with Effusion, D. J. Lim, C. D. Bluestone, J. O. Klein, and J. D. Nelson, Eds.: 71–73. Decker. Philadelphia/Toronto.

44. MORTENSEN, E. H., T. LILDHOLT, N. P. GAMMELGARD & P. CHRISTENSEN. 1983. Distribution of ABO blood groups in secretory otitis media and cholesteatoma. Clin. Otolaryngol. **8:** 263–265.

45. GANNON, M. M., C. JAGGER & M. P. HAGGARD. 1994. Maternal blood group in otitis media with effusion. Clin. Otolaryngol. **19:** 327–331.

46. FREIJD, A., V. OXELIUS & B. RYNNEL-DAGOO. 1984. IgG subclass levels in otitis-prone children. *In* Recent Advances in Otitis Media with Effusion, D. J. Lim, C. D. Bluestone, J. O. Klein, and J. D. Nelson, Eds.: 153–155. Decker. Philadelphia/Toronto.

47. PRELLNER, K., O. KALM, G. HARSTEN, J. HELDRUP & V.-A OXELIUS. 1989. Pneumococcal serum antibody concentrations during the first three years of life: A study of otitis-prone and non-otitis-prone children. Int. J. Pediatr. Otorhinolaryngol. **17:** 267–279.

48. SORENSEN, C. H. & L. K. NIELSEN. 1988. Plasma IgG, IgG subclasses and acute-phase proteins in children with recurrent acute otitis media. APMIS **96:** 676–680.

49. STENFORS, L.-E. & S. RAISANEN. 1993. Secretory IgA-, IgG- and C3b-coated bacteria in the nasopharynx of otitis-prone and non-otitis-prone children. Acta Otolaryngol. (Stockholm) **113:** 191–195.

50. PRELLNER, K., O. KALM & F. K. PEDERSEN. 1984. Pneumococcal antibodies and complement during and after periods of recurrent otitis. Int. J. Pediatr. Otorhinolaryngol. **7:** 39–49.

51. KALM, O., K. PRELLNER, A. FREIJD & B. RYNNEL-DAGOO. 1986. Antibody activity before and after pneumococcal vaccination of otitis-prone and non-otitis-prone children. Acta Otolaryngol. (Stockholm) **101:** 467–474.

52. KALM, O., K. PRELLNER & F. K. PEDERSEN. 1984. Pneumococcal antibodies in families with recurrent otitis media. Int. Arch. Allergy Appl. Immun. **75:** 139–142.

53. SHURIN, P., S. PELTON, I. TAGER & D. KASPER. 1980. Bactericidal antibody and susceptibili-

ty to otitis media caused by nontypeable strains of *Hemophilus influenzae*. J. Pediatr. **97:** 364–367.

54. YAMANAKA, N. & H. FADEN. 1993. Antibody response to outer membrane protein of nontypeable *H. influenzae* in otitis prone children. J. Pediatr. **122:** 212–218.

55. YAMANAKA, N., M. HOTOMI, J. SHIMADA & A. TOGAWA. 1997. Immunological deficiency in "otitis-prone" children. This issue.

56. PRELLNER, K., G. HARSTEN, B. LOFGREN, B. CHRISTENSON & J. HELDRUP. 1990. Responses to rubella, tetanus, and diphtheria vaccines in otitis-prone and non-otitis-prone children. Ann. Otol. Rhinol. Laryngol. **99:** 628–632.

57. HELDRUP, J., O. KALM & K. PRELLNER. 1988. Lymphocyte subpopulations in otitis prone and nonotitis prone children. *In* Recent Advances in Otitis Media, D. J. Lim, C. D. Bluestone, J. O. Klein, and J. D. Nelson, Eds.: 146–149. Decker. Philadelphia/Toronto.

58. PRELLNER, K., T. HALLBERG, O. KALM & B. MANSSON. 1985. Recurrent otitis media: Genetic immunoglobulin markers in children and their parents. Int. J. Pediatr. Otorhinolaryngol. **9:** 219–225.

59. PELTON, S. I., D. W. TEELE, C. B. REIMER, G. G. DELANGE, G. R. SIBER & THE GREATER BOSTON OTITIS MEDIA STUDY GROUP. 1988. Immunologic characteristics of children with frequent recurrences of otitis media. *In* Recent Advances in Otitis Media with Effusion, D. J. Lim, C. D. Bluestone, J. O. Klein, and J. D. Nelson, Eds.: 143–146. Decker. Toronto/Philadelphia.

60. CAMILLERI, A. E., I. R. C. SWAN & R. STURROCK. 1991. Chronic otitis media and ankylosing spondylitis: An HLA association? Clin. Otolaryngol. **16:** 364–366.

61. KALM, O., U. JOHNSON, K. PRELLNER & K. NINN. 1991. HLA frequency in patients with recurrent acute otitis media. Arch. Otolaryngol. Head Neck Surg. **117:** 1296–1299.

62. KALM, O., U. JOHNSON & K. PRELLNER. 1994. HLA frequency in patients with chronic secretory otitis media. Int. J. Pediatr. Otorhinolaryngol. **30:**151–157.

63. PRELLNER, K., A. G. SJOHOLM, G. HARSTEN, J. HELDRUP, O. KALM & R. KORNFALT. 1989. C1q and C1 subcomponent complexes in otitis-prone and non-otitis-prone children. Acta Paediatr. Scand. **78:** 911–917.

64. PRELLNER, K. & O. KALM. 1988. Humoral immune response in acute otitis media. Acta Otolaryngol. (Stockholm) **457**(Suppl.): 133–138.

The Molecular Biology of Bone Resorption Due to Chronic Otitis Media

RICHARD A. CHOLE[a]

Otology Laboratory
Department of Otolaryngology
University of California, Davis
1515 Newton Court #209
Davis, California 95616

INTRODUCTION

Otitis media and the sequelae of otitis media may lead to the destruction of middle- and inner-ear structures, resulting in hearing loss, vestibular abnormalities, as well as intracranial complications. Most of the morbidity associated with chronic otitis media is due to pathological, localized resorption and remodeling of bone. This resorptive process was recognized by Virchow in 1864;[1] Virchow noted that cholesteatomas ". . . extended through the bone to the external auditory canal sometimes also in the cranial cavity. . . ." It was first believed that this erosive process was due to localized bone necrosis due to infection or pressure.[2,3] It was later suggested that an enzymatic process might destroy adjacent bone, and it was suggested that a neutral collagenase may play a role in the resorptive process.[4] In recent years, it has become clear that the erosion of bone due to chronic otitis media with or without cholesteatoma is due to the local action of osteoclasts on the bone of the middle and inner ear.[5] Osteoclast activation has been shown to be associated with chronic inflammatory processes, as well as localized pressure and adaptive bone remodeling. The resorption of bone in chronic otitis media occurs in the immediate microenvironment of the ruffled border of the osteoclasts. Blair and colleagues[6] identified a cathepsin-like proteolytic enzyme in the area of the ruffled border of the osteoclast that has maximal activity at pH 4.0. In the acid environment and in the presence of proteases, the organic and inorganic components of bone are resorbed. The neutral collagenases that have been found in the vicinity of the resorptive process[7,8] may play a role in activating osteoclasts by their activity upon the lining cells or the organic surface of bone.[9,10]

OSTEOCLAST CELLULAR BIOLOGY

Osteoclasts are derived from mononuclear bone-marrow precursors. A process of osteoclastogenesis leads to the recruitment of precursors and the development of the polykaryotic cell at a local site. Osteoclastogenesis fails in an osteoporotic mouse

[a]Phone: 916/754-5040; fax: 916/754-5046; e-mail: RACHOLE@UCDAVIS.EDU

(op/op) with a mutation in the monocyte colony stimulating factor (M-CSF)(CSF-1) gene[11] and is corrected by the administration of M-CSE.[12,13] As the osteoclast differentiates at a local bone site, its peripheral clear zone adheres to the bone matrix. This matrix adherence seems to be essential for multinucleation. This process is dependent upon the integrins $\alpha_v\beta_3$ and $\alpha_v\beta_5$, and is blocked by anti-$\alpha_v\beta_3$ antibody.[14]

Once attached to bone, the peripheral clear zone, or "sealing zone," separates the microenvironment beneath the ruffled border from the general extracellular fluid. The ruffled-border region is acidified by a vacuolar H^+-ATPase. This proton pump may be similar to the proton pump in the intercalated cell of the kidney.[15] Acidification allows mineral mobilization as well as providing a milieu for the action of acidic proteases such as cathespin B and G and acid collagenase.[6,16] Electrical neutrality is preserved by a membrane Cl^- channel on the antiresorptive surface of the osteoclast, which is charge coupled to the H^+-ATPase.[6] The preosteoclast contains H^+-ATPase-containing vesicles. Once attached to the bone matrix, these vesicles move into the osteoclast plasma membrane at the on-the-bone surface side, forming the ruffled border. Since microtubules play a role in polarized vesicular transport in neuronal cells and have been hypothesized to be important of vesicular transport within the osteoclast, it has been hypothesized that the binding at the "sealing zone" by integins polarizes the cell, causing linkages with other intracellular proteins, ultimately forming cytoskeletal polarization, which allows for the migration of the H^+-ATPase-containing vesicles to the resorptive zone (ruffled border).[17] This process is dependent upon the integrity of the microtubules. Calcitonin, a powerful osteoclast inhibitor, acts by altering osteoclast microtubules.[18]

CELLULAR CONTROL OF OSTEOCLASTS

While much is understood of the mechanism by which osteoclasts erode bone, comparatively little is known of the regulation of bone resorption. Numerous cytokines, lymphokines, growth factors, ecosanoids, neuropeptides, and enzymes may be important regulators of esteoclastic activity. Much of our knowledge of the regulation of osteoclasts has come from *in vitro* studies that may or may not replicate events that occur *in vivo*.

ECOSANOIDS

Ecosanoids (arachidonic acid metabolites) play a significant role in the local control of bone resorption, and localized bone resorption is dependent upon at least one of the arachidonic pathways (cyclooxygenase) and possibly others. Ecosanoids are found in significant quantities in all inflammatory processes. Jung reported increased levels of both cyclooxygenase and lipoxygenase metabolites in effusions from children with otitis media.[19] The exact role of ecosanoids in bone remodeling is unclear, although in most experimental systems, bone resorption seems to be dependent upon prostaglandins.[20–24] Arachidonic acid is released from membrane phospholipids by the action of phospholipase in response to specific stimuli.

Prostaglandins

Prostaglandins are produced from the cyclooxygenase pathway of arachidonic acid metabolism and are rapidly metabolized physiologically; for example, PGE_2 is almost completely inactivated in one passage through the lungs. Hence, most studies have been focused on the more stable metabolites. Prostaglandins of the E series stimulate bone resorption.[20,25] In a neonatal mouse calvarial system, Il-1- and TGF-α-induced resorption appears to be prostaglandin dependent, while PTH or 1,25-dihydroxyvitamin D_3-stimulated resorption are not inhibited by indomethacin.[26] Indomethacin blocks not only the prostaglandin pathway but also the prostacyclin and thromboxane pathways. Tashjian and colleagues[27] blocked only the prostacyclin pathway with minoxidil, but failed to inhibit TGF-α-induced resorption *in vitro*. In addition to prostaglandins of the E series, $PGF_{2\alpha}$ is produced by bone cells and exogenous $PGF_{2\alpha}$ causes bone resorption.[24] Therefore, it appears that some pathways leading to bone resorption (localized?) are prostaglandin dependent and others are not (systemic?). A number of forms of localized bone loss have been shown to be prostaglandin dependent, such as rheumatoid arthritis,[28] periodontal disease,[29] and malignancy.[30] It is reasonable to conclude that the chronic inflammatory process in chronic otitis media leads to the production of prostaglandins that include localized osteoclastic activity.[19]

In addition to localized inflammation, mechanical loading, or strain, leads to physiological and pathological modeling. Aural cholesteatomas exert enough pressure on adjacent bone to initiate the modeling process.[31] Prostacyclin and PGE_2 are released from bone that is mechanically loaded.[23] Bone resorption due to mechanical loading in the middle ear, *in vivo*, has been shown to be inhibited by two cyclooxygenase inhibitors: indomethacin[22,32] and ibuprofen.[33]

Leukotrienes

Leukotrienes, 5-lipoxygenase metabolites of arachidonic acid, are potent inflammatory mediators. The peptidoleukotrienes known as LTC_4, LTD_4, and LTE_4 stimulate isolated osteoclasts to accumulate tartrate-resistant acid phosphatase and form resorption pits as well as cause osteoclastic bone resorption.[34] However, the role of leukotrienes in cholesteatoma and chronic otitis media is not clear.

CYTOKINES AND GROWTH FACTORS

Cytokines, lymphokines, and growth factors appear to play a major role in the pathophysiology of chronic otitis media with and without cholesteatoma. These factors are released by macrophages, lymphocytes, monocytes, epithclial cells, endothelial cells, and many other cells at the site of infection. Many cytokines and growth factors have been implicated in bone resorption such as interleukin-1 (IL-1α and β) and 6 (IL-6), colony stimulating factor 1 (CSF-1), transforming growth factor α (TGFα), platelet-derived growth factor (PDGF), and tumor necrosis factor α (TNFα). Other factors are important in the control of bone resorption by their effects on bone deposition since these two processes appear to be inextricably coupled. Factors leading to bone deposition are transforming growth factor β (TGFβ) and bone morphogenetic protein-2 (BMP-2) which lead to osteoid production and mineralization, respectively.[35,36] TGFβ may initiate bone formation by recruitment and proliferation of osteoblast precursor and lead to osteoid deposition, whereas BMP-2 appears to be important in inducing differentiation and mineralization. TBFβ mediates matrix formation and stimulates numerous matrix proteins such as collagen, laminin, and fibronectin.

Interleukin 1

Interleukin 1 (IL-1) is a family of cytokines: IL-1α, IL-1β, and IL-1 receptor antagonist (IL-1ra). Il-Lα and IL-1β have similar biological characteristics, but vary in their affinity for the known receptors (IL-1RI and IL1RII)[37,38] (see Dinarello[37] for review). IL-1 is a very powerful stimulator of bone resorption. (Oritinally, Il-1β was called "osteoclast activating factor.") At concentrations as low as 10^{-10} M, IL-1 will stimulate osteoclasts in organ culture. Minute amounts of IL-1 injected systemically induce resorption[39] and profound hypercalcemia.[40] IL-1α and IL-1β induce bone resorption in most *in vitro* models by increasing PGE_2 production. IL-1 stimulates proliferation of osteoclast precursors,[41] and it may activate mature osteoclasts to resorb bone but only in the presence of osteoblasts.[42] The production and activity of members of the IL-1 family are tightly regulated by gene transcription,[43] protein translation, and secretion, and by the production of surface receptors, soluble receptors, and the receptor antagonist IL-1ra.[37] Human recombinant IL-1 receptor antagonist is more effective in blocking bone resorption in mouse calvaria due to IL-1β than IL-1α.[38] Interestingly, IL-1ra appears to block adaptive bone remodeling,[44] suggesting that IL-1 is an important physiological mediator of bone modeling and remodeling.

The role of IL-1 has been investigated in middle-ear disease; however, most of these studies demonstrate the presence of IL-1 in inflammatory tissues and the ability of the involved inflammatory cells and epithelium to secrete IL-1. Yellon and colleagues[45] found increased levels of IL-1 in the early stages of chronic otitis media with effusion. Interleukin-1 was found in cholesteatoma matrix[46] and was shown to stimulate fibroblasts and macrophages to produce PGE_2 and collagenase.[47] Cultured cholesteatoma specimens were shown to produce IL-1α.[48] IL-1α and IL-1β have been found in cholesteatoma tissue;[49] however, IL-1α may have a more significant role in cholesteatoma.[43,50]

Interleukin 6

Interleukin 6 (IL-6) was identified by its capacity to stimulate B-cell growth.[51] It has been shown to be produced by bone cells in culture, but its role is controversial. Its effects in cultured bone are conflicting. Ishimi and colleagues[52] showed that IL-6 stimulated osteoclasts in fetal murine metatarsal bones, while Gowen[53] failed to demonstrate resorption in more mature bone culture systems. Therefore, IL-6 may be more active against osteoclast precursors than the mature cells. IL-6 has been identified in some cholesteatoma tissues by immunohistochemistry.[54]

Tumor Necrosis Factor α and β

Tumor necrosis factor α (cachectin) (TNFα) and β (lymphotoxin) (TFNβ) are two related cytokines produced mainly by macrophages in response to stimuli such as endotoxin. Both TNFα and TNFβ are potent stimulators of bone resorption.[55] TNFβ was found to be produced by cultured myeloma cells and is thought to be responsible for the bone resorption seen in that disease.[56] Like IL-1, TNF has little direct effect on isolated osteoclasts in culture, but stimulates osteoclastic resorption in the presence of osteoblasts.[57] Yellon and colleagues[45] found increased levels of TNFα in the latter stages of chronic otitis media with effusion; children who had myringotomy performed previously had higher levels of TNFα. Like IL-1, TNF may play a significant role in the recruitment and activation of osteoclasts in chronic otitis media with and without cholesteatoma.

Macrophage Colony Stimulating Factor

In 1986, MacDonald and colleagues[58] found that recombinant CSF-1 enhanced the formation of osteoclast-like cells (polykaryons) in long-term marrow cultures. Yoshida and colleagues[11] found that there was a point mutation in the coding region of the CSF-1 gene in op/op mice with osteopetrosis; these mice are deficient in osteoclasts. The osteopetrosis is reversible by treatment with recombinant CSF-1.[12,13] The requirement of CSF-1 appears to be transient and not required for remodeling in the mature animal. A role of CSF-1 in chronic otitis media has not been established, although it is probably required for the recruitment of precursors to a local site.

Platelet-derived Growth Factor

Platelet-derived growth factor (PDGF) stimulates bone resorption in mouse calvaria by a prostaglandin-dependent mechanism.[59] In human cholesteatoma tissue, Fujioka and Huang[60] reported PDGF stimulated monocytes to form multinucleated osteoclast-like cells, but a direct role in otitis-related bone remodeling has not been determined.

Transforming Growth Factor

Transforming growth factor β (TGFβ) is a powerful stimulator of bone formation. It is stored within bone in a latent form. The activation of latent transforming growth factor β (1TGFβ) by a variety of processes leads to a cascade of events that results in new bone formation. TGFβ is a family of four proteins TGFβ1, TGFβ2, TGFβ4, and

TGFβ5; there is high homology between the mature regions, and there are subtle differences in the functions of each with differing affinities to the known TGFβ receptors.

Osteoblasts make two latent forms of TGFβ. One is a 100-kD precursor that contains a 25-kD homodimer (the active form of TGFβ) and a 75-kD precursor peptide. The second form of 1TGFβ consists of the 100-kD latent form with a 190-kD binding protein, the function of which is unknown.[36] Latent TGFβ is a significant component of the noncollagen protein of bone and can be activated by a number of physiological and pathological processes.

TGFβ activation occurs by cleavage of the mature homodimer from the precursor peptide. Latent TGFβ can be activated by exposure to an acid environment *in vitro* and within the ruffled border of the osteoclast; active TGFβ is released by osteoclasts. Latent TGFβ has also been shown to be activated by activated macrophages,[61] FGF treated mesenchymal cells,[62] and in cocultures with pericytes or smooth muscle cells.[63] In the latter conditions, plasmin is generated that has been shown to digest the precursor peptide of TGFβ-activating 1TGFβ.[64] We have observed that tissue plasminogen activator (tPA) leads to a net calcium accumulation in cultured mouse calvaria, which is likely due to the activation of 1TGFβ stored within the calvarial bone[65] (see the "Plasminogen Activator" section).

When injected into bone defects *in vivo*, TBFβ initiates a cascade of events that results in new bone formation.[66] The release of TGFβ at a local site leads to the activation of local osteoblasts, which, in turn, leads to the formation of osteoid at that site. While TGFβ induces osteoid formation, it may suppress mineralization.[67] Mineralization probably requires the activation of another bone protein, bone morphogenic protein-2 (BMP-2), to complete the process of new bone deposition.[68]

It is likely that TGFβ plays an important role in the "coupling" seen between osteoclastic resorption and osteoblastic bone formation observed in all modeling and remodeling systems. In chronic otitis media, with or without cholesteatoma, one observes bone formation and destruction in adjacent regions. Because of its bone-generating potential, Marenda and Aufdemorte[69] suggested that TGFβ-1 and -2 may potentially slow the proliferation and tissue destruction associated with human cholesteatoma. Even in the absence of inflammation, as in mechanical loading, bone formation is seen in areas adjacent to resorption.[70] These molecular events may explain the common clinical findings of erosion of bone in one area of the mastoid with sclerosis in other regions.

ENZYMES

Neutral Collagenase

Collagenases play an important role in the mechanisms of local invasion by aural cholesteatoma.[4,8] It was originally hypothesized that neutral collagenase, formed in the inflammatory tissue of cholesteatomas, could erode the organic matrix of bone directly. While it is now clear that the bone resorption seen with chronic otitis media is due to the action of osteoclasts, it is also evident that the neutral and acid collagenases play important roles in the process (see the section on "Osteoclast Cell Biology").

Neutral collagenase may stimulate osteoclastic resorption by degrading the osteoid surface of bone, thus allowing osteoclastic activity.[9,10] Neutral collagenase has not been found within osteoclasts[71] but it has been localized in the vicinity of resorbing bone.[8] Acid collagenase and other proteases are produced within the ruffled border of the osteoclast.[6]

Plasminogen Activator

There is evidence that the local control of plasmin may have profound effects on bone remodeling. Plasminogen is activated to plasmin by two serine proteases found in many cell types, a tissue-type (tPA) and a urokinase-type (uPA) plasminogen activator. Plasminogen activators are metabolically controlled by two inhibitors. Plasminogen inhibitor type-1 (PAI-1) inhibits uPA and PAI-2 inhibits tPA. Both tPA and uPA have a growth-factor domain at their amino-terminal region.[72] In the case of uPA, the growth-factor domain can bind to a specific receptor on the plasma membrane of a number of cells.[73] The binding of uPA, and possibly tPA, may localize their enzymatic activity at a specific site.

Two separate lines of research indicate that activation of the plasminogen cascade may mediate bone resorption in chronic otitis media, especially when keratinizing epithelium is present, as in the case of cholesteatoma. First, plasminogen activator activity has been detected in proliferating epithelium and in cholesteatomas. Increased expression of tPA and uPA have been shown in keratinocytes undergoing proliferation, migration, and differentiation.[74] The PA found in epidermis is a result of increased PA mRNA transcription within keratinocytes. These proteinases appear to play an important role in proliferative skin diseases such as psoriasis,[75] pemphigus, and pemphigoid.[76] Nakamura and colleagues[77] demonstrated both types of PA in two of six tissue extracts of human cholesteatoma and tPA in all six specimens. Control tissues were not analyzed, but one might expect that normal epidermis will not express tPA.[74] It is also likely that the plasminogen cascade is activated within the inflammatory tissues of the middle ear and mastoid in cases of chronic otitis media.

Secondly, there is evidence that the plasminogen cascade may play a role in the local control of bone resorption and deposition.[78] mRNA for uPA and its receptor, PAI-1, have been detected in human embryonic bone[79] and in giant cell tumors ("osteoclastomas") of bone.[80] Plasminogen activators may affect bone by at least two mechanisms. First, the conversion of plasminogen to plasmin by tPA or uPA may activate collagenase locally. In the collagenase cascade, procollagenase is activated to collagenase by plasmin. It is generally felt that bone-resorbing factors induce retraction of osteoblasts lining the bone surface, which in turn gives osteoclasts access to the bone matrix. Kahn and Partridge[10] suggested that the production of neutral collagenase by local osteoblasts acts upon the lining surface of bone and acts as a signal for the initiation of osteoclast recruitment and activation. Plasmin may activate procollagen in the vicinity of osteoblasts to initiate the resorptive process. The osteoclast itself may play a role in its own control since there is evidence of the production of tPA and uPA in isolated rat osteoclasts.[81]

There is direct experimental evidence that the PA cascade modulates bone remodeling. Hamilton and colleagues[82,83] reported that plasminogen activator production and secretion from normal and malignant osteoblastic cells was stimulated by three bone resorption-inducing agents: parathyroid hormone, prostaglandin E_2, and 1,25-dihydroxyvitamin D_3. A possible role for plasminogen activators in bone resorption is further supported in recent studies by Hoekman and colleagues,[84,85] who demonstrated the activation of fetal osteoclasts *in vitro* by tPA and the production of tPA and uPA by osteoblasts that are stimulated by cytokines. While Hoekman's model measures only Ca^{45} loss from previously labeled bone explants, we determined *net* calcium changes in calvarial explants due to incubation of tPA and uPA.[65] We found a decrease in medium calcium, indicating a net bone deposition. We speculate that tPA and uPA at high concentrations (10^{-6}M) may act upon latent TGFβ within the calvarial bone, converting it to the active form that leads to bone deposition. Allan and colleagues[86] showed that latent TGFβ (an osteoblast product) was activated by plasmin by cleavage of the mature homodimer, the active form, from the precursor peptide (see the "TGFβ" section). Active TGFβ in turn can stimulate osteoblast-like cells to produce the PA inhibitor PAI-1, which inhibits its own activation from the precursor (see FIGS. 1 and 2). Control of this mechanism could explain the precise temporal and spacial control of osteoblastic and osteoclastic activity seen in normal modeling and remodeling of bone. Perturbations in this mechanism by chronic inflammation could explain the pathological bone erosion and deposition seen in chronic otitis media.

NITRIC OXIDE

Nitric oxide (NO) is a short-lived ($t_{1/2} = 3$–50 s) autocoid product of L-arginine metabolism in a number of cells types.[87] Nitrous oxide is a free radical that is produced

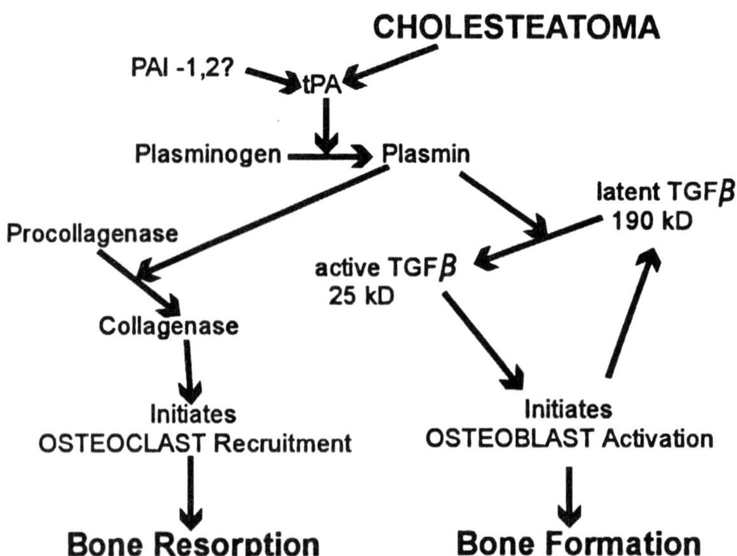

FIGURE 1. Cellular mechanisms of osteoclast resorption of bone (see text for details).

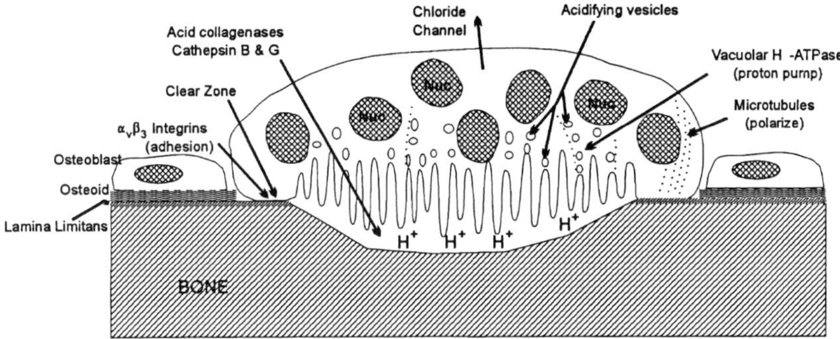

FIGURE 2. It is likely that the plasminogen activators (tPA and uPA) play an important role in bone remodeling in chronic otitis media. This cascade is supported by a number of lines of inquiry (see text).

by the action of nitric acid synthase (NOS) on L-argnine, forming NO and L-citrulline. There is some evidence that cytochrome P-450III may provide an alternative pathway for the production of NO.[88,89] Nitric oxide has been shown to be an important mediator of cell-to-cell interactions. It mediates neurotransmission and smooth muscle relaxation by stimulating the production of cyclic guanosine monophosphate (cGMP).[87] Macrophages, neutrophils, and endothelial cells, which are present in the inflammatory tissues seen in chronic otitis media, have been shown to produce NO when stimulated by endotoxin and a variety of cytokines.[87,90,91] There are at least three known isoforms of NOS: neuronal NOS (nNOS), endothelial NOS (eNOS), and inducible NOS (iNOS). The neural and endothelial forms of NOS are constitutively expressed and continuously produce picomoles of NO.[92] Nitric oxide production by neutrophils and macrophages is catalyzed by iNOS and may be the most important isoform operant in middle-ear disease. Bell and colleagues[93] showed that a NOS inhibitor, L-NAME, significantly diminished the development of experimental middle-ear effusions induced in the rat with endotoxin (lipopolysaccharide). They also showed a significant decrease in subepithelial edema and inflammation within the middle-ear mucosa in L-NAME-treated animals. Since it is likely that much of the inflammatory process seen in chronic otitis media (COM) is mediated through endotoxin or similar inflammatory agents, it is likely that the pathological processes seen in COM are NOS dependent. There is currently increasing evidence that NO is a significant mediator of localized bone resorption and remodeling.

Nitric oxide has profound effects on the recruitment and activation of osteoclasts; however, experimental observations of these effects appear to be conflicting. For example, high concentrations of NO seem to inhibit isolated osteoclast-like cells,[94] resorption in organ culture,[95] and an inhibitor potentiates resorption *in vivo*.[96] However, paradoxically, cytokines associated with chronic inflammation (IL-1 and TNF) are associated with increased NO production[89,97] and increased bone resorption.[98] Recently, Ralston and colleagues,[99] used the newborn mouse calvarial model to explore the role of NO in cytokine-induced resorption. They found that IL-1 + IFN-induced resorption and TGFβ + IL-1-induced resorption were blocked with 200-μM LMMA, a specific NOS inhibitor. Ralston and colleagues[99] showed that NO at low concentrations may have a stimulatory effect on bone resorption; SNAP, a NO donor, potentiated IL-1-induced resorption. There is evidence that NO may mediate bone remodeling due to mechanical loading. Since mechanical loading is at least one of the factors mediating bone resorption in cholesteatomas,[31] these observations may be pertinent to pathological processes within the ear. Pitsillides and colleagues[100] showed that mechanical loading of bone *in vitro* led to increased nitrite release into the culture medium and increased expression of nNOS and iNOS mRNA in canine and rat bone. Pilot studies in our laboratory indicate that L-NAME, an NOS inhibitor, profoundly inhibits bone modeling *in vivo* due to mechanical loading of the bulla wall of the gerbil in the absence of an inflammatory process.[101]

Therefore, in spite of conflicting findings by published studies, NO appears to be an important mediator of bone modeling *in vitro* and *in vivo*. At high concentrations NO appears to inhibit osteoclastic activity, while there is evidence that it is a physiological inducer of bone resorption and lower concentrations.

NEUROTRANSMITTERS

The periosteum of the bone of the middle ear and mastoid is richly innervated by autonomic and sensory nerves. Some investigators have suggested that adaptive bone remodeling may be under neural control. Neuropeptides and vasoactive amines may play an important role in bone resorption and remodeling.

Surgical sympathectomy results in localized bone resorption.[102,103] These effects are not necessarily direct since catecholamines have little effect on resorption in mouse calvarial cultures (personal observation). Other substances related to the autonomic innervation of bone are able to stimulate resorption *in vitro*. For example, vasoactive intestinal peptide (VIP)[104] and C-type natriuretic peptide[105] and substance-P[106] can stimulate bone resorption *in vitro*. It has been shown that the localized bone resorption induced by chemical or pharmacological sympathectomy could be blocked by capsaicin, indicating that the effect is modulated through substance-P.[107,108] Blockage of substance-P by capsaicin was shown to block adaptive bone modeling *in vivo*.[109]

Therefore, although there is substantial evidence that neurotransmitters affect bone modeling and remodeling, their role in bone erosion due to chronic otitis media has not been established.

REFERENCES

1. VON TROLTSCH, A. 1864. William Wood. New York.
2. McKENZIE, D. 1930. The pathology of cholesteatoma. Proc. R. Soc. Med. **24:** 332–362.
3. WALSH, T. E., W. P. COVELL & J. H. OGURA. 1951. The effect of cholesteatosis on bone. Ann. Otol. Rhinol. Laryngol. **60:** 1100–1113.
4. ABRAMSON, M. 1969. Collagenase activity in middle ear cholesteatoma. Ann. Otol. Rhinol. Laryngol. **80:** 177–185.
5. CHOLE, R. A. 1984. Cellular and subcellular events of bone resorption in human and experimental cholesteatoma: The role of osteoclasts. Laryngoscope **94:** 76–95.

6. BLAIR, H. C., S. L. TEITELBAUM & H. L. TAN. 1991. Passive chloride permiability charge coupled to H$^+$ ATPase of avian osteoclast ruffled membrane. Am. J. Physiol. **260:** C1315–C1324.

7. ABRAMSON, M. & C. C. HUANG. 1977. Localization of collagenase in human middle ear cholesteatoma. Laryngoscope **87:** 771–779.

8. MORIYAMA, H., Y. HONDA, C. C. HUANG & M. ABRAMSON. 1987. Bone resorption in cholesteatoma: Epithelial-mesenchymal cell interaction and collagenase production. Laryngoscope **97:** 854–859.

9. CHAMBERS, T. J., J. A. DARBY & K. FULLER. 1985. Mammalian collagenase predisposes bone surfaces to osteoclastic resorption. Cell Tiss. Res. **241:** 671–675.

10. KAHN, A. J. & N. C. PARTRIDGE. 1987. New concepts in bone remodeling; An expanding role for the osteoblast. J. Bone Min. Res. **8:** 258–264.

11. YOSHIDA, H., S. HAYASHI & T. KUNISADA. 1990. The murine mutation osteopetrosis is in the coding region of macrophage colony stimulating factor gene. Nature **345:** 442–444.

12. FELIX, R., M. CECCHINI & H. FLEISH. 1990. Macrophage colony stimulating factor restores in vivo bone resorption in the op/op osteopetrotic mouse. Endocrinology **127:** 2592–2594.

13. KODAMA, H., A. YAMASAKI, M. ABE, S. NIIDA, Y. HAKEDA & H. KAWASHIMA. 1991. Congenital osteoclast deficiency in osteopetrotic (op/op) mice is cured by injection of macrophage colony-stimulating factor. J. Exp. Med. **173:** 269–272.

14. ROSS, F. P., *et al.* 1993. Interactions between the bone matrix proteins osteopontin and bone sialoprotein and the osteoclast integrin potentiate bone resorption. J. Biol. Chem. **268:** 9901–9907.

15. MATTSSON, J. P., P. H. SCHLESINGER & D. J. KEELING. 1994. Isolation and reconstruction of a vacuolar-type proton pump of osteoblast membranes. J. Biol. Chem. **269:** 2479–2482.

16. SASAKI, T. & E. UENO-MATSUDA. 1993. Cystein-proteinase localization in osteoclasts: An immunocytochemical study. Cell Tiss. Res. **8:** S121.

17. TEITELBAUM, S. L., Y. ABU-AMER & F. P. ROSS. 1995. Molecular mechanisms of bone resorption. J. Cell. Biochem. **59:** 1–10.

18. WARSHAFSKY, B. & M. SHEETZ. 1985. Cytoplasmic microtubule associated motors. Ann. Rev. Biochem. **62:** 429–451.

19. JUNG, T. T. K. 1989. Prostaglandins, leukotrienes and other arachidonic acid metabolites in the pathogenesis of otitis media. Laryngoscope **98:** 980–989.

20. TASHJIAN, A. H., J. E. TICE & K. SIDES. 1977. Biological activities of prostaglandin analogues and metabolites on bone in organ culture. Nature **266:** 645–646.

21. VOELKEL, E. F., A. H. TASHJIAN & L. LEVINE. 1980. Cyclooxygenase products of arachidonic acid metabolism by mouse bone in organ culture. Biochem. Biophys. Acta. **620:** 418–428.

22. ADACHI, K., R. A. CHOLE & J. YEE. 1991. Indomethacin inhibition of middle ear bone resorption. Arch. Otolaryngol. Head Neck Surg. **117:** 267–269.

23. RAWLINSON, S. C., A. J. EL-HAJ, S. L. MINTER, J. I. A. TAVARES, A. BENNETT & L. E. LANYON. 1991. Loading related increases in prostaglandin production in cores of adult canine cancellous bone in vitro: A role for prostacyclin in adaptive bone remodelling. J. Bone Mineral Res. **6:** 1345–1351.

24. RAISZ, L. G., C. B. ALANDER, P. M. FALL & H. A. SIMMONS. 1990. Effect of prostaglandin F2a on bone formation and resorption in cultured neonatal mouse calvariae: Role of prostaglandin E2 production. Endocrinology **126**(2): 1076–1079.

25. KLEIN, D. C. & L. G. RAISZ. 1970. Stimulation of bone resorption in tissue culture. Endocrinology **86:** 1436–1440.

26. GARRETT, I. R. & G. R. MUNDY. 1989. Relationship between interleukin-1 and prostaglandins in resorbing neonatal calvaria. J. Bone Min. Res. **4**(5): 789–794.

27. TASHJIAN, A. H., T. J. BOSMA & L. LEVINE. 1988. Use of minoxidil to demonstrate that

prostacyclin is not the mediator of bone resorption stimulated by growth factors in mouse calvariae. Endocrinology. **123:** 969–974.

28. ROBINSON, D. R., A. H. TASHJIAN & L. LEVINE. 1975. Prostaglandin-stimulated bone resorption by rheumatoid synovia—Possible mechanism for bone destruction in rheumatoid arthritis. J. Clin. Invest. **56:** 1181–1187.

29. HARRIS, M., M. V. JENKINS, A. BENNETT & M. R. WILLS. 1973. Prostaglandin production and bone resorption by dental cysts. Nature **45:** 213–215.

30. MINKIN, C., R. S. FREDRICKS & S. POKRESS. 1981 Bone resorption and humoral hypercalcemia of malignancy-stimulation of bone resorption in vitro by tumor extracts is inhibited by prostaglandin synthesis inhibitors. J. Clin. Invest. **53:** 941–947.

31. ORISEK, B. S. & R. A. CHOLE. 1987. Pressures exerted by experimental cholesteatomas. Arch. Otolaryngol. **113:** 386–391.

32. CHUMBLEY, A. B. & O. C. TUNCAY. 1987. The effect of indomethacin (an aspirin-like drug) on the rate of orthodontic tooth movement. Am. J. Orthodont. **89:** 312–314.

33. JUNGKEIT, M. C. & R. A. CHOLE. 1991. Ibuprofen inhibits localized bone resorption in the middle ear. Calcif. Tiss. Int. **48:** 267–271.

34. GALLWITZ, B., M. WITT, U. R. FOLSCH, W. CREUTZFELDT & W. E. SCHMIDT. 1993. Binding specificity and signal transduction of receptors for glucagon-like peptide-1(7-36)amide and gastric inhibitory polypeptide on RINm5F insulinoma cells. J. Molec. Endocrinol. **10**(3): 259–268.

35. MUNDY, G. R. 1993. Cytokines and growth factors in the regulation of bone remodeling. J. Bone Mineral Res. **8**(Suppl. 2): s505–s510.

36. BONEWALD, L. F. & S. L. DALLAS. 1994. Role of active and latent transforming growth factor β in bone formation. J. Cell. Biochem. **55:** 350–357.

37. DINARELLO, C. A. 1996. Biologic basis for interleukin-1 in disease. Blood **87**(6): 2095–2147.

38. CHOLE, R. A., S. P. TINLING & B. T. FADDIS. 1994. Human recombinant interleukin-1 receptor antagonist blocks bone resorption induced by interleukin-1β but not interleukin-1α. Calcif. Tiss. Int. **55:** 12–15.

39. BOYCE, B. F., I. R. AUFDEMORTE, A. J. GARRETT, P. YATES & G. R. MUNDY. 1989. Effects of interleukin-1 on bone turnover in normal mice. Endocrinology **125:** 1142–1150.

40. SABATINI, M., B. BOYCE, T. AUFDEMORTE, L. BONEWALD & G. R. MUNDY. 1988. Infusions of recombinant human interleukin-1 [81] and β cause hypercalcemia in normal mice. Proc. Natl. Acad. Sci. USA **85:** 5235–5239.

41. PFEILSCHIFTER, J., C. CHENU, A. BIRD, G. R. MUNDY & G. D. ROODMAN. 1989. Interleukin-1 and tumor necrosis factor stimulate the formation of human. J. Bone Min. Res. **4**(1): 113–118.

42. THOMSON, B. M., J. SAKLATVALA & T. J. CHAMBERS. 1986. Osteoblasts mediate interleukin-1 stimulation of bone resorption by rat osteoclasts. J. Exp. Med. **164:** 104–112.

43. BUJIA, J., C. KIM, D. BOYLE, C. HAMMER, G. FIRESTEIN & E. KASTENBAUER. 1996. Quantitative analysis of interleukin-1 alpha gene expression in middle ear cholesteatoma. Laryngoscope **106:** 217–220.

44. CHOLE, R. A., B. T. FADDIS & S. P. TINLING. 1995. In vivo inhibition of localized bone resorption by human recombinant interleuki-1 receptor antagonist. J. Bone Min. Res. **10**(2): 281–284.

45. YELLON, R., F. LEONARD, *et al.* 1991. Characterization of cytokines present in middle ear effusions. Laryngoscope **101:** 165–169.

46. AHN, J., C. C. HUANT & M. ABRAMSON. 1990. Localization of interleukin 1 in human cholesteatoma. Am. J. Otolaryngol. **11:** 71–77.

47. AHN, J., C. C. HUANT & M. ABRAMSON. 1990. Interleukin-1 causing bone destruction in middle ear cholesteatoma. Otolaryngol. Head Neck Surg. **103:** 527–534.

48. KURIHARA, A., M. TOSHIMA, R. YUASA & T. TAKASAKA. 1991. Bone destruction mechanisms in chronic otitis media with cholesteatoma. Ann. Otol. Rhinol. Laryngol. **100**(12): 989–998.

49. SCHILLING, V., A. HILLY, J. BUJIA, P. SCHULTZ & E. KASTENBAUER. 1995. High levels of fibronectin in the stroma of aural cholesteatoma. Am. J. Otolaryngol. **16**: 232–235.

50. KAKIUCHI, H., K. KINOSHITA, Y. KATO & T. TABATA. 1992. Interleukin-1 of cholesteatomatous keratinocytes. Ann. Otol. Rhinol. Laryngol. **101**(Suppl.): 32–38.

51. BATAILLE, R., M. JOURDAN, X. G. ZHANG & B. KLEIN. 1989. Serum levels of interleukin-6, a potent myeloma cell growth factor, as a reflection of dyscrasias. J. Clin. Invest. **84**: 2008–2011.

52. ISHIMI, Y., C. MIYAURA, C. H. JIN, T. AKATSU, T. ABE & Y. NAKAMURA. 1990. IL-6 is produced by osteoblasts and induces bone resorption. J. Immunol. **145**: 3297–3303.

53. GOWEN, M. 1991. The bone-resorbing activity of interleukin-6—Reply. J. Bone. Min. Res. **6**: 1145–1146.

54. BUJIA, J., C. KIM, P. OSTOS, E. KASTENBAUER & L. HULTNER. 1996. Role of interleukin-6 in epithelial hyperproliferation and bone resorption. Eur. Arch. Oto-Rhino-Largynol. **253**(3): 152–157.

55. SMITH, D. D. & G. R. MUNDY. 1986. Stimulation of bone resorption and inhibition of bone formation in vitro by human tumorur necrosis factors. Nature **319**: 516–518.

56. GARRETT, I. R., *et al.* 1987. Production of lymphotoxin, a bone resorbing cytokine, by cultured human myeloma cells. New Eng. J. Med. **317**: 526–529.

57. THOMSON, B. M., G. R. MUNDY & T. J. CHAMBERS. 1987. Tumor necrosis factors alpha and beta induce osteoblastic cells to stimulate osteoclastic bone resorption. J. Immunol. **138**: 775–781.

58. MACDONALD, B. R., *et al.* 1986. Effects of human recombinant CSF-GM and highly purified CSF-1 on the formation of osteoclast-like cells. J. Bone Mine. Res. **1**(2): 227–233.

59. TASHJIAN, A. H., E. L. HOHMANN, H. N. ANTONIADES & L. LEVINE. 1982. Platelet-derived growth factor stimulates bone resorption via a prostaglandin mediated mechanism. Endocrinology **111**: 118–123.

60. FUJIOKA, O. & C. C. HUANG. 1994. Platelet-derived growth factor in middle ear cholesteatoma. Eur. Arch. Otorhinolaryngol. **251**(4): 199–204.

61. TWARDZIK, D. R., J. A. MIKOVITS, J. E. RANCHALIS, A. F. PURCHIO, L. ELLINGSWORTH & F. W. RUSCETTI. 1990. Gamma interferon-induced activation of latent transforming growth factor β by human monocytes. Ann. N.Y. Acad. Sci. **593**: 276–284.

62. ROWLEY, D. R. 1992. Glucocorticoid regulation of transforming growth factor β activation in urogenital sinus mesenchymal cells. Endocrinology **131**: 471–478.

63. SATO, Y. & D. B. RIFKIN. 1989. Inhibition of endothelial cell movement by pericytes and smooth muscle cells: Activation of a latent transforming growth factor-β1-like molecule by plasmin during co-culture. J. Cell. Biol. **109**: 309–315.

64. LYONS, R. M., L. E. GENTRY, A. F. PUCHIO & H. L. MOSES. 1990. Mechanism of activation of latent recombinant transforming growth factor β by plasmin. J. Cell. Biol. **100**: 1361–1367.

65. CHOLE, R. A., S. P. TINLING, M. C. JUNGKEIT & K. CHOLE. 1996. Tissue plasminogen activator (tPA) causes bone deposition in mouse calvarial cultures. In preparation.

66. BECK, L. S., L. DEGUZMAN & W. P. LEE. 1991. TGF induces closure of skull defects. J. Bone Min. Res. **6**: 1257–1265.

67. KATO, Y., M. IWAMOTO, T. KOIKE, F. SUZUKI & Y. TAKANO. 1988. Terminal differentiation and calcification in rabbit chondrocyte cultures. Proc. Natl. Acad. Sci. USA **85**(24): 9552–9556.

68. GHOSH-CHOUDNURY, N., M. A. HARRIS, J. Q. FENG, G. R. MUNDY & S. E. HARRIS. 1990.

Expression of the BMP-2 gene during bone cell differentiation. Crit. Rev. Eukaryotic Gene Expression **4:** 345–355.

69. MARENDA, S. A. & T. B. AUFDEMORTE. 1995. Localization of cytokines in cholesteatoma tissue. Otolaryngol. Head Neck Surg. **112:** 359–368.

70. CHOLE, R. A. & D. E. CHAN. 1989. Rapid induction of localized bone resorption in the auditory bulla of the Mongolian gerbil, Meriones unguiculatus, by increased air pressure. Calcif. Tiss. Int. **45**(5): 318–323.

71. SAKAMOTO, S. & M. SAKAMOTO. 1982. Biochemical and immunochemical studies on collagenase in resorbing bone in tissue culture. J. Periodontal. Res. **17:** 523–526.

72. RABBANI, S., *et al.* 1992. Structural requirements for the growth factor activity of the amino-terminal domain of urokinase. J. Biol. Chem. **267:** 14151–14156.

73. BLASI, F., J. VASSALI & K. DANO. 1987. Urokinase-type plasminogen activator: Proenzyme, receptor and inhibitors. J. Cell. Biol. **104:** 801–804.

74. LAZARUS, G. S. & P. J. JENSEN. 1991. Plasminogen activators in epithelial biology. Semin. Thromb. and Hemostasis **17**(3): 210–216.

75. JENSEN, P. J., *et al.* 1990. Tissue plasminogen activator in psoriasis. J. Invest. Dermatol. **95:** 13s–14s.

76. BLAIR, H. C., S. L. TEITELBAUM & L. E. GROSSO. 1993. Extracellular matrix degredation at acid pH: Avian osteoclast acid collagenase isolation and characterization. Biochem. J. **290:** 873–884.

77. NAKAMURA, M., *et al.* 1995. Plasminogen activators in tissue extract of aural cholesteatoma. Laryngoscope **105:** 305–310.

78. MARTIN, T. J., E. H. ALLAN & S. FUKUMOTO. 1993. The plasminogen activator and inhibitor system in bone remodeling. Growth Reg. **3**(4): 209–214.

79. HÄCKEL, C., K. RADIG, I. ROSE & A. ROESSNER. 1995. The urokinase plasminogen activator (uPA) and its inhibitor (PAI-1) in embryo-fetal bone formation in the human: An immunohistochemical study. Anat. Embryol. **192:** 363–368.

80. ZHENG, M., *et al.* 1995. Detection of mRNAs for urokinase-type plasminogen activator, its receptor, and type 1 inhibitor in giant cell tumors of bone with in situ hybridization. Am. J. Pathol. **147:** 1559–1566.

81. GRILLS, B. L., J. A. GALLAGHER & E. H. ALLAN. 1990. Identification of plasminogen activator in osteoclasts. J. Bone Mine. Res. **5:** 499–505.

82. HAMILTON, J. A., S. R. LINGELBACH, N. C. PARTRIDGE & T. J. MARTIN. 1984. Stimulation of plasminogen activator in osteoblast-like cells by bone resorbing hormones. Biochem. Biophys. Res. Commun. **122:**2 30–236.

83. HAMILTON, J., S. R. LINGELBACH, N. C. PARTRIDGE & T. J. MARTIN. 1985. Regulation of plasminogen activator production by bone resorbing hormones in normal and malignant osteoblasts. Endocrinology **116:** 2186–2191.

84. HOEKMAN, K., W. G. LOWIK, M. RUIT, O. L. BIJVOET, J. H. VERHEIJEN & S. E. PAPAPOULOS. 1991. Regulation of the production of plasminogen activators by bone resorption enhancing and inhibiting factors in three types of osteoblast-like cells. Bone Min. **14:** 189–204.

85. HOEKMAN, K. *et al.* 1992. The effect of tissue type plasminogen activator on osteoclastic resorption in embryonic mouse long-bone explants: A possible role for the growth factor domain of tPA. Bone Min. **17:** 1–13.

86. ALLAN, E. H., R. ZEHEB & T. D. GELEHRTER. 1991. Transforming growth factor beta inhibits plasminogen activator (PA) activity and stimulates production of urokinase-type PA, PA inhibitor-1 mRNA, and protein in rat osteoblast-like cells. J. Cell. Physiol. **149:** 34–43.

87. MONCADA, S. & A. HIGGS. 1993. The L-arginine: Nitric oxide pathway. New Eng. J. Med. **329:** 2002–2012.

88. KUO, P. C., K. Y. ABE & D. C. DAFORE. 1995. Cytochrome P450IIIA activity and cytokine-mediated synthesis of nitric oxide. Surgery **118**(2): 310–317.

89. Kuo, P. C. & K. Y. Abe. 1995. Cytokine-mediated production of nitric oxide in isolated rat hepatocytes is dependent on cytochrome P-450III activity. FEBS Lett. **360:** 10–14.

90. Stuehr, D. J. & C. F. Nathan. 1989. Nitric oxide. A macrophage product responsible for cytostasis and respiratory inhibition in tumor target cells. J. Exp. Med. **169:** 1543–1555.

91. McCall, T. B., N. K. Boughton-Smith, R. M. Palmer, B. J. Whittle & S. Moncada. 1989. Synthesis of nitric oxide from L-arginine by neutorphils. Biochem. J. **261:** 293–296.

92. Moncada, S., R. M. Palmer & E. A. Higgs. 1991. Nitric oxide: Physiology, pathophysiology and pharmacology. Pharmacol. Rev. **43:** 109–142.

93. Ball, S. S., J. Prazma, D. Dais, K. W. Rosbe & H. C. Pillsbury. 1996. Nitric oxide: A mediator of endotoxin-induced middle ear effusions. Laryngoscope **106**(8): 1021–1027.

94. MacIntyre, I., et al. 1991. Osteoclastic inhibition: An action of nitric oxide not mediated by cyclic GMP. Proc. Natl. Acad. Sci. USA **88:** 1223–1227.

95. Lowik, C. W., P. H. Nibbering, M. van de Ruit & S. E. Papapoulos. 1994. Inducible production of nitric oxide in osteoblast-like cells and in fetal. J. Clin. Invest. **93**(4): 1465–1472.

96. Kasten, T. P., et al. 1994. Potentiation of osteoclastic bone resorbing activity by inhibition of nitric oxide synthase. Proc. Natl. Acad. Sci. USA **91:** 3569–3573.

97. Farrell, A. J., D. R. Blake, R. M. Palmer, J. & S. Moncada. 1992. Increased concentrations of nitrite in synovial fluid and serum samples suggest increased nitric oxide synthesis in rheumatic diseases. Ann. Rheum. Dis. **51:** 1219–1222.

98. Gowen, M., B. R. MacDonald, D. E. Hughes, H. Skojdt & R. G. Russell. 1986. Immune cells and bone resorption. Adv. Exp. Med. Biol. **208:** 261–273.

99. Ralston, S. H., L. P. Ho, M. H. Helfrich, P. S. Grabowski, P. W. Johnston & N. Benjamin. 1995. Nitric oxide: A cytokine-induced regulator of bone resorption. J. Bone Min. Res. **10**(7): 1040–1049.

100. Pitsillides, A. A., S. Rawlinson, R. F. Suswillo, S. Bourrin, G. Zaman & L. E. Lanyon. 1995. Mechanical strain-induced NO production by bone cells: A possible role in adaptive bone (re)modeling? FASEB J. **9:** 1614–1622.

101. Chole, R. A., S. P. Tinling, E. Leverentz & M. D. McGinn. 1997. Inhibition of nitric oxide synthase blocks osteoclastic resorption in bone remodeling. J. Bone Min. Res. In press.

102. Sandhu, H. S., M. S. Herskovits & I. J. Singh. 1987. Effect of surgical sympathectomy on bone remodeling at rat incisor and molar root sockets. Anat. Rec. **219**(1): 32–38.

103. Sherman, B. E. & R. A. Chole. 1996. In vivo effects of surgical sympathectomy on intramembranous bone resorption. Am. J. Otol. **17:** 343–346.

104. Hohmann, E. L., L. Levine & A. H. Tashjian. 1983. Vasoactive intestinal peptide stimulates bone resorption via a cyclic adenosin 3′5,′ -monophosphate dependent mechanism. Endocrinology **112:** 1233–1239.

105. Holliday, L., A. D. Dean, J. E. Greenwald & S. L. Glucks. 1995. C-type natriuretic peptide increases bone resorption in 1,25-dihydroxyvitamin D3-stimulated mouse bone marrow cultures. J. Bio. Chem. **270**(32): 18983–18989.

106. Davidovitch, Z., Z. T. Rosol & J. Shanfeld. 1990. Direct effects of neurotransmitters on bone resorption in vitro. J. Dent. Res. **69:** 206–211.

107. Hill, E. L., R. Turner & R. Elde. 1991. Effects of neonatal sympathectomy and capsaicin treatment on bone remodeling in rats. Neuroscience **44**(3): 747–755.

108. Sherman, B. E. & R. A. Chole. 1995. A mechanism for sympathectomy-induced bone resorption in the middle ear. Otolaryngol. Head Neck Surg. **113**(11): 569–581.

109. Chole, R. A. & S. P. Tinling. 1997. Adaptive bone remodeling in the middle ear is substance-p dependent. Abstracts 20th Annu. Res. Meet. of the Association for Research in Otolaryngology, Feb. 2–6, G. R. Podelka, Ed.: 48.

Interactions Between the Middle Ear and the Inner Ear: Bacterial Products

STEN HELLSTRÖM,[a] PER-OLOF ERIKSSON, YONG-JOO YOON AND ULF JOHANSSON

Department of Otorhinolaryngology
University of Umeå
S-901 87 Umeå, Sweden

INTRODUCTION

One major issue in ear research is: Can an infectious condition of the middle ear cause a dysfunctioning inner ear? This question is addressed in this review, which is focused on (a) which inflammatory conditions of the middle ear may interact with the inner ear? (b) which bacteria and bacterial products could exert such effects? (c) which are the structural and permeability properties of the barrier between the middle ear and the inner—the round window membrane? and (d) possible inner-ear effects on the cochlear structure and function.

BACTERIA AND BACTERIAL PRODUCTS

Encounters between the human body and bacteria occur many times each day. Yet bacterial infection after such contacts tends to be the exception rather than the rule. In the middle ear the cavity is lined with a mucous membrane. An important protection of the mucosal membranes is the layer of mucus that covers these membranes and that will trap bacteria before they can reach the membrane itself. Within the mucous there are substances—lysozyme, lactoferrin, and lactoperoxidase—that either kill the bacteria or inhibit their growth. At the epithelial surface the bacteria have to cope with the rapidly dividing mucosal cells and the specific mucosal immune system, including antibodies like secretory IgA. Invading the tissue they will meet a nonspecific as well as a specific defense system that will try to erradicate the infection. The nonspecific defense system is represented by phagocytes, transferrin, and complement, whereas the specific defense system involves antibodies and recruiting of T cells. If now the bacteria reach the membrane and overcome the surface and tissue defense systems, which bacterial products could initiate damage to the middle and inner ear tissues? The answer should be exotoxins, endotoxins, other toxic bacterial cell wall components, and hydrolysing enzymes.

[a]Author for correspondence. Phone: 46 90 7851460; fax: 46 90 777684; e-mail: sten. hellstrom@ent.umu.se

Exotoxins[1] are toxic proteins produced by a variety of bacteria, including gram-positive as well as gram-negative bacteria. Exotoxins vary considerably in their activity and the host cell types they attack.

Endotoxin[1] is a lipopolysacharide that is an integral component of the outer membrane of gram-negative bacteria. The lipid portion, lipid A, is embedded in the outer membrane, with the core antigen portions extending outward from the bacterial surface. Lipid A is the toxic portion of the molecule. Because it is embedded in the outer membrane of intact bacteria, it exerts its effects only when bacteria lyse. The toxicity of lipid A resides primarily on its ability to activate complement and to stimulate the release of bioactive host proteins such as cytokines.

Gram-positive bacteria do not have endotoxin, but the presence of these bacteria in tissue provokes inflammatory responses that are identical to that evoked by gram-negative endotoxins. These effects of gram-positive cell wall remnants[1] are most probably mediated through peptidoglycan fragments and teichoic acids.[1]

Many pathogenic bacteria produce hydrolytic enzymes,[1] such as hyaluronidase and proteases, that degrade the extracellular matrix components and thus disrupt host tissue structure. It is, however, difficult to distinguish the action of the hydrolyzing enzymes derived from the bacteria from those derived from phagocytes, because phagocytes produce the same types of hydrolytic enzymes.

INFLAMMATORY CONDITIONS OF THE MIDDLE EAR

The inflammatory conditions of the middle ear that involve bacteria are acute otitis media (AOM), chronic suppurative otitis media (CSOM), and secretory otitis media (SOM).[2] By definition acute otitis media is the condition with an acute onset of ear pain, fever, and a pus-filled middle-ear cavity. Chronic suppurative otitis media is a chronic purulent otitis media with episodes of purulent discharge. Secretory otitis media was until the early 1960s believed to possess a sterile effusion material.[3] However, long-standing secretory otitis media or more commonly called otitis media with effusion (OME) is very often sterile. More recent studies have shown that secretory otitis media contains bacteria and bacterial toxins in the majority of cases,[4] but usually early in the resolution of acute otitis media and not in long-standing cases. It is now well accepted that there is no distinct difference between the three inflammatory conditions mentioned and that secretory otitis media is often the result of an AOM.[5]

Which bacteria/bacterial products related to these inflammatory conditions could be candidates for causing dysfunction of the inner ear? The common bacteria involved in the various types of otitis media conditions are listed in TABLE 1.

Having defined the bacteria involved in the various inflammatory conditions of the middle ear one has to consider how the bacteria or bacterial products would enter the inner ear.

THE ROUND-WINDOW MEMBRANE

Although there could be other routes for the passage of noxious substances from the middle ear to the inner ear, such as hematogenic spread or through lymphatic ves-

TABLE 1. The Bacteria/Bacterial Products Involved in the Various Middle-ear Inflammatory Conditions (Molecular Weight in Parentheses)

Inflammatory Condition	Bacteria	gram–/gram+	Bacterial Products
AOM	*S. pneumoniae*	Gram+	Exotoxin (53,000) (pneumolysin)
			Outer cell wall components
			Autolysin
	Nontypeable *H. influenzae*	Gram–	Endotoxin
	M. catarrhalis	Gram–	Endotoxin
CSOM	*S. aureus*	Gram+	Exotoxin (12,000)
	S. epidermidis	Gram+	Exotoxin
	P. aeruginosa	Gram+	Exotoxin A, enzymes
	P. mirabilis	Gram–	Endotoxin
	P. vulgaris	Gram–	Endotoxin
SOM (early)	*S. pneumoniae*	Gram+	Exotoxin
			Autolysin
	nontypeable *H. influenzae*	Gram–	Endotoxin
	M. catarrhalis	Gram–	Endotoxin

sels, the only soft-tissue barrier between these compartments is the round-window membrane (RWM).[6–10] It is feasable to assume that the RWM is the major route through which the bacterial toxins influence cochlear function in otitis media.

The RWM consists of three layers: the outer, the middle, and the inner. The outer layer consists of a single layer of epithelial cells facing the middle-ear cavity. There is an extensive interdigitating of the lateral walls of the epithelial cells, with tight junctions occurring close to the surface.[9,11] Microvilli are observed on the free surface of the epithelial cells, and micropinocytotic vesicles are observed at both the apical and the basal sides of the epithelial cells. Beneath the outer epithelial layer is a continuous basis lamina.

The middle connective tissue layer consists of collagen fibers, elastic fibers, and fibroblasts. A gradual increase in the number of tissue constituents, in particular the elastic fibers, is seen toward the inner epithelium. Beneath the basal lamina of the outer layer, in the subepithelial connective tissue, is an area in which blood vessels, nerves, melanocytes, and fibroblasts are found.

The inner epithelial layer consists of large flat cells with long lateral extensions overlapping each other. These mesothelial cells are contiguous with the cells lining the scala tympani. No basal cells can be distinguished between the mesothelial cells and the connective tissue layer, and microvilli are few or absent on the cell surfaces toward the scala tympani. Micropinocytotic vesicles are found on both the apical and the basal side.

The average thickness of the RWM in humans varies between 40 and 70 μm, irrespective of age.[9,11] In commonly used animals for ear research, for example, chinchilla and rat, the RWM is much thinner, 10 to 15 μm.[8,10]

RWM PERMEABILITY

As the port of entry for various substances from the middle ear to the inner ear, the permeability of the RWM under normal and pathological conditions has attracted increasing interest. Substances that can traverse the RWM under normal conditions are low molecular-weight substances such as water, sodium, and iodide ions and tracers like horseradish peroxidase (HRP, MW 45,000),[12,13] whereas albumin (MW 70,000) does not pass under normal conditions, but is shown to penetrate into the inner ear during inflammation.[14,15] Thus permeability may vary depending on the degree of inflammatory condition and in which state of the inflammatory condition the RWM is exposed to the noxious agent.[16–18]

THE RWM WHEN SUBJECTED TO BACTERIA/BACTERIAL PRODUCTS

Our knowledge of the tissue reactions and permeability changes of the RWM when the middle-ear cavity is challenged by bacteria or bacterial products rests on studies on human temporal bones and animal experiments. The number of studies of the RWM in pathological conditions is, however, remarkably few.

It has been shown that various exotoxins, like staphylococcal[18] and Pseudomonas[19] exotoxins, as well as endotoxins from *Haemophilus influenzae*[20] and *Escherichia coli*[21] can traverse the RWM. It should be noted that several endotoxin studies related to the RWM and the inner ear have been performed by use of endotoxins obtained from bacterial species not commonly found in middle-ear inflammatory conditions. Although many similarities exist among the lipid moieties of endotoxins from various microorganisms, the chemical and biological heterogeneity of endotoxin is not identical.[22]

RWM IN *STREPTOCOCCUS PNEUMONIAE* INFECTIONS

The RWM undergoes several characteristic changes that parallel the changes in the middle-ear mucosa. In a recent study we inoculated type-3 *S. pneumoniae* in the middle-ear cavity and monitored the structural effects on the RWM for 3 weeks (Johansson *et al.*, in preparation). RWM specimens were collected for histology at 1, 3, 6, 10, and 20 days after inoculation. We could show that *S. pneumoniae* not only had immediate effects on the epithelial lining facing the middle-ear cavity but also caused more slowly developing changes in the connective tissue layer. In the early stage the RWM became extremely edematous and increased several times in thickness. Abundant inflammatory cells, mainly polymorphnuclear leucocytes (PMLs), but also macrophages, occurred in the subepithelial space immediately below the outer epithelial layer. The most striking effect, an interrupted basal lamina, occurred in the interface area between the outer epithelium and the connective-tissue layer noticed within 24 h after the bacterial challenge (FIG. 1). At day 3 the basal lamina appeared thickened with no interruptions (FIG. 2). The dynamic changes of the basal lamina should significantly affect the permeability of the RWM, as it may act as a fil-

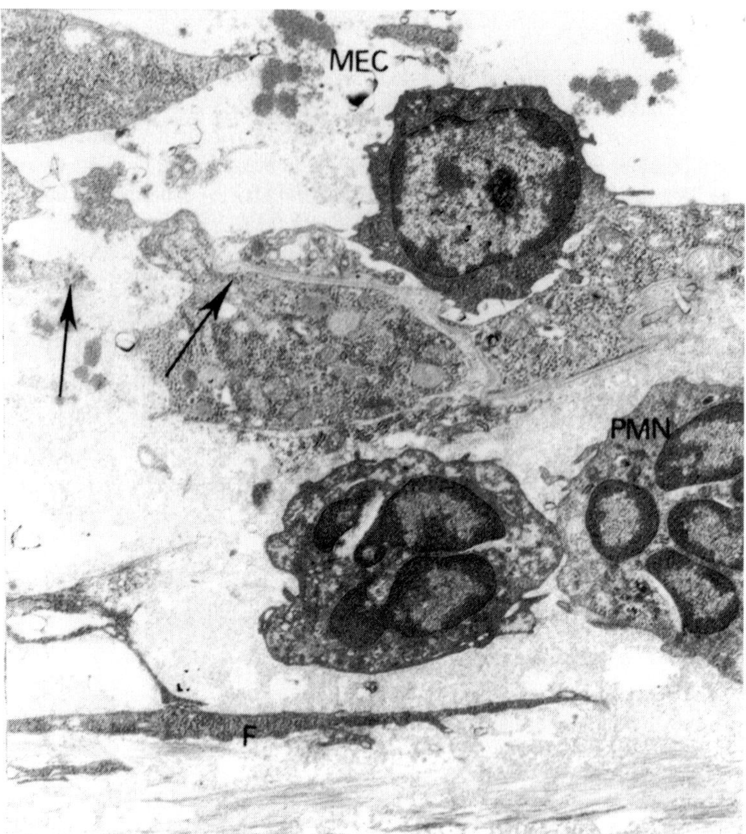

FIGURE 1. Electron micrographs of RWM on day 1 of PnC-induced otitis media. (a) Abundant inflammatory cells, PMNs and macrophages (M) are present in the subepithelial space of the outer layer. The basal lamina (*arrows*) shows distinct changes. It is partly interrupted when in contact with inflammatory cells. ×3000.

ter between the epithelial layer and the connective-tissue layer. The widening and multiple foldings of the basal lamina during the infectious condition may indicate a strengthened barrier mechanism against bacteria and its by products. Later on the RWM decreased in thickness and the connective tissue layer exhibited an increased number of fibroblasts with collagenous fibers of a higher density. Thus fibroblasts and collagen fibers, the principal elements of the connective-tissue layer, may constitute a second layer of defense. The elongated fibroblasts are in contact with one another and form a network. Large molecules should have difficulties in traversing this network. During the inflammatory condition the fibroblasts expand, forming an even denser network.

The elastic fibers could not be distinguished in the light microscope, but were de-

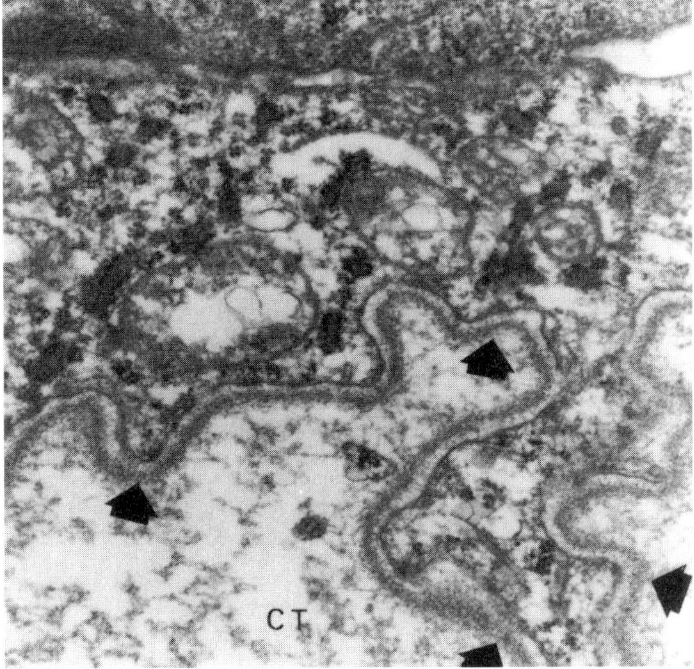

FIGURE 1. (b) A thickened and deeply folded basal lamina below the outer epithelial cell layer. ×15,000.

tected by the electron microscope. The elastic febers were shown to be located predominantly in the region close the inner mesothelial layer. The occurrence of elastic fibers was most pronounced toward the mesothelial layer in the resolution stage of pneumococcal otitis media. These elastic fibers may participate in the barrier function of the RWM and could be involved in the reduced permeability reported during later stages of inflammation.[14–16]

Our structural observations coincide with results from permeability studies,[16] which have shown that bacterial toxins, exotoxins as well as endotoxins, initially could promote an increased permeability of the RWM through tissue-degrading enzymes. This stage parallels the early accumulation of leucocytes in the RWM from which, for example, lysosomal enzymes should derive and further potentiate the degrading activity. Recently Streptolysin 0, the major exotoxin elaborated by *S. pyogenes A* was shown to directly alter the permeability characeristics of the RWM.[23] Streptolysin is the prototype of a large family of bacterial cytolysins that bind to cholesterol and form large pores in the lipid bilayer of erythrocytes. One can suggest that similar pores are created in the membranes of epithelial cells lining the tympanal side of the RWM. Since *S. pneumoniae* manufacture a homologous and functionally similar exotoxin, an analogous process may operate in otitis media caused by this agent.

RWM AND ENDOTOXINS

Regarding effects of endotoxins on the RWM structure, notably few studies have focused on this subject. Kim and Kim (1995)[24] showed a marked thickening of the RWM after exposure to *E. coli* endotoxin. Furthermore, several authors have shown that endotoxin will pass the RWM and be recovered in the perilymph.

BACTERIAL PRODUCTS AND INNER-EAR DAMAGE

Sensorineural hearing loss as a sequel to various types of otitis media has been proposed by many investigators,[25–28] although others have a different opinion.[29–31.]

As we have learned from the RWM permeability studies, the question posed is no longer whether toxins pass into the inner ear but what happens when they get there. Exotoxin derived from *S. pneumoniae* has been shown to be toxic toward hair cells of guinea pig cochlea.[32] Similarly, a study by Lundman *et al.* (1992)[19] on *Pseudomonas aeruginosa* exotoxin A used electrophysiological and morphological techniques to trace inner-ear damage. The highest concentrations of exotoxin A (50 μg/mL) caused a considerable loss of outer hair cells and inner hair cells. Summarized action potential threshold recordings showed no activity of the ear that had been exposed to the exotoxin.

In a more recent study we compared the cochlear function by using a frequency-specific brain stem audiometry technique in two of our otitis media models—the noninfectious serous otitis media obtained through blockage of the eustachian tube and the purulent otitis media caused by clefting of the soft palate (Johansson and Hellström, in preparation). Both otitis media models demonstrated impaired ABR thresholds 3 weeks after the induction of the otitis media condition. The ABR thresholds of the noninfectious inflammatory condition immediately returned to normal, whereas those of the purulent ears remained unchanged except in the low-frequency range, 2 to 6 kHz.

Several studies have focused on cochlear effects of endotoxins. *E. coli* endotoxin was shown to alter the brainstem audiometry response in a study by Spandow *et al.* (1989).[21] The largest threshold impairments occurred in the high-frequency area, anatomically corresponding to the cochlear region located close to the RWM. The changes were transient except at 31.5 kHz. No morphological alterations could be seen at the light microscopical level, which was somewhat surprising, as Kawauchi *et al.* (1988)[33] in an earlier study on *Salmonella typhimurium*-derived endotoxin described disarray of stereocilia and a marked swelling of nerve endings adjacent to hair cells. More recent studies by Kim and Kim (1995)[24] on cochlear effects of *E. coli* endotoxin and a study by Anniko *et al.* (personal communication) on *H. influenzae* type-B endotoxin showed minor effects on the brainstem audiometry thresholds and no structural effects on the cochlear sensory cells.

FUTURE STUDIES TO BE DIRECTED IN THIS FIELD

To summarize, inflammatory conditions of the middle ear caused by bacteria will affect the inner ear. The major route of passage from the middle ear into the inner ear is the RWM. Obviously the RWM is a dynamic structure that will change its permeability properties throughout the infectious condition. Bacterial products reaching the inner ear will cause an impaired cochlear function, and in the case of exotoxins, structural damage to hair cells. Endotoxins appear to evoke transient effects on the electrophysiological thresholds and less structural damage.

Considerable knowledge is lacking concerning the interaction between the middle ear and inner ear in bacterial infections of the middle ear, and many questions remain to be answered, for example: Are there differences regarding persistent functional impairment of the cochlea between exotoxin effects and those of endotoxins? How does the endotoxin influence the structural components of the RWM? Are there alterations of other cochlear elements than hair cells when exposed to bacterial products?

SUMMARY

The round-window membrane (RWM) is extremely thin and is the only soft-tissue barrier between the middle ear and the inner ear. Under inflammatory conditions of the middle ear the various layers of the triple-layered RWM undergo characteristic changes parallel to the changes of the middle-ear mucosa. Several studies report that bacterial products, exo- and endotoxins, from bacteria invading the middle ear may result in profound inflammatory changes in the inner ear, followed by severe damage to the inner-ear function.

The present review, in which we summarized experimental and clinical observations, on bacterial products in interactions between the middle and inner ear, focused on:

1. Bacteria and bacterial products in an inflamed middle ear that may influence inner-ear function.
2. RWM structure and RWM permeability under the influence of bacteria and bacterial products.
3. Morphological and functional inner-ear effects of bacterial infection of the middle ear, and the possible mechanisms involved.
4. Future studies to be directed in this field.

REFERENCES

1. SALYERS, A. A. & D. D. WHITT, Eds. 1994. Bacterial Patahogenesis. A Molecular Approach. ASM Press. Washington, D.C.
2. BLUESTONE, C. D. 1984. State of the art: Definitions and classifications. *In* Recent Advances in Otitis Media with Effusion, D. J. Lim, Bluestone, C. D., Klein, J. O., and J. D. Nelson, Eds.:1–4. Decker, Philadelphia.
3. SENTURIA, B. H., C. F. GESSEN & C. D. CARR. 1960. Middle ear effusions: Causes and treatment. Trans. Am. Acad. Ophthalmol. Otolaryngol. **64:**60–75.
4. LIU, Y. S., D. J. LIM, R. LANG & H. BIRCK. 1976. Microorganisms in chronic otitis media with effusion. Ann. Otol. Rhinol. **85**(Suppl. 25): 245.
5. GIEBINK, G. S. 1984. Epidemiology and natural history of otitis media. *In* Recent Advances in Otitis Media with Effusion, D. J. Lim, C. D. Bluestone, J. O. Klein, and J. D. Nelson, Eds.: 5–9. Decker, Philadelphia.

6. RICHARDSON, T. L., E. ISHIYAMA & W. KAELS. 1971. Submicroscopic studies of the round window membrane. Acta Otolaryngol. (Stockholm) **71:** 9–21.
7. SCHACHERN, P. A., M. M. PAPARELLA, A. J. DUVALL III & Y. B. CHOO. 1984. The human round window membrane. An electron microscopic study. Arch. Otolaryngol. **110:** 15–21.
8. GOYCOOLEA, M. V., A. M. CARPENTER & D. MUCHOW. 1987. Ultrastructural studies of the round window membrane of the cat. Arch. Otolaryngol. Head Neck Surg. **113:** 617–624.
9. CARPENTER, A. M., D. MUCHOW & M. V. GOYCOOLEA. 1989. Ultrastructural studies of the human round window membrane. Arch. Otolaryngol. Head Neck Surg. **115:** 585–590.
10. JOHANSSON, U., S. HELLSTRÖM & M. ANNIKO. 1993. Round window membrane in serous and purulent otitis media. Structural study in the rat. **102:** 227–235.
11. NOMURA, Y. 1984. Otological significance of the round window. *In* Advances in Oto-Rhino-Laryngology, C. R. Pfaltz, Vol. 33, Ed.:1–162. Karger. Basel.
12. GOYCOOLEA, M. V., D. MUCHOW, G. MARTINEZ, P. B. AGUILA, H. G. GOYCOOLEA, P. SCHACHERN & W. KNIGHT. 1988. Permeability of the human round window membrane to cationic ferritin. Arch. Otolaryngol. Head Neck Surg. **114:** 1247–1251.
13. JUHN, S. K., Y. HAMAGUCHI & M. V. GOYCOOLEA. 1988. Review of round window membrane permeability. Acta Otolaryngol. (Stockholm) **457**(Suppl.): 43–48.
14. GOYCOOLEA, M. V., M. M. PAPARELLA, B. GOLDBERG & A. M. CARPENTER. 1980. Permeability of the round window membrane in otitis media. Arch. Otolaryngol. **106:** 430–433.
15. IKEDA, K., M. SAKAGAMI, T. MORIZONO & S. K. JUHN. 1990. Permeability of the round window membrane to middle-sized molecules in purulent otitis media. Arch. Otolaryngol. Head Neck Surg. **116:** 57–60.
16. IKEDA, K. & T. MORIZONO. 1988. Changes of the permeability of round window membrane in otitis media. Arch. Otolaryngol. Head Neck Surg. **114:** 895–897.
17. SCHACHERN, P., M. M. PAPARELLA, M. GOYCOOLEA, A. J. DUVALL II & Y.-B. CHOO. 1987. The permeability of the round window membrane during otitis media. Arch. Otolaryngol. Head Neck Surg. **113:** 625–629.
18. GOYCOOLEA, M. V., M. M. PAPARELLA, B. GOLDBERG, P. M. SCHLIEVERT & A. CARPENTER. 1980. Permeability of the middle ear to staphylococcal pyrogenic exotoxin in otitis media. Int. J. Pediatr. Otorhinolaryngol. **1:** 301–308.
19. LUNDMAN, L., T. HARADA, P. A. SANTI, S. K. JUHN, T. MORIZONO & D. BAGGER-SJÖBÄCK. 1992. Inner ear damage and passage through the round window membrane of pseudomonas aeruginosa exotoxin A in a chinchilla model. Ann. Otol. Rhinol. Laryngol. **101:** 37–441.
20. LUNDMAN, L., S. K. JUHN, D. BAGGER-SJÖBÄCK & C. SVANBORG. 1992. Permeability of the normal round window membrane to Haemophilus influenzae type B endotoxin. Acta Otolaryngol. (Stockholm) **112:** 524–529.
21. SPANDOW, O., M. ANNIKO & S. HELLSTRÖM. 1989. Inner ear disturbances following inoculation of endotoxin into the middle ear. Acta Otolaryngol. (Stockholm) **107:** 90–96.
22. NOWOTYN, A. 1983. In search of the active sites in endotoxins. *In*: Beneficial Effects of Endotoxins, A. Nowotyn, Ed.: 1–55. Plenum Press, New York.
23. ENGEL, F., R. BLATZ, J. KELLNER, M. PALMER, U. WELLER & S. BHAKDI. 1995. Breakdown of the round window membrane permeability barrier evoked by streptolysin O: Possible etiologic role in development of sensorineural hearing loss in acute otitis media. Infect. Immun. **63:** 1305–1310.
24. KIM, C.-S. & H.-J. KIM. 1995. Auditory brain-stem response changes after application of endotoxin to the round window membrane in experimental otitis media. Arch. Otolaryngol. Head Neck Surg., **112:** 557–565.
25. PAPPAS, D. G. 1983. Hearing impairments and vestibular abnormalities among children with subclinical cytomegalvirus. Ann. Otol. Rhinol. Laryngol. **92:** 552–557.

26. PAPARELLA, M. M., T. MORIZONO, C. T. LE, F. MANICINI, P. SIPILÄ, Y. B. CHOO, G. LIDÉN & C. S. KIM. 1984. Sensorineural hearing loss in otitis media. Ann. Otol. Rhinol. Laryngol. **93:** 623–629.

27. SORRI, M. & P. RANTAKALLIO. 1988. Secretory otitis media and hearing loss. Acta Otolaryngol. (Stockholm) **457**(Suppl.): 94–99.

28. LÖPPÖNEN, H., M. SORRI, R. PEKKALA & J. PENNA. 1992. Secretory otitis media and high-frequency hearing loss. Acta Otolaryngol. (Stockholm) **493**(Suppl.): 99–107.

29. BROWNING, G. G. & S. GATEHOUSE. 1989. Hearing in chronic suppurataive otitis media. Ann. Otol. Rhinol. Laryngol. **98:** 245–250.

30. RAHKO, T., P. KARMA & M. SIPILÄ. 1989. Sensorineural hearing loss and acute otitis media in children. Acta Otolaryngol. (Stockholm) **108:** 107–112.

31. KARMA, P., P. SIPILÄ & T. RAHKO. 1993. Hearing and history of acute otitis media in childhood. *In* Recent Advances in Otitis Media, D. J. Lim, C. D. Bluestone, J. O. Klein, J. D. Nelson, P. L. Ogram, Eds.: 552–554. Decker, Philadelphia.

32. COMIS, S.-D., M. P. OSBORNE, J. STEPHEN, M. TARLOW, T. L. HAYWARD, T. J. MICHELL, P. E. ANDREW & G. J. L. BOULNOIS. 1993. Cytotoxic effects on hair cells of guinea pig cochlea produced by pneumolysin, the thil-activated toxin of Streptococcus pneumoniae. Acta Otolaryngol. (Stockholm) **113:** 152–159.

33. KAWAUCHI, H., T. F. DE MARIA & D. J. LIM. 1988. Endotoxin permeability through the RW. Acta Otolaryngol. (Stockholm) **457:** 100–115.

Effect of Streptomycin and Gentamicin on the Inner Ear

DAN BAGGER-SJOBACK[a]

Department of Otorhinolaryngology
Karolinska Institute
Karolinska sjukhuset
171 76 Stockholm
Sweden

The aminoglycoside antibiotics have been in clinical use since the mid-1940s, and can thus be regarded to be among the early antibiotics in clinical use. In 1944, Waksman *et al.*[1] derived streptomycin from the soil organisms *Actinomyces griseus*. The drug proved to be the first antibiotic that could be successfully used against tuberculosis and soon received widespread use. As a result of this initial success, many studies addressed new and more potent antibiotics with similar characteristics. Unfortunately, it became evident that streptomycin had several severe side effects. These could be acute or more chronic in character, the foremost being inner-ear disturbances, including temporary or permanent hearing loss and vestibular deficits, as well as irreversible kidney damage. Hinshaw and Feldman,[2] one year after the first presentation of streptomycin, reported on these severe side effects. Three years later Causse *et al.*[3] could show structural damage on the vestibular apparatus.

A new aminoglycoside antibiotic, dihydrostreptomycin was developed. This did not have the vestibulotoxic effects of streptomycin, but was considerably more cochleotoxic, resulting in severe cochlear disturbances that often resulted in total deafness. This side effect was considered so serious that dihydrostreptomycin was subsequently permanently withdrawn from the market and has been so ever since.[4,5]

Neomycin was developed in 1949. This drug proved to be successful against gram-negative organisms, and was often used in the form of a powder that could be dispersed in an open abdominal cavity, and over large skin burns.[6] Although very potent as an antibiotic, neomycin also proved to be ototoxic; however, not to the same extent as dihydrostreptomycin.[7] The drug has therefore defended its role in clinical practice, but must be used with caution and monitored so that damage to the inner ear does not occur.

A new group of aminoglycoside antibiotics derived from *Actinomyces micromonospora* appeared in the 1960s. Gentamicin was introduced in 1963, followed by tobramycin.[8,9] Amikacin, which was developed in 1972, was the first semisynthetic aminoglycoside antibiotic. It was followed by netilmicin.[10,11] One of the characteristics of these later-developed aminoglycoside antibiotics is that they have a lower ototoxic potential. It has, however, not been possible to develop an antibiotic within this family that is totally devoid of ototoxic effects that depends on the number of free amino- or methylaminogropys that appear on the glycoside structure. The three

[a]Phone: 46-87-29-2000; fax: 46-832-4278.

aminocyclitol rings with 3–5 amine groups are thus thought to determine the nature of the drug.

The aminoglycoside antibiotics are highly water soluble.[12] Their electrical charge results in a slow passage into the cells over the plasma membrane by diffusion mechanisms. This electrical charge also facilitates binding to anions to such a large extent that the drugs act as efficient competitors for cations like calcium and magnesium.[12] The aminoglycoside antibiotics as a whole are also excreted by the kidneys, this being the result of their water solubility and electrical charge. Several different mechanisms have been blamed for their ototoxic potential, one of the foremost being an interaction with protein synthesis.[13]

All aminoglycoside antibiotics are poorly absorbed from the gastrointestinal canal. They therefore must be given by the parenteral mode or topically. They also do not readily pass the blood–brain barrier.[14] Thus the cerebrospinal fluid concentrations of the drug are much lower than what is found in serum. All aminoglycoside antibiotics are excreted into the urine by glomerular filtration.[15] Thus kidney failure rapidly affects the serum and tissue levels of the drugs. This was earlier thought to be one of the main reasons for the development of cochlear and vestibular damage, since the drug levels would increase both in perilymph and in endolymph. This mechanism has, however, been debated and criticized by Henley and Schact, who claimed that there was no clear correlation between ototoxic effects and drug concentrations in inner-ear fluids.[15] Clinical data, however, confirm that patients with manifest kidney failure develop inner-ear damage in conjunction with aminoglycoside therapy much faster and after lower drug doses as compared to normal subjects.

The toxic effects exerted by aminoglycoside antibiotics can be separated into acute and chronic effects.[12] Although the chronic effects pose a major clinical problem, the acute effects also should be mentioned. These effects are usually reversible and include such entities as neuromuscular blockade and acute reversible hearing impairment.[16] The symptoms usually disappear after the administration of calcium, which indicates that a competitive action between the aminoglycoside antibiotic and calcium could be responsible for these events.[16] It should be emphasized that these acute reactions probably are quite separate from the chronic reaction patterns seen after aminoglycoside administration. The chronic effects are not influenced by calcium administration, and usually cause permanent damage to the individual.[17]

The chronic toxicity profile is dominated by damage inflicted on the kidney and the inner ear. Different drugs exert different effects on these target organs. Thus, some compounds appear more cochleotoxic, that is, dihydrostreptomycin, as compared to others that are supposed to be more vestibulotoxic, that is, gentamicin.[4,5] The reason for this diversity is not known, but it has been postulated that even minor changes within the aminoglycoside molecule may totally change the pattern of side effects.

It was already speculated early on that the toxic effects exerted by the aminoglycoside antibiotics were due to accumulation of the drug in the inner-ear fluids, that is, perilymph and endolymph.[18] In the study performed by Tran Ba Huy *et al.*,[19] however, it was found that the inner-ear fluid drug concentrations never reached or exceeded the peak serum levels. It was also found that the tissue concentration of the drug could not be correlated with the ototoxic damage pattern. It was thus shown that the inner-ear tissues were saturated with gentamicin within three hours after the administration. In spite of this, no signs of otoxocity were evident until after three weeks of daily injections.[20] Another finding that contradicts the old accumulation hypothesis is that, when comparing different drugs with different toxicity profiles, that is, cochleotoxicity or vestibular toxicity, no correlation could be seen between the tissue concentration in the various inner-ear tissues and the development of toxic effects on the particular tissue.[21,22] In another study performed at the cellular level, it was shown that although gentamicin was present in the sensory cells and remains there for a long time, no electrophysiologic signs of inner-ear impairment or hair-cell dysfunction could be demonstrated in the experimental animals.[23]

Currently, it has been postulated that the aminoglycoside antibiotics may have to be metabolized before they can exert their potential for developing inner-ear damage. Thus, Takada *et al.* proposed that a toxic metabolite of the drugs could be the damaging stimulus for the inner ear.[24] This hypothesis was later supported by other experimental studies. These studies show that the aminoglycoside antibiotics in their non-metabolized form do not affect isolated outer hair cells *in vitro*.[25] On the other hand, when matabolized gentamicin was present in the culture medium, the cells showed signs of devitalization and cell destruction.[26,27] Several different aminoglycoside antibiotics were shown to produce a similar reaction. The exact mode of action of the aminoglycoside antibiotics on the cell level is not known. Thus, a number of different mechanisms have been proposed to be responsible for the deleterious effect on the inner ear. Among these are interactions with DNA, RNA, and protein synthesis, metabolism of different components as well as interaction with the energy metabolism and fluid and ion balance.[12] It is conceivable that several of these actions may exist in conjunction with aminoglycoside ototoxicity, but to what extent they represent primary or secondary events remains unknown. Schacht pointed out early that the aminoglycoside antibiotics have a specific affinity to bind to phosphatidylinositol-4-5-disphospate.[28] This lipid component that is present in the plasma membrane belongs to the transmembrane signaling system, which interacts with a number of events such as transport of hormones, neurotransmittors, and other related substances.[12] Drug interaction with phospatidyl inositide metabolism could also change the membrane permeability and membrane transport systems, with a subsequent effect at the cell and subcell level.[12] Phosphoinositides are also involved in the synthesis of prostaglandin and leukotrienes. These important compounds may thus be inhibited by the presence of aminoglycoside antibiotics.[29] While these general effects seem to prevail in many different types of cells in the body, the so-called dark cells of the inner ear seem to be a specific target for the aminoglycoside antibiotics.[30,31] These dark cells are secretory cells that are present in the utricle and the cristae of the semicircular canals. Secretory cells are also present in the stria vascularis of the cochlea. The secretory cells are thought to be involved in the important ion-transport events that are necessary for normal inner-ear function. Hawkins and coworkers proposed that the aminoglycoside antibiotics would interact with the secretory cells, resulting in changes in the homeostasis mechanisms of the inner ear.[32] These changes could then lead to secondary changes within the sensory epithelia and the sensory hairy cells. This possible effect on the secretory cells of the inner ear is one of the reasons that the ototoxic potential of the aminoglycoside antibiotics has been used in order to alter inner-ear function in patients with diseases emanating from the inner ear, such as Meniere's disease.

The idea to utilize aminoglycoside antibiotics such as streptomycin for treatment of inner-ear symptoms in patients with Meniere's disease was initially launched by Hawkins in 1947.[33] Hawkins assumed that the proven vestibulotoxic effects exerted by streptomycin could be used in a therapeutic way for these patients. The first clinical description of a patient material having had treatment for their vertigo with systemic administration of streptomycin was given by Fowler in 1948.[34] He reported that four patients who, after having been given streptomycin by intramuscular injections, experienced relief from their vertigo. This study was later followed by Hamberger *et al.* in 1949.[35] He reported that four patients had been successfully treated with systemic streptomycin administration.[35] In 1951, Ruedi as well as Hansson also published the results of studies utilizing only a few patients.[36] The treatment schemes utilized in these reports were similar in that the drug was given until the caloric responses using ice water were abolished. This would imply that the vestibular function in the affected ear was destroyed. It is worth noting that the total doses utilized in these reports varied greatly between different patients. This is a prerogative for the current regimes utilizing local drug administration into the affected ear. The reason for this great interindividual variability in sensitivity to ototoxic antibiotics is not known and is thought to depend on a number of variables. A common finding in these early series, however, was that the patients developed ataxia and often severe oscillopsia posttreatment, which caused them considerable distress. The hearing was affected more in some cases and less in others.

The first more systematic attempt to utilize systemic administration of aminoglycoside antibiotics as a treatment modality for Meniere's disease was performed by Schuknecht, who in 1956 reported on a large number of patients that were given streptomycin in intramuscular injections twice daily until the ice water caloric response was abolished.[38] The total doses utilized in this report ranged from 13.5 to 89 g, with a mean of 39 g. Twenty patients being treated in this way were followed for a long time, and Schuknecht in 1991 reported good vertigo control in 95% of them.[39] Approximately one-third of the patients had some degree of ataxia and 15% had persistent oscillopsia. The hearing was remarkably unaffected and a large majority of the patients (90%) thus had stable hearing.

While these former regimes were thought to drastically reduce or even abolish the vestibular function, usually in both ears, the so-called titration or subtotal treatment regimes aimed at only causing minor damage to the vestibular end organs. It was believed that this destruction of the dark cells also reduced the afferent nerve impulses giving rise to dysequilibrium and vertiginous attacks. Such schemes were almost simultaneously published by Silverstein *et al.* as well as by Graham and Kemink in 1984.[40,41] In these protocols the patients were treated with repeated injections of streptomycin until they either produced signs of vestibular toxicity, that is, spontaneous nystagmus, or experienced relief from their vertiginous symptoms. Langman *et al.*, in a long time study, followed 19 patients who had been given titration therapy with streptomycin.[42] In this protocol about one-third of the patients who had experienced good control of vertigo initially reported different degress of dysequilibrium or pure vertigo attacks at the end of the study period. Oscillopsia was reported in a small proportion of the patients, while mild unsteadiness was present in a little over half of them.

It soon became apparent that systemic treatment of patients with Meniere's disease and disabling vertigo, although providing good vertigo control in a majority of cases, was accompanied by several undesirable side effects, such as risk of hearing loss, in a healthy ear, and, in a number of cases, persistent ataxia and/or oscillopsia. These side effects were to some extent reduced by the introduction of the titration or subtotal treatment regimes, but still persisted to a degree that motivated a search for other ways of administrating the drugs. In 1957 Schuknecht published articles on eight patients who had been given streptomycin by local injection in the affected ear.[43] This was done through a small plastic catheter that was placed in the external ear canal, with an extension into the middle ear through the posterior, inferior quadrant of the tympanic membrane. Streptomycin was given in daily injections ranging from one to seven days until the patient lost the caloric response for ice water in the affected ear as well as showing signs of the effects of the drug on the vestibular end organ, that is, a sensation of dysequilibrium or vertigo. The amoung of streptomycin given to this small group of patients also varied widely between 150 and 600 mg/day. Five of the eight treated patients experienced good control of their vertigo, however, paying the price of losing their hearing in the affected ear. The remaining three patients retained their hearing but also their pretreatment vertigo. In view of later findings, it seems reasonable to believe that the three patients who did not achieve vertigo control probably would have required larger doses of the drug or more likely presented with local middle-ear conditions that impeded or even blocked drug entry into the inner ear. It seems likely that the drug administration resulted in some kind of pharmacological or toxic labyrinthectomy in the five successful cases.

In view of this fact, this type of local treatment mode did not gain widespread use until Lange in 1978 stated that patients could be treated with intratympanic injections of streptomycin and ozothin oil, a compound that in animal experments had been shown to protect the cochlea from damage after streptomycin challenge.[44] In addition to good vertigo control the hearing ability remained unchanged in a large proportion of the patients. Lange thus proposed that he produced a more selective impairment of the vestibular end orgams as compared to the cochlear sensory epithelium. Inner-ear studies revealed that gentamicin provided a safer way to selectively affect the vestibular apparatus while saving cochlear function as compared to streptomycin. This led the German investigators to employ gentamicin even in an intratympanic mode on a larger scale that previously. In 1977 and in 1981 Lange presented his results on 67 patients who had been followed up for up to 13 years.[45,46] Ninety-five percent of the patients had no further vertigo attacks, and 76% reported that their hearing was unchanged or even better. While the tinnitus was cured or improved in 35%, the feeling of pressure had disappeared in almost half of the patients (43%). The drug was delivered through a small transtympanic polyethylene tube fixed in place surgically. Only 0.1 mL of gentamicin was given every 5 h until signs of vestibular reaction were evident (dizziness or nystagmus). At the same time, Beck and Schmidt utilized a similar protocol in 112 patients, who were followed up for several years.[47] In this protocol, 0.4 mL of gentamicin was tiven twice daily until signs of nystagmus appeared. Their success rate was comparable to that of Lange with regard to vertigo control and hearing, while the control of tinnitus and the feeling of pressure was reported to be considerably better in Beck and Schmidt's material.[47] Their conclusion was that with this regime, they could affect the secretory epithelium in the vestibular apparatus, while at the same time maintaining the essential function of the vestibular apparatus as well as the cochlea. Whether this alleged dark-cell effect resulted in true changes in the ion and fluid balance in the inner ear has not been proven.

In an attempt to clarify the mode of action of gentamicin on the inner ear, Bagger-Sjoback *et al.* in 1990 presented two patients who had undergone subtotal labyrinthectomy due to persistent vertigo after having been previously given gentamicin intratympanically.[48] Both patients were treated with an older protocol, wherein a large number of gentamicin injections were given until nystagmus appeared. Both patients had severely impaired hearing before starting the gentamicin treatment, and were clinically deaf after the repeated injections. It was thus possible not only to remove the vestibular sensory epithelia, but also parts of the cochlea during the surgery. In both cases the cristae of the semicircular canals and the otolith organs, including the dark-cell regions were quite well preserved, whereas the cochlea presented with severe changes, that is, the whole organ of Corti was entirely missing in the basal and middle coils. Although this type of finding could be anticipated in these patients, who retained their vertigo but who had previously lost their hearing, this is not what generally could be expected after gentamicin therapy. Gentamicin has been considered to be more vestibulotoxic than ototoxic, and the reason why the vestibular sensory epithelia did not present with more severe changes as compared to the cochlea remains unknown. It should be pointed out, however, that both patients received much larger doses of gentamicin than what is currently given according to the current protocol.

In an attempt to administer the aminoglycoside antibiotic therapy directly into the inner ear, Shea and Norris introduced a technique whereby a fenestra in the lateral semicircular canal is created after a standard mastoidectomy procedure.[49] Dissolved streptomycin was then allowed to slowly diffuse into the perilymphatic space via the fenestra. The exact amount of streptomycin that actually reached the membraneous labyrinth and the sensory epithelia of the inner ear is not known. Shea initially claimed to have good results with this technique, and in 1989 a multicenter study was designed in the United States in order to evaluate this infusion protocol. A majority of the patients achieved control of their vertigo, but almost 20% required yet another therapeutical procedure, indicating that their vertigo control was far from satisfactory.[50] A majority of the patients (57%) lost useful hearing in the affected ear. An apparent finding was that patients with poor hearing pretreatment were also at greater risk of having their hearing worsen after the streptomicin infusion. A similar trend has been noted by Bergenius (personal communication), who claims that the better condition the inner ear is in before gentamicin is given in intratympanic injections, the smaller the risk of sustaining a permanent cochlear dysfunction posttreatment. It also became apparent that a majority of the surgeons taking part in the multicenter study in the United States did not feel that this approach could be advocated in the future, due to the great risk of cochleotoxicity and severe hearing loss.[50] Regarding the choice of aminoglycoside antibiotic, Shea recommends the use of streptomycin rather than gentamicin for treatment of disabling vertigo and Meniere's disease based on the findings of Norris and coworkers who demonstrated that streptomycin, while being equally vestibulotoxic as gentamicin, seemed to be much less cochleotoxic.[51]

A modification of the more direct inner-ear approach was presented by Shea in 1994 when he introduced the drug into the round-window niche by a routine tympanotomy.[33] This was done by incising the tympanic membrane in the posteroinferior quadrant. The round-window niche could then be inspected and obstructing adhesions removed. Using a small syringe, streptomycin dissolved in 0.5 mL of hyaluronan was injected down into the niche. The injections were repeated on the second and third days after the initial surgery. Shea reported good vertigo control in 96% and a hearing ability that had either improved or remained unchanged in 96%. Only 4% of the patients displayed worse hearing than preoperatively. It must be emphasized, however, that these results come from 24 cases that were followed for only 3–8 months postoperatively.[33] This technique is certainly much less invasive compared to the opening of the lateral semicircular canal, and it remains to be seen whether Shea's results are stable, and also whether they can be repeated by other investigators.

At present the general trend seems to be to reduce the number of injections, and thus the total drug dose given to the patient. The rationale for this type of protocol is that one wants to achieve inhibition of the secretory epithelia of the inner ear, that is, the dark cells in the vestibular end organs and possibly also the stria vascularis in the cochlea without inflicting damage to the sensory structures in the end organs. In this way hearing and the sense of equilibrium can be maintained in an inner ear that has been treated with an aminoglycoside antibiotic, with the aim of impeding or influencing fluid turnover and hydrops. Such protocols are currently in use in Sweden. Odkvist and Magnusson thus utilized the quadruple intratympanal gentamicin treatment in 22 patients with disabling Meniere's disease.[52] Four single doses of the drug were proven to be sufficient for treatment of vertigo in 18 out of the 22 patients who remained free from vertiginous attacks. Hearing loss due to the treatment regime was infrequent. In a further attempt to reduce the amount of drug given, Odkvist and Magnusson compared a dual-application technique with the quadruple regime.[52] In the dual-treatment regime the patients were given one injection into the middle ear daily for two consecutive days. In their first trial this was done with 16 patients. All patients but two experienced a short posttreatment period of vertigo. Following a period of rehabilitation, the patients were free from ataxia and vertigo attacks. Most patients demonstrated a diminished or even lost caloric response in the treated ear. In regard to hearing, most patients experienced some improvement—the median improvement was five decibels. None of the patients lost their hearing. It thus seems relevant to draw the conclusion that gentamicin can be given in smaller doses as compared to earlier protocols and achieve vertigo relief for most patients. It is also quite apparent that the risk for permanent damage to the cochlea and subsequent hearing loss is greatly reduced with this type of regime. In the few cases where the level of vertigo control is unsatisfactory, one or two further injections can safely be given.

Aminoglycoside antibiotics have been in clinical use for more than 50 years. Although they are still used in some specific infection treatment protocols, less toxic antibiotics have been developed that can safely be used when treating infections caused by gram-negative microorganisms. Quite uniquely, however, it has been possible to utilize one of the most serious adverse effects of the drugs—the potential for inner-ear damage—for the treatment of inner-ear diseases, such as Meniere's disease. Active treatment of inner-ear disorders is a new field that is expanding rapidly, and it is quite conceivable that this type of drug interaction with the inner ear only marks the beginning of a new era where pharmacological treatment of inner-ear disorders will be a logical and natural choice of treatment for these diseases.

REFERENCES

1. WAKSMAN, S. A., E. BUGIE & A. SCHATZ. 1944. Isolation of antibiotic substances from soil microorganisms with special reference to streptothricin and streptomycin. Proc. Staff Meet. Mayo Clin. **19:** 537.
2. HINSHAW, H. C. & W. H. FELDMAN. 1945. Streptomycin in treatment of clinical tuberculosis: A preliminary report. Proc. Staff Meet. Mayo Clin. **20:** 313.
3. CAUSSE, R., I. GONDET & B. VALLANCIEN. 1948. Actione vestibulaire de la streptomycine chez la souris. C.R. Soc. Biol. (Paris) **142:** 747.
4. HAWKINS, J. E., JR & M. H. LURIE. 1953. Ototoxicity of dihydrostreptomycin and neomycin in cat. Ann. Otol. Rhinol. Laryngol. **62:** 1128–1148.
5. SHAMBAUGH, S. F., D. L. DERLACHI, W. H. HARRISON, *et al.* 1959. Dihydrostreptomycin deafness. J. Am. Med. Assoc. **170:** 1657–1658.
6. WAKSMAN, S. A., E. KATZ & H. LECHAVALIER. 1950. Antimicrobial properties of neomycin. J. Lab. Clin. Med. **36:** 93–99.
7. GIBSON, W. S. 1967. Deafness due to orally administered neomycin. Arch. Otolaryngol. **86:** 57–59.
8. WEINSTEIN, M. J., G. M. LEUDEMANN, E. M. ODEN, *et al.* 1963. Gentamicin: A new broad spectrum antibiotic complex. Antimicrob. Agents Chemother. **3:** 1.
9. HIGGINS, C. C. & R. E. KASTNERS. 1967. Nebramycin—A new broad spectrum antibiotic complex. II. Description of Streptomyces tenebrarius. Antimicrob. Agents Chemother. **7:** 324.
10. KAWAGUCHI, H., J. NAITO, S. NAKAGAWA, *et al.* 1972. BB-K8. A new semisynthetic antibiotic. J. Antibiot. **25:** 695.
11. WRIGHT, J. J. 1976. Synthesis of 1-N-ethyl sisomycin: A new broad spectrum semisynthetic aminoglycoside antibiotic. Chemo. Commun. **206:**
12. SCHACHT, J. 1993. Biochemical basis of aminoglycoside ototoxicity. Otolaryngol. Clin. North Am. **26**(5): 845–856.
13. DAVIS, B. D. 1987. Mechanism of bactericidal action of aminoglycosides. Microbiol. Rev. **51:** 341–350.
14. SANDE, M. A. & G. L. MANDELL. 1990. Antimicrobial agents. *In* Goodman and Gilman's: The Pharmacological Basis of Therapeutics, 8th ed., A. G. Gilman, T. W. Rall, A. S. Nies, *et al.*, Eds.: 1098–1116. Pergamon Press. New York.
15. HENLEY, C. M., III & J. SCHACHT. 1988. Pharmacokinetics of aminoglycoside antibiotics in inner ear fluids and their relationship to ototoxicity. Audiology **27:** 137–147.
16. CORRADO, A. P., I. P. DEMORAIS & W. A. PRADO. 1989. Aminoglycoside antibiotics as a tool for the study of the biological role of calcium ions: Historical overviw. Acta Physiol. Pharmacol. Latinoam. **39:** 419–430.
17. WAGMAN, G. H., J. A. MARQUEZ & M. J. WEINSTEIN. 1968. Chromatographic separation of the components of the gentamicin complex. J. Chromatogr. **34:** 210–215.
18. HENLEY, C. M. & J. SCHACHT. 1988. Pharmacokinetics of aminoglycoside antibiotics in blood, inner ear fluids and tissues and their relationship to ototoxicity. Audiology **27:** 137–146.
19. TRAN BA HUY, P., C. MANUEL, A. MEULEMANS, *et al.* 1981. Pharmacokinetics of gentamicin in perilymph and endolymph of the rat as determined by radioimmunoassay. J. Infect. Dis. **143:** 476–486.

20. TRAN BA HUY, P., P. BERNHARD & J. SCHACHT. 1986. Kinetics of gentamicin uptake and release in the rat: Comparison of inner ear tissues and fluids with other organs. J. Clin. Invest. **77:** 1492–1500.
21. OHTANI, I., K. OHTSUKI, T. AIKAWA, *et al.* 1984. Mechanism of protective effect of fosfomycin against aminoglycoside ototoxicity. Auris Nasus Larynx **11:** 119–124.
22. OHTSUKI, K., I. OHTANI, T. AIKAWA, *et al.* 1982. The ototoxicity and the accumulation in the inner ear of the various aminoglycoside antibiotics. Ear Res. Jpn. **13:** 85–87.
23. HIEL, H., H. BENNANI, J.-P. ERRE, *et al.* 1992. Kinetics of gentamicin in cochlear hair cells after chronic treatment. Acta Otolaryngol. **112:** 272–277.
24. TAKADA, A., S. BLEDSOE & J. SCHACHT. 1985. An energy-dependent step in aminoglycoside ototoxicity: Prevention of gentamicin ototoxicity during reduced endolymphatic potential. Hear. Res. **19:** 245–251.
25. DULON, D., G. ZAJIC, J.-M. ARAN, *et al.* 1989. Aminoglycoside antibiotics impair calcium-entry but not viability and motility of cochlear outer hair cells. J. Neurisci. Res. **24:** 338–3346.
26. CRANN, S. A., M. Y HYANG, J. D. McLAREN, *et al.* 1992. Formation of a toxic metabolite from gentamicin by a hepatic cytosolic fraction. Biochem. Pharmacol. **43:** 1835–1839.
27. HUANG, M. Y. & J. SCHACHT. 1990. Formation of a cytotoxic metabolite from gentamicin by liver. Biochem. Pharmacol. **40:** R11–R14.
28. SCHACHT, J. 1979. Isolation of an aminoglycoside receptor from guinea pig inner ear tissues and kidney. Arch. Otorhinolaryngol. **24:** 129–134.
29. ESCOUBET, B., P. AMSALLEM, E. FERRARY, *et al.* 1985. Prostaglandin synthesis by the cochlea of the guinea pig: Influence of aspirin, gentamicin and acoustic stimulation. Prostaglandins **29:** 589–599.
30. PARK, J. & G. COHEN. 1982. Vestibular ototoxicity in the chick: Effects of streptomycinon equilibrium and on ampullary dark cells. Am. J. Otolaryngol. **6:** 117–127.
31. PENDER, D. 1985. Gentamicin tympanoclysis: Effects on the vestibular secretory cells. Am. J. Otolaryngol. **6:** 789–809.
32. HAWKINS, J. E., N. J. RAHWAY & M. H. LURIE. 1952. The ototoxicity of streptomycin. Ann. Otol. Rhinol. Laryngol. **61:** 789–809.
33. SHEA, J. J. & X. GE. 1994. Streptomycin perfusion of the labyrinth through the round window plus intravenous streptomycin. Otolaryngol. Clin. North Am. **27(2):** 317–324.
34. FOWLER, E. P. 1948. Streptomycin treatment of vertigo. Trans. Am. Acad. Opthalmol. Laryngol. **52:** 239–301.
35. HAMBERGER, C.-A., H. HYDEN & H. KOCH. 1949. Streptomycin bei der Menierschen Krankheit. Arch. Ohren-Nasen Kehlkopfh. **155:** 667–682.
36. RUEDI, L. 1951. Therapeutic and toxic effects of streptomycin in otology. Laryngoscope **61:** 613–636.
37. HANSON, H. V. 1951. The treatment of endolymphatic hydrops (Meniere's disease) with streptomycin. Ann. Otol. Rhinol. Laryngol. **60:** 676–691.
38. SCHUKNECHT, H. F. 1956. Ablation therapy for the relief of Meniere's disease. Laryngoscope **66:** 859–870.
39. SCHUKNECHT, H. F. 1991. Ablation of vestibular function with intramuscular streptomycin (Op. Tech.). Otolaryngol. Head Neck Surg. **21:** 38–40.
40. SILVERSTEIN, H. 1984. Streptomycin treatment for Meniere's disease. Ann. Otol. Rhinol. Laryngol. **93(Suppl. 122):** 44–48.
41. GRAHAM, M. D., R. T. SATALOFF & J. L. KEMINK. 1984. Titration streptomycin therapy for bilateral Meniere's disease: A preliminary report. Otolaryngol. Head Neck Surg. **92:** 440–447.
42. LANGMAN, A. W., J. L. KEMINK & M. D. GRAHAM. 1990. Titration therapy for bilateral Meniere's disease, follow-up report. Ann. Otol. Rhinol. Laryngol. **99:** 923–926.

43. SCHUKNECHT, H. F. 1957. Ablation therapy in the management of Meniere's disease. Acta Otolaryngol. (Stockholm) **132**(Suppl.): 1–42.

44. LANGE, G. 1978. Isolierte medikamentose Ausschaltung eines Gleichgewichtsorganes beim Morbus Meniere mit Steptomycin-Osothin. Arch. Klin. Exp. Ohren-Nasen-Kehlkopfheilk. **191**: 545.

45. LANGE, G. 1977. Die intratympanale Behandling des Morbus Meniere mit ototoxischen Antibiotika. Laryngol. Rhinol. Otol. **56**: 409.

46. LANGE, G. 1981. Transtympanic treatment for Meniere's disease with gentamicin sulfate. *In* K. H. Vosteen, H. Schuknecht, C. R. Pfaltz, *et al.*, Eds.: 208. Georg Thieme Verlag, Stuttgart.

47. BECK, C. & C. L. SCHMIDT. 1978. Ten years of experience with intratympanally applied streptomycin (gentamicin) in the therapy of Morbus Meniere. Arch. Otorhinolaryngol. **221**: 149.

48. BAGGER-SJOBACK, D., J. BERGENIUS & A.-M. LUNDBERG. 1990. Inner ear effects of topical gentamicin treatment in patients with Meniere's disease. Am. J. Otol **11**(6): 406–410.

49. SHEA, J. J. & C. H. NORRIS. 1989. Streptomycin perfusion of the labyrinth. *In* Proceedings of the Second International Symposium on Meniere's Disease, J. B. Nadol, Ed. Kugler & Ghedini. Amsterdam.

50. MONSELL, E. M., C. SHELTON, P. F. ANTHONY, *et al.* 1992. Labyrinthotomy with streptomycin infusion: Early results of a multicenter study. Am. J. Otol. **13**: 416–442.

51. NORRIS, C. H., A. AUBERT & J. J. SHEA. 1993. Comparison of cochleotoxicity and vestibulotoxicity of streptomycin and gentamicin. *In* Proceedings of the Third International Symposium on Meniere's Disease. Kugler. Dortrecht, The Netherlands. In Press.

Effects of Inflammatory Mediators on Middle Ear Pathology and on Inner Ear Function

S. K. JUHN,[a,d] TIMOTHY T. K. JUNG,[b]
JIZHEN LIN,[a] AND C. K. RHEE[c]

[a]Department of Otolaryngology
University of Minnesota
Lions Research Building
2001 6th Street SE
Minneapolis, Minnesota 55455

[b]Department of Otolaryngology
Loma Linda University
Loma Linda, California 92354

[c]Department of Otolaryngology
Dankook University
College of Medicine
Choongnam, Korea

INTRODUCTION

Inflammatory mediators released in the middle-ear cavity appear to play an important role in the pathogenesis of otitis media (OM) and can cause functional as well as morphological changes in the inner ear. Inflammatory mediators can be defined as biochemical components (peptide, glycoproteins, phospholipids, and others) produced by epithelial cells, infiltrating inflammatory cells, and endothelial cells, which mediate inflammatory reactions in a sequential manner.

In the beginning, the only known target was microcirculation. In the late 1930s, Menkin[1] showed that the accumulation of leukocytes could be explained in terms of mediators. As the number of known mediators has grown, the number of targets has also grown. At the present time, any cell is known to be a fair target of mediators, including epithelial cells, mast cells, fibroblasts, smooth muscles, endothelium, and white cells. As the number of known cell targets has increased, so has the number of possible cell responses, because every cell, when stimulated, will react according to its particular receptors and metabolism. All cells are known to exist in two forms, namely, resting and activated. Activated cells can produce many materials, including new mediators. According to Majno *et al.*,[2] inflammatory mediators represent the basic language of cells. Cells must communicate through chemical messengers, whether they are resting or activated. The reason for so many mediators may be that

[d]Author to whom correspondence should be addressed. Phone: 612/626-9879; fax: 612/626-9871; e-mail: Juhnx001@maroon.tc.umn.edu

inflammation is essential for survival. Mucus production in response to infection may be an initial protective mechanism, preventing viral and bacterial admittance to the epithelial cells. As seen in many pathophysiologic conditions, excessive protective mechanisms can become deleterious. In the case of excessive mucus production in the middle ear, mucocilliary clearance becomes impaired. Thus, continued production of mucous glycoproteins contributes to the pathogenesis of middle-ear disease.

Several inflammatory mediators have been identified in middle-ear effusions (MEEs). Some mediators have specific effects on the secretion of mucous glycoproteins in cultured middle-ear epithelial cells *in vitro*. Several inhibitors are known to cause middle-ear inflammation. Some mediators can penetrate the round-window membrane and cause inner-ear dysfunction and even morphological damage. Therefore, inflammatory mediators play a significant role in middle-ear and inner-ear pathology, and further understanding of their roles may facilitate advancement toward the prevention of middle- and inner-ear disorders.

INFLAMMATORY MEDIATORS IN MIDDLE-EAR EFFUSIONS

The composition of MEE reflects the inflammatory events taking place in the middle-ear cavity. Many inflammatory mediators have been identified and quantified in MEE.

Histamine, a potent pharmacologic mediator of inflammation generally derived from mast cells, can increase vascular permeability. Histamine has been detected in most MEEs, and appears to be produced by mast cells in the middle-ear cavity that have been stimulated by nonallergic stimuli such as immune complexes.[3] Chonmaitree *et al.*[4] reported that histamine content in MEE was higher in bacteria-positive than in bacteria-negative fluid, and was higher in samples from patients with viral infections than in those without viral infection.

The ability of the middle-ear mucosa and cultured epithelial cells to convert arachidonic acid to PGE_2, 6-keto-PGF1α, and PGD_2 has been reported.[5,6] Various metabolites of arachidonic acid (AA) have been found in human MEE and in the MEE of animals with experimentally produced otitis media.[7–9] Arachidonic acid metabolism through two pathways is shown in FIGURE 1. In human MEE, higher levels of prostaglandins (PGs) and leukotrienes (LTs) were found in purulent MEE than in serous or mucoid effusion. Concentrations of LTB_4 and LTE_4 were observed to be higher in culture-positive than culture-negative effusions. It has been inferred from animal experiments that metabolites produced in the lipoxygenase pathway play a more important role in the pathogenesis of OM than metabolites produced in the cyclooxygenase pathway.[9] It has also been suggested that LTC_4 and LTD_4 are involved in the damage in the mucociliary transport system and in the production of MEE in the middle-ear cavity.[10,11] In animal studies, topical application of several inflammatory mediators (histamine, LTC_4, LTD_4, and PAF) on the eustachian tube caused a rapid increase of tubal resistance and opening pressure.[11] Eicosanoids and PAF have also been shown to affect the ciliary clearance of the eustachian tube.[10–12]

Cytokines are proteins that mediate immunologic, physiologic, and metabolic changes associated with inflammation and the host defense system. Platelet-activating factor (PAF), a low-molecular-weight phospholipid, is a strong mediator of in-

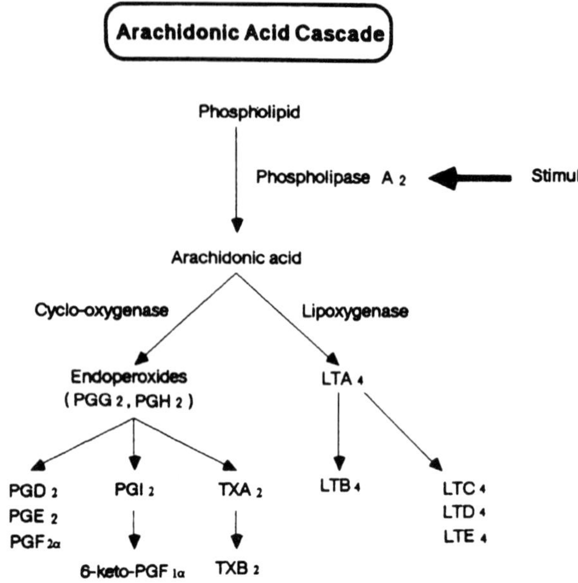

FIGURE 1. Arachidonic acid metabolism demonstrating the production of prostaglandins, thromboxane, and leukotrienes.

flammation. This potent chemotactic factor is produced by a variety of cells and has been found in MEE.[13,14] Intratympanic administration of PAF caused reduced ciliary activity and prolonged the mucociliary clearance time of the tubotympanum. Presence of a MEE was reported 3–6 days after PAF administration. Intrabullar injection of PGE_2, LTB_4, AA, LTC_4, or PAF alone caused inflammation in middle-ear mucosa and induced MEE in chinchillas.[9,15]

The polypeptide cytokines, interleukin-1 (IL-1), and tumor necrosis factor (TNF) affect nearly every tissue and organ system, including the middle ear. IL-1 and TNF are key mediators of biologic responses to bacterial lipopolysaccharide (LPS), infection, and inflammatory stimulants. Catanzaro et al.[16] reported the production of middle-ear effusion in guinea pigs by transtympanic injection of IL-1, IL-2, and TNF. Recently, several cytokines (IL-1, IL-2, IL-6, IL-8, TNF, and interferon) have been identified in MEE.[17–20] Although interactions between cytokines exist, and higher levels tend to be found in purulent MEE than in other types of effusion, the significance of these differences is not known. One example showing the difference of mediators in different types of effusions is shown in TABLE 1.[21]

Higher levels of cytokines have been reported in younger age groups than in older ones.[17,18,22] Since numerous developmental changes occur in the immune system throughout childhood, maturational changes may play a role in the differences in cytokine levels in these age groups.

TABLE 1. Levels of Biochemical Parameters in Different Types of Middle-ear Effusion

	Effusion Type		
Mediator	Purulent ($N = 13$)	Mucoid ($N = 39$)	Serous ($N = 18$)
Collagenase (μg/mg TP)	40.41 ± 10.88	13.98 ± 2.68	15.92 ± 3.58
IL-1β (pg/mg TP)	176.82 ± 81.72	29.84 ± 7.19	8.08 ± 3.35
TNFα (pg/mg TP)	29.38 ± 10.17	11.02 ± 3.10	6.62 ± 2.32

Data are mean $\pm$ SEM; quantity per milligrams of total protein (TP).

EFFECT OF INFLAMMATORY MEDIATORS ON THE SECRETION OF MUCUS GLYCOPROTEINS FROM THE CULTURED EPITHELIAL CELLS

Hypersecretion from middle-ear secretory epithelium together with an increase in mucus glycoproteins appears to play an important role in the pathogenesis of OM and in delayed resolution of inflammatory changes within the middle-ear cavity. Increased mucus in the middle-ear cavity increases viscoelasticity of the MEE and impairs mucociliary clearance in the middle ear and eustachian tube.

In an attempt to characterize the role of inflammatory mediators on the secretion of mucus glycoproteins from the cultured middle-ear epithelial cells, middle-ear epithelial cells have been successfully cultured from rats and chinchillas.[23,24] Interleukin-1β (IL-1β), PAF, TNFα, and arachidonic acid metabolites have been shown to stimulate mucus glycoprotein (MGP) production and secretion.[25,26] At a concentration of 100 mM, PAF significantly stimulated MGP secretion (FIG. 2). When PAF receptor inhibitor, WEB2170Bs, was applied, it significantly inhibited the PAF-stimulated MGP secretion (FIG. 3). It did not, however, affect MGP secretion stimulated by IL-1β. This finding suggests that WEB2170BS specifically inhibits PAF-stimulated MGP secretion.[27] Lin *et al.*[28] reported that the stimulatory effect of TNF-α on MGP secretion was attenuated by addition of TNF-α monoclonal antibody. These findings suggest the possibility that application of MGP inhibitors or antibodies may reduce hypersecretion of MGP.

ROUND-WINDOW MEMBRANE PERMEABILITY

The round-window membrane (RWM) is the only soft-tissue structure separating the middle ear from the inner ear. It consists of an outer layer, middle layer, and inner layer. The outer layer is made up of epithelial cells contiguous with the mucus membrane of the promontory, and a subepithelial connective-tissue layer that lies between the epithelial layer and the middle layer. Blood vessels and nerve fibers are found

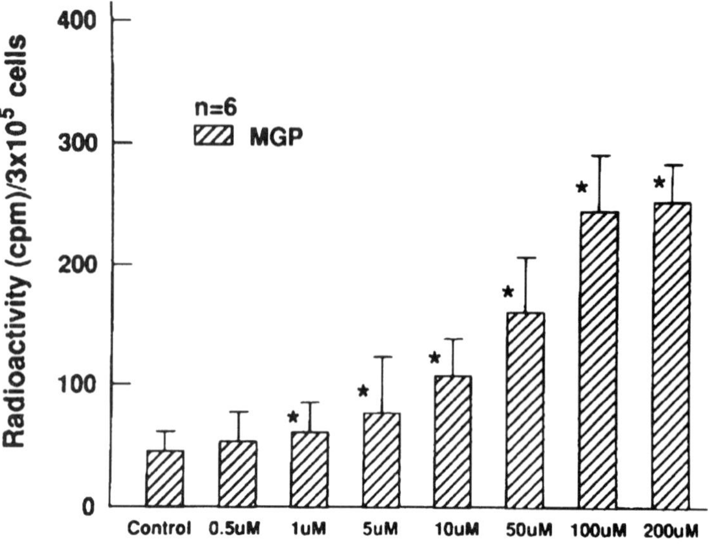

FIGURE 2. Effect of PAF on secretion of mucous glycoprotein by chinchilla middle-ear epithelial cells over a 2-h period. A gradual increase was seen with increased concentrations of PAF from 0.5 to 200 μm, demonstrating stimulated mucous glycoprotein secretion in a concentration-dependent manner.

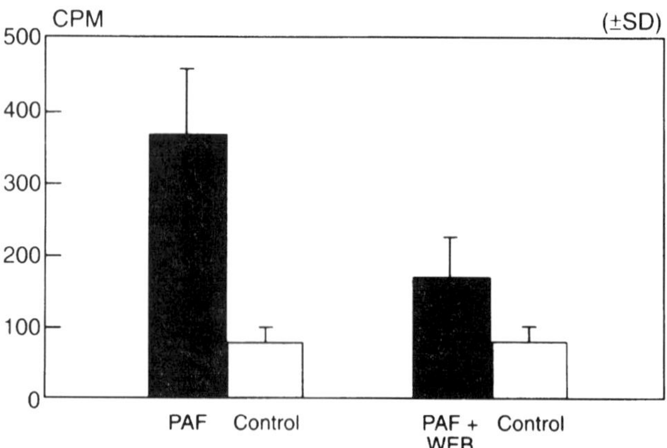

FIGURE 3. WEB 2170 BS at a concentration of 2000 μm significantly inhibited PAF-stimulated MGP secretion (PAF vs. PAF + WEB, $p < 0.05$).

within this layer. The middle layer lies between the subepithelial connective-tissue layer and the inner layer. It is connective tissue consisting mainly of fibroblasts, collagen, and elastic fibers. The inner layer is basically a continuation of the mesothelial cells lining the scala tympani of the cochlea. The cell junctions are usually loose and the intercellular spaces are wide.[29]

Permeability of the RWM to various substances is an area of research important to understanding of inner-ear pathology and sensorineural hearing loss associated with OM or administration of ototopic drugs. Past studies on the permeability of the RWM are summarized in FIGURES 4 and 5. This middle-ear–inner-ear barrier is quite permeable to most substances. Even macromolecular proteins can pass through the membrane by pinocytosis (FIG. 4).[30–32]

An increase in RWM permeability has been observed in experimental OM, possibly due to degenerative changes in the epithelial layer of the membrane.[33] Harris and Ryan[34] observed an increase of antikeyhole limpet hemocyanin (KLH) in perilymph after the middle-ear cavity was challenged with KLH. They discussed the possibility of diffusion of antibody from the middle ear through the RWM, and local production of antibody within the inner ear by antigen diffused across the RWM. An increase in permeability to human serum albumin (HSA) has been observed in antigen-induced OM by measuring HSA levels in the perilymph. Transport of HSA into perilymph was reduced when triamicinolone, an anti-inflammatory agent, was applied. This action may be due to suppression of antigen-induced OM by the corticosteroid.[35]

Transient functional changes measured by auditory brainstem recording were noted after repeated application of hyaluronic acid in the middle-ear cavity.[36] A decrease in perilymph osmolality was observed when diluted Healon was instilled into the middle-ear cavity, suggesting the possibility of alteration of perilymph osmotic pressure via the middle ear cavity and RWM.[31]

Endotoxin has been found in the inner ear after application to the middle ear.[37,38] Staphylococcal pyrogenic exotoxin has been reported to pass through the RWM into

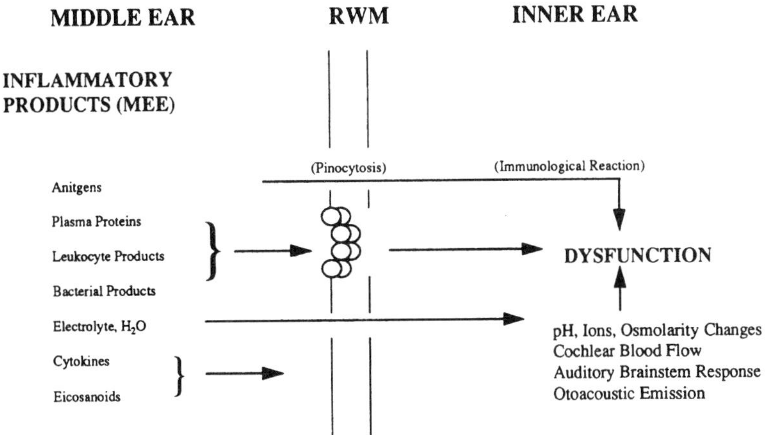

FIGURE 4. Possible factors from the middle ear responsible for inner-ear dysfunction.

the inner ear.[39] Passage of *Pseudomonas aeruginosa* exotoxin into the perilymph through the RWM has been observed to cause substantial hair-cell loss at a concentration of 50 ng/mL.[40]

EFFECTS OF INFLAMMATORY MEDIATORS ON COCHLEAR FUNCTION

Among those diseases attributable to interaction between the middle and inner ear, sensorineural hearing loss (SNHL) induced by OM is one of the more frequently seen entities.[41] However, the mechanisms of SNHL associated with OM are not well understood. Bacterial infections, endotoxins, inflammatory products, and immune responses have been suggested as factors involved in SNHL in OM.[42–44] Many substances involved in middle-ear inflammation have been shown to enter into the inner-ear space through the RWM.[39,43,45] Inflammatory mediators produced in the middle-ear cavity following middle-ear inflammation may be responsible for hearing loss. They are known to increase vascular permeability and secretory activity of the middle-ear mucosa, and to remain in the middle-ear cavity during the period of middle-ear inflammation. Among the inflammatory mediators detected in MEE, prostaglandins, leukotrienes, and PAF appear to be important in the pathogenesis of OM with effusion (OME).[13] Local effects of PAF and PAF-receptor antagonists on the guinea pig inner ear have been reported.[46,47] Gloddeck *et al.*[48] reported an elevation of interleukin-2 (IL-2) in MEE and a perilymph-marked decrease of auditory-evoked potential and increase of latency time three days after the immunological challenge of middle ear with KLH.

Attempts have been made to investigate the effects of inflammation mediators on cochlear function after application on the RWM.[49] Small pieces of Gelfoam soaked in various concentrations of PGE_2, LTC_4, and PAF in 5 μL of normal saline each, and Gelfoam soaked in 5 μL of saline as a control were applied to the RWM. Half of the animals treated with LTC_4 were pretreated with 2 mg/kg of LT blocker given orally. Skin incisions were closed, and Gelfoam was left in place for various time intervals and then removed. Auditory brain stem response (ABR), transient evoked otoacoustic emissions (TEOAEs), and cochlear blood flow (CoBF) were then measured. In the PGE_2 group, 5-dB hearing loss was recorded and returned to 0 dB within 2 h, while LTC_4 caused an elevation in ABR ranging from 10 dB to 33 dB during the 8-h experiment and peaked (33 dB) at 1 h after the application (FIG. 5). The group treated with 200 ng of PAF developed a 28.3-dB hearing loss after 4 and 8 h, and total hearing loss after 24 h. There was no evidence of recovery of hearing loss within 96 h in any of the experimental groups. The saline control group showed no sign of hearing loss. CoBF changes after application of saline, PGF_2, LTC_4, and PAF to the RWM were compared to the initial pretest value (100%). No significant changes in CoBF was observed in the saline control group. In the PGE_2 group, a significant increase in CoBF both at 120 min and 150 min after application was observed. On the other hand, a significant decrease in CoBF was observed at 90, 120, and 150 min after the application in LTC_4 group (FIG. 6). In the PAF group, there was a slight increase in CoBF at one half hour, followed by a 30% decrease after 6 h.

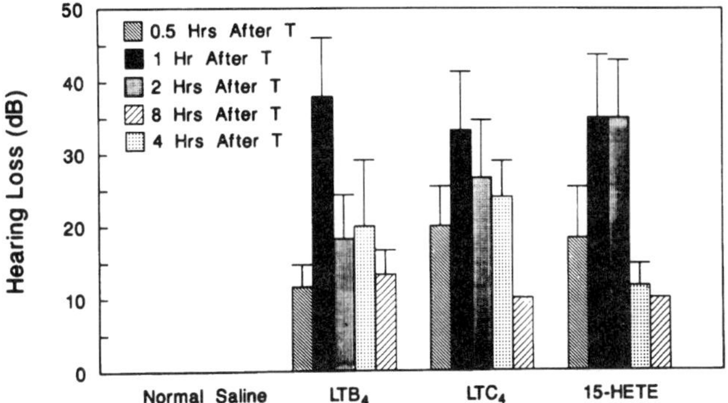

FIGURE 5. ABR thresholds (dB SPL) after application of normal saline, LTB$_4$, LTC$_4$, and HETE at 0.5, 1, 2, 4, and 8 h.

After obtaining highly reproducible and stable TEOAEs in chinchillas, the data on various experimental groups were compared. In the PGE$_2$ group there was no significant drop in the mean response below the baseline response, while the best frequency response significantly decreased. In the LTC$_4$ group there was a decrease in mean response below the baseline response. In those animals pretreated with LT blockers, no significant drop below the baseline response was observed. The best frequency response after application of LTC$_4$ significantly decreased, peaking at 6 h. In the PAF group, there was a decrease in mean response, and the best frequency response also dropped significantly.

The effects of inflammatory mediators on ABR can be summarized as follows: minimal hearing loss in the PGE$_2$ group; moderate and reversible hearing loss in the LTC$_4$ group; and moderate to profound irreversible hearing loss in the PAF group.

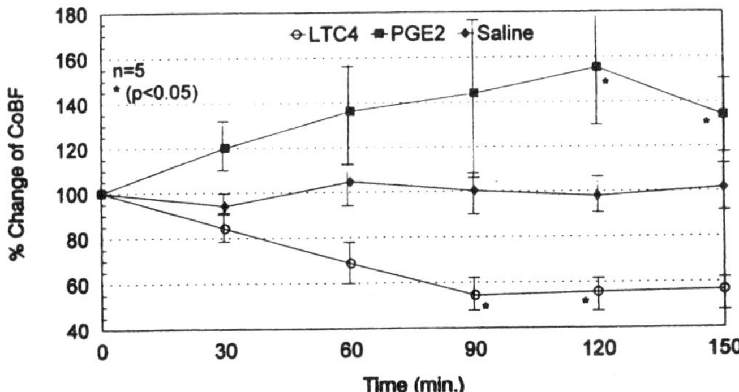

FIGURE 6. CoBF changes with time after application of PGE$_2$, LTC$_4$, and saline on the RWM.

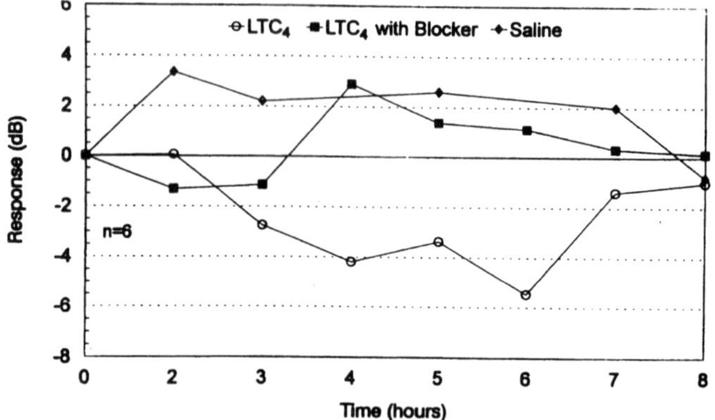

FIGURE 7. Mean response (FIG. 6) and best frequency (FIG. 7) of TEOAEs following RWM application of saline or LTC₄ with or without LT-blocker (Sch 3724).

Based on this information, it seems quite possible that inflammatory mediators like PAF in the MEE of chronic OM can induce sensorineural hearing loss. LTC_4 may induce transient hearing loss. In previous studies, it was observed that ototoxic doses of salicylate either systemically or by application to the RWM decreased PG levels and increased LT levels in perilymph. Decreased cochlear blood flow has been suggested as a possible cause of sudden hearing loss, presbycusis, noise trauma, and salicylate ototoxicity. Since PGE_2 is a known vasodilator and LTC_4 a vasoconstrictor, it is interesting to observe the blood-flow changes after application of these vasoactive compounds. However, the reduction in CoBF observed after the application of LTC_4 and PAF may be one of the many factors responsible for hearing loss secondary to OM.

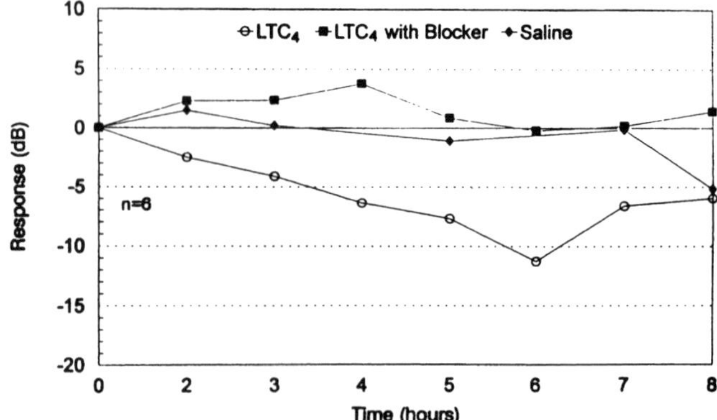

FIGURE 8. Mean response (FIG. 6) and best frequency (FIG. 8) of TEOAEs following RWM application of saline or LTC₄ with or without LT-blocker (Sch 3724).

TEOAEs are known to reflect an active response of the cochlea to a sound stimulation. The response of the TEOAEs is believed to be produced and transmitted by the outer hair cells. Application of PGE_2, LTC_4, or PAF to the RWM all resulted in a significant decreases in TEOAEs, most significantly with PAF, followed by LTC_4 and PGE_2, suggesting that more outer hair cells were damaged by PAF treatment than with LTC_4 or PGE_2. Mean response and best frequency of TEOAEs following RWM application of LTC_4 with or without LT-blocker (Sch 37224) are shown in FIGURES 7 and 8. It is interesting to observe the effect of LT-blocker on the TEOAEs. These findings provide certain possibilities for ameliorating the inner ear disorders caused by toxic substances when underlying pathology is identified and mechanisms of disorders are clarified.

CONCLUSION

Knowledge about inflammatory mediators has increased tremendously in the last few years. These ubiquitous agents probably have an effect on all cells and systems of the body, and their role in middle-ear disease is just now being studied. It has been shown that inflammatory mediators are present in the middle-ear cavity during inflammation, and are most prevalent during purulent infection. These inflammatory mediators have an effect on middle-ear inflammation, chemotaxis, vascular permeability, production of mediators, and synthesis and secretion of mucous glycoproteins. The RWM is permeable to many substances, including inflammatory mediators during infections. The round window pathway is the mechanism by which middle-ear inflammation can affect inner-ear function, as shown by auditory brain-stem response, cochlear microphonics, otoacoustic emissions, and cochlear blood flow.

These are complex relationships. Studies have shown that application of inhibitors or blockers of inflammatory mediators can reduce middle-ear inflammation or inner-ear dysfunction. The initial response caused by the inflammatory mediators is very likely protective. The challenge will be to determine at which point the inflammatory response can, and should, be abrogated. Success in this endeavor will hopefully prevent the middle ear and inner ear disorders caused by inflammatory mediators.

REFERENCES

1. MENKIN, V. 1938. Studies on inflammation. SV. Concerning the mechanism of cell migration. J. Exper. Med. **67:** 145–146.
2. MAJNO, G., G. A. HIGGS & T. J. WILLIAMS, Eds. 1989. Inflammatory mediators: Where are they going? *In* Inflammatory Mediators: 1–6. VCH.
3. BERGER, G., M. HAWKE, D. W. PROOPS, N. S. RANADIVE & D. WONG. 1984. Histamine levels in middle ear effusions. Acta Otolaryngol. (Stockholm) **98:** 385–390.
4. CHONMAITREE, T., J. A. PATEL, M. A. LETT-BROWN, T. UCHIDA, R. GAROFALO, M. J. OWEN & V. M. HOWIE. 1994. Virus and bacteria enhance histamine production in middle ear fluids of children with acute otitis media. J. Infect. Dis. **169:** 1265–1270.
5. SMITH, D. M., T. T. K. JUNG & S. K. JUHN. 1979. Prostaglandins in experimental otitis media. Arch Otolaryngol. **225:** 207–209.
6. HARADA, T., S. K. JUHN, Y. KIM & Y. SAKAKURA. 1993. Arachidonic acid metabolism by

isolated and cultured middle ear epithelial cells from the chinchilla. Eur. Arch. Otorhinolaryngol. **250:** 220–223.

7. BERNSTEIN, J. M., T. OKAZAKI & R. E. REISMAN. 1976. Prostaglandins in middle ear effusion. Arch. Otolaryngol. **102:** 257–258.

8. JUNG, T. T. K. 1988. Prostaglandins, leukotrienes and other arachidonic acid metabolites in the pathogenesis of otitis media. Laryngoscope **98:** 980–993.

9. JUNG, T. T. K., Y. M. PARK & D. SCHLUND. 1990. Effect of prostaglandin, leukotriene, and arachidonic acid on experimental otitis media with effusion in chinchillas. Ann. Otol. Rhinol. Laryngol. **99:** 28–32.

10. GAMBO, T., S. SHIMOMURA, S. HORIGUCHI, I. NOZAWA & K. HISAMATSU. 1994. The effect of leukotriene C4, D4 and prostaglandin E2 on cillary clearance of the eustachian tube. *In* Recent Advances in Otitis Media (Proc. 2nd Extraordinary Int. Symp.), G. Mogi *et al.*, Eds.: 667–669. Kugler. Amsterdam.

11. MINAMI, T., N. KUBO, K. TOMODA & T. KUMAZAWA. 1992. Effects of various inflammatory mediators on eustachian tube patency. Acta Otolaryngol. (Stockholm) **112:** 680–685.

12. SUGIURA, Y., Y. OHASHI, Y. OHNO, H. OKAMOTO, A. TANAKA & Y. NAKAI. 1994. The influence of platelet activating factor on the mucocilliary system of the tubotympanum. *In* Recent Advances in Otitis Media (Proc. 2nd Extraordinary Int. Symp.), G. Mogi *et al.*, Eds.: 687–694. Kugler. Amsterdam.

13. JUNG, T. T. K., C. K. RHEE, J. A. HEEINRICH, S. J. HWANG & D. J. TAMBUNAN. 1993. Profile of arachidonic acid metabolites and platelet activation factor in human middle ear effusion. *In* Recent Advances in Otitis Media (Proc. 5th Int. Symp.), D. J. Lim, C. D. Bluestone, J. O. Klein, J. D. Nelson, and P. L. Ogra, Eds.: 415–419. Decker Periodicals. Ont., Canada.

14. TACHIBANA, F., T. SHIMADA, Y. HORI, Y. WADA, Y. ISHITANI & Y. KOIKE. 1996. Platelet-activating factor and leukotrienes in acute otitis media, secretory otitis media and chronic otitis media on the acute excerbation. Auris Nasus Larynx (Tokyo) **23:** 20–25.

15. RHEE, C., T. T. K. JUNG, S. MILLER & D. WEEKS. 1993. Experimental otitis media with effusion induced by platelet activating factor. Ann. Otol. Rhinol. Laryngol. **102:** 600–605.

16. CATANZARO, A., A. RYAN, S. BATCHER & S. I. WASSERMAN. 1991. The response to human rIL-1, rIL-2, and rTNF in the middle ear of guinea pigs. Layrngoscope **101:** 271–275.

17. JUHN, S. K., C. T. TOLAN, W. J. GARVIS, D. S. CROSS & G. S. GIEBINK. 1992. The levels of IL-1β in human middle ear effusions. Acta Otolaryngol. (Stockholm) **493**(Suppl.): 37–42.

18. YELLON, R. F., G. LEONARD, P. MARUCHA, J. SIDMAN, R. CARPENTER, J. BURELSON, J. CAARLSON & D. KREUTZER. 1992. Demonstration of interleukin 6 in middle ear effustions. Arch. Otolaryngol. Head Neck Surg. **118:** 745–748.

19. JOHNSON, M. D., J. E. FITZGERALD, G. LEONARD, J. A. BURLESON & D. L. KREUTZER. 1994. Cytokines in experimental otitis media with effusion. Laryngoscope **104:** 191–196.

20. HOTOMI, M., T. SAMAKAWA & N. YAMANAKA. 1994. Interleukin-8 in otitis media with effusion. Acta Otolaryngol. (Stockholm). **114:** 406–409.

21. JUHN, S. K., W. J. GARVIS, C. LEES, C. T. LE & C. S. KIM. 1994. Determining otitis media severity from middle ear fluid analysis. Ann. Otol. Rhin. Laryngol. **103**(5) (Pt. 2, Suppl. 163): 43–45.

22. YELLON, R. F., L. GERALD & P. T. MARUCHA. 1991. Characterization of cytokines present in middle ear effusions. Laryngoscope **101:** 105–109.

23. VAN BLITTERSWIJK, C., M. PONEC, G. N. P. VAN MUIJEN, M. C. WIJSMAN, H. K. KOERTEN & J. J. GROTE. 1986. Culture and characterization of rat middle-ear epithelium. Acta Otolaryngol. (Stockholm) **101:** 453–466.

24. AMESARA, R., Y. KIM, S. SANO, T. HARADA & S. K. JUHN. 1992. Primary culture of middle ear epithelial cells from chinchilla. Eur. Arch. Otorhinolaryngol. **249:** 164–167.

25. AMESARA, R., Y. KIM & S. K. JUHN. 1993. Effects of arachidonic acid metabolites on mucous glycoprotein production in middle ear epithelial cell culture. *In* Recent Advances in Otitis Media (Proc. 5th Int. Symp.), D. J. Lim, C. D. Bluestone, J. O. Klein, J. D. Nelson, and P. L. Ogra, Eds.: 411–413. Decker Periodicals. Ont., Canada.

26. LIN, J., Y. KIM, C. LEES & S. K. JUHN. 1995. Effect of platelet-activating factor on secretion of mucous glycoprotein from chinchilla middle ear epithelial cells in vitro. Eur. Arch. Otorhinolaryngol. **252:** 92–96.

27. LIN, J., Y. KIM, C. LEES & S. K. JUHN. 1996. Effects of platelet-activating factor (PAF) receptor blockage on mucous glycoprotein secretion in cultured chinchilla middle ear epithelium. Acta Otolaryngol. (Stockholm) **116:** 69–73.

28. LIN, J., Y. KIM & S. K. JUHN. 1997. TNF-α increases mucous glycoprotein secretion via a protein kinase C-dependent mechanism in cultured chinchilla middle ear epithelial cells. Ann. Otol. Rhinol. Laryngol. In press.

29. HELLSTROM, S., U. JOHANSSON & M. ANNIKO. 1988. Structure of the round window membrane. Acta Otolaryngol. (Stockholm) **457** (Suppl.): 33–42.

30. NOMURA, Y. 1984. Otological significance of the round window. *In* Advances in Oto-rhinolaryngology, Vol. 33, C. R. Pfaltz, Ed.: 63–72. Karger. New York.

31. JUHN, S. K., Y. HAMAGUCHI & M. GOYCOOLEA. 1988. Review of round window membrane permeability. Acta Otolaryngol. (Stockholm) **457** (Suppl.): 43–48.

32. OKUNO, T. & Y. NOMURA. 1984. Permeability of the round window membrane. Arch. Otorhinolaryngol. **240:** 103–106.

33. GOYCOOLEA, M. V., M. M. PAPARELLA, B. GOLDBERG & A. M. CARPENTER. 1980. Permeability of the round window membrane in otitis media. Arch. Otolaryngol. **106:** 430–433.

34. HARRIS, J. P. & A. F. RYAN. 1985. Effect of middle ear immune response on inner ear antibody levels. Ann. Otol. **94:** 202–206.

35. HAMAGUCHI, Y., T. MORIZONO & S. K. JUHN. 1988. Round window membrane permeability to human serum albumin in antigen-induced otitis media. Am. J. Otolaryngol. **8:** 34–40.

36. LAURENT, C., S. HELLSTROM & M. ANNIKO. 1988. Inner ear effects of exogenous hyaluronan in the middle ear of the rat. Acta Otolaryngol. (Stockholm) **105:** 273–280.

37. KAWAUCHI, H., T. F. DEMARIA & D. J. LIM. 1988. Endotoxin permeability through the round window. Acta Otolaryngol. (Stockholm) **457** (Suppl.): 100–115.

38. SPANDOW, O., M. ANNIKO & S. HELLSTROM. 1989. Inner ear disturbances following inoculation of endotoxin into the middle ear. Acta Otolaryngol. (Stockholm) **107:** 90–96.

39. GOYCOOLEA, M. V., M. M. PAPARELLA, B. GOLDBERG, *et al.* 1980. Permeability of the middle ear to staphylococcal pyogenic exotoxin in otitis media. Int. J. Pediat. Otorhinolaryngol. **1:** 301–308.

40. LUNDMAN, L., P. A. SANTI, T. MORIZONO, T. HARADA, S. K. JUHN & D. BAGGER-SJOBACK. 1992. Inner ear damage and passage through the round window membrane of *Pseudomonas aeruginosa* exotoxin in a chinchilla model. Ann. Otol. Rhinol. Laryngol. **101:** 437–444.

41. PAPARELLA, M. M., P. A. SCHACHERN & T. H. YOON. 1988. Survey of interactions between the middle ear and inner ear. Acta Otolaryngol. (Stockholm), **457** (Suppl.): 9–24.

42. MORIZONO, T., G. S. GIEBINK, M. M. PAPARELLA, M. A. SIKORA & D. SHEA. 1985. Sensorineural hearing loss in experimental purulent otitis media due to *Streptococcus pneumoniae*. Arch. Otolaryngol. **111:** 794–798.

43. SUZUKI, M., H. KAWAUCHI, T. FUJIYOSHI & G. MOGI. 1989. Round window membrane and perilymph in experimental otitis media with effusion. Ann. Otol. Rhinol. Laryngol. **98:** 980–987.

44. MORIZONO, T. & T. TONO. 1991. Middle ear inflammatory mediators and cochlear function. Otolaryngol. Clin. N. Am. **24:** 835–843.

45. LEE, S. H., H. Y. WOO, T. T. K. JUNG, C. LEE, S. K. MILLER, Y. M. PARK & S. K. HWANG.

1992. Permeability of arachidonic acid metabolites through the round window membrane in chinchillas. Acta Otolaryngol. (Stockholm) **493** (Suppl.): 165–169.

46. ERNST, A., J. SYKA, A. RIEDEL & H. J. MEST. 1989. Local effects of PAF in guinea-pig inner ear. J. Lipid Mediators **1:** 297–301.

47. ERNST, A. & H. O. HEUER. 1991. PAF receptor antagonists influence asphyxia-induced changes of the inner ear. J. Lipid Mediators **4:** 327–332.

48. GLODDECK, B., K. LAMM & K. HASLOV. 1992. Influence of middle ear immune response on the immunologic state and function of the inner ear. Laryngoscope **102:** 177–181.

49. JUNG, T. T. K., C. K. RHEE, D. K. CHOI, J. ARRUDA, Y. S. PARK & D. WEEKS. 1996. Effects of inflammatory mediators in middle ear effusions on cochlear function. Recent Advances in Otitis Media. In press.

Role of Viruses in Middle-ear Disease[a]

TASNEE CHONMAITREE[b] AND TERHO HEIKKINEN

Department of Pediatrics
Division of Infectious Diseases
University of Texas Medical Branch
Galveston, Texas 77555-0371

INTRODUCTION

Acute otitis media (AOM) is generally considered a bacterial infection because pathogenic bacteria can be isolated from the middle-ear effusion (MEE) in approximately 70% of cases of AOM.[1,2] In clinical practice, patients diagnosed with AOM are usually treated with antibiotics. However, a substantial proportion of AOM cases do not have a proven bacterial etiology. This fact, together with extensive clinical experience connecting AOM with viral respiratory tract infections, has led investigators to search for the role of viruses in AOM.

To date, ample evidence supports a crucial role for respiratory viruses in the etiopathogenesis of AOM. This evidence is derived from numerous studies ranging from animal experiments to clinical and epidemiologic studies in children. Viruses not only play a role in the etiology and pathogenesis of AOM, but they may also have profound effects on the outcome of this disease. These findings have prompted intense research on viral–bacterial interactions, because a better understanding of these mechanisms might lead to innovative strategies to improve treatment of otitis media (OM).

ASSOCIATION OF VIRAL RESPIRATORY INFECTION WITH ACUTE OTITIS MEDIA: EPIDEMIOLOGIC STUDIES

Clinical experience indicates that AOM is closely associated with viral respiratory infections. Otitis media usually occurs concurrently with, or just after, a viral upper respiratory-tract infection (URI), and the peak incidence of the disease coincides with the age when viral infections are prevalent. The incidence of AOM is also notably higher during the winter respiratory viral season than in the summer.[3] Further, day-care attendance, which significantly increases the frequency of respiratory-tract infections in children, is also a major risk factor for AOM.[4,5]

The important association between viral respiratory infection and the occurrence of AOM was first reported in 1982 in an extensive 14-year study among children in day care.[6] Viral infections were shown to increase the risk of AOM even more than

[a]This work is supported in part by Research Grant 1 R01 DC 02620-01 from the National Institute of Deafness and Other Communication Disorders, National Institutes of Health.

[b]Author to whom correspondence should be addressed. Phone: 409/772-2798; fax: 409/747-1753.

did colonization of the nasopharynx with *Streptococcus pneumoniae* or *Haemophilus influenzae*. In a subsequent study, viral cultures obtained on the day of, or within the 14 days preceding, the diagnosis of AOM were positive in 43% of all the episodes of AOM.[7] The tight association between viral respiratory infections and AOM was further confirmed in a large hospital-based study, which showed a significant correlation between the monthly occurrence of AOM and recovery of respiratory viruses from nasopharyngeal specimens of children.[3]

Concurrent respiratory virus infection has been documented in nasopharyngeal specimens of 30 to 50% of children with AOM.[8–14] It is obvious that limitations in currently available techniques result in underdetection of viruses in nasopharyngeal specimens. In a study of 363 children with AOM, only 42% of the patients showed evidence of viral infection in nasopharyngeal specimens, even though clinical symptoms clearly indicating a viral URI were observed in 94% of these children at the time of the diagnosis of AOM.[13]

Although AOM can be considered a complication of a viral URI, types of respiratory viruses may vary in their ability to predispose to AOM. For example, a large clinical study showed that AOM was diagnosed in 57% of children with respiratory syncytial virus (RSV) infection, but in only 10% of children with parainfluenza virus type 2 infection.[3] Yet the relative ability of different respiratory viruses to predispose the subject to AOM is difficult to determine because the development of AOM depends on multiple factors. In particular, the age of the child is an important confounding factor that has not been controlled in many studies. However, some studies that did control for child age have reported that RSV, and especially RSV group B, may be the type of virus most likely to predispose a child to AOM.[15,16]

CONTRIBUTION OF VIRUSES TO THE PATHOGENESIS OF OTITIS MEDIA

Animal Studies

Although results obtained in animal studies should be extrapolated cautiously to humans, animal experiments have provided valuable information on viral contribution to the pathogenesis of OM because they allow strict control over the multiple factors of the disease process. The majority of this work has been carried out in chinchillas. In one of the first studies, conducted in the early 1980s, OM developed in 67% of chinchillas inoculated intranasally with both influenza A virus and *S. pneumoniae*, compared with only 4% of animals inoculated with influenza A virus alone, and 21% of animals inoculated with *S. pneumoniae* alone.[17] Further, intranasal inoculation with influenza A virus induced negative middle-ear pressure and polymorphonuclear leukocyte (PMN) dysfunction, which were not observed after inoculation with *S. pneumoniae* alone.[18] The highest incidence of pneumococcal OM occurred when the bacteria were inoculated 4 days after the virus, that is, just before the time of the virus-induced PMN dysfunction. A further histopathologic study demonstrated epithelial damage in the eustachian tube (ET), and accumulation of cellular and mucous debris in the tubal lumen in association with the development of negative middle-ear pressure during experimental influenza A virus infection.[19]

Recently, a synergistic effect of adenovirus type 1 and nontypeable *H. influenzae* was reported in chinchillas.[20] While the study demonstrated that all animals inoculated intranasally with both pathogens developed OM of greater severity than animals receiving either pathogen alone, the most severe and prolonged episodes of OM were induced by initial inoculation with adenovirus, followed 7 days later by inoculation with *H. influenzae*. However, a similar synergy was not observed in a subsequent experiment using adenovirus type 1 and *Moraxella catarrhalis*.[21]

Direct inoculation of adenovirus type 1 into the middle ears of chinchillas caused severe tympanic membrane inflammation within 48 h of the inoculation.[22] Similarly, inoculation of influenza A virus into the middle ear of chinchillas resulted in capillary engorgement, subepithelial hemorrhage, tissue edema and inflammatory cell infiltration within 1 to 2 days.[23] The greatest damage in the ET occurred in ciliated epithelial cells; restoration of the mucosal architecture was not seen until 28 days postinoculation. In studies of chinchillas, guinea pigs, and ferrets, impairment of both ET transport function and ciliary activity of ET mucosal epithelium has been shown after inoculation of influenza A virus or adenovirus type 1, either intranasally or directly into the middle ear.[22,24–26] In guinea pigs, inoculation with influenza A virus and endotoxin together induced epithelial cell injury, mucociliary dysfunction, and MEE, while neither the virus nor the endotoxin alone produced these effects.[27]

In addition to their direct effects on the ET and middle-ear epithelium, viruses may also affect bacterial colonization of the nasopharynx. A study in cotton rats showed that colonization with nontypeable *H. influenzae* increased significantly within 4 days of RSV infection.[28] Data on the effect of viruses on bacterial adherence to epithelial cells of animals are controversial. While studies in cotton rats and epithelial cells from chinchillas documented no virus-induced augmentation of bacterial adhesion, a study in ferrets inoculated with influenza A virus showed a significant increase in bacterial adherence to the respiratory mucosa.[28–30] These animal experiments clearly suggest that, by various mechanisms, viruses predispose the middle ear to bacterial infection.

Human Studies

Eustachian-tube Function during Viral Respiratory-tract Infection

Dysfunction of the ET is considered the most important factor in the pathogenesis of AOM. This abnormal function results in (1) impairment of pressure equilibration between the nasopharynx and the middle ear; (2) loss of protective function of the ET; and (3) impairment of clearance function of the ET.[31] There is strong evidence supporting a causal role for respiratory viruses in the disruption of normal ET function. Deterioration of tubal function in children with URI has been well documented.[32–34] Among preschool children, significant middle-ear underpressure developed in 75% of URIs.[33] Most of the abnormalities were detectable by the second day of illness; an interesting finding, considering that a clinical study among children aged 1 to 4 years showed that the peak incidence of AOM was on day 3 after the onset of symptoms of URI.[35]

Most data on ET dysfunction during URIs in humans have come from experimental studies carried out in adult volunteers. A marked impairment of tubal function and development of middle-ear underpressure have been observed after intranasal challenge with rhinovirus and influenza A virus.[36–39] Similar alterations occurred during natural rhinovirus infections.[40] In these studies, the most profound middle-ear underpressures developed by days 2–5 after viral infection. Furthermore, even though the subjects were adults, some developed AOM.[37–39]

Virus-induced Alteration of Host Immune and Inflammatory Responses

Recent studies have disclosed potential mechanisms by which respiratory viruses may cause ET dysfunction. There is accumulating evidence that respiratory viruses are capable of inducing a release of cytokines and inflammatory mediators from target cells in the nasopharynx. A variety of mediators, for example, histamine, bradykinin, interleukin(IL)-1β, IL-6, IL-8, leukotriene C4, and tumor necrosis factor have been detected in human nasopharyngeal secretions in response to a viral infection, and after intranasal challenge, many of these substances have been shown to provoke ET dysfunction.[41–47]

Numerous *in vitro* studies have documented the increased production of cytokines by human epithelial cells, and our knowledge of host immune and inflammatory responses to viral infection is rapidly increasing. For instance, both RSV and rhinovirus infection stimulate the production of IL-8, and rhinovirus infection also induces the release of IL-6 and granulocyte-macrophage colony-stimulating factor from respiratory epithelial cells.[46,48,49] In addition to producing cytokines, many respiratory viruses increase the expression of intercellular adhesion molecule-1 (ICAM-1), which not only functions as an important endothelial adhesion molecule for immune cells, but also serves as the major cell surface receptor for rhinoviruses.[50–52] Many of these cellular events are mediated by a chain of factors affecting each other. Enhanced expression of ICAM-1 by RSV infection, for instance, is mediated primarily by IL-1α.[53] Also, IL-1 and tumor necrosis factor have been shown to stimulate the production of IL-8, which, in turn, increases the PMN adhesion and migration through epithelial cells.[48,54,55] These few examples demonstrate the complexity of host response mechanisms triggered by a viral infection, and it is likely that many essential factors contributing to the inflammatory process in human respiratory epithelium remain to be identified.

Viral infections may also increase the host's susceptibility to secondary infection by several other mechanisms. Suppression of PMN function following influenza A virus infection has been shown in humans.[56–58] Also, alteration of cell-mediated immune function has been observed during RSV and rhinovirus infections.[59–61] In an experimental study in adult volunteers, influenza A virus infection promoted colonization of the oropharynx by *S. pneumoniae*.[62] Influenza A virus and adenovirus have also been shown to increase the adherence of bacteria to human epithelial cells, permitting enhanced bacterial proliferation and invasion into normally sterile tissues.[63,64] All these effects initiated by viral infection could compromise host defenses and increase the susceptibility to secondary bacterial infection.

Presence of Viruses in Middle-ear Effusion

One piece of evidence suggesting a role for viruses in the pathogenesis of AOM is the presence of the virus, with or without bacteria, in the MEEs of children with

AOM. Since the 1950s, investigators have attempted to isolate viruses from MEEs. Although data from a few studies performed during viral outbreaks demonstrated isolation of virus from the MEE, the overall detection rate of viruses during the 1950s and 1960s was only 5%.[65–72] The failure to isolate viruses prompted investigators to search for more sensitive detection methods. In 1982, use of enzyme immunoassays for RSV, influenza A virus, adenovirus, and rotavirus enabled the detection of viral antigens in the MEE of 25% of 53 patients.[8] Since then, several studies have documented the presence of viruses or viral antigens in the MEEs of children with AOM (TABLE 1.). Evidence of virus in MEEs, either alone or combined with bacterial pathogens, has been found in 19% of children with AOM.

The failure to isolate viruses from MEEs in the earlier studies was probably due to the poor sensitivity of the culture techniques, but rapid antigen detection also has problems. The disadvantage of this technique is that specific antibody against each virus is required and, therefore, the number of viruses that can be tested is limited. In addition, many clinically important viruses, for example, rhinoviruses and enteroviruses, have numerous serotypes, which makes antigen detection techniques impractical. Given that the sensitivities of viral detection techniques are limited, use of both viral culture and antigen detection is recommended to maximize the number of viral types detected.

The use of polymerase chain reaction (PCR) has further increased the rate of viral detection in MEE. In a recent report, RSV genomic sequences were found in 53% of 44 MEEs tested.[51] Further, the RSV sequences were detected in more than 80% of the MEEs from children in whom RSV could be cultured in nasopharyngeal secretions. In another PCR study, DNA from human herpesvirus 6 was recovered in 71%

TABLE 1. Detection of Viruses from Middle-ear Effusions in Cases of Acute Otitis Media Since 1982[a]

| | | | Virus-positive Cases | | | |
| | | | Total[b] | | Virus Alone | |
Reference	Year	Number of Patients	n	%	n	%
Klein et al.[8]	1982	53	13	25	8	15
Sarkkinen et al.[73]	1983	84	7	8	NA	
Sarkkinen et al.[9]	1985	137	24	18	10	7
Chonmaitree et al.[10]	1986	84	17	20	2	2
Arola et al.[11]	1988	143	16	11	7[c]	6
Arola et al.[12]	1990	88	17	19	NA	
Chonmaitree et al.[74]	1990	58	11	19	0	0
Chonmaitree et al.[14]	1992	271	66	24	16	6
Chonmaitree et al.[75]	1996	106	19	18	5	5
Total		1024	190	19	48	6

[a]Detection of viruses by cell cultures and/or rapid viral antigen detection.
[b]With or without bacteria.
[c]Of 116 children without antibiotic treatment.
NA = not available

of MEEs of 49 children with AOM.[76] Such high detection rates inevitably raise the question of whether viral nucleic acids detected in MEEs by PCR techniques represent viruses with a pathogenetic role in the middle ear, or if they represent viral materials that have migrated passively from the nasopharynx to the middle ear.

The types of viruses found in MEE vary from study to study, depending on the patient population, the virologic methods used, and the timing of the study in regard to major viral outbreaks. However, the most common viruses identified are RSV, influenza virus, parainfluenza virus, rhinovirus, and adenovirus, which are the same viruses that have been found to be closely associated with AOM in epidemiologic studies.[8–12,14,74] In addition, enteroviruses, cytomegalovirus, herpes simplex virus, human herpesvirus 6, and rotavirus have been detected in the MEEs of children with AOM.[8,10,14,76,77]

In most AOM cases when virus is found in the MEE, bacteria can also be isolated, indicating a mixed infection. As presented in TABLE 1, virus as the only pathogen in MEE has been detected in 6% of AOM cases, using the best virologic detection methods currently available. However, this percentage may not represent the true occurrence of exclusively viral AOM, because a substantial proportion of AOM cases still have no provable microbiologic etiology. Although it has been suggested that the bacteriologic techniques routinely used to evaluate MEEs are not sensitive enough for optimal detection of bacteria, it is obvious that underdetection of viruses is even more common.[78] Therefore, the actual proportion of exclusively viral AOM may be even greater than 6%. PCR techniques have also been shown to significantly increase the detection rates of bacterial pathogens in the MEEs of children with OM.[79,80] Positive bacterial PCR results from MEE specimens should, however, be interpreted with the same caution as positive viral PCR results, since detection of bacterial DNA fragments in MEEs does not necessarily prove the activity, or even the viability, of those bacteria in the middle ear.

Viral Vaccines in the Prevention of Acute Otitis Media

Because of the strong evidence suggesting a role for viruses in the etiopathogenesis of AOM, viral vaccines have been used for prevention of viral respiratory infection in order to prevent the development of AOM. In a prospective clinical study of 374 children in day care, investigators in Turku, Finland, administered influenza vaccine to half of the children before an expected outbreak.[81] During the subsequent influenza A epidemic, the incidence of AOM associated with influenza A was reduced by 83% in the vaccinees, and a significant 36% reduction in the overall morbidity due to AOM was observed in the vaccine group. The efficacy of this approach to prevention of AOM was further confirmed in another day-care study performed in North Carolina; influenza vaccine was shown to produce significant protection against AOM during a subsequent influenza A epidemic.[82]

The preceding findings serve to confirm the importance of viruses in the pathogenesis of OM. At present, influenza vaccine is the only commercially available vaccine for the control of viral respiratory infections. An obvious inference is that effective vaccines against other viruses that commonly predispose children to AOM would also reduce the incidence of this disease.

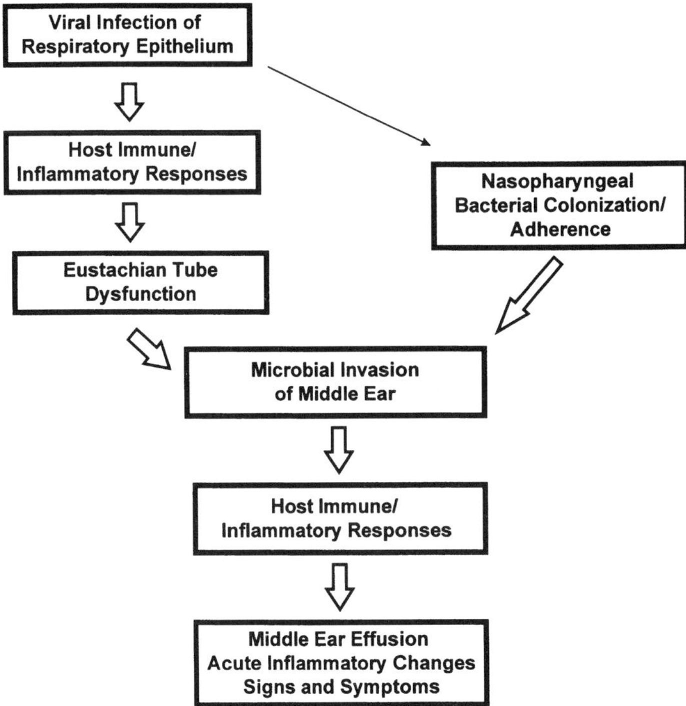

FIGURE 1. The cascade of events in the pathogenesis of otitis media following respiratory viral infection.

Summary

Taken together, there is ample evidence suggesting a role for viruses in the pathogenesis of OM. This evidence comes from numerous studies performed in animals and *in vitro* cell cultures, as well as in adults and children with URI and OM. Viruses induce host immune and inflammatory responses that result in pathology of the ET and the middle ear, and predispose the host in various ways to secondary bacterial infection. A suggested mechanism for the pathogenesis of OM following respiratory viral infection is presented in FIGURE 1.

ROLE OF VIRUSES IN FAILURE OF OTITIS MEDIA TREATMENT

Although several investigators have reported that viruses are frequently found in the MEE during AOM, the importance of this finding has been questioned because viral replication in the human middle ear during the AOM process has not been demonstrated. However, recent studies on the outcome of combined viral-bacterial

OM, as well as studies on certain inflammatory mediators, strongly suggest an active role for viruses in middle-ear infection.

In clinical practice, despite the availability and use of broad-spectrum antibiotics, poor clinical response to treatment of AOM is a common phenomenon. When this happens, the physician generally prescribes a different antibiotic, assuming that the cause of the failure is bacterial resistance to the initial antibiotic. However, a few studies have shown that resistant bacteria, in fact, account for only a small proportion of cases of treatment failure. In 1981, it was reported that the immediate cause of poor response to at least 36 h of antibiotic therapy was unidentifiable in 81% of 43 children with AOM.[83] Only 19% of the MEE isolates were resistant to the antibiotic used, and bacteria susceptible to the initial therapy were discovered in 24% of the children. Therefore, in the majority of the cases, resistant bacteria did not explain the observed lack of response to therapy. Similar results were obtained in a recent study of 137 children with persistent AOM.[84] In this study, no pathogenic bacteria were found in MEEs from 49% of the children, and in only 22% of the cases could the persistence of infection be attributed to resistant bacteria. Viral diagnostic tests were not performed in either of these two studies.

In an investigation of the effect of viruses on AOM outcome, 58 children with AOM were studied at the University of Texas Medical Branch, Galveston, Texas. MEEs were obtained before and 2 to 4 days after initiation of antibiotic treatment.[74] At the latter visit, even though the etiologic bacteria were susceptible to the antibiotic used, bacteriologic failure was observed in 33% of the children who had both bacteria and virus in their initial MEE, compared with 3% of the patients with only bacteria in the MEE. The effect of concurrent viral infection on the course of OM was also supported by a subsequent, larger study of 271 children with AOM, in which persistent otitis was noticed in a significantly higher proportion of patients with combined bacterial and viral infection, compared to those with bacteria alone in the MEE.[14] Investigators at the University of Turku, Finland, have reported similar findings. In a study of 22 children with AOM who had failed to improve clinically after at least 48 h of antimicrobial therapy, bacteria were isolated from MEEs of only four patients; two of the isolates were susceptible to the antibiotic used.[12] Viruses were recovered from MEEs of 32% of these 22 children, compared with 15% of 66 children in a comparison group with newly diagnosed, untreated AOM. All these studies indicate that the presence of virus in the MEE at the time of AOM diagnosis may contribute strongly to the poor response to antimicrobial therapy observed in some patients. Rhinoviruses have been suggested to be more commonly associated with bacteriologic failure than other respiratory viruses.[85]

The mechanisms by which viruses might interfere with bacteriologic response to antibiotics are still unclear. One hypothesis is that viral infection of the middle ear epithelium causes local inflammation that interferes with the penetration of antibiotics into the middle ear, resulting in lower antibiotic concentrations. Some support for this hypothesis is derived from an experimental pharmacokinetic study in chinchillas, which showed that influenza A virus significantly decreased antimicrobial elimination from the middle ear as a marker of decreased middle-ear antibiotic penetration.[86] Other potential mechanisms include delayed killing and clearance of bacteria from the middle ear due to virus-induced PMN dysfunction, and damage to the ciliated epithelial cells caused by viral infection.[18,23,25,58]

Recently, much attention has focused on the role of various inflammatory mediators in recovery from bacterial and viral OM. Numerous cytokines and mediators—for example, IL-1β, IL-2, IL-6, IL-8, tumor necrosis factor, histamine, leukotrienes, and prostaglandins—have been detected in MEEs from patients with OM.[87–89] Histamine is a potent inflammatory mediator produced by mast cells or peripheral blood basophils. *In vitro* data have shown that respiratory viruses are capable of enhancing IgE-mediated histamine release.[90] A study of MEEs from 248 children with AOM showed higher histamine concentrations in patients with evidence of concurrent viral infection than in those without.[91] Virus and bacteria also appeared to have an additive effect on histamine production in the MEE, and antibiotic treatment for 3 to 5 days did not decrease the amount of this potent mediator. A study of tryptase concentrations in MEEs suggested that histamine may be generated by both mast cells and basophils, and that viral infection is an essential trigger for histamine production.[92] Two chemokines, macrophage inflammatory protein-1-α and monocyte chemotactic protein-1-α, which are considered histamine-releasing factors, have also been found in higher concentrations in MEEs containing both bacteria and virus, compared to MEEs with bacteria alone.[93]

Leukotriene B4 (LTB4), another potent inflammatory mediator released by PMNs, and IL-8, a potent PMN chemotactic cytokine, have also been detected in MEEs of AOM patients with viral and/or bacterial infection.[75] The highest concentrations of LTB4 and IL-8 were found in MEEs containing both bacteria and virus. High concentrations of LTB4 at the time of AOM diagnosis and initiation of antibiotic therapy were also strongly correlated with an increased rate of treatment failure. Antibiotic treatment did not reduce the concentrations of these mediators.

These findings, taken together, suggest that active viral infection plays a significant role in the production of these cytokines and mediators which, in turn, may enhance or prolong the inflammation in the middle ear, long after the elimination of bacteria. Therefore, treatment of OM with antibiotic alone may not be adequate to stop these inflammatory cascades.

Like the etiopathogenesis of AOM, the process of recovery from OM is apparently very complex, involving numerous contributing factors. It is likely that several mediators of inflammation play important roles in the delayed recovery from OM, as well as in the development of recurrent and chronic OM. Viral infection of the respiratory tract and the middle ear appears to be a major contributor to these processes. Further studies are needed to elucidate the influence of viral–bacterial interactions on the outcome of OM, and for the development of new strategies to improve recovery from this disease.

CONCLUSION

There is growing evidence that the etiopathogenesis of AOM is very complicated, involving a network of factors, some probably not yet identified, which affect each other in a time-dependent manner. Respiratory viruses appear to play a decisive role in the initiation of a cascade of events that finally leads to development of AOM. The role of viruses is not limited to the etiopathogenesis of AOM; it appears that viral infection of the middle ear may also have a profound effect on the outcome of this disease. Therefore, the relative importance attributed to respiratory viruses, viral–bacterial interactions, and inflammatory mediators in the study and treatment of OM is likely to increase. Major improvements in the management of OM, such as the use of adjuvant therapies, antiviral drugs, or viral vaccines, will depend on the knowledge gained from further examination of these viral–bacterial interactions.

ACKNOWLEDGMENT

We thank Constance D. Baldwin, Ph.D., for reviewing and editing the manuscript.

REFERENCES

1. KLEIN, J. O. 1981. Microbiology and antimicrobial treatment of otitis media. Ann. Otol. Rhinol. Laryngol. **90** (Suppl. 3, Pt. 3): 30–36.
2. CHONMAITREE, T. & V. M. HOWIE. 1987. Bacteriology of otitis media. *In* Immunology of the Ear. J. M. Bernstein & P. L. Ogra, Eds.: 231–247. Raven Press. New York.
3. RUUSKANEN, O., M. AROLA, A. PUTTO-LAURILA, J. MERTSOLA, O. MEURMAN, M. K. VILJANEN & P. HALONEN. 1989. Acute otitis media and respiratory virus infections. Pediatr. Infect. Dis. J. **8:** 94–99.
4. WALD, E. R., B. DASHEFSKY, C. BYERS, N. GUERRA & F. TAYLOR. 1988. Frequency and severity of infections in day care. J. Pediatr. **112:** 540–546.
5. ALHO, O. P., M. KOIVU, M. SORRI & P. RANTAKALLIO. 1990. Risk factors for recurrent acute otitis media and respiratory infection in infancy. Int. J. Pediatr. Otorhinolaryngol. **19:** 151–161.
6. HENDERSON, F. W., A. M. COLLIER, M. A. SANYAL, J. M. WATKINS, D. L. FAIRCLOUGH, W. A. CLYDE, JR. & F. W. DENNY. 1982. A longitudinal study of respiratory viruses and bacteria in the etiology of acute otitis media with effusion. New Eng. J. Med. **306:** 1377–1383.
7. CLEMENTS, D. A., F. W. HENDERSON & E. C. NEEBE. 1993. Relationship of viral isolation to otitis media in a research day-care center 1978-1988. *In* Recent Advances in Otitis Media. D. J. Lim, C. D. Bluestone, J. O. Klein, J. D. Nelson & P. L. Ogra, Eds.: 27–29. Decker Periodicals.
8. KLEIN, B. S., F. R. DOLLETE & R. H. YOLKEN. 1982. The role of respiratory syncytial virus and other viral pathogens in acute otitis media. J. Pediatr. **101:** 16–20.
9. SARKKINEN, H., O. RUUSKANEN, O. MEURMAN, H. PUHAKKA, E. VIROLAINEN & J. ESKOLA. 1985. Identification of respiratory virus antigens in middle ear fluids of children with acute otitis media. J. Infect. Dis. **151:** 444–448.
10. CHONMAITREE, T., V. M. HOWIE & A. L. TRUANT. 1986. Presence of respiratory viruses in middle ear fluids and nasal wash specimens from children with acute otitis media. Pediatrics **77:** 698–702.
11. AROLA, M., T. ZIEGLER, O. RUUSKANEN, J. MERTSOLA, K. NÄNTÖ-SALONEN & P. HALONEN. 1988. Rhinovirus in acute otitis media. J. Pediatr. **113:** 693–695.
12. AROLA, M., T. ZIEGLER & O. RUUSKANEN. 1990. Respiratory virus infection as a cause of prolonged symptoms in acute otitis media. J. Pediatr. **116:** 697–701.
13. AROLA, M., O. RUUSKANEN, T. ZIEGLER, J. MERTSOLA, K. NÄNTÖ-SALONEN, A. PUTTO-LAURILA, M. K. VILJANEN & P. HALONEN. 1990. Clinical role of respiratory virus infection in acute otitis media. Pediatrics **86:** 848–855.
14. CHONMAITREE, T., M. J. OWEN, J. A. PATEL, D. HEDGPETH, D. HORLICK & V. M. HOWIE. 1992. Effect of viral respiratory tract infection on outcome of acute otitis media. J. Pediatr. **120:** 856–862.

15. UHARI, M., J. HIETALA & H. TUOKKO. 1995. Risk of acute otitis media in relation to the viral etiology of infections in children. Clin. Infect. Dis. **20:** 521–524.

16. HEIKKINEN, T., M. WARIS, O. RUUSKANEN, A. PUTTO-LAURILA & J. MERTSOLA. 1995. Incidence of acute otitis media associated with group A and B respiratory syncytial virus infections. Acta Paediatr. **84:** 419–423.

17. GIEBINK, G. S., I. K. BERZINS, S. C. MARKER & G. SCHIFFMAN. 1980. Experimental otitis media after nasal inoculation of *Streptococcus pneumoniae* and influenza A virus in chinchillas. Infect. Immun. **30:** 445–450.

18. ABRAMSON, J. S., G. S. GIEBINK & P. G. QUIE. 1982. Influenza A virus-induced polymorphonuclear leukocyte dysfunction in the pathogenesis of experimental pneumococcal otitis media. Infect. Immun. **36:** 289–296.

19. GIEBINK, G. S., M. L. RIPLEY & P. F. WRIGHT. 1987. Eustachian tube histopathology during experimental influenza A virus infection in the chinchilla. Ann. Otol. Rhinol. Laryngol. **96:** 199–206.

20. SUZUKI, K. & L. O. BAKALETZ. 1994. Synergistic effect of adenovirus type 1 and nontypeable *Haemophilus influenzae* in a chinchilla model of experimental otitis media. Infect. Immun. **62:** 1710–1718.

21. BAKALETZ, L. O., D. M. MURWIN & J. M. BILLY. 1995. Adenovirus serotype 1 does not act synergistically with *Moraxella (Branhamella) catarrhalis* to induce otitis media in the chinchilla. Infect. Immun. **63:** 4188–4190.

22. BAKALETZ, L. O., R. L. DANIELS & D. J. LIM. 1993. Modeling adenovirus type 1-induced otitis media in the chinchilla: Effect on ciliary activity and fluid transport function of eustachian tube mucosal epithelium. J. Infect. Dis. **168:** 865–872.

23. CHUNG, M. H., S. R. GRIFFITH, K. H. PARK, D. J. LIM & T. F. DEMARIA. 1993. Cytological and histological changes in the middle ear after inoculation of influenza A virus. Acta Otolaryngol. **113:** 81–87.

24. OHASHI, Y., Y. NAKAI, Y. ESAKI, Y. OHNO, Y. SUGIURA & H. OKAMOTO. 1991. Influenza A virus-induced otitis media and mucociliary dysfunction in the guinea pig. Acta Otolaryngol. **486**(Suppl.): 135–148.

25. PARK, K., L. O. BAKALETZ, J. M. COTICCHIA & D. J. LIM. 1993. Effect of influenza A virus on ciliary activity and dye transport function in the chinchilla eustachian tube. Ann. Otol. Rhinol. Laryngol. **102:** 551–558.

26. BUCHMAN, C. A., J. D. SWARTS, J. T. SEROKY, N. PANAGIOTOU, F. HAYDEN & W. J. DOYLE. 1995. Otologic and systemic manifestations of experimental influenza A virus infection in the ferret. Otolaryngol. Head Neck Surg. **112:** 572–578.

27. OHASHI, Y., Y. NAKAI, Y. OHNO, Y. SUGIURA, H. OKAMOTO, H. SAKAMOTO & M. HAYASHI. 1993. Influenza A modification of endotoxin-induced otitis media with effusion in the guinea pig. Eur. Arch. Otorhinolaryngol. **250:** 27–32.

28. PATEL, J., H. FADEN, S. SHARMA & P. L. OGRA. 1992. Effect of respiratory syncytial virus on adherence, colonization and immunity of non-typable *Haemophilus influenzae*: Implications for otitis media. Int. J. Pediatr. Otorhinolaryngol. **23:** 15–23.

29. BAKALETZ, L. O., T. M. HOEPF, T. F. DEMARIA & D. J. LIM. 1988. The effect of antecedent influenza A virus infection on the adherence of *Hemophilus influenzae* to chinchilla tracheal epithelium. Am. J. Otolaryngol. **9:** 127–134.

30. SANFORD, B. A. & M. A. RAMSAY. 1987. Bacterial adherence to the upper respiratory tract of ferrets infected with influenza A virus. Proc. Soc. Exp. Biol. Med. **185:** 120–128.

31. BLUESTONE, C. D. 1996. Pathogenesis of otitis media: Role of eustachian tube. Pediatr. Infect. Dis. J. **15:** 281–291.

32. BLUESTONE, C. D., E. I. CANTEKIN & Q. C. BEERY. 1977. Effect of inflammation on the ventilatory function of the eustachian tube. Laryngoscope **87:** 493–507.

33. SANYAL, M. A., F. W. HENDERSON, E. C. STEMPEL, A. M. COLLIER & F. W. DENNY. 1980. Ef-

fect of upper respiratory tract infection on eustachian tube ventilatory function in the preschool child. J. Pediatr. **97:** 11–15.

34. BYLANDER, A. 1984. Upper respiratory tract infection and eustachian tube function in children. Acta Otolaryngol. **97:** 343–349.

35. HEIKKINEN, T. & O. RUUSKANEN. 1994. Temporal development of acute otitis media during upper respiratory tract infection. Pediatr. Infect. Dis. J. **13:** 659–661.

36. MCBRIDE, T. P., W. J. DOYLE, F. G. HAYDEN & J. M. GWALTNEY, JR. 1989. Alterations of the eustachian tube, middle ear, and nose in rhinovirus infection. Arch. Otolaryngol. Head Neck Surg. **115:** 1054–1059.

37. DOYLE, W. J., D. P. SKONER, F. HAYDEN, C. A. BUCHMAN, J. T. SEROKY & P. FIREMAN. 1994. Nasal and otologic effects of experimental influenza A virus infection. Ann. Otol. Rhinol. Laryngol. **103:** 59–69.

38. BUCHMAN, C. A., W. J. DOYLE, D. SKONER, P. FIREMAN & J. M. GWALTNEY. 1994. Otologic manifestations of experimental rhinovirus infection. Laryngoscope **104:** 1295–1299.

39. BUCHMAN, C. A., W. J. DOYLE, D. P. SKONER, J. C. POST, C. M. ALPER, J. T. SEROKY, K. ANDERSON, R. A. PRESTON, F. G. HAYDEN, P. FIREMAN & G. D. EHRLICH. 1995. Influenza A virus-induced acute otitis media. J. Infect. Dis. **172:** 1348–1351.

40. ELKHATIEB, A., G. HIPSKIND, D. WOERNER & F. G. HAYDEN. 1993. Middle ear abnormalities during natural rhinovirus colds in adults. J. Infect. Dis. **168:** 618–621.

41. WELLIVER, R. C., D. T. WONG, M. SUN, E. MIDDLETON, JR, R. S. VAUGHAN & P. L. OGRA. 1981. The development of respiratory syncytial virus-specific IgE and the release of histamine in nasopharyngeal secretions after infection. New Eng. J. Med. **305:** 841–846.

42. NACLERIO, R. M., D. PROUD, L. M. LICHTENSTEIN, A. KAGEY-SOBOTKA, J. O. HENDLEY, J. SORRENTINO & J. M. GWALTNEY. 1988. Kinins are generated during experimental rhinovirus colds. J. Infect. Dis. **157:** 133–142.

43. VOLOVITZ, B., H. FADEN & P. L. OGRA. 1988. Release of leukotriene C4 in respiratory tract during acute viral infection. J. Pediatr. **112:** 218–222.

44. NOAH, T. L., F. W. HENDERSON, I. A. WORTMAN, R. B. DEVLIN, J. HANDY, H. S. KOREN & S. BECKER. 1995. Nasal cytokine production in viral acute upper respiratory infection of childhood. J. Infect. Dis. **171:** 584–592.

45. MATSUDA, K., H. TSUTSUMI, Y. OKAMOTO & C. CHIBA. 1995. Development of interleukin 6 and tumor necrosis factor alpha activity in nasopharyngeal secretions of infants and children during infection with respiratory syncytial virus. Clin. Diagn. Lab. Immun. **2:** 322–324.

46. ZHU, Z., W. TANG, A. RAY, Y. WU, O. EINARSSON, M. L. LANDRY, J. GWALTNEY, JR. & J. A. ELIAS. 1996. Rhinovirus stimulation of interleukin-6 in vivo and in vitro. J. Clin. Invest. **97:** 421–430.

47. DOYLE, W. J., S. BOEHM & D. P. SKONER. 1990. Physiologic responses to intranasal dose-response challenges with histamine, methacholine, bradykinin, and prostaglandin in adult volunteers with and without nasal allergy. J. Allergy Clin. Immunol. **86:** 924–935.

48. BECKER, S., H. S. KOREN & D. C. HENKE. 1993. Interleukin-8 expression in normal nasal epithelium and its modulation by infection with respiratory syncytial virus and cytokines tumor necrosis factor, interleukin-1, and interleukin-6. Am. J. Respir. Cell Mol. Biol. **8:** 20–27.

49. SUBAUSTE, M. C., D. B. JACOBY, S. M. RICHARDS & D. PROUD. 1995. Infection of a human respiratory epithelial cell line with rhinovirus. J. Clin. Invest. **96:** 549–557.

50. TOSI, M. F., J. M. STARK, A. HAMEDANI, C. W. SMITH, D. C. GRUENERT & Y. T. HUANG. 1992. Intercellular adhesion molecule-1 (ICAM-1)-dependent and ICAM-1-independent adhesive interactions between polymorphonuclear leukocytes and human airway epithelial cells infected with parainfluenza virus type 2. J. Immunol. **149:** 3345–3349.

51. OKAMOTO, Y., K. KUDO, K. ISHIKAWA, E. ITO, K. TOGAWA, I. SAITO, I. MORO, J. A. PATEL & P.

L. OGRA. 1993. Presence of respiratory syncytial virus genomic sequences in middle ear fluid and its relationship to expression of cytokines and cell adhesion molecules. J. Infect. Dis. **168:** 1277–1281.

52. STAUNTON, D. E., V. J. MERLUZZI, R. ROTHLEIN, R. BARTON, S. D. MARLIN & T. A. SPRINGER. 1989. Cell adhesion molecule, ICAM-1, is the major surface receptor for rhinoviruses. Cell **56:** 849–853.

53. PATEL, J. A., M. KUNIMOTO, T. C. SIM, R. GAROFALO, T. ELIOTT, S. BARON, O. RUUSKANEN, T. CHONMAITREE, P. L. OGRA & F. SCHMALSTIEG. 1995. Interleukin-1α mediates the enhanced expression of intercellular adhesion molecule-1 in pulmonary epithelial cells infected with respiratory syncytial virus. Am. J. Respir. Cell Mol. Biol. **13:** 602–609.

54. MOLINA, E., N. NAKAJIMA, Z. JIANG, T. CHONMAITREE & J. A. PATEL. 1996. Role of IL-8 and ICAM-1 in polymorphonuclear leukocyte (PMN) migration through respiratory syncytial virus (RSV)-infected pulmonary epithelial cells. J. Invest. Med. **44:** 72A.

55. NAKAJIMA, N., E. MOLINA, Z. JIANG & J. A. PATEL. 1996. Upregulation of Mac-1 on polymorphonuclear leukocytes (PMNs) by IL-8 produced by RSV-infected pulmonary epithelium. J. Invest. Med. **44:** 72A.

56. SAWYER, W. D. 1969. Interaction of influenza virus with leukocytes and its effect on phagocytosis. J. Infect. Dis. **119:** 541–556.

57. RUUTU, T. & T. U. KOSUNEN. 1971. Phagocytic activity of neutrophilic leukocytes of A2 influenza patients. Acta Pathol. Microbiol. Scand. **79:** 67–72.

58. LARSON, H. E. & R. BLADES. 1976. Impairment of human polymorphonuclear leucocyte function by influenza virus. Lancet **1:** 283.

59. RUUSKANEN, O. & P. L. OGRA. 1993. Respiratory syncytial virus. Curr. Probl. Pediatr. **23:** 50–79.

60. HSIA, J., A. L. GOLDSTEIN, G. L. SIMON, M. SZTEIN & F. G. HAYDEN. 1990. Peripheral blood mononuclear cell interleukin-2 and interferon-gamma production, cytotoxicity, and antigen-stimulated blastogenesis during experimental rhinovirus infection. J. Infect. Dis. **162:** 591–597.

61. SKONER, D. P., T. L. WHITESIDE, J. W. WILSON, W. J. DOYLE, R. B. HERBERMAN & P. FIREMAN. 1993. Effect of rhinovirus 39 infection on cellular immune parameters in allergic and nonallergic subjects. J. Allergy Clin. Immunol. **92:** 732–743.

62. WADOWSKY, R. M., S. M. MIETZNER, D. P. SKONER, W. J. DOYLE & P. FIREMAN. 1995. Effect of experimental influenza A virus infection on isolation of *Streptococcus pneumoniae* and other aerobic bacteria from the oropharynges of allergic and nonallergic adult subjects. Infect. Immun. **63:** 1153–1157.

63. FAINSTEIN, V., D. M. MUSHER & T. R. CATE. 1980. Bacterial adherence to pharyngeal cells during viral infection. J. Infect. Dis. **141:** 172–176.

64. HÅKANSSON, A., A. KIDD, G. WADELL, H. SABHARWAL & C. SVANBORG. 1994. Adenovirus infection enhances in vitro adherence of *Streptococcus pneumoniae*. Infect. Immun. **62:** 2707–2714.

65. YOSHIE, C. 1955. On the isolation of influenza virus from mid-ear discharge of influenza otitis media. JPN J. Med. Sci. Biol. **8:** 373–377.

66. GRÖNROOS, J. A., A. E. KORTEKANGAS, L. OJALA & M. VUORI. 1964. The aetiology of acute middle ear infection. Acta Otolaryngol. **58:** 149–158.

67. LAXDAL, O. E., R. M. BLAKE, T. CARTMILL & H. E. ROBERTSON. 1966. Etiology of acute otitis media in infants and children. Can. Med. Assoc. J. **94:** 159–163.

68. BERGLUND, B., A. SALMIVALLI & P. TOIVANEN. 1966. Isolation of respiratory syncytial virus from middle ear exudates of infants. Acta Otolaryngol. **61:** 475–487.

69. BERGLUND, B., A. SALMIVALLI & J. A. GRÖNROOS. 1967. The role of respiratory syncytial virus in otitis media in children. Acta Otolaryngol. **63:** 445–454.

70. TILLES, J. G., J. O. KLEIN, R. L. JAO, J. E. HASLAM, JR., M. FEINGOLD, S. S. GELLIS & M.

FINLAND. 1967. Acute otitis media in children. Serologic studies and attempts to isolate viruses and mycoplasmas from aspirated middle-ear fluids. New Eng. J. Med. **277:** 613–618.

71. HALSTED, C., M. L. LEPOW, N. BALASSANIAN, J. EMMERICH & E. WOLINSKY. 1968. Otitis media: Clinical observation, microbiology, and evaluation of therapy. Am. J. Dis. Child. **115:** 542–551.

72. GRÖNROOS, J. A., L. VIHMA, A. SALMIVALLI & B. BERGLUND. 1968. Coexisting viral (respiratory syncytial) and bacterial (pneumococcus) otitis media in children. Acta Otolaryngol. **65:** 505–517.

73. SARKKINEN, H. K., O. MEURMAN, T. T. SALMI, H. PUHAKKA & E. VIROLAINEN. 1983. Demonstration of viral antigens in middle ear secretions of children with acute otitis media. Acta Paediatr. Scand. **72:** 137–138.

74. CHONMAITREE, T., M. J. OWEN & V. M. HOWIE. 1990. Respiratory viruses interfere with bacteriologic response to antibiotic in children with acute otitis media. J. Infect. Dis. **162:** 546–549.

75. CHONMAITREE, T., J. A. PATEL, R. GAROFALO, T. UCHIDA, T. SIM, M. J. OWEN & V. M. HOWIE. 1996. Role of leukotriene B4 and interleukin-8 in acute bacterial and viral otitis media. Ann. Otol. Rhinol. Laryngol. **105:** 968–974.

76. CONE, R. W., T. CHONMAITREE, M. W. HUANG, V. M. HOWIE & M. J. OWEN. 1993. Human herpesvirus 6 variant B in acute otitis media (Abstract 165). Clin. Infect. Dis. **17:** 558.

77. CHONMAITREE, T., M. J. OWEN, J. A. PATEL, D. HEDGPETH, D. HORLICK & V. M. HOWIE. 1992. Presence of cytomegalovirus and herpes simplex virus in middle ear fluids from children with acute otitis media. Clin. Infect. Dis. **15:** 650–653.

78. DEL BECCARO, M. A., P. M. MENDELMAN, A. F. INGLIS, M. A. RICHARDSON, N. O. DUNCAN, C. R. CLAUSEN & T. L. STULL. 1992. Bacteriology of acute otitis media: A new perspective. J. Pediatr. **120:** 81–84.

79. VIROLAINEN, A., P. SALO, J. JERO, P. KARMA, J. ESKOLA & M. LEINONEN. 1994. Comparison of PCR assay with bacterial culture for detecting *Streptococcus pneumoniae* in middle ear fluid of children with acute otitis media. J. Clin. Microbiol. **32:** 2667–2670.

80. POST, J. C., R. A. PRESTON, J. J. AUL, M. LARKINS-PETTIGREW, J. RYDQUIST-WHITE, K. W. ANDERSON, R. M. WADOWSKY, D. R. REAGAN, E. S. WALKER, L. A. KINGSLEY, A. E. MAGIT & G. D. EHRLICH. 1995. Molecular analysis of bacterial pathogens in otitis media with effusion. JAMA **273:** 1598–1604.

81. HEIKKINEN, T., O. RUUSKANEN, M. WARIS, T. ZIEGLER, M. AROLA & P. HALONEN. 1991. Influenza vaccination in the prevention of acute otitis media in children. Am. J. Dis. Child. **145:** 445–448.

82. CLEMENTS, D. A., L. LANGDON, C. BLAND & E. WALTER. 1995. Influenza A vaccine decreases the incidence of otitis media in 6- to 30-month-old children in day care. Arch. Pediatr. Adolesc. Med. **149:** 1113–1117.

83. TEELE, D. W., S. I. PELTON & J. O. KLEIN. 1981. Bacteriology of acute otitis media unresponsive to initial antimicrobial therapy. J. Pediatr. **98:** 537–539.

84. PICHICHERO, M. E. & C. L. PICHICHERO. 1995. Persistent acute otitis media: I. Causative pathogens. Pediatr. Infect. Dis. J. **14:** 178–183.

85. SUNG, B. S., T. CHONMAITREE, L. D. BROEMELING, M. J. OWEN, J. A. PATEL, D. C. HEDGPETH & V. M. HOWIE. 1993. Association of rhinovirus infection with poor bacteriologic outcome of bacterial-viral otitis media. Clin. Infect. Dis. **17:** 38–42.

86. JOSSART, G. H., D. M. CANAFAX, G. R. ERDMANN, M. J. LOVDAHL, H. Q. RUSSLIE, S. K. JUHN & G. S. GIEBINK. 1994. Effect of *Streptococcus pneumoniae* and influenza A virus on middle ear antimicrobial pharmacokinetics in experimental otitis media. Pharm. Res. **11:** 860–864.

87. BERGER, G., M. HAWKE, D. W. PROOPS, N. S. RANADIVE & D. WONG. 1984. Histamine levels in middle ear effusions. Acta Otolaryngol. **98:** 385–390.

88. BRODSKY, L., H. FADEN, J. BERNSTEIN, J. STANIEVICH, G. DeCASTRO, B. VOLOVITZ & P. L. OGRA. 1991. Arachidonic acid metabolites in middle ear effusions of children. Ann. Otol. Rhinol. Laryngol. **100:** 589–592.

89. YELLON, R. F., W. J. DOYLE, T. L. WHITESIDE, W. F. DIVEN, A. R. MARCH & P. FIREMAN. 1995. Cytokines, immunoglobulins, and bacterial pathogens in middle ear effusions. Arch. Otolaryngol. Head Neck Surg. **121:** 865–869.

90. CHONMAITREE, T., M. A. LETT-BROWN, Y. TSONG, A. S. GOLDMAN & S. BARON. 1988. Role of interferon in leukocyte histamine release caused by common respiratory viruses. J. Infect. Dis. **157:** 127–132.

91. CHONMAITREE, T., J. A. PATEL, M. A. LETT-BROWN, T. UCHIDA, R. GAROFALO, M. J. OWEN & V. M. HOWIE. 1994. Virus and bacteria enhance histamine production in middle ear fluids of children with acute otitis media. J. Infect. Dis. **169:** 1265–1270.

92. GAROFALO, R., I. ENANDER, M. NILSSONS, V. M. HOWIE, M. J. OWEN & T. CHONMAITREE. 1996. Mast cell degranulation in the middle ear of children with acute otitis media. *In* Recent Advances in Otitis Media, D. J. Lim, C. D. Bluestone, M. Casselbrant, J. O. Klein, and P. L. Ogra, Eds.: 191–193. Decker. Hamilton, Ont., Canada.

93. PATEL, J. A., T. SIM, M. J. OWEN, V. M. HOWIE & T. CHONMAITREE. 1996. Influence of viral infection on middle ear chemokine response in acute otitis media. *In* Recent Advances in Otitis Media, D. J. Lim, C. D. Bluestone, M. Casselbrant, J. O. Klein, and P. L. Ogra, Eds.: 178–179. Decker. Hamilton, Ont., Canada.

Summary: Recent Developments in the Immunology of Otitis Media

PEARAY L. OGRA[a]

Department of Pediatrics
Children's Hospital
University of Texas Medical Branch
301 University Blvd.
Galveston, Texas 77555-0351

INTRODUCTION

During the past 25 years, significant advances have been made in understanding the natural history, pathogenesis of, and immune mechanisms associated with the evolution of otitis media in childhood. Information reviewed during this Congress highlighted recent developments in several facets of human middle-ear disease. These include new advances in (1) basic framework of mucosal immune system, including the middle-ear mucosa; (2) etiologic aspects of otitis media; (3) outcome of antigenic exposure relative to the development of specific systemic and mucosal responses; (4) immunologically mediated complications of otitis media; and (5) other amplifying mechanisms that contribute to the natural history and/or outcome of middle-ear infection. This report is based on about 20 presentations on middle-ear disease delivered during the course of this conference.

BASIC FRAMEWORK OF THE MUCOSAL IMMUNE SYSTEM

Recent studies carried out in a number of laboratories have provided extensive characterization of the important components of mucosa-associated lymphoid tissue (MALT), antigen-sensitized cells, antigen processing and presentation, cell traffic, and mucosal cytokines. Brandtzaeg and Bernstein provided a comprehensive and critical analysis of the information related to the development of immunologic reactivity in the middle ear. Although normal middle-ear mucosa appears to be devoid of any organized lymphoid follicles, the middle-ear mucosal epithelium participates with other sites of common mucosal immune system in the expression of local immune responses in the middle ear during otitis media.

Immunological defense of the upper airway mucosa depends primarily on secretory antibodies. The responsible B cells are initially stimulated in organized MALT, including the tonsils and the adenoid. From these inductive sites, both memory B and T cells migrate to mucosal effector sites where they extravasate in a partly tissue-spe-

[a]Phone: 409/772-1594; fax: 409/747-4995.

TABLE 1. Functional Role of Different Cytokines in the Mucosal Tissues, Including Possibly in the Middle Ear

Function	Participating Cytokine
Regulation of inflammation and immune response	IL-1α, IL-β, IL-6, IL-10, TNF-γ, LIF, TGF-β, IL-2, IFN-γ
Growth differentiation	IL-1α, IL-β, IL-3, IL-7, LIF, TGF-β, G, CSF, GM-CSF
Cellular recruitment and chemotaxis	IL-8, MCP-1, RANTES, MIP-1α
Epithelial cell transformation	IL-1, TGF-α, β, IL-6
TH$_1$	IL-2, IFN-γ
TH$_2$	IL-4, IL-5, IL-6, IL-10, IL-13
Bone resorption	IL-1, TNF-γ, EGF, IL-6, VIP, SP
Bone formation	TGF-β

cific manner determined by adhesion molecules on microvascular endothelial cells. The primed B cells undergo terminal differentiation in the mucosal lamina propria to immunoglobulin (lg) -producing blasts and plasma cells. Locally produced lg consists mainly of J-chain-containing dimers and larger polymers of IgA (collectively called plgA) that are selectively transported through epithelial cells by a receptor called secretory component (SC) or the plg receptor. The resulting secretory IgA antibodies are designed to perform immune exclusion at the mucosal surface. IgG can contribute to such surface defense because it reaches the secretions by passive diffusion. However, its proinflammatory properties render IgG antibodies of immunopathological importance when mucosal elimination of antigens is unsuccessful. T-helper (TH) cells activated locally may, by a Th2 cytokine profile, promote persistent mucosal inflammation with extravasation and priming of inflammatory cells, including eosinophils. This development may be considered as "pathotopic potentiation" of local defense. It appears to be part of the late-phase allergic reaction, perhaps initially driven by interleukin-4 (IL-4) released from mast cells subjected to IgE-mediated or other types of degranulation, and subsequently maintained by further Th2-cell stimulation. Eosinophils are potentially tissue-damaging, particularly after priming with IL-5. Various cytokines upregulate adhesion molecules on endothelial and epithelial cells, thereby enhancing accumulation of eosinophils and perhaps in addition, causing aberrant immune regulation within the epithelium. Soluble antigens bombarding the epithelial surfaces normally appear to induce various immunosuppressive mechanisms, but such homeostasis seems to be less potent in the airways than oral tolerance to dietary antigens operating in the intestinal immune system.

A major portion of the discussion at the conference focused on the role of cytokines and chemokines in the development of immunity and possible immunopathology in the middle ear. The diverse functions of cytokines present constitutively or induced after infection are summarized in TABLE 1.

ETIOLOGIC SPECTRUM OF ACUTE OTITIS MEDIA

It is apparent that acute middle-ear infections are etiologically related to bacterial pathogenesis, namely *Streptococcus pneumoniae, Moraxella catarrhalis*, nontypeable *Haemophilus influenzae* (NTHI), and less commonly, to other pathogens. Faden reviewed the historical data on the bacteriology of otitis media (OM), and discussed the implications of local immune responses and the mechanisms of protection. Evidence was presented to suggest that OM continues to be the most common illness encountered by children. The highest incidence of disease occurs in the first few years of life. By the age of two years, 85% of children will have experienced at least one episode, and 5% of the population will have experienced seven or more episodes. Acute otitis media (AOM) accounts for the majority of episodes, while OM with effusion, often sterile represents most other episodes.

Bacteria cause 75% of episodes, and viruses are associated with more than 50% of AOM episodes. Thus, many episodes of AOM are concurrently due to both bacteria and viruses. Susceptibility to infection with middle-ear pathogens is associated with the absence of specific antibody. Serum antibody enters the middle-ear space during acute inflammatory changes to eradicate the infecting organism. Subsequently, the middle-ear space is protected against challenge with the same organism. Most of the protective antibody appears to belong to the IgG class of immunoglobulins. Local production of specific IgA antibody occurs during recurrent or persistent infections. The role of IgA in the middle-ear space remains unknown. An alarming increase in the frequency of antibiotic resistant otitis-producing bacterial pathogens has been observed in the last few years. In some studies, 20 to 40% of middle-ear isolates of *S. pneumoniae* have been found to be resistant to antibiotics. Those predictable problems of antibiotic use underscore the need for development of effective vaccines against otitis-producing pathogens.

Studies of Bernstein and colleagues have recently demonstrated specific interaction between purified nasopharyngeal mucin and the outer membrane proteins of *S. pneumoniae*, NTHI, *M. catarrhalis*, and *Pseudomonas aeruginosa*. A high degree of specificity exists for the outer-membrane protein components to bind to purified nasopharyngeal mucin. *S. pneumonia* binds primarily with a 17 Kd protein, nontypeable *H. influenzae* binds specifically with P2 and P5 in almost all cases. In addition, a higher molecular-weight protein and a protein close to P6 also bind in occasional strains. A single 57 Kd protein of *M. catarrhalis* has been shown to bind to purified mucin. Finally, *P. aeruginosa* binds with a nonpilis protein in the vicinity of 16 Kd.

Bernstein also summarized the observations that suggest that secretory IgA is the most important immunoglobulin locally produced in the nasopharynx and nasal mucosa. It has been suggested by Faden and colleagues that otitis-prone children tend to make less secretory IgA against the conserved P6 outer membrane protein of NTHI. Furthermore, work from other laboratories has also demonstrated that local production of secretory IgA against *S. pneumonia* occurs early in life and is directed against the carbohydrate moiety of the capsule of *S. pneumoniae*.

Another mechanism that is potentially protective is bacterial interference. Viridans streptococci appear to be the most important commensal organisms in the nasopharyngeal lymphoid tissue. A mechanism of inhibition by viridans streptococci against NTHI has recently been suggested. It involves both the release of an acid pH and the production of hydrogen peroxide. It is independent of any synthesis of a bacterial toxin. These three mechanisms offer new opportunities to examine cell–pathogen interaction in OM. Thus, specific outer-membrane protein–mucin interaction, specific secretory IgA, and bacterial interference, may be responsible for the inhibition of bacterial colonization with potential pathogens in the upper airway and middle-ear mucosa.

In related studies, Murphy and colleagues discussed pathogen-directed immunological mechanisms that may relate to development of recurrent OM. Children with OM experience recurrent episodes of disease due to NTHI. A protective immune response occurs following infection, but this response is specific for the infecting strain, leaving the child susceptible to infection by other strains of NTHI. Little is known about the mechanism by which a strain-specific antibody response occurs in nonencapsulated bacteria. To explore the mechanism by which strain-specific responses occur, animals were inoculated with whole bacterial cells and the antibody response was studied. The immunologic activity was predominantly directed to a highly strain-specific, immunodominant surface loop on the major outer membrane protein, P2. This exquisitely restricted immune response leaves the host susceptible to recurrent infections by many strains of NTHI. The ability of the bacterium to direct the host to make a strain-specific antibody response has important implications in understanding the immune response to OM due to HTHI and in designing strategies for vaccine development.

Chonmaitree reviewed the role of respiratory viruses in the development of otitis, either as single etiological agents and/or as pathogens that contribute to the subsequent invasions of the middle-ear cavity by bacterial pathogens. Recent evidence suggests that viruses play an important role in AOM, both in the pathogenesis and outcome of the disease. AOM usually occurs concurrently with, or just after a viral respiratory infection, and the peak incidence of the disease coincides with the age when viral infections are prevalent. As was pointed out earlier, concomitant viral infection has been documented in up to half of infants and children with AOM. Studies of middle-ear fluids from patients with AOM have shown the presence of bacteria alone in approximately 55% of cases, bacteria and viruses in 15%, and viruses alone in 5% of cases. Other evidence suggesting a role for viruses in the pathogenesis includes the demonstrated effect of viruses on the middle-ear epithelium in animal models; the effect of viruses on eustachian-tube function; and successful prevention of AOM with some viral vaccines. The role of viruses in the mechanism underlying the pathogenesis of AOM may thus be critical under certain clinical situations.

Viruses have been shown to interfere with the clearance of bacterial infections in a notable proportion of AOM episodes. Viruses not only affect the nasopharyngeal and eustachian-tube mucosa, but may also directly affect the middle-ear mucosal homeostasis. Some recent data suggest that viral-induced changes in the middle ear are partially responsible for the high rate of unresponsiveness of AOM to antimicrobial therapy, and probably contribute to the frequency of relapses, recurrences, or chronicity of the disease. Major changes in the management of AOM, such as the use of adjuvant therapies, antiviral drugs, or vaccines, will clearly depend on further characterization of viral–bacterial interactions *in situ* in the middle-ear cavity.

Other observations reported at this meeting provided evidence of a strong relationship between induction of cell adhesion molecules, such as MHC class I and II, and regulation of antigen processing and presentation during viral infection of the mucosal epithelial cells.

Studies reported by Mogi and colleagues and by Bernstein and colleagues have suggested that allergen-induced dysfunction of eustachian tubes may underlie many aspects of immunologically mediated or allergy-induced damage to middle-ear cavity. However, all middle-ear disease is not allergic, although allergic diathesis may represent an important risk factor in the expression of OM with effusion in man.

OUTCOME OF ANTIGENIC EXPOSURE

Evidence was presented to suggest that OM is associated with the appearance of pathogen-specific immune responses in the serum as well as in the middle-ear cavity. Specific immunologic reactivity is observed for IgG, IgA, IgM, and IgE, as well as for T-lymphocytes. It appears that chronic middle-ear disease is more often associated with prominent secretory IgA responses. However, its role in the mechanisms of pathogenesis or protection against middle-ear disease remains to be determined.

Several investigators have explored the induction and role of cytokines in OM. It appears that presence of cytokines in middle ear represent a constitutive as well as an inductive process, based on the observations reviewed by Rynnel-Dagöö and by Van Canwenberge. Il-4, IL-6, IL-1β, IL-3, IFN-γ, IL-2, and Il-8 are frequently expressed in different forms of middle-ear effusions (MEE). However, little information is available about their origin or function. A brief report by Nassif *et al.* suggested that IL-8 is consistently present in MEE, and its concentration predicts the total number and proportion of neutrophils in MEE. IL-8 concentration and the total number of neutrophils often correlated positively with the type of effusion. These results support the hypothesis that IL-8 may mediate recruitment of neutrophils to the middle ear. Other cytokines may similarly act as mediators of proinflammatory or immunoregulatory functions in the middle-ear cavity during AOM.

COMPLICATIONS

A number of observations on immunopathology of bone resorption were highlighted in the reports by DiMuzio and Chole. Several factors seem to contribute to the sequence of events in the pathogenesis of OM and development of cholesteatoma. It is clear that the inflammatory response plays a key role in the bone resorption and subsequent architectural changes that accompany chronic forms of these diseases.

Resorption is carried out by osteoclasts, which are specialized multinucleated cells of hematopoietic origin. Bone resorption takes place under a specialized area of the osteoclast called the *ruffled border*, which is composed of a sealed lysosomal compartment where the acidic pH solubilizes the mineral and the proteolytic enzymes digest the matrix. The osteoclast has been carefully scrutinized with an array of immunological techniques. Monoclonal antibodies have provided tools to explore the relationship of osteoclasts to other mononuclear phagocytes and identified a group of plasma membrane proteins, such as mannose-6-phosphate receptor, ATPase ion transport systems of the potassium, hydrogen ion, and calcium. These enzymes are thought to contribute to the acidification, proteolytic activation, mineral dissolution, and calcium translocation associated with the resorption process.

The cellular events that compose the balanced remodeling sequence are controlled by cytokines and growth factors which are generated in the microenvironment of the bone. However, under conditions of stress (e.g., hypocalcemia), the osteoclasts can respond by increasing in number and activation frequency, which will then functionally alter bony structures and ultimately organ functions. The signals that initiate this cascade of destruction are called *coupling factors*, and involve cytokines derived from mononuclear cells, resident bone cells, and, in the presence of an inflammatory response, from expanding granulation tissue components. In part, these factors can act directly or are incorporated into the bone matrix and released in biologically active forms during periods of bone resorption. Evidence is accumulating that the cytokines and growth factors, notably IL-1, IL-6, IL-8, TNF-α, and the TGF~ family, as well as other factors, such as oxygen radicals and nitric oxide, play important role not only in physiological bone remodeling but also in localized inflammatory diseases, such as OM and cholesteatoma.

Chole reviewed additional recent data that suggest that following acute infection, OM may enter a stage of chronicity due to persistence of bacteria, their metabolic products, or the presence of cholesteatoma within the middle ear and mastoid spaces. One of the most destructive effects of this inflammatory process is bone remodeling due to the local activation of osteoclasts and osteoblasts. Thus, bone resorption and remodeling as it relates to chronic OM is regulated by complex molecular events within a highly localized region. The pathologic process is highly dependent upon arachidonic acid metabolites. The process is prostaglandin dependent, and recent evidence has shown that it may be more specifically dependent upon the cytochrome p450 branch of the arachidonic acid cascade.

A number of cytokines can induce bone resorption *in vivo* and *in vitro*, and are present in COM with or without cholesteatoma. IL-1β is probably the most potent osteoclast stimulator and is present in the inflamed mucosa of COM and within the keratinocytes of cholesteatomas. Other cytokines are osteoclast stimulators. These include TNF-α, and β, TGF-α, EGF, IL-1α, and possibly IL-6. There is some evidence that neuropeptides such as substance-P and vasoactive intestinal peptide (VIP) are also stimulators of bone resorption. Nitric oxide synthetase is present within osteoblasts and may be responsible for IL-1- and TNF-mediated bone resorption.

The role of immunologic responses in the evolution of cholesteatoma remains to be determined. Investigations reported by Bellusi, and Chang *et al.*, suggest that IL-1, TGF-β and IL-6, and other epithelial-cell-transforming cytokines may play a key role in the development of cholesteatomas.

AMPLIFYING MECHANISMS

Genetic studies reported by Prellner have raised the possibility of a link between the presence of HLA-A2 antigen profile and the occurrences of recurrent OM. Such a link shows that population groups with a high frequency of this antigen are at increased risk for contracting recurrent AOM. Another indication of the importance of the HLA-A2 antigen in connection with its possible association with recurrent AOM is provided by the generally lower incidence of AOM in some racial groups with low frequency of HLA-A2 antigen profiles.

Another important study by Yamanaka *et al.*, suggested a role for immunologic deficiency in OM. As mentioned earlier, NTHI and *S. pneumoniae* are frequently associated with recurrent and chronic episodes of middle-ear disease. P6, outer membrane protein of NTHI highly conserved among strains, appears to serve as a target for bactericidal antibody, and has been proposed as a possible vaccine candidate. The serum antibody response to P6 and pneumococcal polysaccharide antigens were studied in otitis-prone and normal children. IgG2 subtype, which contributes to antibody against capsular polysaccharides, was also measured. Anti-P6 antibody levels increased sevenfold in the normal group compared with less than threefold for the otitis-prone group, and were significantly higher in the normal children after the age of 18 months ($p < 0.05$). Over 70% of otitis-prone children elicited total IgG2 over the cutoff value (100 mg/dL), whereas pneumococcal polysaccharide-specific IgG2 antibody in 85% and P6-specific IgG antibody in 80% of the subjects were below the cutoff value. The failure to recognize P6 and/or pneumococcal polysaccharides as specific immunogens may thus account for recurrent infections in this population.

CONCLUDING REMARKS

The observations summarized at this meeting have provided a wealth of new information regarding immunologic aspects of OM and the mucosal immune system. There is sufficient evidence, as reviewed by Giebink, to suggest that AOM can be prevented by vaccination. Pneumococcal conjugate vaccines are being developed to circumvent T-independence of these antigens and provide durable immunity at a very young age. Protein conjugated to the capsular polysaccharides associates with cell-surface major histocompatibility complex (MHC) molecules, which trigger T-helper cells to promote effective B-cell antibody responses. Conjugate vaccine technology has proven highly successful in *H. influenzae* type-B disease prevention. Six pneumococcal conjugate vaccines are currently in various phases of clinical testing. As discussed by Murphy, potential vaccine antigens for NTHI include outer membrane proteins (OMP), high molecular-weight proteins (HMW), pili, and fimbriae. Many OMPs show extensive homology among strains, but surface determinants are highly variable so that antibodies to surface epitopes of one strain will not bind to surface epitopes of another. Several *M. catarrhalis* OMP and HMW antigens have vaccine potential, but no functional correlates of protection have been identified, and there is no clear evidence, to date, that bactericidal antibody to *M. catarrhalis* is associated with protection against AOM.

Otitis-prone children experience recurrent episodes of OM due to NTHI. A protective immune response occurs following infection, but his response is specific only for the infecting strain, leaving the child susceptible to infection by other strains. Little is known about the mechanisms by which a strain-specific antibody response occurs with nonencapsulated bacteria. To explore the mechanism by which strain-specific response occurs, animals have been inoculated with whole bacterial cells and the antibody response was studied. The response was predominantly directed to a highly strain-specific, immunodominant surface loop on the major outer membrane protein, P2. This exquisitely restricted immune response leaves the host susceptible to recurrent infections by many strains of NTHI. The ability of the bacterium to direct the host to make a strain-specific antibody response may thus have important implications in understanding the immune response to OM due to NTHI and in designing strategies for vaccine development.

In view of the emerging role of respiratory viruses in the evolution of bacterial OM, vaccine for these viruses, most notably RSV, will have a major impact on prevention of OM in childhood. Attenuated viral vaccines hold promise of preventing childhood OM. Two clinical trails with killed influenza vaccines have shown a significant reduction in OM among vaccine recipients compared to control children during periods of high influenza disease activity in the community.

Finally, passive immunoprophylaxis also appears to hold potential for preventing OM. Human bacterial polysaccharide immune globulin was protective for pneumococcal AOM in children and in the chinchilla model. High-dose respiratory syncytial virus-enriched immunoglobulin reduced the incidence and severity of RSV lower respiratory tract infection in high-risk children. Passive immunoprophylaxis may also be effective in children with specific immune deficiencies, such as IgG2 deficiency, and patients who fail to respond to active immunoprophylaxis.

On a personal note, it is gratifying to recognize the remarkable growth of knowledge in and interest of the scientific community in the immunologic aspects of OM during the past two decades. We have come a long way toward understanding the basis of middle-ear immunity since early 1970, when Bernstein (one of the organizers of the conference) and his colleagues first proposed a role for secretory IgA in the mucosa of middle ear during OM. This conference has added much to the field and to the understanding of immunology and immunopathology of middle-ear disease.

Immunopathology of the Inner Ear: An Update

JEFFREY P. HARRIS,[a] JENNIFER HEYDT, ELIZABETH M. KEITHLEY, AND MIEN-CHI CHEN

Division of Otolaryngology
Department of Surgery
University of California, San Diego
9350 Campus Point Drive, 0970,
La Jolla, California 92037

THE INNER-EAR IMMUNE RESPONSE

The central nervous system (CNS), and the inner ear by extension, were originally thought to be immunoprivileged sites through the actions of the blood–brain barrier and blood–labyrinthine barrier, respectively. It is now known that the inner ear, as well as the CNS, is capable of mounting an immune response.

The sequence of events that make up this immune response in the inner ear have recently been well characterized. Interestingly, the inner ear contains immunoglobulin, and the endolymphatic sac contains immunocompetent cells in the resting state. Immunoglobulin crosses the blood–labyrinthine barrier and is present in perilymph at a level of 1/1000 the concentration found in serum.[1,2] The water resorptive properties of the inner ear may also be responsible for the increased concentration of immunoglobulin there relative to the levels in the CNS.[1,2] Levels of IgG appear to predominate, with lesser amounts of IgM and IgA present.[2,3] This immunoglobulin-rich environment is assumed to assist in protecting the inner ear from pathogens through their roles in neutralization, opsonization, and complement fixation. The two latter functions require the actions of immunocompetent cells in conjunction with immunoglobulin. Although the quiescent cochlea contains no ascertainable cells, the endolymphatic sac has been shown to contain a variety of T cells, macrophages, and B cells bearing IgM, IgG, and IgA.[4] Macrophages and certain classes of T cells are capable of processing and presenting antigen as well as opsonization of bacteria and viruses. Cytotoxic T cells are capable of the direct killing of cells expressing foreign antigen. T-helper cells are believed to facilitate B-cell responsiveness through the release of cytokines, and T-suppresser cells are associated with the down regulation of immune responses. Finally, activated B cells secrete various classes of immunoglobulin that aid in neutralization, opsonization, and complement fixation. Nonspecific T cells and helper T cells appeared to predominate with the existence of minimal T-suppresser cells in the endolymphatic sac. Of immunoglobulin-bearing cells, IgM was the most common class, followed by IgG, and small amounts of IgA.[4] Thus, the non-challenged inner ear not only appears to derive protection through diffusion of im-

[a]Author to whom correspondence should be addressed. Phone: 619/657-8590; fax: 619/657-8682; e-mail: jpharris@ucsd.edu

munoglobulin from the systemic circulation and the CNS, but contains a full complement of immunocompetent cells in the endolymphatic sac, which presumably allows for a local immune response.

For a local immune response to be generated in the inner ear, antigen must gain access to the immunocompetent cells in the endolymphatic sac. We have shown that antigen, namely horseradish peroxidase (HRP), does diffuse to the sac after scala tympani injection, and its concentration in the sac lumen, epithelial cells, subepithelial tissue, and perisaccular connective tissue (FIG. 1) as compared to labeling of cochlear endolymphatic tissues, suggests movement through perilymph and the perisaccular tissues as opposed to movement in the endolymphatic space. The dense staining of the spiral ligament with HRP reaction product in this study also supports the hypothesis that perilymph is resorbed from the inner ear by the spiral ligament and its dense network of small venules.[5] The importance of the endolymphatic sac in initiating an immune response was supported by the evidence of phagocytosed antigen in macrophages of the endolymphatic sac lumen within hours of injection, while no labeled cells appeared in the cochlea during the study period. By 72 h following the HRP challenge, the cochlea, vestibule, and endolymphatic sac were completely cleared of HRP.[5] This was also seen in a previous study where keyhole limpet hemocyanin (KLH), a potent stimulator of cellular immunity, was used to investigate the development of inner-ear immunocompetent cells. Both macrophages with phagocytosed antigen and T-helper cells appeared in the endolymphatic sac before they appeared in the cochlea.[6] Hence, antigen does gain access to the endolymphatic sac and this appears to be the initial site of the immune response.

Models of the immune response *in vivo* as well as *in vitro* have established the

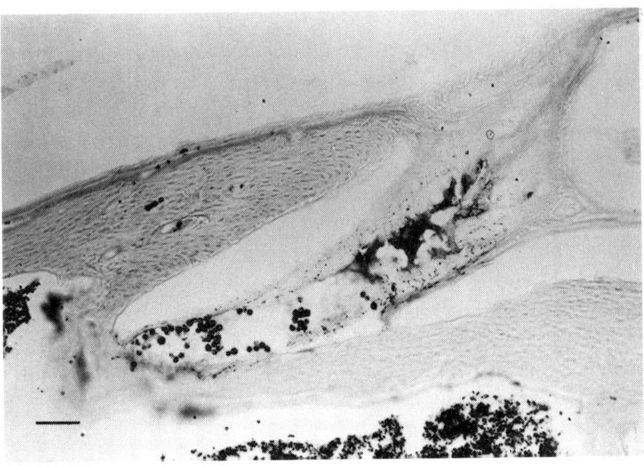

FIGURE 1. Photomicrograph of horseradish-peroxidase (HRP) -labeled fluid and cells in the endolymphatic sac lumen. Because the endolymphatic structures in the cochlea are not labeled, it is hypothesized that antigen diffused to the endolymphatic sac area in the perilymphatic connective tissue and was transported into the lumen where it is phagocytosed by the labeled cells illustrated here. *Scale bar*, 120 μm

role of numerous chemicals elaborated by cells involved in the immune response as important mediators of the inflammatory event. A host of cytokines, namely interleukins, interferons, and tumor necrosis factors, as well as growth factors have been characterized. The interleukin IL-2 and transforming growth factor β (TGF-β) have been studied with respect to the inner-ear inflammatory response. IL-2 is regarded as an early mediator and is released by T-helper cells upon stimulation from IL-1, a lymphokine released by activated macrophages. IL-2 is felt to have a myriad of functions: activation of T-helper, T-cytotoxic, and T-suppresser cells;[7] activation of B cells;[8] enhancement of natural killer activity;[9] chemoattraction for polymorphonuclear cells, monocytes, and lymphocytes;[10,11] and immunoregulation for prevention of autoimmune disease.[12] IL-2 is not present in perilymph in the resting state, but is a component of the inner-ear immune response. Following inner-ear challenge of the scala tympani with KLH, IL-2 was measurable at 6 h, peaked at 18 h, and declined over 5 days.[13] The time frame of this response suggests that the lymphokine is generated by T cells residing in the endolymphatic sac, and that it plays a comparable role in the inner ear as noted in other inflammatory sites. The early egress of polymorphonuclear leukocytes and lesser amounts of monocytes and lymphocytes in this study may be secondary to the actions of IL-2, as this is one of its roles elsewhere in the body. TGF-β has also been identified as a mediator in the inner-ear immune response. Following scala tympani challenge with KLH, leukocytes within the scala tympani and scala vestibuli were labeled with mRNA probes to TGF-β1. This label was detected at one day, peaked at three days, and had decreased by one week.[14] Its role in inflammation appears to be a combination of proinflammatory and negative-feedback molecule. TGF-β has been purported to be chemoattractant for monocytes, T cells, and neutrophils, while increasing levels of IL-1, IL-6, and platelet-derived growth factor. However, TGF-β also interferes with the IL-2 response, deactivates macrophages, and inhibits production of interferon gamma and tumor necrosis factor alpha (TNF-α) A multitude of other cytokines and growth factors undoubtedly play a role in the full response, but these have not yet been characterized in the inner ear.

Despite the importance of the endolymphatic sac in contributing immunocompetent cells and inflammatory mediators to the inner-ear immune response, the inner ear also receives systemic immune cells for protection against viral and bacterial antigens. Both KLH challenge and viral inoculation of the inner ear cause massive cellular infiltration in both the scala tympani and to a lesser extent the scala vestibuli. The spiral modiolar vein (SMV) appears to play a key role in this cellular infiltration.[15] Egress of lymphocytes from the circulation into lymph nodes has long been known to occur at specialized postcapillary venules that have a unique morphology and histochemistry, earning them the name high endothelial venules (HEV).[16–18] Somewhat surprisingly, the SMV has been shown to undergo an HEV-like transformation during the inflammatory response. This transformation consists of endothelial cells with large nuclei and increased cytoplasm, and is present at day two following inner-ear inoculation of virus and continues to progress to day six. Additionally, lymphocytes can be seen adherent to and within the vascular wall[19] (FIG. 2). Hence, HEV-like morphology can apparently be acquired during an acute inflammatory condition in the cochlea. Additionally, at least one adhesion molecule, intercellular adhesion molecule-1 (ICAM-1), has been demonstrated in the SMV and collecting venules in the acute phase of inner-ear inflammation.[20] ICAM-1 is expressed in

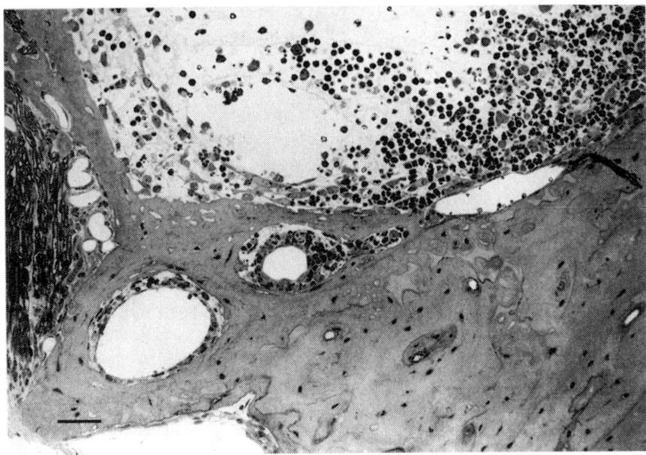

FIGURE 2. Photomicrograph of the spiral modiolar vein during an inflammatory response induced by inoculation of guinea-pig-specific cytomegalovirus into the scala tympani of an adult guinea pig. An HEV-like transformation consisting of endothelial cells with large nuclei and increased cytoplasm is present as early as two days following inner-ear inoculation. Extravasated lymphocytes fill the space between the vessel wall and the bony channel in which the vessel runs. *Scale bar*, 120 μm

HEVs of humans, mice, and rats and is involved in the interactions between leukocytes and endothelial cells, and ultimate extravasation of cells.[21–23] In a study of KLH-induced inner-ear inflammation in rats, staining for ICAM-1 was found within 6 h postchallenge on the epithelium of SMVs and collecting venules, reaching a maximum by day two, and then fading gradually. In contrast, cellular extravasation was observed to peak between days three and seven in the cochlea. ICAM-1 was also found at 12 and 24 h on the epithelium of the endolymphatic sac and perisaccular region, while cellular infiltration lagged by two to three days.[20] Whether or not the HEV-like changes seen in the SMV are part and parcel of the expression of adhesion molecules such as ICAM-1 is still undetermined; however, it is clear that the inner ear is able to mount an immune response and recruit systemic immunocompetent cells through changes in its venous drainage morphology.

The type and timing of cells that enter the cochlea have also been characterized. Macrophages and granulocytes are observed as early as 6 h postchallenge in the cochlea and endolymphatic sac and rapidly increase thereafter. T-helper cells gradually increase in the endolymphatic sac, peaking at two to three weeks, while their presence in the cochlea is noted on day one and continues to increase. Increased levels of T-suppresser cells are not detected in the cochlea or endolymphatic sac until three weeks postchallenge. Additionally, immunoglobulin-bearing cells are seen early in the response. IgG cells are seen in the endolymphatic sac by day one, and IgM follows shortly after with a rise on day two. IgA cells do not appear until three weeks postchallenge.[4] Inflammatory cells in the endolymphatic sac and cochlea continue to proliferate *in situ* during the response and active proliferation is noted a full six weeks following challenge.[24,25] This suggests the absence of strong immunosuppressive mechanisms of the inner ear despite the aforementioned infiltration of T-suppresser cells. The actual quantities of cells derived from endolymphatic sac proliferation versus extravasation is unknown. However, the pattern of rise in cellular constituents is consistent with the roles proposed for each class. The early response of PMNs results in antigen clearing, while the egress of macrophages allows for antigen processing and presentation. T-helper cells also arrive early, presumably in order to potentiate/regulate the response and accentuate the development of arriving B cells into immunoglobulin-secreting plasma cells. The late appearance of T-suppresser cells would be consistent with its proposed function as an immune down-regulator.

A fairly late event in the immune response is the production of antigen-specific antibody in the inner ear. Direct challenge of the perilymph with KLH results in an anti-KLH antibody rise in the perilymph, which peaks between four and seven weeks, and is not due to increased vascular permeability, serum contamination during the sampling process, or from CSF contributions via the cochlear aqueduct.[1,26] Numerous plasma cells are noted in the scala tympani and endolymphatic sac during the response. An important aspect of the timing and magnitude of this response is the animal's immunization status. When a systemically KLH-sensitized animal receives inner-ear challenge with KLH, the secondary humoral immune response is faster, peaking at two weeks, and tenfold larger than the primary response.[1,26] This suggests the egress of KLH-specific plasma cells from the circulation during the response. This rise in anti-KLH antibody was also seen following direct inoculation of the endolymphatic sac. Cellular infiltrates in and around the sac were deemed responsible for the increase in antibody in the perilymph of the cochlea in this study, again suggesting the importance of this structure in sending signals and immune components to the inner ear during challenge.[27] Secretion of antigen-specific antibody is a mechanism of immune response utilized by the inner ear that occurs relatively late in the response and is greatly modified by previous immunization status. Previous immunization therefore undoubtedly has an effect on the final outcome of an inner-ear immune response.

Concomitant with this cellular proliferation is a steady increase in extracellular matrix. Both suppurative and sterile labyrinthitis are known to result in the formation of a dense extracellular matrix and eventual ossification in the cochlea.[1,28,29] The cells responsible for this outcome are now coming to light. Ki-67 immunoassay has revealed that already by day one postchallenge fibroblast and endosteal cells lining the scala tympani are proliferating. The numbers of these cells continue to increase and signs of their proliferation are still present six weeks postchallenge. Fibrotic tissue becomes visible for the first time at one week and ossification is present by three weeks.[25] Ossification of the normally fluid-filled cochlear scalae is a common result of inner-ear inflammation (FIG. 3). A variety of insults result in labyrinthitis ossificans, including purulent labyrinthitis,[28] sterile labyrinthitis,[1] advanced otosclerosis, autoimmune inner-ear disease, temporal bone trauma, labyrinthectomy, meningitis,[30,31] and cochlear implant.[32] The inner ear seems particularly incapable of clearing this extracellular matrix during an immune response, which over time results in osteoneogenesis. The endosteal cells lining the scala tympani now appear to be a key component in this chain of events.

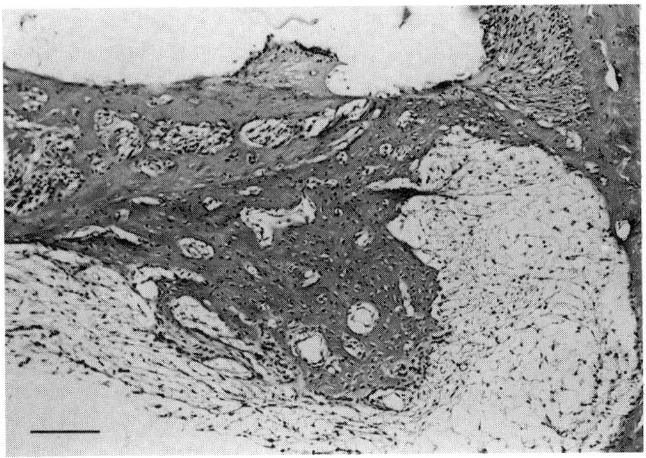

FIGURE 3. Photomicrograph of a guinea pig cochlea 6 weeks following inoculation with guinea-pig-specific cytomegalovirus. Fibrosis and ossification of the inflamed perilymphatic scala that begins at 4 weeks is severe at 6 weeks. *Scale bar*, 120 μm

Unfortunately, this elaborate chain of events, intended to protect the inner ear against pathogens, can often lead to hearing loss. Early studies on the effect of virally induced labyrinthitis revealed severe hearing loss in animals not previously exposed to the pathogen. A full 70% of these seronegative animals had profound elevations of the cochlear microphonic (CM) and eighth nerve N1 compound action potential (CAP) thresholds.[33,34] Further research has revealed that the immune response may be in part responsible for the negative effect on hearing. Investigation of the inner-ear histopathology following virally induced labyrinthitis resulted in consistent findings of degeneration in the organ of Corti, stria vascularis, and spiral ganglion with mild endolymphatic hydrops.[35] What argues for the role of the immune system in this damage is the fact that a variety of viruses can infect the inner ear at different sites and cell types; yet, degeneration of these same structures appears to occur irrespective of the site of viral infection.[35] Additionally, negative effects on histopathology and hearing have been found with sterile labyrinthitis and the amount of damage was associated with the magnitude of the immune response. KLH systemic sensitization prior to secondary inner-ear challenge resulted in a much larger antibody response, greater histopathology, and more significant hearing loss as evidenced by CM and CAP when compared to animals receiving only primary inner-ear challenge.[36] Thus, the more robust immune response appears to result in greater damage to the inner ear. How the immune response damages the aforementioned structures is currently being elucidated. The apparent lack of clearing of the extracellular matrix and subsequent ossification appears to be in part due to activation of the endosteal cells.[26] The degeneration of the spiral ganglion appears to be independent of this ossification, but the mechanism is not yet understood.[29] The degeneration of the stria vascularis has a proposed immune-mediated etiology. Although these cells never express viral antigens in our model, the damage is likely caused by edema secondary to the egress of cells in the downstream venules, creating venous stasis and eventually capillary stasis in the strial vessels. The danger of an inflammatory response in the inner ear therefore seems analogous to infections with pathogens at other sites in the body: pneumonia results in scarring and fibrosis secondary to immune system intervention; immunocompetent cells destroy healthy bone around an osteomyelitis; inflammatory infiltrates cause increased intracranial pressure in meningitis. Unfortunately, the inner ear seems particularly sensitive and incapable of controlling the deleterious effects of an inflammatory response.

AUTOIMMUNE IMMUNOPATHOLOGY

In addition to the damage that may be incurred during an immune response to invading pathogens, the inner ear may also suffer insults from autoimmune phenomena. The three primary mechanisms for autoimmune disease are autoantibodies against tissue antigens, deposition of antigen–antibody immune complexes in tissue, and infiltration and destruction of tissue by specific cytotoxic T cells. There is evidence that the inner ear can be affected in a variety of non-organ-specific autoimmune diseases. Polyarteritis nodosa has been associated, although rarely, with cochlear injury. Although SNHL may be a rare complication of the disease,[37] hearing loss may be the only presenting symptom,[38–40] and histopathologic analysis has revealed ischemic changes as the likely etiology.[41–43] Likewise, Wegener's granulomatosis has been associated with both middle- and inner-ear pathology.[44–47] The improvement of some of these patients with SNHL with prednisone therapy underscores the autoimmune nature of the disease. Otologic manifestations have also been seen with systemic lupus erythematosis, including chronic otitis media with necrotizing vasculitis and progressive SNHL or disequilibrium.[48] Although otologic pathology has been reported in patients with rheumatoid arthritis,[49–51] no temporal bone studies have been reported, and the relationship of rheumatoid arthritis to inner ear disease has not been confirmed. Cogan's syndrome, characterized by interstitial keratitis and vestibuloauditory dysfunction,[52–54] may blur the distinction between non-organ-specific and organ-specific autoimmune disease. The syndrome is thought to be a hypersensitivity response to one or more infectious agents associated with vasculitis;[55] yet, lymphocyte transformation on exposure of patient's lymphocytes to corneal antigen[56,57] and inner-ear antigen has been reported,[58] suggesting possible specific autoimmunity. However, this evidence of specific autoimmunity directed against the eye and ear may merely be a secondary result of the nonspecific vasculitis.

Evidence does exist that the inner ear may be a site of organ-specific autoimmunity. Lehnhardt[59] suggested that cases of bilateral deafness were caused by anticochlear antibodies, and McCabe[48] reestablished this hypothesis as a line of inquiry. Anti-collagen type II antibody has received considerable attention as an animal model of autoimmune inner-ear disease. Several authors have found extensive damage to inner-ear structures, and some hearing loss following initiation of type II collagen autoimmunity;[60–64] however, others have not.[65,66] Initiation of autoimmune inner ear dysfunction has been accomplished with exposure of animals to heterologous cochlear tissue[67,68] with 32% of animals showing significant hearing loss in one study.[66] Interestingly, despite the species of animal used in the study, analysis of sera from the hearing-impaired animals by Western blot revealed an antibody against an inner-ear antigenic epitope with a molecular weight of approximately 68,000 daltons.[68,69] Even more compelling is the finding that some patients (33%) with progressive SNHL show evidence of this same 68,000-dalton anticochlear antibody in their serum on Western blot.[69] This observation has been confirmed by Moscicki[70] in 11 patients who demonstrated this antibody on Western blot analysis and whose hearing improved with immunosuppressive therapy. Humoral autoantibodies are also implicated as a cause of autoimmune SNHL by studies that have shown immunofluorescent labeling following incubation of serum from patients with suspected autoimmune SNHL onto sections of nonrelated, healthy human temporal bones.[71–75] Unfortunately, interpretation of these results remains difficult, as antigen degradation does occur with prolonged decalcification, and HLA differences between the patients and the cadavers may account for the labeling. Alternately, some authors propose cell-mediated immunity as a source of autoimmune inner-ear disease.[76,77] Unfortunately, the specificity and sensitivity of the lymphocyte migration inhibition assay[76] have been questioned, and the lymphocyte transformation assay has also been found to be fairly insensitive.[69] Despite the difficulty in proving the presence and mechanism of organ-specific autoimmunity in the inner ear, the profound response of some patients with rapidly progressive SNHL to immunosuppressives and the clear existence of otologic pathology in some non-organ-specific autoimmune diseases supports this as a clinical entity.

EXPERIMENTAL PARADIGMS

Understanding the mechanisms of immunopathology in the inner ear will hopefully direct our efforts to prevention of this immune-mediated damage. Several studies have revealed that interference with the predictable order of events is possible. As previously mentioned, the normal cochlea contains no observable immunocompetent cells, while the endolymphatic sac appears to contain the cells necessary to initiate an immune response. Several studies have supported the importance of the endolymphatic sac in this function. Challenge of the cochlea with KLH in systemically immunized animals following endolymphatic sac obliteration, resulted in markedly reduced perilymph antibody levels and cellular infiltrates in the cochlea when compared to controls.[78,79] Additionally, this effect was found not to be secondary to surgical trauma.[79] Furthermore, direct KLH challenge of the endolymphatic sac resulted in increased levels of perilymph antibody, and this response was abrogated by prior endolymphatic duct obstruction.[27] Hence, the endolymphatic sac appears to be crucial in antigen processing and appears to be the site from which perilymph antibody emanates. Direct inoculation of the endolymphatic sac with guinea pig cytomegalovirus (GPCMV) in animals with systemic immunity to GPCMV resulted in marked inflammatory cell infiltration in the region of the sac and mild endolymphatic hydrops, but no hearing loss or viral antigen production.[80] Thus, the sac can protect the inner ear structures, but at the expense of some damage to itself. Further evidence of the detrimental effects of the immune response on the inner ear come from Darmstadt *et al.*[81] It was demonstrated that immunosuppression with cyclophosphamide prior to GPCMV inoculation into the scala tympani actually reduced the amount of hearing loss as measured by CAP thresholds when compared to controls. The amount of GPCMV antigen detected in the cochleas did not correlate with the CAP thresholds. However, the greater the inflammatory response to GPCMV in the cochlea, the higher the CAP threshold and thus the greater the hearing loss.[81] The inflammatory response to GPCMV may be more important than direct cytopathic effects of the virus in producing SNHL in GPCMV-induced labyrinthitis. As previously noted, the expression of ICAM-1 in the SMV and its collecting ducts increases during inflammation and undoubtedly has effects on cell trafficking.[20] A modest decrease in this trafficking was accomplished with the use of monoclonal antibodies to ICAM-1 during inner-ear inflammation.[82] Despite this decrease in cellular infiltrates, anti-ICAM-1-treated animals did not show sparing of hearing when compared to controls.[82] Due to the modest decrease in cellular infiltrates, lymphokines, and/or other adhesion molecules yet to be described in the inner ear must play a major role. Thus from these experiments we have been able to determine that inner-ear inflammation can be manipulated by interfering with both the afferent and efferent limbs of the immune response and in doing so not only provide an increased understanding of the pathogenesis of many inner-ear diseases but also help to open new avenues of treatment.

SUMMARY

We have reviewed the events of an inner-ear immune response. The perilymph contains antibody, presumably derived from the systemic circulation and CSF, which would allow for neutralization and help with opsonization and complement fixation. The endolymphatic sac contains immunocompetent cells capable of processing and presenting viral or bacterial antigen, potentiating the immune response, attacking the invaders directly or attacking infected cells, and developing immunoglobulin responses *in situ*. The early release of mediators such as IL-2 likely emanate from the endolymphatic sac and result in potentiation and regulation of the response and may assist in changes in the SMV, including expression of ICAM-1, which aid in the egress of immune cells from the systemic circulation. PMNs arrive first, followed by T cells and B cells, with secretion of specific antibody a relatively late event. Concomitant with the increase in cellular constituents is the formation of a dense extracellular matrix. The inner ear appears to have remarkable difficulty in clearing this matrix, ultimately resulting in ossification. The immune response is unfortunately deleterious to the inner ear, resulting in degeneration of the organ of Corti, stria vascularis, and spiral ganglion. Hearing loss is consistently seen following sterile and virally induced labyrinthitis.

The inner ear also appears to be a target for autoimmune disease. While inner-ear damage has been described as part of non-organ-specific autoimmune disease, specific disease against the hearing apparatus is also likely. Experimental paradigms have allowed alterations of both the afferent and efferent limbs of this response; ultimately, with the hope that we can alter the course of the response and the subsequent damage in patients.

REFERENCES

1. HARRIS, J. P. 1983. Immunology of the inner ear: Response of the inner ear to antigen challenge. Otolaryngol. Head Neck Surg. **91:** 17.
2. MOGI, G., D. LIM & N. WATANABE. 1982. Immunologic study on the inner ear. Arch. Otol. **108:** 270.
3. PALVA, T. & V. RAUNIO. 1981. Disc electrophoretic studies of human perilymph. Ann. Otol. Rhinol. Laryngol. **76:** 23.
4. TAKAHAHSI, M. & J. P. HARRIS. 1988. Anatomic distribution and localization of immunocompetent cells in normal mouse endolymphatic sac. Acta Otolaryngol. **106:** 409.
5. YEO, S. W., S. GOTTSCHLICH, J. P. HARRIS & E. M. KEITHLEY. 1995. Antigen diffusion from the perilymphatic space of the cochlea. Laryngoscope **105:** 623.
6. TAKAHASHI, M. & J. P. HARRIS. 1988. Analysis of immunocompetent cells following inner ear stimulation. Laryngoscope **98:** 1133.
7. MERTELSMANN, R. & K. WELT. 1986. Human interleuken-2: Molecular biology, physiology, and clinical possibilities. Immunobiology **172:** 400.
8. WEYAND, C. M., J. GORONZ, M. J. DALLMAN & C. G. FATHMAN. 1986. Administration of recombinant interleukin-2 in vivo induces a polyclonal IgM response. J. Exp. Med. **163:** 1607.
9. HENNEY, C. S., K. KURIBAYASHI, D. E. KERN & S. GILLIS. 1981. Interleukin-2 augments natural killer cell activity. Nature **291:** 335.
10. DINARELLO, C. A. & J. W. MIER. 1986. Interleukins. Ann. Rev. Med. **37:** 173.
11. MIOSSEC, P., C.-L. YU & M. ZIFF. 1984. Lymphocyte chemotactic activity of human interleukin-1. J. Immunol. **133:** 2007.
12. MIYASAKA, N., T. NAKAMURA, I. J. RUSSEL & N. TALAI. 1984. Interleukin-2 deficiencies in rheumatoid arthritis and SLE. Clin. Immun. Immunopath. **31:** 109.
13. GLODDEK, B. & J. P. HARRIS. 1989. Role of lymphokines in the immune response of the inner ear. Acta Otolaryngol. **108:** 68.
14. YEO, S. W. & A. F. RYAN. 1994. Transforming growth factor-beta (TGF-β) mRNA expression in the rat cochlea during experimental immune labyrinthitis. *In* Immunobiology in Otorhinolaryngology, G. Mogi, J. Veldman, and J. Harris, Eds.: 181–188. Kugler. Amstelveen, The Netherlands.
15. HARRIS, J. P., S. FUKUDA & E. M. KEITHLEY. 1990. Spiral modiolar vein: Its importance in inner ear inflammation. Acta Otolaryngol. **110:** 357.
16. GOWANS, J. L. & E. J. KNIGHT. 1964. The route of recirculation of lymphocytes in the rat. Proc. Soc. Exp. Biol. Med. **159:** 257.
17. ANDERSON, A. O. & N. D. ANDERSON. 1976. Lymphocyte emigration from high endothelial venules in rat lymph nodes. Immunology **31:** 731.
18. FREEMONT, A. J. & C. J. P. JONES. 1983. Light microscopic, histochemical and ultrastructural studies of human lymph node paracortical venules. J. Anat. **136:** 349.
19. STEARNS, G. S., E. M. KEITHLEY & J. P. HARRIS. 1993. Development of high endothelial venule-like characteristics in the spiral modiolar vein induced by viral labyrinthitis. Laryngoscope **103:** 890.
20. SUZUKI, M. & J. P. HARRIS. 1995. Expression of intercellular adhesion molecule-1 during inner ear inflammation. Ann. Otol. Rhinol. Laryngol. **104:** 69.

21. JALKANEN, S. T., R. F. BARATZE, L. R. HERRON & E. C. BUTCHER. 1986. A lymphocyte surface glycoprotein involved in endothelial cell recognition and lymphocyte in man. Eur. J. Immunol. **16:** 1195.

22. STREETER, P. R., B. T. ROUSE & E. C. BUTCHER. 1988. Immunohistologic and functional characterization of a vascular addressin involved in lymphocyte homing into peripheral lymph nodes. J. Cell Biol. **107:** 1853.

23. TAMATANI, T. & M. MIYASAKA. 1990. Identification of monoclonal antibodies reactive with the rat homologue of ICAM-1, and evidence for a differential involvement of ICAM-1 in the adherence of resting versus activated lymphocytes to high endothelial cells. Int. Immunol. **2:** 167.

24. TAKAHASHI, M. & S. TOMIYAMA. 1995. Cell proliferation in the endolymphatic sac in situ after inner ear immunostimulation. Acta Otolaryngol. **115:** 396.

25. CHEN, M. C., E. M. KEITHLEY & J. P. HARRIS. 1997. Immunohistochemical analysis of proliferating cells in a sterile labyrinthitis animal model. Laryngoscope. In press.

26. HARRIS, J. P. 1984. Immunology of the inner ear: Evidence of local antibody production. Ann. Otol. Rhinol. Laryngol. **93:** 157.

27. TOMIYAMA, S & J. P. HARRIS. 1989. Elevation of inner ear antibody levels following direct antigen challenge of the endolymphatic sac. Acta Otolaryngol. **107:** 202.

28. PAPARELLA, M. M. & S. SUGIURA. 1967. The pathology of suppurative labyrinthitis. Ann. Otol. **76:** 554.

29. KEITHLEY, E. M. & J. P. HARRIS. 1996. Late sequelae of cochlear infection. Laryngoscope **106:** 341.

30. BALKANY, T., B. J. GANTZ, R. L. STEENERSON & N. L. COHEN. 1996. Systematic approach to electrode insertion in the ossified cochlea. Otolaryngol. Head Neck Surg. **114:** 4.

31. NADOL, J. B. 1984. Histological considerations in implant patients. Arch. Otolaryngol. **110:** 160.

32. IBRAHIM, R. A. & F. H. LINTHICUM. 1980. Labyrinthine ossificans and cochlear implants. Arch. Otolaryngol. Head Neck Surg. **106:** 111.

33. HARRIS, J. P., N. K. WOOLF, A. F. RYAN, D. M. BUTLER & D. D. RICHMAN. 1984. Immunologic and electrophysiological response to cytomegaloviral inner ear infection in the guinea pig. J. Infect. Dis. **150:** 523.

34. WOOLF, N. K., J. P. HARRIS, A. F. RYAN, D. M. BUTLER & D. D. RICHMAN. 1985. Hearing loss in experimental cytomegalovirus infection of the guinea pig inner ear: Prevention by systemic immunity. Ann. Otol. Rhinol. Laryngol. **94:** 350.

35. KEITHLEY, E. M., N. K. WOOLF & J. P. HARRIS. 1989. Development of morphological and physiological changes in the cochlea induced by cytomegalovirus. Laryngoscope **99:** 409.

36. WOOLF, N. K. & J. P. HARRIS. 1986. Cochlear pathophysiology associated with inner ear immune responses. Acta Otolaryngol. **102:** 353.

37. MALAMUD, N. & O. B. FOSTER. 1941. Periarteritis nodosa: A clinicopathological report with special reference to the central nervous system. Arch. Neurol. Psychiatry **47:** 828.

38. BAKAAR, L. G. 1978. Polyarteritis nodosa presenting with nerve deafness. J. R. Soc. Med. **71:** 144.

39. PEITERSEN, E. & B. H. CARLSEN. 1966. Hearing impairment as the initial sign of polyarteritis nodosa. Acta Otolaryngol. **61:** 189.

40. WOLF, M., J. KRONENBURG, S. ENGELBERG & G. LEVENTON. 1987. Rapidly progressive hearing loss as a symptom of polyarteritis nodosa. Am. J. Otolaryngol. **8:** 105.

41. GUSSEN, R. 1977. Polyarteritis nodosa and deafness: A human temporal bone study. Arch. Otorhinolaryngol. **217:** 263.

42. JENKINS, H. A., A. M. POLLAK & U. FISCH. 1981. Polyarteritis nodosa as a cause of sudden deafness: A human temporal bone study. Am. J. Otolaryngol. **2:** 99.

43. YANAGITA, N., H. YOKOI, J. KOIDE, M. TORIYAMA & T. ISHII. 1987. Acute bilateral deafness with nephritis: A human temporal bone study. Laryngoscope **97**: 345.

44. MCDONALD, T. J. & R. A. DEREMEE. 1983. Wegener's granulomatosis. Laryngoscope **93**: 220.

45. CAMPBELL, S. M., A. MONTANARO & E. J. BARDANA. 1983. Head and neck manifestations of autoimmune disease. Am. J. Otolaryngol. **4**: 187.

46. KORNBLUT, A. D., S. M. WOLFF & A. S. FAUCI. 1982. Ear disease in patients with Wegener's granulomatosis. Laryngoscope **92**: 713.

47. KEMPF, H. G. 1989. Ear involvement in Wegener's granulomatosis. Clin. Otolaryngol. **14(5)**: 451.

48. MCCABE, B. F. 1979. Autoimmune sensorineural hearing loss. Ann. Otol. Rhinol. Laryngol. **88**: 585.

49. MOFFAT, D. A., R. T. RAMSDEN, J. N. ROSENBERG, J. B. BOOTH & W. P. R. GIBSON. 1977. Oto-admittance measurements in patients with rheumatoid arthritis. J. Laryngol. Otol. **91**: 917.

50. HUGHES, G. B., S. E. KINNEY, B. P. BARNA, R. L. TOMSAK & L. H. CALABRESE. 1983. Autoimmune reactivity in Cogan's syndrome: A preliminary report. Otolaryingol. Head Neck Surg. **91**: 24.

51. MCCABE, B. F. 1987. Autoimmune inner ear disease. *In* Immunology of the Ear, J. Bernstein and P. Ogra, Eds. New York. Raven Press.

52. CODY, D. T. & D. A. SONES. 1971. Relapsing polychondritis: Audiovestibular manifestations. Laryngoscope **81**: 1208.

53. COGAN, D. G. 1945. Syndrome of nonsyphilitic interstitial keratitis and vestibuloauditory symptoms. Arch. Opthalmol. **33**: 144.

54. HAYNES, B. F., M. I. KAISER-KUPFER, P. MASON & A. S. FAUCI. 1980. Cogan's syndrome: Studies in thirteen patients, long-term follow-up, and a review of the literature. Medicine **56**: 426.

55. CHESON, B. P., W. Z. BLUMING & J. ALROY. 1976. Cogan's syndrome: A systemic vasculitis. Am. J. Med. **60**: 549.

56. BRINKMAN, C. J. & R. M. BROEKHUYSE. 1978. Cell-mediated immunity after retinal detachment as determined by lymphocyte stimulation. Am. J. Ophthalmol. **86**: 260.

57. CHAR, D. H., D. G. COGAN & W. K. SULLIVAN. 1975. Immunologic study of nonsyphilitic interstitial keratitis with vestibuloauditory symptoms. Am. J. Opththalmol. **80**: 491.

58. HUGHES, G. B., S. E. KINNEY, B. P. BARNA & L. H. CALABRESE. 1983. Autoimmune reactivity in Meniere's disease: A preliminary report. Laryngoscope **93**: 410.

59. LEHNHARDT, E. 1958. Plotzliche Horstorungen, auf beiden Seiten gleichzeitig oder nacheinander aufgetreten. Z. Laryngol. Rhinol. Otol. **37**: 1.

60. YOO, T. J., K. TOMOKA, J. M. STUART, A. J. KANG & A. S. TOWNES. 1983. Type II collagen-induced autoimmune otospongiosis: A preliminary report. Ann. Otol. Rhinol. Laryngol. **92**: 103.

61. YOO, T. J., K. TOMODA, J. M. STUART, M. A. CREMER, A. S. TOWNES & A. J. KANG. 1983. Type II vollagen-induced autoimmune sensorineural hearing loss and vestibular dysfunction in rats. Ann. Otol. Rhinol. Laryngol. **92**: 267.

62. HUANG, C. C., A. X. YI & M. ABRAMSON. 1986. Type II collagen-induced otospongiosis-like lesions in rats. Am. J. Otolaryngol. **7(4)**: 258.

63. OHASHI, T., K. TOMODA & B. YOSHIE. 1989. Electrocochleographic changes in endolymphatic hydrops induced by type II collagen immunization through the stylomastoid foramen. Ann. Otol. Rhinol. Laryngol. **98**: 556.

64. SOLIMAN, A. M. 1990. Type II collagen-induced inner ear disease: Critical evaluation of the guinea pig model. Am. J. Otol. **11(1)**: 27.

65. HARRIS, J. P., N. K. WOOLF & A. F. RYAN. 1986. A reexamination of experimental type II

collagen autoimmunity: Middle and inner ear morphology and function. Ann. Otol. Rhinol. Laryngol. **95:** 176.

66. SOLVSTEN-SORENSEN, M., L. P. NIELSEN, P. BRETLAU & M. B. JORGENSEN. 1988. The role of type II collagen autoimmunity in otosclerosis revisited. Acta Otolaryngol. **105**(3–4): 242.

67. HARRIS, J. P. 1987. Experimental autoimmune sensorineural hearing loss. Laryngoscope **97:** 63.

68. OROZCO, C. R., *et al.* 1990. Experimental model of immune-mediated hearing loss using cross-species immunization. Laryngoscope **100**(9): 941.

69. HARRIS, J. P. & P. SHARP. 1990. Inner ear autoantibodies in patients with rapidly progressive sensorineural hearing loss. Laryngoscope **97:** 63.

70. MOSCICKI, R. 1990. Western blot analysis of serum antibody to inner ear antigens in patients with idiopathic progressive bilateral sensorineural hearing loss. American Neurotology Society Meeting, Palm Beach, Fla., April 27–29.

71. ARNOLD, W., R. PFALTZ & H. J. ALTERMATT. 1985. Evidence of serum antibodies against inner ear tissues in the blood of patients with certain sensorineural hearing disorders. Acta Otolaryngol. **99:** 437.

72. GEBBERS, J. O., H. J. ALTERMATT, W. ARNOLD & J. A. LAISSUEL. 1987. Binding of serum immunoglobulins to human inner ear tissue in inner ear hearing loss: Methodologic limits. HNO **35:** 487.

73. SOLIMAN, A. M. 1988. An improved technique for the study of immunofluorescence using non-decalcified frozen guinea pig cochlea. J. Laryngol. Otol. **103**(3): 215.

74. SOLIMAN, A. M. 1988. A comparative immunofluorescent study of fixed decalcified tissue from the guinea pig cochlea. Arch. Otol. Rhinol. Laryngol. **244**(6): 337.

75. SOLIMAN, A. M. & F. ZANETTI. 1988. Improvements of a method for testing autoantibodies in sensorineural hearing loss. Adv. Otol. Rhinol. Laryngol. **39:** 13.

76. HUGHES, G. B., B. P. BARNA, L. H. CALABRESE, S. E. KINNEY & N. L. NALEPA. 1986. Predictive value of laboratory tests in autoimmune inner ear disease: Preliminary report. Laryngoscope **96:** 502.

77. BERGER, P., S. KOFA, M. ROGOWSKI & M. VOLLRATH. 1989. The lymphocyte transformation test for detecting immunologic inner ear deafness. HNO **37:** 153.

78. TOMIYAMA, S. & J. P. HARRIS. 1986. The endolymphatic sac: Its importance in experimental cytomegalovirus infection of the guinea pig inner ear: Prevention by systemic immunity. Ann. Otol. Rhinol. Laryngol. **94:** 350.

79. TOMIYAMA, S. & J. P. HARRIS. 1987. The role of the endolymphatic sac in inner ear immunity. Acta Otolaryngol. **103:** 182.

80. FUKUDA, A., E. M. KEITHLEY & J. P. HARRIS. 1988. The development of endolymphatic hydrops due to CMV infection of the endolymphatic sac and associated anti-viral inner ear immune responses. Laryngoscope **98:** 439.

81. DARMSTADT, G. L., J. P. HARRIS & E. M. KEITHLEY. 1990. Effects of cyclophosphamide on the pathogenesis of cytomegalovirus-induced labyrinthitis. Ann. Otol. Rhinol. Laryngol. **99**(12): 960.

82. TAKASU, T. & J. P. HARRIS. 1996. Reduction of inner ear inflammation by treatment with anti-ICAM-1 antibody. Sendai Ear Symposium, Syozankan, Sendai, Japan, May 11.

Immune-mediated Sensorineural Hearing Loss with or without Endolymphatic Hydrops: A Clinical and Experimental Approach

JAN E. VELDMAN[a]

Department of Otorhinolaryngology
University Hospital Utrecht
P.O. Box 85500
3508 GA Utrecht
The Netherlands

INTRODUCTION

Since 1979, when McCabe[1] described a pattern of bilateral sensorineural hearing loss (SNHL), characterized by a rapid progression over days to weeks, we are still struggling with the postulated issue of an "auto"-immune inner-ear disorder. [2] A clinical diagnosis, based on the responsiveness of hearing restoration after immunosuppresive treatment, is only circumstantial evidence for an immune-mediated disease, but not sufficient to prove the issue of organ-specific autoimmunity. Various attempts have been made to develop the best assays that will clinically confirm the diagnosis and help to identify those patients who may respond to therapy.[3,4] Yamanobe and Harris, [5] Veldman *et al.*,[6] and Cao *et al.*[7] have used the Western blot (W-B) assay to demonstrate that patients with rapidly progressive sensorineural hearing loss have circulating antibodies that cross-react with different inner-ear antigens of heterologous origin (cow;[4,6] swine;[6] guinea pig[7]). Antigens of interest that show up as a positive band in a W-B assay have a molecular weight ranging between 15–27, 40, 45, 50, 65–68, and 80 kD.

Interspecies differences may exist in these assays (cow, swine versus guinea pig). It was first thought that the discrete positive bands in this assay were unique for this inner-ear disease. However, detailed analyses revealed that the same patients' sera will also cross-react in an identical manner with other tissues protein extracts.[6,7] Furthermore, 65% of our patients with idiopathic sudden deafness (S.D.), that is, *unilateral* sensorineural hearing loss of 30 dB in at least three frequences within 24 h after onset, had also circulating antibodies that cross-react in the same W-B assay with various antigens of similar molecular weight. Immunosuppressive therapy seems to be as effective in S.D. cases as in the presumed "autoimmune" group of patients.[6] In the most recent literature,[4,8] arguments are put forward that the antibody to the 65–68-kD protein is closely associated with this particular form of rapidly progressive SNHL and correlates with the disease activity and responsiveness to immunosuppressive (corticosteroid) therapy. Based on the amino-acid sequence of this protein of interest (65–68 kD), it has been postulated that it is a so-called heat-shock

[a]Phone: +31 30 2506645; fax: +31 30 2541922.

protein (hsp 70).[9] Whether these proteins are instrumental in the etiopathogenesis of this particular inner-ear disease, or that release of hsp(s) elicits antibody formation as a consequence of the underlying disease is still not clear.

Rapidly progressive SNHL and sudden deafness present clinically in a different manner than those cases with SNHL associated with systemic autoimmune disease. In the latter cases, the SNHL is either a result of an immune-complex-induced vasculitis, or even more rarely, a defect secondary to other immunological complications of immune defense such as postvaccination serum sickness. Corticosteroid treatment has proven to be beneficial in these cases and leads to partial or total restoration of audiovestibular function.[10,11]

Another category of patients who may suffer from immune-mediated inner-ear disease are those with "serous" labyrinthitis. Their SNHL is also rapidly progressive, occasionally fluctuating and nearly always accompanied by disabling vertigo. They often complain of tinnitus and pressure in one or both ears. The latter may reflect endolymphatic hydrops. The underlying cause is usually an infectious disease-state in the direct vicinity of the inner-ear complex. Biologic mediators of inflammation released during an immune-reaction around the inner ear (e.g., cholesteatoma cases with a labyrinthine fistula), may gain access to the labyrinthine compartments as soon as the natural protective barriers are "broken." A *perilabyrinthitis* can thus interfere with the inner ear's fluid and electrolyte homeostasis, subsequently leading to immune-mediated endolymphatic hydrops and severe but reversible SNHL. Recent experimental data support this concept.[12]

The fundamental immune mechanisms in all three inner-ear disease categories— (1) "auto-immune" organ-specific SNHL, (2) SNHL as part of a systemic autoimmune disorder; and (3) immune-mediated SNHL with endolymphatic hydrops due to perilabyrinthitis—are different. Immunosuppressive treatment responses are as effective in all three categories, at least in the initial stage of the disease. Organ-specific vestibuloauditory autoimmunity remains of all these clinical entities the most controversial one.

ORGAN-SPECIFIC AUTOIMMUNE INNER-EAR DISEASE?

Organ-specific autoimmune diseases are characterized by the frequent presence of autoantibodies against antigens of the involved organs (e.g., Hashimoto's disease thyroid; uveitis eye; glomerulonephritis kidney). Cell-mediated immunity may be involved, but is more difficult to prove. If disease expression occurs in tissues, accessible for biopsies, modern immunohistological analyses may reveal T-lymphocyte involvement in the disease process. In general, however, inner-ear disorders are hampered by the inaccessability for adequate tissue research during the active phase of the disease. Thus the final diagnosis is often based on circumstantial clinical evidence.

We have studied sera from 127 patients. A clinical diagnosis of rapidly progressive SNHL (N=33), unilateral sudden deafness (N=53) as well as patients with a variety of causes for their SNHL (N=41; mixed group) were analyzed by Western blot assays. To establish organ specificity in these tests, different sera from patients with one or more positive bands also ran in a similar assay against protein extracts from dissected swine vestibular, and cochlear membrane protein, cranial nerves (VII & VIII), kidney and brain. Immunosuppressive treatment responses in the rapidly progressive SNHL group were evaluated and compared with the final outcome of the W-B assays.

MATERIAL AND METHODS

Patients

Sera from 127 patients with an uni- or bilateral idiopahtic SNHL were collected and stored (1985–1995) at the Department of Otorhinolaryngology, Utrecht University, Utrecht, The Netherlands. Within this total group 33 patients with a *rapidly progressive SNHL* were separated for serological analyses. Their hearing loss (uni- or bilateral) was defined as ≥30 dB in at least three frequencies by toneburst and speech audiometry, and was progressive over weeks to months.

Another category, not presented in this paper but referred to, are unilateral *sudden deafness* cases (*N*=53), whose onset of SNHL is acute and within 24 hours. Both groups may present with tinnitus and/or vertigo. Forty-one patients were designed as a *mixed group*. All patients had a general physical and ENT examination. An extensive audiovestibular, radiological, microbiological, and immunological work-up was performed according to an earlier reported protocol.[11]

Western Blot Assays

Fresh swine temporal bones, kidney, and brain tissue were obtained from a local slaughter house. Surgical dissection was immediately carried out. The cochlear and vestibular membranous proteins, cranial nerves (VII and VIII), kidney, and brain tissue were subsequently extracted with 1% sodiumdodecyl sulfate (SDS) and placed in boiling water for 5 minutes. After centrifuging, the supernatant was mixed with equal volumes of sample buffer (10 mM tris,10 mM $MgCl_2$, and 0.1 mM $CaCl_2$) and stopmix (bromophenol blue 0.001%, glycerol 10%, SDS 2%, and tris-HCL buffer, pH 6.8, 62.5 mM, 1.85% α-iodoacetamide).

The total amount of protein was measured according to Bradford. Electrophoresis in SDS and 12% polyacrylamide (SDS-PAGE) was performed. Proteins were tranferred onto Immunobilon-P® membranes (Millipore Corp., Badford, Mass.) by semidry electroblotting with a Transblot® cell and power supply from Biorad (Richmond, Calif.). After incubation in blocking solution (5% nonfat dry milk, 0.2% Tween-20® and 0.01% Antifoam-A® emulsion (Sigma, St.Louis, Mo.), and 0.02% sodium azide) the membranes were placed in an incubation tray (Accutran Cross Blot®, Schleicher and Schnell, Dassel, Germany) and incubated with blocking-solution-diluted patient sera for 2 h at room temperature. After washing in PBS (pH 7.4) with 0.2% Tween-20, membranes were incubated with peroxidase conjugated goat-antihuman IgG, IgM, or IgA, and finally developed with 3.3′-diaminobenzidine.

Immunosuppressive Therapy

Rapidly Progressive SNHL-group (N = 33)

Immunosuppressive therapy (2 mg prednisone/kg body weight; $N = 17$); prednisone (2 mg/kg body weight), and cyclophosphamide (Endoxan®) (2 mg/kg body weight; $N = 10$) was started on pure clinical grounds. Endoxan was added if prednisone alone was not effective within 2 weeks after starting the initial therapy. Six patients received neither medication. At the time of initial therapy the results of the W-B assays were not known. Treatment responses were afterwards compared with the outcome of the W-B assay (positive/negative?) and possibly related to particular W-B profiles per individual patient.

RESULTS

Of those patients who met the clinical criteria to be included in the rapidly progressive SNHL group ($N = 33$), 45% had a positive W-B assay with one or more bands, but 55% were negative (TABLE 1). Positive bands were found with a molecular weight of 15, 20, 25, 27, 40, 44–45, 50, 55, 65–68, and 80 kD.

TABLE 2 represents the results of immunosuppressive therapy in both W-B-positive and -negative patients. Those patients considered to belong to the rapidly progressive SNHL group had a positive treatment response in 45% of the cases (with a W-B + profile) (TABLES 2 and 3). However, also 33% *positive responses* were noticed in cases with W-B-negative profiles. Immunosuppressive therapy appeared to be most effective in the 65–68-kD positive patients: restoration of SNHL with ≥25 dB in at least three frequencies. Whether or not vestibular symptoms or function loss as part of the disease were present did not interfere with the effects of therapy.

The 65–68-kD protein is apparently not "inner ear" specific since W-B assays with other protein extracts from kidney and brain showed up with similar discrete positive bands. Also within the inner ear itself these proteins of interest are as well found in the cochlear, as in the vestibular and neural partition. Determination of the immunoglobulin class showed that these circulating cross-reacting antibodies were either of the IgG or IgA class.[6]

TABLE 1. Results of Western Blot Assays in Different Patients Groups

Patient Group	N	Wetern Blot +	Western Blot −
Rapidly progressive SNHL	33	15 (45%)	18 (55%)
Sudden deafness	53	21 (40%)	32 (60%)
Mixed group	14	21 (51%)	20 (49%)

TABLE 2. Rapidly Progressive SNHL: Western-blot-profile-positive Patients

	+	−
Prednisone ($N = 7$)[a]	3	3
Prednisone/endoxan ($N = 5$)	2	3
− ($N = 3$)	—	3

[a]Follow-up of one patient was lost.

DISCUSSION AND COMMENTS

Evaluation of the diagnostic and therapeutic modalities in this particular group of patients with idiopathic rapidly progressive SNHL remains difficult. The number of patients is still small and the workup lacks the prospective randomized double-blind/placebo-controlled clinical-trial criteria. The group of patients with this tentative diagnosis remains small per individual clinic. Even in a referal center such as ours only 33 patients who meet the inclusion criteria of presumed autoimmune organ-specific inner-ear disease are seen, analyzed, and treated over a period of approximately 10 years. It is questionable whether on medical ethical grounds randomized placebo-therapy is any more acceptable in this population of patients who face severe irreversible SNHL unless treated with high doses of immunosuppressive medication. The results of our retrospective study indicate that 3 out of 10 patients with a W-B-negative laboratory outcome still benefit from corticosteroid therapy. In the W-B-positive group corticosteroid therapy has been effective in 3 out of 6 cases, whereas adding Endoxan medication as a combined therapy leads to beneficial effects in another 2 out of 5 cases. In the W-B-negative cases additional Endoxan medication does not lead to better hearing. Witholding therapy in both W-B-positive and -negative patients led to an irreversible progression of the SNHL. This is in contrast to the earlier published data on the effectiveness of corticosteroid treatment in sudden deafness cases. Corticosteroid therapy is more effective in this latter group than no therapy, whatever the outcome is in a W-B assay. Spontaneous recovery also occurs, but only in those cases with a positive W-B profile.[6]

It appears that the antigenic epitopes with a molecular weight of interest are not unique for the cochlea. They are also found in other tissue extracts. Whether or not the presence of circulating antibodies to a 65–68-kD constituent of bovine[4,5] and swine inner-ear extract[6] serve as unique markers for organ-specific autoimmune au-

TABLE 3. Rapidly Progressive SNHL: Western-blot-profile-negative Patients

	+	−
Prednisone ($N = 10$)	3	7
Prednisone/endoxan ($N = 5$)	—	5
− ($N = 3$)	—	3

diovestibular dysfunctioning is still a matter of interpretation and discussion. Its presence suggests a correlation with disease activity (= inner-ear destruction?). A positive response to immunosuppressive therapy is obvious in these cases. However, in our material, this is not exclusively restricted to these patients. Those who had positive bands of another molecular weight and even patients with a negative W-B profile did respond to immunosuppressive therapy (TABLES 2 and 3), although to a lesser extent. It should be noted further that reversible progression of SNHL was never observed in cases with a 65–68-kD band who did not receive medical treatment (6 out of 41 in the so-called mixed SNHL group). We may have misdiagnosed these patients on pure clinical grounds. Their SNHL developed over months to years. They did not meet the inclusion criteria of the other two catagories, that is, rapidly progressive SNHL or sudden deafness.

IMMUNE-MEDIATED ENDOLYMPHATIC HYDROPS

Does endolymphatic hydrops always accompany immune-mediated/autoimmune inner-ear disease as it does in Meniere's disease? For example, can immune-mediated SNHL also develop without endolymphatic hydrops? Human temporal bone studies of autoimmune cases—mainly with Cogan's disease—illustrate that endolymphatic hydrops and destroyed or damaged sensory epithelia are present at the same time. The same may hold for inner-ear-specific autoimmune disease[13,14]

Recent experimental data show that an aspecific immune reaction (mononuclear cell infiltrate)—elicited around the endolymphatic sac in the guinea pig—leads to a moderate endolymphatic hydrops within 1–2 weeks. The microanatomy of the membranous labyrinth is undisturbed in this animal model, but fluctuating hearing loss is present. This is presumably a consequence of the production and release of biomediators into the endolymph and perilymph. SNHL appears to be reversible in this particular experimental model. Hearing comes back to the normal threshold under conditions where endolymphatic hydrops persists. The sensory epithelium remains intact.[12]

Systemic challenge with swine inner-ear protein antigens leads within 2 weeks in guinea pigs to a negative summating potential and decreased combined action potential. It is present in the majority of the animals, some with and some without an endolymphatic hydrops (unpublished data). These latter experiments challenge the concept of organ-specific (auto-)immune inner-ear disease. Although in both animal models fundamental immune mechanisms operate, their basic targets at a cellular level (endolymphatic sac, stria vascularis, organ of Corti, neural elements?) is very likely a different one.

Future basic and clinical research will hopefully bring immune-mediated inner-ear diseases into the correct perspectives of clinical otology.

SUMMARY

Since 1979, when McCabe first described a pattern of bilateral sensorineural hearing loss (SNHL) characterized by a rapid progression over days to weeks, the postulated autoimmune basis of this disease remains unknown. Various attempts have been made to develop the best assays that will clinically confirm the diagnosis and will help identify those patients who may respond to immunosuppressive therapy. The Western blot assay has now been widely applied by different research groups. It has been suggested that antibody to the 68-kD protein is most closely associated with this disorder. Recent analyses suggest that the protein of interest is probably a heat-shock protein (hsp 70) with this molecular weight.

This disease pattern of rapidly progressive bilateral SNHL presents itself clinically as a different disease than endolymphatic hydrops with fluctuating SNHL, and it is most often associated with vertigo and roaring tinnitus. Meniere's disease may be also immune-mediated, but lacks an autoimmune basis. Its etiopathogenesis is different. A critical review of our own Western blot analyses from patients with either idiopathic rapidly progressive SNHL ($N = 33$), sudden deafness ($N = 53$), or other SNHL forms ($N = 71$) is presented. Immuno-suppressive treatment responses were evaluated.

A new concept of immune-mediated endolymphatic hydrops was also further developed on the basis of recent experimental data and earlier clinical observations in order to focus on another aspect of this most intriguing inner-ear disease.

REFERENCES

1. McCabe, B. F. 1979. Autoimmune sensorineural hearing loss. Ann. Otol. Laryngol. **88:** 585–590.
2. Veldman, J. E. 1991. Immune-mediated inner ear disorders: An otoimmunologist's view. *In* Bearing of Basic Research on Clinical Otolaryngology, C. R. Pfaltz, W. Arnold, and O. Kleinsasser, Eds. Adv. Otorhinlaryngol. **46:** 71–1. Karger. Basel.
3. Hughes, G. B. & B. P. Barba. 1991. Autoimmune inner ear disease: Fact or fantasy? *In* Bearing of Basic Research on Clinical Otolaryngology, C. R. Pfaltz, W, Arnold, and O. Kleinsasser, Eds. Adv. Otorhinlaryngol. **46:** 82–91. Karger. Basel.
4. Moscicki, R.A., J. E. San Martin, C. H. Quintero, S. D. Rauch, J. B. Nadol & K. J. Bloch. 1994. Serum antibody to inner ear proteins in patients with progressive hearing loss. JAMA **272:** 611–616.
5. Yamanobe, S. & J. P. Harris. 1993. Inner ear-specific autoantibodies. Laryngoscope **103:** 319–325.
6. Veldman, J. E., T. Hanada & F. Meeuwsen. 1993. Diagnostic and therapeutic dilemmas in rapidly progressive sensorineural hearing loss and sudden deafness. Acta Otolaryngol. (Stockholm) **113:** 303–306.
7. Cao M. Y., N. Deggoui, M. Gersdorff & J. P. Tomassi. 1996. Guinea pig inner ear antigens: Extraction and application to the study of human autoimmune inner ear disease. Laryngoscope **106:** 207–212.
8. Harris, J. P. & A. F. Ryan. 1995. Fundamental immune mechanisms of the brain and inner ear. Otolaryngol. Head Neck Surg. **112:** 639–653.
9. Billings, P. B., E. M. Keithley & J. P. Harris. 1995. Evidence linking the 68 kD antigen associated with progressive sensorineural hearing loss with the highly inducable hsp 70. Ann. Otol. Rhinol. Laryngol. **104:** 181–188.
10. Veldman, J. E., J. J. Roord, A. F. O'Connor & J. J. Shea. 1984. Autoimmunity and inner ear disorders: An immune-complex mediated sensorineural hearing loss. Laryngoscope **94:** 501–507.

11. VELDMAN, J. E. 1987. Immune-mediated inner ear disorders. New syndromes and their etiopathogenesis. *In* Otoimmunology, J. E. Veldman and B. F. McCabe, Eds.: 125–138. Kugler. Amsterdam/Berkley.

12. BOUMAN, H., S. F. L. KLIS, J. C. M. J. DE GROOT, G. F. SMOORENBURG, E. H. HUIZING & J. E. VELDMAN. 1997. Induction of an immune-mediated endolymphatic hydrops by perisaccular deposition of sepharose beads with and without immune complexes. Hearing Research. In press.

13. SCHUKNECHT, H. F. 1993. Disorders of the immune system. *In* Pathology of the Ear, 2nd ed. Chap. 10: 345–365. Lea & Febiger, Philadelphia.

14. IURATO, S. & J. E.VELDMAN, EDS. 1997. Progress in Human Auditory and Vestibular Histopathology. 1–193. Kugler. Amsterdam/New York.

Systemic Autoimmune Diseases Associated with Hearing Loss

WOLFGANG ARNOLD[a]

Department of Otorhinolaryngology, Head and Neck Surgery
Technical University of Munich
Klinikum rechts der Isar
Ismaninger Str. 22, D-81675 München, Germany

INTRODUZIONE

Autoimmune disease is characterized by production of either antibodies that react with host tissue or immune effector T cells that are autoreactive to endogenous self-peptides. Since B-cell responses in humans generally require inducer T cells, a B-cell autoantibody response directly implies disordered T-cell immunoregulatory control. In some instances, autoantibodies may arise by a normal T- and B-cell response activated by foreign organisms or substances that contain antigens, particularly polysaccharides, that cross-react with similar self-antigens in body tissues. This phenomenon is called *molecular mimicry.* Examples of clinically relevant autoantibodies are antibodies against acetylcholine receptors in *myasthenia gravis* and anti-DNA, antierythrocyte, and antiplatelet antibodies in *systemic lupus erythematosus* (SLE).

The unique portion of the variable region of the immunoglobulin molecule where antigen binds is called the *idiotype,* and an antibody that reacts specifically with that region is called an *anti-idiotype antibody.* Anti-idiotype antibodies may arise during the course of the normal immune response. For example, anti-idiotypes against antitetanus antibodies develop during normal immunization of humans to tetanus toxoid, and serve to deliver "off" signals to B cells secreting antitetanus antibodies. Such antibodies are thus an important component of the normal immunoregulatory network. Anti-idiotype antibodies also may be relevant to two types of autoimmunity: (1) dysfunction of the idiotype–anti-idiotype antibody system could lead to B-cell hyperreactivity by failure to generate off signals for B-cell differentiation, and (2) some antireceptor antibodies produced in autoimmune diseases (antiacetylcholine receptor antibodies in myasthenia gravis, anti-insulin receptor antibodies in forms of type I diabetes mellitus, and antithyrotropin receptor antibodies in autoimmune thyroid disease) may be anti-idiotype antibodies made against the antibody-combining site (idiotype) of an autoantibody.[1,2]

Genetic factors likely play a role in the genesis of autoimmune disease, either by selecting for inherent B-cell hyperreactivity and tendency toward autoantibody formation or, in the case of MHC antigen association with autoimmune diseases, by presentation of self- or foreign peptides that stimulate an inappropriate antiself response. Myasthenia gravis, autoimmune thyroid disease, and pernicious anaemia are all asso-

[a]Phone: 00 49-89-41 40-23 70; fax: 00 49-89-41 40-48 53; e-mail: W. Arnold @ lrz.tu. muenchen.de

187

TABLE 1. Organ-*specific* Autoimmune Diseases with Ear Symptoms

Endocrine system	∅
Skin	∅
Hematologic system	∅
Neuromuscular system	Myasthenia gravis Acute disseminated encephalomyelitis
Hepatobiliary system	∅
Gastrointestinal tract	Inflammatory bowel disease

ciated with HLA-B8 (MHC class I) and -DR3 (MHC class II) expression, and are also associated with certain immunoglobulin heavy chain markers. There is also a strong association of certain DR types with the development of rheumatoid arthritis and ulcerative colitis.[2–4]

Whereas *organ-specific autoimmune diseases* are likely the result of the combined effects of several factors that lead to inappropriate targeting of a particular organ or system to immune damage (TABLE 1), *nonorgan-specific autoimmune diseases,* such as SLE, can be thought of as diseases in which there is episodic breakdown of immunologic tolerance to self molecules (TABLE 2). Recent studies have demonstrated that in a mouse model of autoimmunity (the MRL mouse), the cause of autoimmune disease is a defect in a cell surface molecule (fas/APO-1) on T cells that is required for the intrathymic death of autoreactive T lymphocytes. The defective fas/APO-1 molecule prevents negative selection of autoreactive T cells, leading to seeding of peripheral lymphoid organs with excessive numbers of autoreactive T cells. Interestingly enough MRL-mice reveal severe cochlear damage at early stages of the systemic disease.[5,6]

TABLE 2. Organ-*nonspecific* Autoimmune Diseases with Ear Symptoms

Connective tissue diseases	Systemic lupus erythematosus? Sjögren's syndrome Rheumatoid arthritis Reactive arthritides Vogt–Koyanagi–Harada syndrome Behçet's syndrome? Relapsing polychondrities

Vasculitis syndromes	Systemic necrotizing vasculitides
	   Polyarteritis nodosa
	   Giant cell vasculitis
	Wegener's granulomatosis
	Cogan's syndrome
	Behçet's syndrome?
	Systemic lupus erthematosus?

TEMA CON VARIAZIONI

Although precise details of the autoimmune response are incompletely understood, the outcome of antigenic stimulation, whether antibody formation or activated T cells or tolerance, seems to depend on the same factors with autoantigens as with exogenous antigenes. Four possible mechanisms for the developing an immune response to autoantigenes are recognized:

1. Hidden or sequestered antigens (e.g., intracellular substances) may not be recognized as "self"; if released into the circulation they may induce an immune response. This occurs in sympathetic ophthalmia with the traumatic release of an antigen normally sequestered within the eye. The same seems to be valid for the sympathetic cochleopathia, which at least clinically can be described as a sudden or progressive sensorineural hearing loss in the last hearing ear many years following infectious or traumatic deafness of the contralateral ear.[7] This may be an example for a possible, but not proven organ-specific autoimmunity of the ear since there is no further involvement of other organs of the body. McCabe established the term autoimmune sensorineural hearing loss in 1979.[8] Although immunologic mechanisms were implicated in pathogenesis within McCabe's case report, autoimmunity was not proven, but interpreted because of the excellent response on an immunosuppresive therapy.

2. The self-antigenes may become immunogenic because of chemical, physical, or biologic alteration. This is valid in contact dermatitis, hypersensitivity to drugs, or physically (photosensitivity) induced autoallergy.

3. Foreign antigens may induce an immune response that cross-reacts with normal self-antigens; for example, the cross-reaction that occurs between streptococcal M. protein and human heart muscle; the encephalitis that can follow rabies vaccination in which an autoimmune cross-reaction probably is initiated by animal brain tissue in the vaccine. As far as I know there is no example of sensorineural hearing loss based on mechanism 2 or 3.

4. Autoimmune phenomena may be epiphenomena, and the primary pathogenesis the result of an immune response to an obscure antigen (e.g., virus). As known from virus-infected cells a viral infection of inner-ear tissue should be able to alter the antigenic characteristics of certain cells or cell-components, in a way that the locally induced immune response is directed against inner-ear tissue (on the understanding that the immune defense system of the endolymphatic sac[9,10] is provided ("triggered") with the capacity of antibody production against proteins of the infectious agents).

In contrast to these—until now—more or less hypothetical organ-specific autoimmune diseases of the inner ear there are a number of nonorgan-specific (systemic) autoimmune diseases that affect the ear. The amazing personal observation that gets support by the literature is that the ear disease can be the first symptom of the later developing systemic autoimmune disease and vice versa. Examples are given in the following subsections.

Variazione 1

Relapsing Polychondritis

Relapsing polychondritis (RP) is an autoimmune disease with an unknown etiology causing inflammatory reactions in the cartilaginous tissues of nose, ears, eyes, trachea, and joints, where collagen type II is the major protein.[11] Acute painful swelling and redness of the external ear (FIG. 1) are the first symptoms of the disease in about 40% of all patients. Later in the course of the disease more than 80% experience these symptoms. About 40% of the patients experience vestibular or auditory abnormality of varying degrees from probable vasculitis of the internal auditory artery, although the pathomechanism is not known.[12] Over 30% of patients have an associated disorder, including Sjögren's syndrome, rheumatoid arthritis, SLE, systemic vasculi-

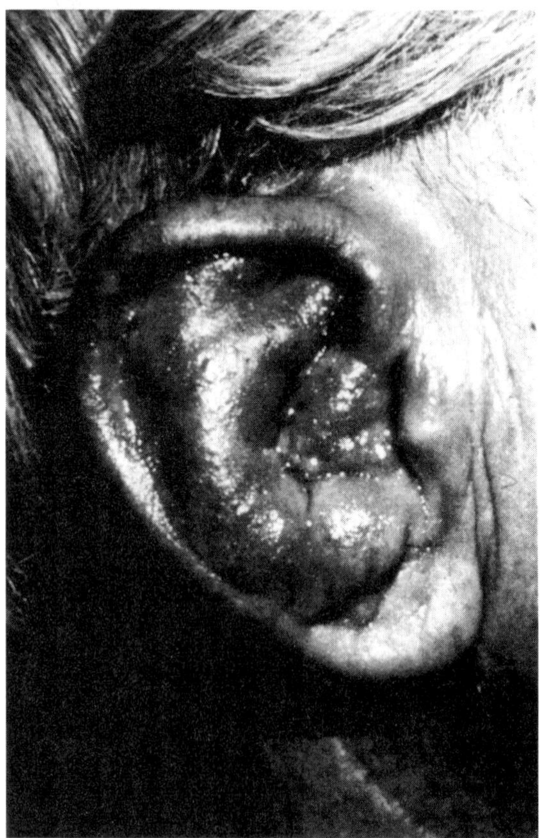

FIGURE 1. Relapsing polychondritis. Sixty-three-year-old woman with recurrent painful swelling of her right auricle extending to the cartilagineous part of the external auditory canal. She had rheumatoid arthritis and a both side severe sensorineural hearing loss.

tis, overlapping connective tissue disorders, psoriasis vulgaris, spondyloarthro-pathies, dysmyelopoietic syndrome, Hodgkin's disease, or diabetes mellitus.[11] The pathology shows destructive changes in the fibrocartilaginous junction that are mediated by mononuclear cells, particularly CD4+ lymphocytes.[13] Evidence of local complement activation was observed and an elevated level of anticollagen antibodies and cell-mediated immunity to cartilage components was also found.[14] It is likely that RP belongs to the connective tissue autoimmune diseases, since antibodies against collagen type II are serologic markers.

Among 40 cases with RP reported by Cody *et al.*[15] profound deafness in four cases progressed rapidly within 24 h. Most cases of inner ear disturbance associated with RP show audiovestibular symptoms, including hearing loss that can be bilateral or unilateral, conductive and/or sensorineural, sudden and profound in onset or rapidly or slowly progressive, and vertigo.[15,16] The conductive hearing loss can be explained by the involvement of the cartilageous structures of the middle ear (joints of ossicles or eustachian tube) in the inflammatory process. Because there is no cartilage in the inner ear, it can be assumed that the inner-ear pathology is caused by obliterative vasculitis of the labyrinthine artery or its branches. The globuli interossei or the enchondral bony labyrinth consist of islands of calcified cartilage, which probably would not generate an antigenic response.[16] Temporal bone findings in a case of sudden deafness and RP[17] revealed severe degeneration of the membranous labyrinth and a fibro-osseous reaction within the basal turn of the cochlea and lateral semicircular canal. There was no endolymphatic hydrops.

Variazione 2

Systemic Vasculitis

Systemic vasculitis is characterized by clinical evidence of blood vessel inflammation that produces ischemic changes in any or all organ systems and by histopathologic evidence of necrosis in vessel walls and in perivascular tissue, including inflammatory cell infiltrate. Vasculitis includes a broad spectrum of disorders, such as *Wegener's granulomatosis* (WG), *polyarteritis nodosa* (PAN), and SLE. Any size or type of blood vessel can be involved in systemic vasculitis, and most kinds of systemic vasculitis can be associated with immunopathogenic mechanisms.

Involvement of the ear is not unusual in systemic vasculitis, and many cases of otitis media or changes in the middle ear have been described.[18–22] Hearing loss is commonly reported as a presenting otologic symptom of WG,[23,24] PAN,[16,25,26] and SLE.[27–29] The nature of the hearing loss is usually mixed or of the fluctuating sensorineural type, suggesting that endolymphatic hydrops might play a role in the pathomechanism of sensorineural hearing loss.[29] Yoon *et al.*[30] studied 16 temporal bones from eight patients to determine histopathologic changes that occur in systemic vasculitis. Three persons had WG, two had PAN, and three had SLE. Otitis media was seen in 15 ears, with 10 ears showing chronic middle-ear changes and two fibrotic inner-ear changes. In WG granulation tissue was observed around the eustachian tube and protympanum (FIG. 2), and in PAN inflammatory cell infiltrate and thickened plugged vessels were observed around the facial nerve. In SLE there was severe fi-

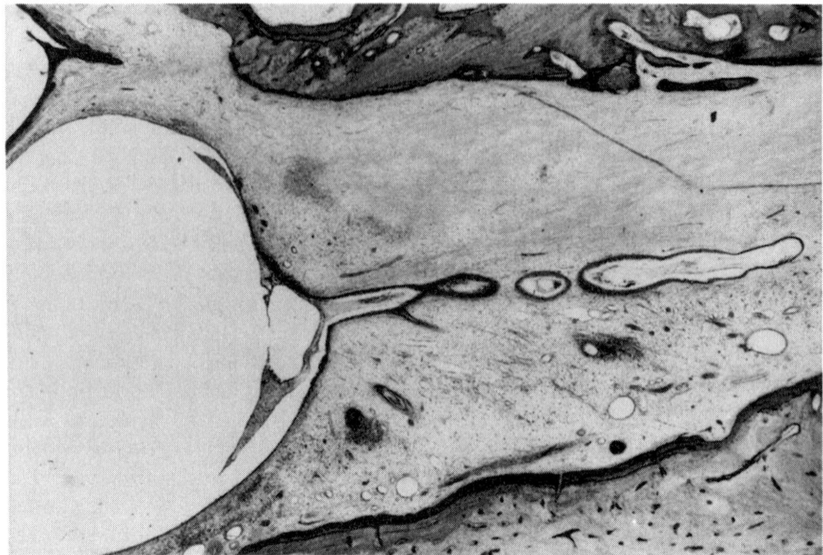

FIGURE 2. Wegener's granulomatosis. One year before death from terminal renal failure, this patient developed a bilateral acute otitis media. The submucosal layer of the middle ear and mastoid is thickened by deposition of fibrous tissue with a leucozytic infiltration, especially around necrotizing vessels. This is most pronounced in the protympanum and has caused Eustachian tube obstruction.

brosis and new bone formation throughout the inner ear. In WG, involvement of the middle ear is mentioned with an incidence ranging from 35% to 47%.[31,32] The same seems to be valid for PAN.[22]

Loss of hearing has commonly been observed as an initial symptom in systemic vasculitis. Although mixed conductive hearing loss and sensorineural loss have been reported in WG and PAN, most reported cases of PAN and all reported cases of SLE have included sensorineural hearing loss.[32] In animal experiments it has been demonstrated that after systemic immunization followed by local exposition of the antigen, the inner ear reacts with an inflammation of the spiral modiolar vein with severe leukocyte infiltration at this point, leading to fibrosis and new bone formation in the cochlea.[33] Fibrotic changes and formation of new bone in the inner ear have been observed in humans who have systemic vasculitis, including WG and PAN.[19,25,34] It may be suggested that there is a common ethiopathogenesis in the development of similar histopathologic changes in the various types of systemic vasculitis.

Variazione 3

Cogan's Syndrome, as originally described by Cogan,[35] consists of nonsyphilitic interstitial keratitis with audiovestibular symptoms, occasionally associated with irits and subconjunctival hemorrhages. Two types of this syndrome have been recognized, the "localized" and the "systemic" type.[15,36] The localized Cogan's syndrome causes chronic inflammation of the cornea and a Ménière's like complex of symptoms, including sudden hearing loss, tinnitus, and severe vertigo, in most cases resulting in deafness. In the majority of the reported cases there was an underlying systemic process resembling polyarteritis nodosa. About 20% of the patients had fatal or near-fatal aortic valvular disease, or other systemic manifestations, including congestive heart failure, systemic necrotizing vasculitis, gastrointestinal hemorrhage, adenopathy, glomerulonephritis, splenomegaly, hypertension, musculoskeletal involvement, and eosinophilia.[37] It is worth noting that similar symptoms and findings have been described in systemic vasculitis, as mentioned before. According to Cheson *et al.,*[38] of 18 reported vessel or muscle biopsies in patients with Cogan's syndrome, 10 specimens (56%) showed inflammatory vascular changes, of which 4 were thought to be diagnostic of polyarteritis.

IgG and IgA antibodies binding to human cornea (FIG. 3) and IgG antibodies binding to vessels of the human inner ear (stria vascularis, lamina spiralis ossea, FIG. 4) were identified in the serum of patients with Cogan's syndrome by the indirect immunofluorescence method.[39,40] These findings and the recognized vascular lesions described by various authors have been interpreted as the effect of an underlying autoimmune mechanism also operating in Cogan's syndrome.[41,42]

The temporal bone pathology in Cogan's syndrome shows changes that are similar to those observed in other autoimmune disorders associated with audiovestibular

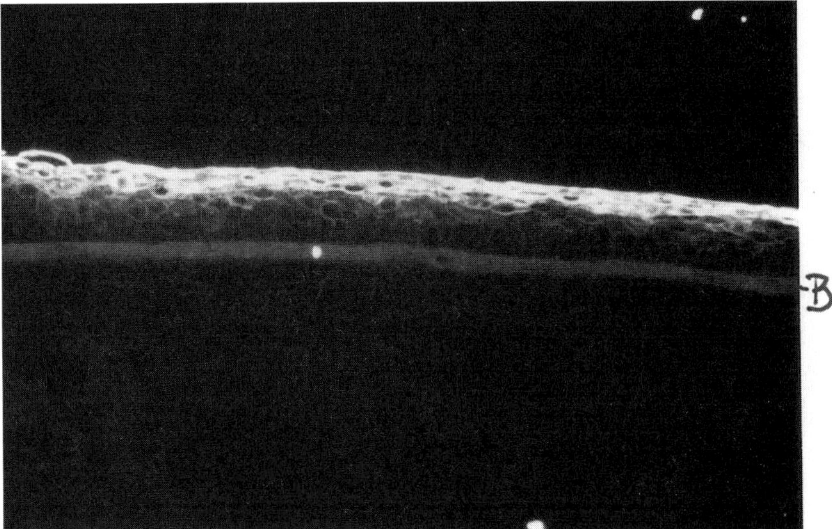

FIGURE 3. Cogan's syndrome. Serum of a 19-year-old female patient with Cogan's syndrome was exposed to healthy human cornea. Fluorescein-conjugated antihuman-IgG antibodies were added. (39). There is an intensive fluorescence of the corneal epithelium. B: Bowman's membrane.

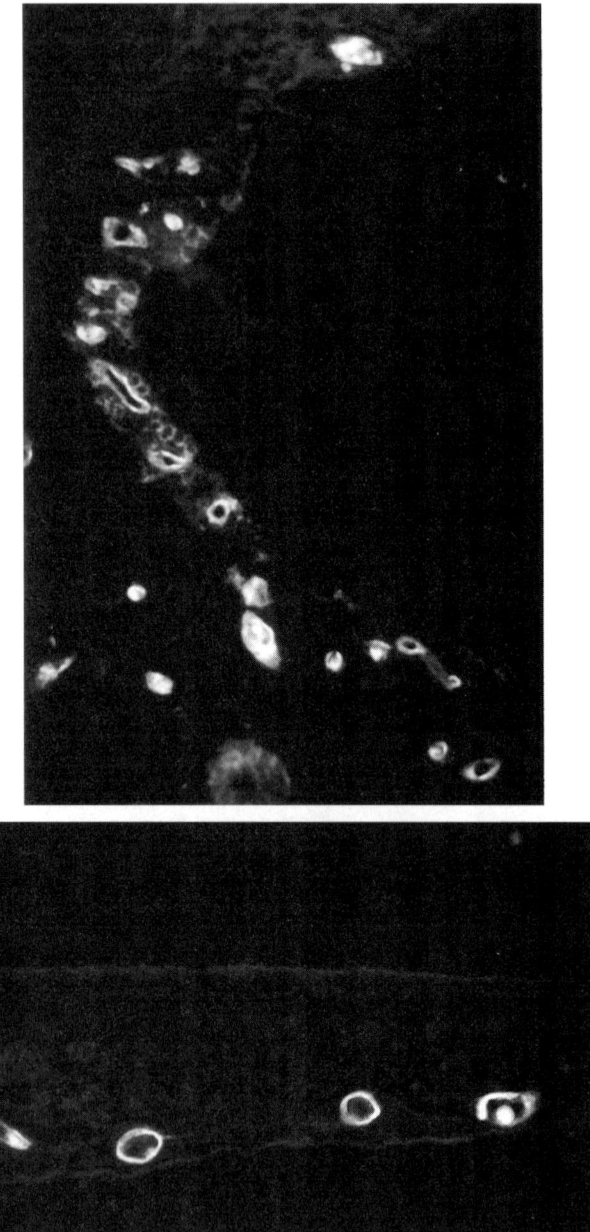

FIGURE 4. (a) Section through the lateral wall of a healthy human cochlea incubated in the serum from a 19-year-old female patient suffering from Cogan's syndrome. The section then was exposed to fluorescein-conjugated antihuman-IgG antibodies from the mouse. There is intensive fluorescence of the vessel walls of the stria capillaries and of vessels from the spiral ligament. **(b)** Sagittal section through the lamina spiralis ossea of a healthy human cochlea incubated in the serum of a 19-year-old patient suffering from Cogan's syndrome. After exposition with fluorescein-conjugated antihuman-IgG antibodies from the mouse, a selective fluorescence of the vessel walls is obvious.

dysfunction.[43–45] There is endolymphatic hydrops, fibro-osseous obliteration of the perilymphatic spaces, and vasculitis (FIG. 5).

Variazione 4

Connective Tissue Diseases

Systemic lupus erythematosus (SLE, a disease that in the same way fulfills the criteria of a systemic vasculitis), *rheumatoid arthritis, reactive arthritides, Sjögren's syndrome, Behçet's syndrome,* and probably *Vogt–Koyanagi–Harada syndrome* belong to the group of nonorgan-specific autoimmune diseases probably of the connective tissue where the cochleovestibular system can be affected. Interestingly enough, the histopathologic findings in a temporal bone from SLE revealed the same pathologic alterations as seen in the *vasculitic syndromes.*[30]

Behçet's syndrome is a multisystem, inflammatory, relapsing, and chronic disorder that may include mucocutaneous, ocular, genital, articular, vascular, CNS, and gastrointestinal involvement. Histopathologic vasculitic changes are common to all involved organs. Autoimmune and viral causes and an HLA-related immunogenetic predisposition have been suggested. Whereas in modern medical textbooks[1] Behçet's syndrome is still listed among nonorgan-specific connective tissue autoimmune diseases, others[40] understand Behçet's disease as a vasculitic syndrome. Igarashi *et al.*[46] reported a case of Behçet's disease where the patient had fluctuating hearing loss, tin-

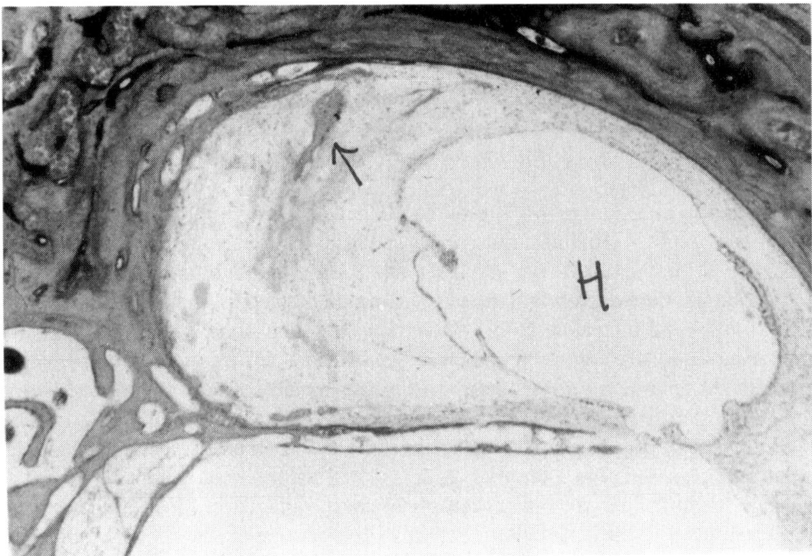

FIGURE 5. Cogan's syndrome. There is evidence of a vasculitis with labyrinthitis ossificans (*arrow*) within the scala vestibuli. H: Hydrops.

nitus, and dizziness. The 37-year-old woman had bilateral hearing loss in low audiometric frequencies. Audiological and vestibular examinations revealed an inner-ear lesion similar to that seen in Ménière's disease. The patient had an enlarged negative-summation potential in the electrocochleogram and a positive glycerol test, which suggested endolymphatic hydrops. The pathological characteristic of Behçet's disease is thought to be vasculitis. So this case suggests an association of autoimmune vasculitis with endolymphatic hydrops.

INTERMEZZO

Myasthenia gravis is characterized by episodic muscle weakness, chiefly in muscles innervated by cranial nerves and characteristically improves by cholinesterase-inhibiting drugs. This disease is caused by an autoimmune attack on the acetylcholine receptor of the postsynaptic neuromuscular junction, resulting in loss or dysfunction of acetylcholine receptors and jeopardizing normal neuromuscular transmission. The initiating event leading to antibody production is unknown. Since the transmitter of the efferent innervation of the outer hair cells in the organ of Corti is acetylcholine, it should be expected that patients suffering from myasthenia gravis will reveal a cochlear hearing loss. But, the acetylcholine receptor of the outer hair cell is encoded by a different gene and has a different molecular structure than the receptor at the neuromuscular junction. It is thus possible that myasthenia gravis could have no effect on the inner-ear receptor. This may explain that there exists only one case report of severe myasthenia gravis, that is, in a 40-year-old woman who presented bilateral progressive sensorineural hearing loss during the evolution of her disease.[47]

SCHERZO

Inflammatory Bowel Disease

A spectrum of inflammatory bowel disorders with overlapping clinical, epidemiologic, and pathologic findings, but without a definite etiology, is listed in Harrison's principles of internal medicine among organ-specific autoimmune disorders.[1] There are two main entities, Crohn's disease (CD, regional enteritis, granulomatous ileitis, or ileocolitis) and ulcerative colitis (UC, a chronic, nonspecific, inflammatory, and ulcerative disease arising in the colonic mucosa, characterized most often by bloody diarrhoea). The etiology of this group of diseases is unknown: immunologic factors have been extensively examined; possible infectious agents have included various enteric bacteria, viruses, and chlamydiae, and attention has most recently focused on measles viruses. There is a familial tendency, and autoimmune epiphenomena have been discussed.[48–50] Extracolonic complications (TABLE 3) in ulcerative colitis include peripheral arthritis, ankylosing spondylitis, sacroileitis, anterior uveitis, erythma nodosum, pyoderma gangrenosum, and episcleritis. The peripheral arthritis, episcleritis, and skin complications often fluctuate with the colitits, whereas the spondylitis, sacroileitis, and uveitis usually follow a course independent of the bowel

TABLE 3. Extracolonic Complications (Mainly Connective-tissue Disorders) in Inflammatory Bowel Disease

For example, ulcerative colitis:	Peripheral arthritis
	Ankylosing spondylitis
	Sacroileitis
	Bechterew's disease
	Hepatic cirrhosis
	Anterior uvetis
	Episcieritis
	Erythema nodosum
	Bullous dermatitis
	Pyoderma gangrenosum
	Sensorineural deafness

disease. There is a strong association with the HLA-antigen B27. Clinically, apparent liver disease may occur in up to 3% of patients. The liver disease may manifest as fatty liver or more seriously as chronic active hepatitis.[51] The association of inflammatory bowel disease and autoimmune disorders is well documented, including autoimmune sensorineural deafness and inflammatory aortitis.[50,52–56] The association of giant cell arteritis and ulcerative colitis has been reported by Jacob *et al.*[50] The precise etiology of sensorineural deafness in ulcerative colitis remains unclear, although in some patients, there is evidence of an immune complex vasculitis.[57,58] It is reported that in two of three cases the hearing loss associated with ulcerative colitis improved with steroids either alone[53] or in combination with cyclophosphamide.[52,59] The problem of deafness in ulcerative colitis is even discussed in psychiatric medicine.[60]

ADAGIO MAESTOSO

Beethoven's Disease

The detailed medical history of Beethoven's illness, as published by Neumayr[61] and discussed by Larkin[62] and Palferman[63] makes it probable that Beethoven suffered from ulcerative colitis with sensorineural hearing loss. The chronicle of the main features of Beethoven's medical history is shown in TABLE 4. The documentation is, of course, no formal medical history in the modern sense, but the contemporary accounts are remarkably consistent. At the age of 19 years (1789) Beethoven had his first attack of severe diarrhea and his life-long history of "colitis" was characterized with symptoms of abdominal pain, diarrhea, and rectal bleeding. It is documented that the chronic diarrhea was associated with abdominal pain, fever, and rheumatic attacks, bronchitis, and sinusitis. Hearing loss started in 1796 at the age of 27. Beethoven's hearing loss was progressive with periods of standstill, and it varied with his health. It was accompanied by severe tinnitus, headache, and deep depression. In 1813 Beethoven became deaf in his right ear and almost deaf in his left ear. In the following years severe rheumatic attacks with fever, keratoconjunctivitis, or iridocyclitis

TABLE 4. Beethoven's Deafness

1770	Born
1789	Fever, abdominal pain, rectal bleeding, rheumatic attacks
1796	First reports about hearing loss, tinnitus
1801	Progressive hearing loss
1802	Depression
1806	Remarkable improvement of hearing, "fluctuating hearing"
1808	Beethoven started lip reading
1813	Complete deafness on the right ear, headache
1818	Complete deafness on both ears, recurrent sinusitis
1823	Persistent conjunctival inflammations, "iridocyclitis"
1825	Recurrent mucosal bleedings from the oral cavity and nose
1826	Ascites, pneumonia
1827, March 26	Death from hepatic coma

(1823) and recurrent mucosal bleedings from the oral cavity and nose (1825) were reported. After the year 1818 he was totally deaf in both ears, and only written communication was possible. Late in the year 1826 there were the first signs of liver dysfunction with ascites, and in March 1827 he died from hepatic coma (TABLE 4).

CONCLUSIONE

Audiovestibular manifestations are a common occurrence in several systemic (nonorgan-specific) autoimmune diseases. While the external and middle ear can be involved, particularly in relapsing polychondritis and Wegener's granulomatosis, where the Eustachian tube is blocked, the more devasting autoimmune phenomena involve the inner ear. The most common nonorgan-specific autoimmune diseases that involve the inner ear are polyarteritis nodosa and Cogan's syndrome. Less commonly, the inner ear may be involved in relapsing polychondritis, Vogt–Koyanagi–Harada syndrome, giant cell arteritis, Takayasu's disease, hypersensitivity vasculitis (small vessel involvement), sarcoidosis, and systemic lupus erythematosus.[16] Independent from the type or character of the nonorgan-specific autoimmune diseases, the pathological features that characterize inner ear pathology are more or less identic. They can be described as *vasculitis, accompanied by diffuse proliferation of fibrous tissue and bone.* Endolymphatic hydrops is a frequent but not constant finding. It is not surprising that sensory structures degenerate under these conditions.[16]

RIASSUNTO

Autoimmune disease is characterized by production of either antibodies that react with host tissue or immune effector T cells that are autoreactive to endogenous self-peptides. Whereas organ-specific autoimmune diseases are likely the result of the combined effects of several factors that lead to inappropriate targeting of a particular organ or system to immune damage (e.g., Hashimoto's thyroiditis, Graves' disease, insulin-dependant diabetes mellitus, immune-mediated infertility, pemphigus vulgaris, autoimmune hemolytic anaemia), generalized, nonorgan-specific autoimmune diseases can be thought of as diseases in which there is episodic breakdown of immunologic tolerance to self-molecules (e.g., systemic lupus erythematosus, rheumatoid arthritis, mixed connective tissue disease, myasthenia gravis). The autoantibodies will then affect all tissues that bear the characteristics of these molecules. If those molecules are also present in certain middle- or inner-ear tissues, then a loss of function should be expected. There are nonorgan-specific autoimmune diseases that during the course of the disease cause hearing loss (e.g., connective tissue diseases, vasculitis syndromes, systemic lupus erythemadosus, myasthenia gravis, relapsing polychondritis, Behçet's disease, ulcerative colitis). But sensorineural hearing loss can also be the first symptom of a later fully developing systemic autoimmune disease (e.g., Cogan's syndrome, rheumatoid arthritis). It is possible that Beethoven's deafness today can be understood in the light of a nonorgan-specific autoimmune disease.

REFERENCES

1. 1994. Harrison's Principles of Internal Medicine, 13th ed. R. G. Petersdorf, R. D. Adams, E. Braunwald, V. J. Isselbacher, J. B. Martin, and J. D. Wilson, Eds. McGraw-Hill. New York.
2. MELCHERS, F. 1991. Immunity and autoimmunity. *In* Advances in Oto-Rhino-Laryngology, Vol. 46, C. R. Pfaltz, W. Arnold, and O. Kleinsasser, Eds.: 17–25. Karger Press. Basel.
3. SELBY, W. S., L. W. POULTER, S. HOBBES, D. P. JEWELL & G. JANOSSY. 1983. Heterogenity of HLA-DR-positive histiocytes in human intestinal lamina propria. J. Clin. Pathol. **36:** 379–384.
4. HERBAY, VON A., J.-O. GEBBERS & H. F. OTTO. 1990. Immunopathology of ulcerative colitis: A review. Hepato-gastroenterology **37:** 99–107.
5. THEOFILOPOULOS, A. N., R. KOFLER, P. A. SINGER & F. J. DIXON. 1989. Molecular genetics of murine lupus models. Adv. Immunol. **46:** 61–109.
6. RUCKENSTEIN, M. J., R. J. MOUNT & R. V. HARRISON. 1993. The MRL-lpr/lpr mouse: A potential model of autoimmune inner ear disease. Acta Otolaryngol. (Stockholm) **113:** 160–165.
7. GLODDEK, B., M. ROGOWSKI & W. ARNOLD. 1994. Adoptive transfer of an autoimmunological labyrinthitis in the guinea pig; Animal model for a sympathetic cochleolabyrinthitis. Clin. Exp. Immunol. **57:** 133–137.
8. MCCABE, B. F. 1979. Autoimmune sensorineural hearing loss. Ann. Otol. Rhinol. Laryngol. **88:** 585–589.
9. ARNOLD, W. & H. J. ALTERMATT. 1995. The significance of the human endolymphatic sac and its possible role in Ménière's disease. Acta Otolaryngol. (Stockholm) **519**(Suppl.): 36–42.
10. Altermatt, H. J., J. O. Gebbers, C. Müller, J. Laissue & W. Arnold. 1992. Immunohistochemical characterization of the human endolymphatic sac. Acta Otolaryngol. (Stockholm) **112:** 229–235.
11. LUTHRA, H. S., & C. J. MICHET. 1984. Relapsing polychondritis. *In* Rheumatology, J. H. Klippel and P. Dieppe, Eds. Mosby. London.
12. ISAAK, B. L., T. J. LIESEGANG & C. R. MICHEL, JR. 1986. Ocular and systemic findings in relapsing polychondritis. Ophthamology **93:** 681–689.

13. RICCICCI, V., A. SPADARO, E. TACCARI & A. ZOPPINI. 1988. A case of relapsing polychondritis: Pathogenetic considerations. Clin. Exp. Rheum. **6:** 95–96.
14. MCKENNA, C. H., H. S. LUTHRA & R. E. JORDAN. 1976. Hypocomplementemic ear effusion in relapsing polychondritis. Mayo Clin. Proc. **51:** 495–497.
15. CODY, D. T. R. & D. A. SONES. 1971. Relapsing polychondritis: Audiovestibular manifestations. Laryngoscope **81:** 1208–1222.
16. SCHUKNECHT, H. F. 1991. Ear pathology in autoimmune disease. *In* Bearing of Basic Research on Clinical Otolaryngology. Advances in Oto-Rhino-Laryngology, Vol. 46, C. R. Pfaltz, W. Arnold, and O. Kleinsasser, Eds.: 50–70. Karger Press. Basel.
17. HOSHINO, T., T. ISHII, A. KODAMA & I. KATO. 1980. Temporal bone findings in a case of sudden deafness and relapsing polychondritis. Acta Otolaryngol. (Stockholm) **90:** 257–261.
18. HERBERTS, G., O. HILLERDAL & S. RANSTRÖM. 1957. Rhinitis, sinusitis and otitis as initial symptoms in periarteritis nodosa (Wegener's granulomatosis). Acta Otolaryngol. (Stockholm) **48:** 205–218.
19. BLATT, I. M. & M. LAWRENCE. 1961. Otologic manifestations of fatal granulomatosis of respiratory tract. Lethal midline granuloma—Wegener's granulomatosis. Arch. Otolaryngol. **73:** 639–643.
20. PER-LEE, I. H. & R. PARSON. 1969. Vasculitis presenting as otitis media. South. Med. J. **62:** 161–165.
21. LINTHICUM, F. H., JR. & J. A. SCHWARTZMAN. 1972. Wegener's granulomatosis appearing initially as otitis media. Trans. Am. Acad. Ophthalmol. Otolaryngol. **72:** 301–307.
22. SERGENT, I. S. & C. CHRISTIAN. 1974. Necrotizing vasculitis after acute serous otitis media. Ann. Intern. Med. **81:** 195–199.
23. FRIEDMANN, I. & F. BAUER. 1973. Wegener's granulomatosis causing deafness. J. Laryngol. Otol. **87:** 449–464.
24. CALONIUS, I. J. & C. K. CHRISTENSEN. 1980. Hearing impairment and facial palsy as initial sign of Wegener's granulomatosis. J. Laryngol. Otol. **94:** 649–657.
25. GUSSEN, R. 1977. Polyarteritis nodosa and deafness. A human temporal bone study. Arch. Otorhinolaryngol. **217:** 263–271.
26. WOLF, M., I. KRONENBERG, S. ENGELBERG & G. LEVENTON. 1987. Rapidly progressive hearing loss as a symptom of polyarteritis nodosa. Am. J. Otolaryngol. **8:** 105–108.
27. CALDARELLI, D. D., I. E. REJOWSKI & I. P. COREY. 1986. Sensorineural hearing loss in lupus erythematosus. Am. J. Otolaryngol. **7:** 210–213.
28. BOWMAN, C. A., F. H. LINTHICUM & R. A. NELSON. 1986. Sensorineural hearing loss associated with systemic lupus erythematosus. Otolaryngol. Head Neck Surg. **94:** 197–204.
29. KATAOKA, H., T. TAKEDA, H. NAKATANI & H. SAITO. 1995. Sensorineural hearing loss of suspected autoimmune etiology: A report of three cases. Auris-Nasus-Larynx **22**(1): 53–58.
30. YOON, T. H., M. M. PAPARELLA & P. A. SCHACHERN. 1989. Systemic vasculitis: A temporal bone histopathologic study. Laryngoscope **99:** 600–609.
31. ILLUM, P. & K. THORLING. 1982. Otological manifestations of Wegener's granulomatosis. Laryngoscope **92:** 801–804.
32. KORNBLUT, A. D., S. M. WOLFF & A. S. FANCI. 1982. Ear disease in patients with Wegener's granulomatosis. Laryngoscope **92:** 713–717.
33. HARRIS, J. P. 1991. Experimental immunology of the inner ear. *In* Bearing of Basic Research on Clinical Otolaryngology. Advances in Otorhinolaryngology, Vol. 46, C. R. Pfaltz, W. Arnold, and O. Kleinsasser, Eds.: 26–33. Karger Press.
34. JENKINS, H. A., A. M. POLLAK & U. FISCH. 1981. Polyarteritis nodosa as a cause of sudden deafness. A human temporal bone study. Am. J. Otol. **2**(2): 99–107.
35. COGAN, D. G. 1945. Syndrome of nonsyphilitic interstitial keratitis and vestibuloauditory symptoms. Arch. Ophthalmol. **33:** 144–149.

36. YEE, R. D. 1982. Atypical Cogan's syndrome: A case report. *In* Nystagmus and Vertigo: Clinical Approaches to the Patient with Dizziness, V. Honrubia, and M. Brazier, Eds.: 157–161. Academic Press. London.

37. BERNHARDT, D., R. VELTMANN, R. DORWALD & R. HUTH. 1976. Cogan's syndrome associated with angiitis of the cerebral nerves, aortitis and glomerulonephritis. Dtsch. Med. Wochenschr. **101:** 373–377.

38. CHESON, B. D., A. Z. BLUMING & J. ALROY. 1976. Cogan's syndrome: A systemic vasculitis. Am. J. Med. **60:** 549–555.

39. ARNOLD, W. & J. O. GEBBERS. 1984. Serum-Antikörper gegen Kornea- und Innenohrgewebe beim Cogan-Syndrom. Z. Laryngol. Rhinol. Otol. (Thieme) **63:** 428–432.

40. HUMBEL, R. L. 1994. Auto-Anticorps et Maladies Auto-Immunes. Editions Scientifiques. Elsevier. Paris.

41. HAYNES, B. F., M. I. KAISER-KUPFER, P. MASON & A. S. FANCI. 1980. Cogan's syndrome: Studies in 13 patients, long-term follow-up and a review of the literature. Medicine **59:** 426–441.

42. MAJOOR, M. H., F. W. ALBERS, R. VAN DER GAAG, F. GMELIG-MEYLING & E. H. HUIZING. 1992. Corneal autoimmunity in Cogan's syndrome? A report of two cases. Ann. Otol. Rhinol. Laryngol. **101**(8): 679–684.

43. SCHUKNECHT, H. F. & J. B. NADOL. 1994. Temporal bone pathology in a case of Cogan's syndrome. Laryngoscope **104:** 1135–1142.

44. FRIEDMANN, I. & W. ARNOLD. 1993. Pathology of the Ear. Churchill Livingstone. Edinburgh/London.

45. NADOL, J. B. & W. ARNOLD. 1987. Ear. *In* Diseases of the Head and Neck: An Atlas of Histopathology, Chap. 2, W. Arnold, J. A. Laissue, I. Friedmann, and H. H. Naumann, Eds. Thieme Medical Publishers. New York.

46. IGARASHI, Y., Y. WATANABE & S. ASO. 1994. A case of Behçet's disease with otologic symptoms. J. Otorhinolaryngol. (ORL) **56**(5): 295–298.

47. AMMAR-KHODJA, A. 1991. Surdité auto-immune et myasthenie. Rev. Laryngol. Otol. Rhinol. (Bordeaux) **112:** 161–163.

48. KRONMAN, B. S. 1971. Ulcerative colitis, autoimmune epiphenomena, and colonic cancer. Cancer **28:** 82–88.

49. WINTER, H. S., P. M. CRUM, N. W. KING, P. K. SEHGAL, & J. K. ROCHE. 1989. Expression of immune sensitization to epithelial cell-associated components in the cotton-top tamarin: A model of chronic ulcerative colititis. Gastroenterology **97:** 1075–1082.

50. JACOB, A., J. G. LEDINGHAM, A.-J. G. KERR & M. J. FORD. 1990. Ulcerative colititis and giant cell arteritis associated with sensorineural deafness. J. Laryngol. Otol. **104:** 889–890.

51. MERCK MANUAL OF DIAGNOSIS AND THERAPY. 1992. 16th ed., Merck Research Laboratories. Rahway, N.J., pp. 834–839.

52. SUMMERS, R. W. & L. MARKER. 1982. Ulcerative colitis and sensorineural hearing loss; Is there a relationship? J. Clin. Gastroenterol **4:** 251–252.

53. WEBER, R. S., H. A. JENKINS & N. J. COKER. 1984. Sensorineural hearing loss associated with ulcerative colitis. A case report. Arch. Otolaryngol. **110:** 810–812.

54. DOWD, A. & W. D. W. REES. 1987. Treatment of sensorineural deafness associated with ulcerative colitis. Brit. Med. J. **295:** 26.

55. GOODIN, D. S. 1989. Neurological sequelae of aortic disease and surgery. *In* Neurology and General Medicine, M. J. Aminoff, Ed.: 23–48. Churchill Livingston. Edinburgh.

56. SNOOK, I. A., H. J. DE SILVA & D. P. JEWELL. 1989. The association of autoimmune disorders with inflammatory bowel disease. Quart. J. Med. **269:** 835–840.

57. KANZAKI, J. & T. O-UCHI. 1983. Circulating immune complexes in steroid-responsive sensorineural hearing loss and the long-term observation. Acta Otolaryngol. (Stockholm) **393**(Suppl.): 77–84.

58. HUNDER, G. G. 1989. Giant cell arteritis and polymyalgia rheumatica. *In* Textbook of

Rheumatology, W. N. Kelly, E. D. Harris, S. Ruddy, and C. Sledge, Eds.: 1200–1208. Saunders. Philadelphia.

59. HOLLANDERS, D. 1986. Sensorineural deafness—A new complication of ulcerative colitis? Postgrad. Med. J. **62:** 753–755.

60. LEVITAN, H. L. 1973. The etiologic significance of deafness in ulcerative colitis. Psychiatry & Med. **4:** 379–387.

61. NEUMAYR, A. 1989. Musik und Medizin, Edition Wien, 121–184. 3. Auflage, J&V Edition. Wien.

62. LARKIN, E. 1971. Beethoven's illness—A likely diagnosis. Proc. R. Soc. Med. **64:** 493–496.

63. PALFERMAN, T. G. 1990. Classical notes: Beethoven's medical history. Variations on a rheumatological theme. J. R. Soc. Med. **83:** 640–645.

Clinical Management of Immune-mediated Inner-ear Disease

STEVEN D. RAUCH[a]

Deptartment of Otolaryngology
Harvard Medical School at
The Massachusetts Eye and Ear Infirmary
Boston, Massachusetts 02114

INTRODUCTION

In 1979, McCabe described 18 patients with idiopathic, rapidly progressive, bilateral sensorineural hearing loss who regained hearing after administration of corticosteroids.[1] He theorized an autoimmune etiology based on the response to immunosuppressive drugs. The next decade saw proliferation of a host of clinical reports, diagnostic tests, and treatment protocols for this entity, few of which have subsequently been validated. The next significant step toward understanding this disorder came in 1990 when Harris and Sharp reported circulating antibodies against inner-ear antigens detected by use of a Western blot technique.[2] Four years later Moscicki and coworkers presented the clinical correlation of idiopathic, progressive, bilateral sensorineural hearing loss (IPBSNHL) with circulating antibodies against a 68 kD protein antigen present in bovine inner-ear and renal extracts.[3] They demonstrated that the presence of these antibodies correlated both with activity of disease and steroid responsiveness. Using different experimental approaches, Billings *et al.* and Bloch *et al.* both identified the 68-kD protein antigen as heat-shock protein 70 (Hsp70) in 1995.[4,5] Whether Hsp70 within the inner ear is the target of these antibodies or simply has a shared epitope with the actual target antigen is unknown. This uncertainty notwithstanding, it is reasonable to refer to these antibodies as anti-Hsp70 antibodies because it is immunoreactivity with Hsp70 that is the basis for their detection in the Western blot assay. This assay for circulating anti-Hsp70 antibodies remains the only diagnostic study with proven prognostic significance in IPBSNHL.

Though the Western blot assay for circulating antibodies reactive with Hsp70 has prognostic significance, its diagnostic value is unproven. The assay has not been widely applied to other inner-ear disorders nor to other autoimmune disorders in order to characterize its sensitivity and specificity. Therefore, IPBSNHL remains a clinical diagnosis based on historic and audiometric criteria. Likewise, there has been no certain confirmation that IPBSNHL is actually an autoimmune disorder. Such confirmation must meet three criteria: (1) identification of antibodies or activated T cells reactive with a "self" protein; (2) identification of a characteristic immune-induced "lesion"; and (3) reproduction of this lesion by introduction of the specific antibodies or activated T cells into a na•ve host. Until these criteria are met, it is more

[a]Address for correspondence: to Steven D. Rauch, MD, 243 Charles Street, Boston, MA 02114. Phone: 617/573-3644; fax: 617/573-3939; e-mail: sdr@epl.meei.harvard.edu

accurate to refer to this entity by its clinical description (i.e., IPBSNHL) or acknowledge the undefined role of the immune system and call it immune-mediated inner ear disease. This paper reviews the details of the clinical presentation of IPBSNHL and describes the diagnostic and treatment protocols now in use at the Massachusetts Eye and Ear Infirmary.

CLINICAL PRESENTATION OF IMMUNE-MEDIATED INNER-EAR DISEASE

The hallmark of the condition originally described by McCabe was the presence of rapidly progressive sensorineural hearing loss; too fast to be age-related degeneration and too slow to be sudden sensorineural hearing loss. This remains the most salient distinguishing feature of the disorder. Moscicki *et al.* articulated a precise clinical description of IPBSNHL, which enabled them to minimize heterogeneity in their study population and, ultimately, correlate this clinical presentation with results of Western blot assays.[3] Specifically, they defined IPBSNHL as a bilateral sensorineural hearing loss of ≥30 dB at any frequency *and* evidence of progression in at least one ear on two serial audiograms performed ≤3 months apart, progression being defined as a threshold shift of ≥15 dB at one frequency, 10 dB at two or more consecutive frequencies, or a significant change in discrimination score. A single episode of threshold shift occurring in less than 72 hs and then stabilizing was classified as sudden sensorineural hearing loss and excluded. Fluctuating hearing loss, however, qualified if there was also progression according to the preceding criteria. This is still the most explicit description of IPBSNHL in the literature. Analogous to Ménière's disease, in the absence of a "gold standard" diagnostic test, adherence to these diagnostic criteria permits comparison of observations and results between different studies.

In the paper by Moscicki *et al.*, demographic features, test results, and treatment outcome were reported for 72 patients with IPBSNHL.[3] Review of 66 new patients evaluated at the Massachusetts Eye and Ear Infirmary for possible immune-mediated inner-ear disease was carried out. Five patients with a diagnosis of Cogan's syndrome, an autoimmune vasculitis characterized by SNHL, vertigo, and interstitial keratitis of the eyes, were excluded, leaving 61 cases for analysis. Results are tabulated in TABLES 1 and 2. IPBSNHL diagnostic criteria were the same as for Moscicki's

TABLE 1. Clinical Features of 61 Patients Evaluated at the Massachusetts Eye and Ear Infirmary for Possible Immune-mediated Inner-ear Disease

IPBSNHL	61
M:F	32:29
Mean age (range)	47 (4–72)
Vestibular symptoms	30 (49.2%)
Ménière's disease	13 (21.3%)
Uni:Bilateral	5:8
Other autoimmune diagnosis	9 (14.8%)

TABLE 2. Relationship of Western Blot Assay for Anti-Hsp70 Antibodies and Response to Corticosteroid Therapy in 61 Patients with IPBSNHL

	Steroid Response		
Western Blot	+	−	No Rx
+	14	11	7
−	5	12	8
?	2	2	—

study. Demographic features and trends in the correlation of Western blot assay with steroid response in the present group of patients are essentially the same as Moscicki's original cohort.

IPBSNHL and idiopathic sudden sensorineural hearing loss are two distinct disorders. IPBSNHL is far rarer than sudden loss. IPBSNHL is by definition bilateral, while sudden hearing loss is virtually always unilateral. Sudden hearing loss develops in $\leq$72 h. In contrast, IPBSNHL progresses over days to months such that serial audiograms on a monthly basis will show continued decline. Sudden hearing loss is an otologic emergency with a treatment of "window" of perhaps two to four weeks during which a short "burst and taper" of corticosteroids must be administered in order to achieve optimum recovery. IPBSNHL is not urgent. Patients with progression over six to twelve months can still achieve significant recovery with administration of a long course of high-dose corticosteroids or other immunosuppressive drugs. Throughout the otolaryngology community there is wide awareness that some cases of sensorineural hearing loss are potentially reversible with corticosteroids. However, unfortunately, there is little awareness of the fact that these two entities are quite different in etiology, presentation, workup, and management. Hasty administration of a short tapering course of steroids can delay diagnosis of IPBSNHL and can confuse interpretation of serologic testing.

Approximately half of IPBSNHL patients also experience vestibular symptoms (see TABLE 1). These can include disequilibrium, motion intolerance, positional vertigo, and episodic whirling vertigo of the Ménière's type. Approximately 20% of IPBSNHL patients have a combination of fluctuating and progressing sensorineural hearing loss and episodic vertigo that meets strict American Academy of Otolaryngology—Head and Neck Surgery diagnostic criteria for Ménière's disease. Rauch *et al.*[6] and Gottschlich *et al.*[7] have reported that approximately one third of classic Ménière's disease patients have a Western blot assay positive for anti-Hsp70 antibodies. This overlap between IPBSNHL and Ménière's disease suggests that a subset of patients falling into both diagnostic categories may share a common pathophysiologic mechanism.

IPBSNHL can occur in combination with other systemic autoimmune diseases. Nearly 15% of IPBSNHL cases have another autoimmune diagnosis (see TABLE 1). These diagnoses include multiple sclerosis, inflammatory bowel disease (ulcerative colitis and Crohn's disease), systemic lupus erythematosis, rheumatoid arthritis, and ankylosing spondylitis. Though not definitely autoimmune, several other IPBSNHL patients listed in TABLE 1 had diabetes or thyroid dysfunction. There are reports of certain HLA subtypes that correlate with immune-mediated inner-ear disease.[8] This suggests the possibility of a genetic predisposition to autoimmune disease that may include IPBSNHL as well as other systemic disorders.

DIAGNOSIS OF IMMUNE-MEDIATED INNER-EAR DISEASE

As noted earlier, the salient feature of IPBSNHL is audiometric evidence of progression over days to months. Serial audiometry performed at an interval of ≤3 months is necessary to confirm the diagnosis. When in doubt, monthly audiograms for several months can be helpful. The pattern of hearing loss is highly variable. As yet, no one has described a characteristic pattern of hearing loss. The loss may be high tone, low tone, up- or downsloping, or predominantly affecting discrimination rather than threshold. Exclusion of retrocochlear disease such as multiple sclerosis or acoustic neuroma is mandatory and can be accomplished by evoked response audiometry and/or gadolinium-enhanced magnetic resonance imaging (MRI).

Routine serologic tests in possible IPBSNHL patients include complete blood count with differential white count, erythrocyte sedimentation rate (ESR), rheumatoid factor, ANA, C3 and C4 complement levels, and Raji cell assay for circulating immune complexes. Serologic workup is aimed at detecting evidence of systemic immunologic dysfunction; none of these tests has been shown to correlate with the diagnosis of IPBSNHL.

Western blot assay for anti-Hsp70 antibodies is a useful adjunct in diagnosis and management of IPBSNHL. As noted before, the sensitivity and specificity of this test has not been validated and it should not be used as the absolute determinant of whether a patient has actual immune-mediated inner-ear disease, nor should it be the sole determinant of whether or not to treat with immunosuppressive drugs. On the other hand, Moscicki *et al.* have shown that the presence of these antibodies is correlated with active disease and with steroid responsiveness.[3] Review of Western blot results in our most recent 61 cases of IPBSNHL reveals similar findings (see TABLE 2). It may therefore be an aid to clinical decision making in difficult cases. For example, a brittle diabetic or patient with peptic ulcer disease may be at considerable risk from treatment with high-dose corticosteroids. Such risk may be more acceptable if one finds a positive Western blot, indicating as much as 75% chance of steroid response. Conversely, a high-risk patient might forgo therapy if the assay is negative, suggesting the chance of response is less than 20%.

In addition to the lack of sensitivity and specificity data, the Western blot assay for anti-Hsp70 antibodies has other shortcomings. It is not a quantitative assay. Because the antigen used is a relatively crude protein extract from bovine renal cells rather than a single purified protein or polypeptide, the exact amount of Hsp70 is not standardized. The test is therefore reported only as antibodies "present" or "absent." Eventually, an ELISA or quantitative Western blot could be developed based on identification of the specific epitope(s) relevant to this disorder. Results would then be reported as an antibody titer, as is currently done in ANA and many other routine immunologic studies. Antibody titers could then be measured serially to monitor progress of the treatment or possibly to herald relapse. Despite its limitations, to date the Western blot assay for anti-Hsp70 antibodies remains the only serologic study with demonstrated prognostic significance in IPBSNHL.

IMMUNOSUPPRESSIVE THERAPY OF IMMUNE-MEDIATED INNER-EAR DISEASE

Corticosteroid therapy for IPBSNHL at the Massachusetts Eye and Ear Infirmary has evolved over the last 15 years based on clinical experience with over 150 IPB-SNHL patients. There have not been any prospective, randomized clinical trials to validate this empirical approach. Initial therapy for adults consists of a therapeutic trial of 60-mg Prednisone daily for four weeks. Pediatric patients receive 1-mg/kg/D Prednisone for four weeks. Although occasional patients may show a response early in the four-week period, many do not begin to improve until late in the month, and shorter courses of treatment usually result in relapse. Patients' hearing is tested at the initiation of therapy and again at four weeks. If the threshold has improved by ≥ 15 dB at one frequency or 10 dB at two or more consecutive frequencies, or if the discrimination is significantly improved, patients are considered steroid responders. Nonresponders are tapered off their medication in 12 days. Responders continue full-dose therapy until monthly audiograms confirm that they have reached a plateau of recovery. They are then slowly tapered over eight weeks to a maintenance dose of 10–20 mg every other day. This maintenance dose is continued for a variable length of time. Clinical observation at the Massachusetts Eye and Ear Infirmary suggests that patients with a total treatment duration of less than six months are at increased risk of relapse compared to those treated for six months or longer.

Patterns of response to corticosteroid therapy vary. Some patients have improvement in threshold, some in discrimination only, and some show benefit to both. Some patients with fluctuation and progression before therapy show stabilization of their hearing without actual improvement. Historically, these cases have been considered nonresponders, but this issue is currently under reassessment. The majority of responders are carried through their slow taper, weaned from steroids, and do well. A subset of IPBSNHL patients relapse while tapering or after discontinuing their medication. In some instances retreatment is effective. However, occasionally the hearing loss becomes refractory to corticosteroids. In such cases alternative immunosuppressive drugs are considered. An occasional patient, especially in the pediatric age group, may show steroid-dependent hearing loss. In other words, they cannot be weaned below a certain level of steroid dosage without decline in hearing. Such patients often develop unacceptable side effects of chronic steroid administration. Recently, we have observed benefit from combining Prednisone with low-dose (15 mg/wk) methotrexate in these steroid-dependent cases. After several weeks of combined therapy, the Prednisone can be tapered and discontinued and the patient maintained on methotrexate alone for an additional two to three months, at which time the last drug is also successfully discontinued.

Corticosteroid therapy has obvious limitations. There are risks of long-term administration that include gastritis and ulcers, fluid retention and weight gain, blood pressure lability, altered blood sugar metabolism and diabetes, mood changes or psychiatric problems, sleep disturbance, accelerated cataract formation, and Cushingoid habitus. Ischemic necrosis of bone is a rare complication more likely to be seen in cases of prolonged high-dose steroid administration, though none of our patients have had this problem.[9] We have observed an overall steroid response rate of approximately 60% in IPBSNHL patients. Some initial responders become refractory at the time of subsequent relapse. Despite these limitations, corticosteroid therapy remains the mainstay of IPBSNHL treatment based on the extensive clinical experience with its use.

Alternatives to systemic corticosteroids include methotrexate and cyclophosphamide. We have found low-dose methotrexate to be especially useful as an adjunct in management of steroid-dependent hearing loss. It is the first-line drug of choice for patients unable to take corticosteroids. A low-dose protocol as for rheumatoid arthritis or psoriasis is used. Methotrexate is administered by mouth in three doses given at 12-h intervals once weekly. The initial dose is 7.5 mg/wk (three doses of 2.5 mg). If this is tolerated without toxicity for two weeks, the dose is doubled to 15-mg/wk. This dose is continued for six to eight weeks as a therapeutic trial. Nonresponders are discontinued; responders are carried on the 15-mg/wk dose for six months. Potential toxicity includes myelosuppression, gastrointestinal upset, oral ulceration, acute pneumonitis, and hepatic fibrosis. This last complication is insidious and generally seen only when methotrexate is given for more than one year. It may be associated with normal liver function tests, and early diagnosis is achieved by liver biopsy. Weekly testing of complete blood count with differential white count, liver function tests, BUN, creatinine, and urinalysis is recommended to monitor for signs of toxicity.

Cyclophosphamide is a potent cytotoxic agent generally used for cancer chemotherapy. It is somewhat selective for B-cell and monocyte-macrophage function.[10] Although some advocate its use as a first line drug,[11] the high risk of toxicity makes it a better choice as a salvage drug or treatment of last resort. We have used it in a small number of patients at an initial dose of 1 mg/kg/d orally for four to six weeks. When no response is apparent, the dose is doubled to 2 mg/kg/d. Responders are treated for six to twelve months. Toxicity includes severe myelosuppression, opportunistic infection, hair loss, cystitis, infertility, and increased risk of malignancies. Weekly monitoring of hematological status is mandatory. Many patients when confronted with the risk of this medication would rather consider cochlear implantation.

Intratympanic steroid therapy, systemic IgG injections, and plasmapheresis are possible treatments with sound theoretical justification. Intratympanic steroid therapy is particularly appealing because it is minimally invasive and enables direct application of drug to the affected site with low risk of systemic effects. There are, however, no published series in which these treatments have been systematically applied. Determination of the best role for any of these treatment modalities remains to be determined.

CONCLUSIONS AND FUTURE DIRECTIONS

The story of IPBSNHL from initial description by McCabe to present therapy routines has been presented here as a simple and direct path. That has not been the actual case. It has been a broad and meandering path with significant contributions by many investigators and numerous interesting and important digressions. It is a story that still has far to go. The clinical description of this disorder is confined to its auditory manifestations. However, as noted earlier, 50% of IPBSNHL patients have vestibular symptoms. This aspect of the illness has not been well characterized clinically. Just as there are many IPBSNHL patients with exclusively auditory symptoms, there may well be an equal number with exclusively vestibular symptoms. Such a presentation has not yet been reported. Until the Western blot assay for anti-Hsp70 antibodies is systematically applied to a wide range of vestibulopathy patients, this possibility will be unexplored.

Little is understood about the underlying pathophysiology of IPBSNHL. The very fact of reversible sensorineural hearing loss flies in the face of accepted dogma that sensorineural hearing loss is not medically recoverable. It is interesting to consider what pathophysiologic mechanism could disable neural signal transduction and/or transmission in the auditory system yet be reversed months later by anti-inflammatory or immunosuppressive drugs. Solution to this puzzle will come from systematic research into the nature of the humoral and cell-mediated immune response of affected patients. As yet there is no good animal model of the IPBSNHL phenomenon in which to carry out such research, and human studies progress slowly due to the rarity of the clinical material. This rarity does not diminish the significance of the topic, however. Understanding the mechanism of IPBSNHL will provide a new level of insight into the role of systemic and organ-specific immune reactions in disease of the inner ear. The fact that 20% of IPBSNHL patients have a clinical presentation overlapping with Ménière's disease and 33% of Ménière's disease patients have evidence of anti-Hsp70 antibodies by Western blot assay is strong evidence of a shared pathophysiologic mechanism. Though IPBSNHL is rare, Ménière's disease is not. In the United States alone there are an estimated 125,000 cases yearly. New ways of understanding Ménière's disease could have great public health benefit.

Diagnosis of IPBSNHL currently relies on clinical factors alone, supplemented by the Western blot assay for anti-Hsp70 antibodies. As stated earlier, the observation that many IPBSNHL patients carry serum antibodies reactive with Hsp70 does not prove that Hsp70 is the actual inner-ear target antigen. Hsp70 may carry an epitope shared with the true target antigen. Alternatively, the antibodies may not be pathogenic at all. They may simply be reactive antibodies, reflecting upregulation of Hsp70 synthesis in inner-ear cells injured by some unknown mechanism. Despite our poor understanding of IPBSNHL pathophysiology, detection of these marker antibodies remains clinically useful. The utility of the assay will be greatly enhanced by development of a quantitative measure enabling clinicians to follow antibody titers by serial testing. In addition, estimation of sensitivity and specificity of the assay must be made by its broad application to a wide variety of ear diseases and immunologic disorders.

Current therapy of IPBSNHL is based upon empirical experience over the last 15 years rather than upon a clear understanding of the underlying pathophysiology. In the future, therapeutic protocols must be informed by expanding knowledge of the pathophysiology of the disorder. Large multicenter studies are necessary to carefully evaluate the best use of corticosteroids and other immunosuppressive drugs. Consensus must be achieved on the clinical diagnostic criteria and treatment regimens in order to enable comparison between studies. Even with strict adherence to rigorous methodology, it may take many years to address these questions. For the foreseeable future, IPBSNHL will remain one of the most interesting, important, and challenging problems confronting otologists and otologic researchers.

ACKNOWLEDGMENTS

The author wishes to acknowledge collaboration of Richard A. Moscicki, José E. San Martin, Stacey B. Weston, Donald B. Bloch, and Kurt J. Bloch in the research and clinical work described in this manuscript.

REFERENCES

1. McCabe, B. F. 1979. Autoimmune sensorineural hearing loss. Ann. Otol. Rhinol. Laryngol. **88**(4): 585–589.
2. Harris, J. P. & P. A. Sharp. 1990 Inner ear autoantibodies in patients with rapidly progressive sensorineural hearing loss. Laryngoscope **100**(5): 516–524.
3. Moscicki, R. A., J. E. San Martin, C. H. Quintero, S. D. Rauch, J. B. Nadol, Jr. & K. J. Bloch. 1994. Specificity of serum antibodies to a 68 kD inner ear antigen in disease associated with hearing loss and responsivity to corticosteroid therapy. JAMA **272**(8): 611–616.
4. Billings, P. B., E. M. Keithley & J. P. Harris. 1995. Evidence linking the 68 kilodalton antigen identified in progressive sensorineural hearing loss patient sera with heat shock protein 70. Ann. Otol. Rhinol. Laryngol. **104**(3): 181–188.
5. Bloch, D. B., J. E. San Martin, S. D. Rauch, R. A. Moscicki & K. J. Bloch. 1995. Serum antibodies to heat shock protein 70 in sensorineural hearing loss. Arch. Otolaryngol. **121**(10): 1167–1171.
6. Rauch, S. D., J. E. San Martin & K. J. Bloch. 1995. Prevalence of anti-heat shock protein 70 (HSP70) antibodies in Ménière's disease (Abstract). Research Forum of the Association for Research in Otolaryngology and the American Academy of Otolaryngology—Head and Neck Surgery, New Orleans.
7. Gottschlich S., P. B. Billings, E. M. Keithley, M. H. Weisman & J. P. Harris. Assessment of serum antibodies in patients with rapidly progressive sensorineural hearing loss and Ménière's disease. Laryngoscope **105**(12): 1347–1352.
8. Cao, M.-Y., J. Thonnard, M. Deggouj, M. Gersdorff, M. Philippe, J.-C. Osselaer & J-P. Tomasi. 1996. HLA Class II-associated genetic susceptibility in idiopathic progressive sensorineural hearing loss. Ann. Otol. Rhinol. Laryngol. **105**(8): 628–633.
9. Zizic, T. M., C. Marcoux, D. S. Hungerford, J.-V. Dansereau & M. B. Stevens. 1985. Corticosteroid therapy associated with ischemic necrosis of bone in systemic lupus erythematosus. Am. J. Otol. **79**: 596–604.
10. Hadden, J. W. & D. L. Smith. 1992. Immunopharmacology: Immunomodulation and immunotherapy. JAMA **268**(20): 2964–2969.
11. McCabe, B. F. 1989. Autoimmune inner ear disease: Therapy. Am. J. Otol. **10**(3): 196–197.

The Cochlear Protein Antigens 28 kd and 30 kd, and Their Antibodies in Ménière's Disease[a]

MIKIO SUZUKI,[b] K.-C. CHENG,[c] H. MATSUOKA,[c] N. S. KIM,[c] M. KRUG,[c] JOEL BERNSTEIN,[d] AND TAI-JUNE YOO[c,e,f]

[b]Shiga University Medical Center
Seta, Otsu
Japan

[c]Department of Medicine, Microbiology and Immunology
Division of Allergy and Immunology
University of Tennessee
956 Court Avenue, Room H300
Memphis, Tennessee 38163

[d]Amherst Otolaryngology Center
Williamsville, NY 14221

[e]Biomedical Research Center
KAIST
Taejon, Korea

INTRODUCTION

Since McCabe first described autoimmune sensorineural hearing loss,[1] now accepted as autoimmune inner-ear disease (AIED),[2] a number of experimental and clinical studies were reported in the field of otoimmunology.[3–7] These reports presented evidence that the etiology and pathogenesis of certain inner-ear diseases, for example Ménière's disease and progressive sensorineural hearing loss (PSNHL), might be related to autoimmunity, but have not yet fully confirmed the autoimmune pathological mechanisms. One of the main reasons for this is that the inner-ear antigens targeted by the immune system either have not been identified or not well characterized, although attempts to find the antigens have been promising. Our laboratory has reported that type II collagen might have a key role in the etiology of Ménière's disease and otosclerosis as the inner-ear antigen.[3,8] Helfgott *et al.* suggested that type II collagen may be important in the pathogenesis of bilateral PSNHL.[9] Joliat *et al.* reported that patients with Ménière's disease had antibodies directed against 30-kd protein extract-

[a]This study is supported by NIH Grant USPHS DC-00652-02. This study was performed in accordance with the PHS Policy on Human care and Use of Laboratory Animals, the NIH Guide for the Care and Use of Laboratory Animals, and the Animal Care and Use Committee (IACUC) of the University of Tennessee.
[f]Author for correspondence. Phone: 901/448:6663; fax: 901/448-5854; e-mail: tjyoo@ut-meml.utmem.edu

ed from human inner ear in western blotting.[8] We focus on Ménière's disease and attempt to define the localization of antigenic epitope and molecular size on western blotting with the proteins extracted from guinea pig inner ear. Recently, using guinea pig inner-ear extracts, Cao *et al.* demonstrated that a 30-kd band was detected in sera from patients with various inner-ear diseases, especially in Ménière's disease and progressive sensorineural hearing loss, in accordance with our study.[10] However, because they used the whole inner ear, including the acoustic nerve in creating the extract to detect the autoantibodies in western blot assay, it is not clear which parts of the inner ear reacted to sera of patients. Guinea pig 30 kd is found to be 30-kd myelin protein PO.[11] In our study we found the PO protein could induce hearing loss in mice.

MATERIALS AND METHODS

Preparation of Patient Sera

Sera from 45 patients with various inner-ear diseases were supplied courtesy of Drs. J. Bernstein and Y. Yazawa. The diagnosis of Ménière's disease was based on the AAO-HNS criteria. All of the patients with Ménière's disease were symptomatic. The sera from patients with other inner-ear diseases were added to the present study to compare their immunoreactivity against inner-ear proteins with that of Ménière's patients' sera and controls. The control subjects without inner-ear diseases were selected according to the medical examination by interview to be a match in age and overall health status other than ear disease; none of these controls had other autoimmune diseases. The patients' diagnoses are presented in TABLE 1. The sera used in the present study were stored at –20°C.

TABLE 1. Patients' Diagnoses and Western Blot Results of Guinea Pig Inner-ear Protein Probed with Sera from Patients with Various Inner-ear Diseases

		Positive Western Blot	
	n	*n*	%
Ménière's disease	25	15	60
Otosclerosis	6	3	50
Hearing loss and tinnitus (diagnosis undetermined)	6	3	50
PSNHL	2	2	100
Cogan's syndrome	1	0	0
Sudden deafness	1	0	0
Strial atrophy	2	0	0
Hereditary hearing loss	1	0	0
Syphilitic labyrinthitis	1	1	100
Control	10	0	0

Preparation of Cochlear Tissue from Guinea Pigs and Humans

The cochlea tissues were obtained from 20 Hartley strain male guinea pigs (300–320 g). Human cochlear tissues were obtained from 19 living patients with acoustic tumors undergoing inner-ear microsurgical dissection (courtesy Dr. Gardner). Specimens were stored frozen at –80°C or in liquid nitrogen until protein extraction. The guinea pig inner-ear tissue was used within 5 days and the human inner-ear tissues were stored from 1 day to 3 years. The majority of human inner-ear samples were used within 1 year. Guinea pigs were sacrificed painlessly under deep anesthesia (intraperitoneal injection of a mixture of ketamine 70 mg/kg and xylazine 70 mg/kg). Each animal was perfused with 0.01-M phosphate buffered saline (pH 7.4; PBS) through the left ventricle. Immediately both temporal bones were removed and kept on crushed ice. The inner ear was divided into two parts under a dissecting microscope. The first part was the membranous labyrinth containing basement membrane, organ of Corti, stria vascularis, spiral ligament, and vestibular epithelium (the membranous part of the inner ear); the other part contained the spiral ganglion and cochlear nerve in the modiolus, and vestibular nerve in the temporal bone (the neural part of the inner ear). The facial nerve, brain, and heart were also obtained from the animals. These tissues were dispersed in 10 volumes of ice-cold lysis buffer (100 mM sodium chloride, 10 mM tris-chloride (pH 7.6), 1 mM ethylenediaminetetraacetate (pH 8.0; EDTA), 0.1% sodium dodecyl sulfate (SDS), 1% Nonidet P-40, 2 μg/mL aprotinin, 100 μg/mL phenylmethylsulfonyl fluoride (PMSF)). The tissues in lysis buffer were sonicated for 20 s (Sonifier cell disruptor model w-185, Heatsystems Ultrasonics, Inc., New York). After 30 min on ice, the homogenates were centrifuged at 10,000 rpm for 10 min. The supernatant was filtered through a 0.22-μm filter and boiled for 5 min in a boiling water bath. The resultant antigen preparations were frozen at –80°C.

SDS–Polyacrylamide Gel Electrophoresis

Electrophoresis was performed in vertical electrophoresis apparatus (Life Technologies, Maryland) utilizing a 12% SDS–polyacrylamide (SDS–PAGE). The acrylamide concentrations of the running gel and the stacking gel were 12% and 5%, respectively. The gel polymerized was placed in the electrophoresis apparatus filled with the buffer (250 mM glycine (pH 8.3), 25 mM tris, and 0.1% SDS). The samples were added the same volume of gel-loading buffer (100 mM tris-chloride (pH 6.8), 4% SDS, 0.2% bromophenol blue, 20% glycerol, and 200 mM dithiothreitol). Prestained proteins (Life Technologies Inc., Maryland) were used as molecular weight standards. The gel was run at 90 V for 14 h. Separated proteins were then stained with Coomassie brilliant blue (BIO-RAD, Melville, New York) and destained with 45% methanol and 10% acetic acid in distilled water. For Western blotting the gel was transferred immediately to polyvinylidene difluoride (PVDF; BIO-RAD, Melville, New York) membrane without gel staining. The dimensions of the gel before transblotting were approximately 11.5 by 16.2 cm with 4 mm thickness.

Transfer of Proteins to PVDF Membranes

The separated proteins were transferred to PVDF membrane using a semidry-type transblot cell (BIO-RAD, Melville, New York) with a transfer buffer (48 mM tris, 39 mM glycine, 20% methanol, 0.0375% SDS; pH 8.3) for 1 h. The PVDF membrane was dried and kept at $-80°C$ until the Western blotting. One piece was stained with protein detection kit (BIO-RAD, Melville, New York) to visualize the transferred proteins.

Western Blotting

Each blotted membrane was washed with tris-buffered saline (TBS; 20 mM Tris, 500 mM sodium chloride; pH 7.5) containing Tween 20 (TTBS; 20 mM tris, 500 mM sodium chloride, and 0.025% Tween 20, pH 7.5). Nonspecific antibody binding was blocked by adding 25% normal goat serum in TTBS containing 0.02% sodium azide and rocking at room temperature for 1 h. The membrane was incubated with patient serum that was diluted to 1:50 with TTBS containing 25% goat serum and 0.02% sodium azide. The paper was rocked overnight at 4°C. The paper was then washed three times with TTBS and one time with TBS for 10 min. The paper was then reacted with a peroxidase-conjugated goat antihuman polyvalent immunoglobulin (Accurate Chemical & Scientific Corp., New York) for 2 h at room temperature (1:2000 dilution in TBS containing 1% goat serum). The membrane was washed two times with TTBS and one time with TBS for 10 min at room temperature. Finally, the paper was stained with 0.05 M tris-HCl (pH 7.6) containing 0.02% 3, 3′-diaminobenzidine (Chemicon International Inc., California) and 0.01% H_2O_2.

RESULTS

Analysis of Proteins by SDS-PAGE

The inner ear was microdissected into membranous and neural portions. The proteins extracted from the membranous part of the inner ear showed five major bands (79, 52, 46, 30, and 28 kd). The proteins from the neural part of the inner ear showed four major bands (79, 52, 46, and 30 kd). Of these bands, the band with 28-kd molecular weight was found only in the membranous part. Although a strong 30-kd band was found in the neural part, two bands with 30- and 28-kd molecular weights were found in the membranous part. Human inner ear showed two major bands (79 and 48 kd) and four distinguishable minor bands (67, 44, 35, and 30 kd). The proteins from the guinea pig facial nerve presented an electrophoresis pattern similar to the neural part of the inner ear. The proteins extracted from heart showed four major bands (52, 46, 44, 42, 40, and 30 kd). The proteins extracted from the heart showed four major bands (79, 67, 52, and 46 kd). The protein with 28-kd molecular weight in the SDS-PAGE analysis was not found in the neural part of the inner ear, the facial nerve, the brain, or in the heart (FIG. 1).

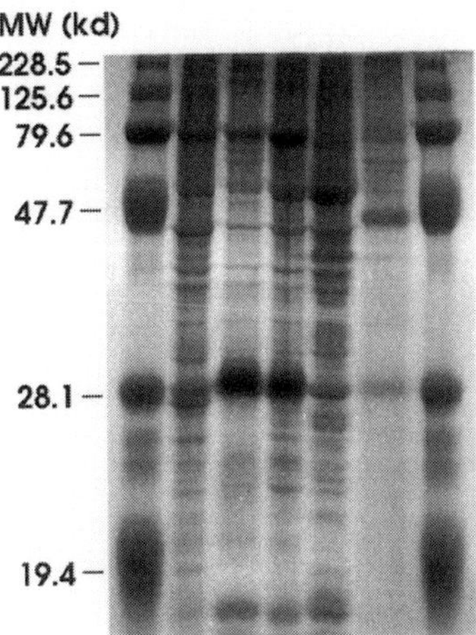

FIGURE 1.

Western Blotting Analysis

Western blotting was carried out with the preceding extracted proteins from guinea pig inner ear, and patient and control sera. In 24 (53%) of 45 patients with various inner-ear diseases, Western blot analysis with the membranous part and/or the neural part of guinea pig inner ear showed at least one positive band (TABLE 1, $p =$ 0.002; chi-square test). In contrast, normal subjects ($n = 10$) did not show any positive reaction to these inner-ear antigens at all. Of 25 patients with Ménière's disease, 15 (60%) showed positive Western blots ($p = 0.001$; chi-square test). The positive bands in patients with inner-ear diseases were distributed widely at 25, 28, 30, 32, 40, 42, 46, 52, 65, and 79 kd (TABLE 2). The most common positive bands were located at 28-, 52-, and 67-kd molecular weights (FIG. 2). Of these ten positively reactive bands, the 28-kd protein was the most common band found in Ménière's disease sera with 7 out of 25 sera reactive ($p = 0.06$; chi-square test compared with control subjects). The 67-kd band was found in 16% of patients with Ménière's disease and 50% of patients with rapidly PSNHL. Of 24 patients who showed at least one positive band in this assay, ten patients showed positive bands only in the membranous part, one patient only in the neural part, and thirteen patients in both (TABLE 3). The marked difference in the Western blotting results between the two parts of the inner ear was the 28-kd protein. This protein was detected only in the membranous part of the guinea pig inner ear. To investigate organ specificity of the reactivity against the 28-kd protein, Western blot analysis was carried out with the tissues of brain and heart and the sera of nine patients with positive reaction against the 28-kd protein. Of the ten control subjects, four sera selected at random were also examined for immunoreactivity against

TABLE 2. Distribution of Positive Bands in the Western Blot Assays

	25 kD	28 kD	30 kD	32 kD	40 kD	42 kD	46 kD	52 kD	67 kD	79 kD
Ménière's disease	2 (8)[a]	7 (28)	2 (8)	0	0	0	1 (4)	5 (20)	4 (16)	1 (4)
Otosclerosis	2 (33)	0	0	0	0	0	0	1 (17)	0	1 (17)
Hearing loss and tinnitus	0	2 (33)	0	0	1 (17)	1 (17)	0	0	0	0
PSNHL	0	0	0	1 (50)	0	1 (50)	0	1 (50)	1 (50)	0
Cogan's syndrome	0	0	0	0	0	0	0	0	0	0
Sudden deafness	0	0	0	0	0	0	0	0	0	0
Strial atrophy	0	0	0	0	0	0	0	0	0	0
Hereditary hearing loss	0	0	0	0	0	0	0	0	0	0
Syphilitic labyrinthitis	0	0	0	0	0	0	0	0	1 (100)	1 (100)
Total	4 (9)	9 (20)	2 (4)	1 (2)	1 (2)	2 (4)	1 (2)	7 (16)	6 (13)	3 (7)

[a]Figures in parentheses indicate percentages.

brain and heart proteins. Of the nine patients' sera, five sera showed reactivity against one or more brain proteins and three against one or more heart proteins (TABLE 4). The numbers in TABLE 4 indicate the number of the sera that showed the positive blots at corresponding molecular weight. However, no positive band at the 28-kd molecular weight was detected in the fractions of brain and heart. The four control sera did not react with the tissues of brain and heart in western blots.

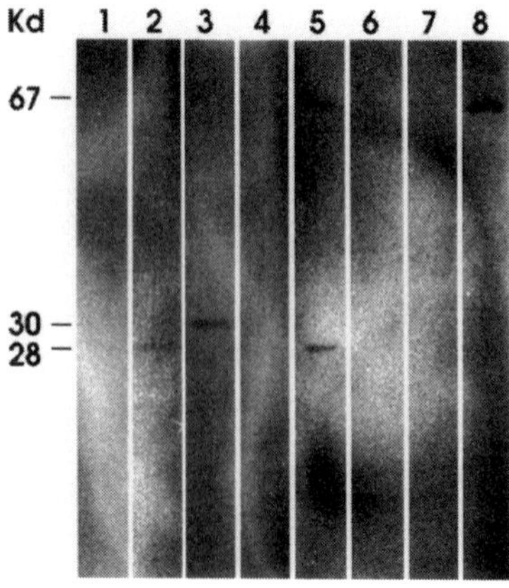

FIGURE 2.

TABLE 3. Difference in the Western Blotting Results Between the Two Parts of the Inner Ear

	25 kD	28 kD	30 kD	32 kD	40 kD	42 kD	46 kD	52 kD	67 kD	79 kD
Membranous part	4	9	1	1	1	2	1	7	6	2
Neural part	0	0	2	1	1	2	1	6	4	0

TABLE 4. Western Blots with the Extracts of Portions of the Inner Ear, Brain, and Heart against Patient Sera that Showed a Positive Reaction against the 28-kD Inner-ear Protein

	25 kD	26 kD	28 kD	42 kD	46 kD	52 kD	67 kD	79 kD
Membranous part	1	—	9	—	1	2	2	1
Neural part	—	—	—	—	1	2	3	—
Brain	—	1	—	1	—	4	—	—
Hearth	—	2	—	1	—	—	1	—

Myelin PO Protein Induce Hearing Loss in Mice

We have purified myelin PO protein from the bovine spinal root and immunized to DBA/1-lac mice. Twenty percent of the PO protein-immunized mice develop hearing loss with prolonged peak I, III, and V wave latency, I–III, III–V interpeak latency, and increased hearing threshold. Mononuclear cell including lymphocytes and macrophages are observed in the cochlear nerve lesion. These results suggest that inflammation in the peripheral nerve induced by PO immunization leads to hearing loss.

DISCUSSION

AIED has been diagnosed based on clinical manifestations, responsiveness to immunosuppressive therapy, and positive immune laboratory test. Some patients with inner-ear diseases, especially Ménière's disease and progressive sensorineural hearing loss, possess evidence of autoimmune involvement. Hughes *et al.* have shown that approximately half of their patients with diagnosed autoimmune inner-ear disease manifest endolymphatic hydrops and Ménière's syndromes.[12] In a previous study, we found that three of six patients with Ménière's disease showed the positive reaction to a protein band around 30-kd molecular weight in Western blotting performed on extracted human inner-ear protein.[8] This report also supported the proposition that a certain population of patients diagnosed with Ménière's disease may be AIED cases.

Several attempts to obtain a specific diagnostic marker of AIED have been made. Initially, the cell-mediated immune responses were employed, for example, lymphocyte migration inhibition test[1,2] and lymphocyte transformation test[13] against inner-ear tissue. However, because of poor reproductivity[7,14] and difficulties of obtaining fresh inner-ear tissue constantly, these tests have been replaced by a test of treatment.[15] To investigate the humoral immune mechanism in AIED, indirect immunofluorescence,[6,16] and Western blotting[7,8,10,17–20] have been employed in clinical investigations. Arnold *et al.* found that 54% of 119 patients' serum with bilateral SNHL had autoantibodies against the inner ear using an indirect immunofluorescence method.[6] They were able to detect not only the autoantibodies against inner ear, but also the localization of targeted antigen within the inner ear. However, this method requires difficult techniques and cannot determine the antigens targeted by the immune system. Therefore we chose to employ a Western blot assay to provide a clue as to the number and sizes of the antigens. These blots were probed with sera from 45 patients with various inner-ear diseases especially Ménière's disease.

Fifty-three percent of patients with various inner-ear diseases had the antibodies against guinea pig inner-ear fraction in the present study, compared with 0% in the control group. In spite of the limited number of patients examined, this result suggests that certain cases of inner-ear diseases might have autoimmune involvement. The positive bands in the guinea pig inner-ear fraction were widely distributed in size, but the most common bands were at 28-, 52-, and 67-kd molecular weight.

Cao *et al.* have reported 30- and 58-kd protein bands reacted with sera from patients with various inner-ear diseases in western blotting using guinea pig.[10] In this study, we found ten proteins with different molecular weights reacted with sera of patients with inner-ear disease. Of these proteins, the 28-kd protein was only found in the membranous part of guinea pig inner ear, and antibodies to it were also frequently found in Ménière's disease patient sera. In a swine inner-ear study, Veldman *et al.* showed that patients with inner-ear diseases have antibodies against 27-, 45-, 50-, 58-, and 80-kd proteins.[18] The positive reaction against the 27-kd protein was found in rapid PSNHL, sudden deafness, and other inner-ear diseases, but they failed to obtain a positive correlation between efficacy of immunosuppressive therapy and positive blot profile.

We found two prominent positive bands (28 and 30 kd) around the 30-kd molecular weight in the guinea pig inner-ear fraction. The 28-kd protein was only found in the membranous part of the inner ear and was reactive with 28% of Ménière's disease patient sera. In contrast, the 30-kd protein was found in both the membranous and neural parts, and the incidence of positive reaction was only 8% of Ménière's disease. In an indirect immunofluorescence study using human temporal bones and sera taken from patients with bilateral PSNHL of unknown etiology, sudden hearing loss and Ménière's disease showed a high positive reaction to inner-ear components: vascular stria (73.4%), organ of Corti (23.4%), spiral ligament (15.6%), and Reissner's membrane (8.2%) were high deposit areas, and the spiral ganglion (1%) and nervous tissue (5.1%) were classified as low incidence.[6] Salomon *et al.* also found specific reaction on the epithelium of the stria vascularis using this method.[16] In our separation of the guinea pig inner ear into two components, the membranous part corresponds to the high antibody-deposition areas and neural part to the low-deposit regions. In our previous study, the membranous part of the human inner ear had only one band around 30-kd molecular weight on SDS-PAGE. The differences in molecular weight between the 28 kd protein from guinea pigs and the 30-kd protein from humans were so small that the 28-kd protein of the guinea pig inner ear may in fact be the guinea pig equivalent of the human 30-kd protein. Further studies are needed to clarify these results. However, results of the 30-kd of guinea pig collagen protein described by Cao *et al.* is found to be PO protein. PO protein induced hearing loss in mice when they were immunized, which suggests that this could be an autoantigen in human hearing loss (Yoo *et al.*, unpublished observation).

In summary, we found that guinea pig inner-ear proteins with various molecular weights showed a positive reaction in Western blots with sera of inner-ear disease cases. Of these proteins, the 28-kd protein was the most common reactive and is specific to the membranous portion of the guinea pig inner ear. Although the importance of this protein is unclear at the present time, the results in this study suggest that it may have a key role as an autoimmune factor in inner-ear diseases, especially Ménière's disease and PSNHL. Further studies, for example, the correlation between the positive blots and disease activity of immunosuppressive therapy and protein sequence, to address these issues are under way.

REFERENCES

1. McCabe B. F. 1979. Autoimmune sensorineural hearing loss. Ann. Otol. Rhinol. Laryngol. **88:** 585–589.
2. McCabe B. F. 1985. Autoimmune inner-ear disease. *In* Immunobiology, Autoimmunity, Transplantation in Otorhinolaryngology, J. E. Veldman, B. F. McCabe, E. H. Huizing, and N. Mygind, Eds.: 107–110. Kugler. Amsterdam.
3. Yoo T. J., J. M. Stuart, A. H. Kang, A. S. Townes, K. Tomoda & S. Dixit. 1982. Type II collagen autoimmunity in otosclerosis and Ménière's disease. Science **217:** 1153–1155.
4. Yoo T. J., Y. Yazawa, K. Tomoda & R. Floyd. 1983. Type II collagen-induced autoimmune endolymphatic hydrops in guinea pig. Science **222:** 65–67.
5. Tomiyama, S. & J. P. Harris. The endolymphatic sac: Its importance in inner ear immune responses. Laryngoscope **96:** 685–691.
6. Arnold W. & C. R. Pfaltz. 1987. Critical evaluation of the immunofluorescence microscopic test for identification of serum antibodies against human inner ear tissue. Acta Otolaryngol. (Stockholm) **103:** 373–378.
7. Harris J. P. & P. A. Sharp. Inner ear autoantibodies in patients with rapidly progressive sensorineural hearing loss. Laryngoscope **100:** 516–524.
8. Joliat T., J. Seyer, J. Bernstein, M. Krug, X. J. Ye, J. S. Cho, T. Fujiyoshi & T. J. Yoo. 1992. Antibodies against a 30 kilodalton cochlear protein and type II and IX collagens in the serum of patients with inner ear diseases. Ann. Otol. Rhinol. Laryngol. **101:** 1000–1006.
9. Helfgott, S. M., R. A. Mosciscki, J. S. Martin, C. Lorenzo, R. Kieval, M. Mckenna, J. Nadol & D. E. Trentham. 1991. Correlation between antibodies to type II collagen and treatment outcome in bilateral progressive sensorineural hearing loss. Lancet **337:** 387–389.
10. Cao M. Y., M. Gersdorff, N. Deggouj, M. Warny & J. P. Tomasi. 1995. Detection of inner-ear disease autoantibodies by immunoblotting. Mol. Cell. Biochem. **146:** 157–163.
11. Cao M. Y., V. J. Dupriez, M. H. Rider, N. Deggouj, M. N. C. H. Gersdorff, G. G. M. Rousseau & J. P. Tomasi. 1996. Myelin protein PO as a potential autoantigen in autoimmune inner-ear disease. FASEB **10:** 1635–1640.

12. HUGHES G., B. P. BARNA, S. M. KINNEY, L. H. CALABRESE, M. A. HAMID & N. J. NALEPA. 1998. Autoimmune endolymphatic hydrops: Five-year review. Otolaryngol. Head Neck Surg. **98:** 221–225.

13. HUGHES G., B. P. BARNA, S. M. KINNEY, L. H. CALABRESE & N. J. NALEPA. 1988. Clinical diagnosis of immune inner-ear disease. Laryngoscope **98:** 251–253.

14. ARNOLD W., R. PFALTZ & H. J. ALTERMATT. 1985. Evidence of serum antibodies against inner ear tissue in the blood of patients with certain sensorineural hearing disorders. Acta Otolaryngol. (Stockholm) **99:** 437–444.

15. MCCABE B. F. 1989. Autoimmune inner-ear disease: Therapy. Am. J. Otol. **10:** 196–197.

16. SALOMON P., R. CHARACHON & J. M. LEJEUNE. 1993. Indirect immunofluorescence in the investigation of rapidly progressive sensorineural hearing loss and Ménière's disease. Acta Otolaryngol. (Stockholm) **113:** 318–320.

17. LEJEUNE J. M. & CHARACHON. 1992. New immunobiological tests in the investigation of Ménière's disease and sensorineural hearing loss. Acta Otolaryngol. (Stockholm) **112:** 174–179.

18. VELDMAN J. E., T. HANADA & F. MEEUWSEN. 1993. Diagnosis and therapeutic dilemmas in rapidly progressive sensorineural hearing loss and sudden deafness. Acta Otolaryngol. (Stockholm) **113:** 303–306.

19. MOSCICKI R. A., J. E. S. MARTIN, C. H. QUINTERO, S. D. RAUCH, J. B. NADOL & K. J. BLOCH. 1994. Serum antibody to inner ear proteins in patients with progressive hearing loss. JAMA **272:** 611–616.

20. GOTTSCHLICH S., P. B. BILLINGS, E. M. KEITHLEY, M. H. WEISMAN & J. P. HARRIS. 1995. Assessment of serum antibodies in patients with rapidly progressive sensorineural hearing loss and Ménière's disease. Laryngoscope **105:** 1347–1352.

Molecular Basis of Type II Collagen Autoimmune Ear Diseases[a]

T.-J. YOO,[b,d,e] TATSUYA FUJIYOSHI,[c] KUANG-CHUAN CHENG,[b]
M. S. KRUG,[b] N. S. KIM,[b] K. M. LEE,[b] T. SHEN,[b]
AND H. MATSUOKA[b]

[b]Department of Medicine, Microbiology and Immunology
Neuroscience Program and VAMC
University of Tennessee
956 Court Avenue, Room H300
Memphis, Tennessee 38163

[c]Kenwakai Otemachi Hospital
Fukuoka 803
Japan

[d]Biomedical Research Center
KAIST
Taejon, Korea

INTRODUCTION

McCabe first coined the term autoimmune sensorineural hearing loss in 1979.[1] Although immunologic mechanisms were implicated in the pathogenesis of McCabe's case report, autoimmunity was not proven. He showed that about one-third of cases had a positive leukocyte migration inhibition test and patients responded to either steroid or other immunosuppression agent(s).[1] However, the identity of the antigen(s) responsible for the production of this immune reaction remained unclear. A number of authors have observed elevated serum titer against the components of inner ear tissue in some patients who have sensorineural hearing loss or other inner ear disorders.[2,3] Those studies suggest the existence of an autoimmune response to native type II, XI collagen or a 30-kd protein extracted from human inner-ear tissue. In an independent study, serum from patients with Ménière's disease and progressive hearing loss contained antibody against a 68-kd protein from bovine inner-ear tissue.[4,5] This bovine inner tissue contains 68-kd protein has been used in experimental autoimmune sensorineural hearing loss in animals.[6]

Monoclonal antibodies against type II collagen-induced hearing loss and auricular chondritis when they were infused in the animal. Recent advances in molecular im-

[a]This study is supported by NIH Grant USPHS DC-00652-02. This study was performed in accordance with the PHS Policy on Human care and Use of laboratory Animals, the NIH Guide for the Care and Use of laboratory Animals, and the Animal care and use Committee (IACUC) of the University of Tennessee

[e]Author for correspondence. Phone: 901/448-6663; fax: 901/448-5854; e-mail: tjyoo@ut-meml.utmem.edu

munology have revealed a key trimolecular interaction of the antigen molecule; the class II major histocompatibility complex; and the T-cell receptor (TCR) molecule. The specific TCR gene repertoire is an important event in the autoimmune responses of both animals and humans. Therefore, such study has an immense potential for intervention via immunotherapy targeting the specific TCR(s) involved in the autoimmune response.[7] The oral tolerance has been successfully applied in the collagen-induced arthritis (CIA).[8,9] CD8+ cells have been implicated in the suppression of this autoimmune disease.[10,11] However, a high dosage of antigen is required to induce tolerance (ranged from 500 μg to 10 mg per mouse). Recently, the conjunction of cholera toxin B subunit (CTB) with myelin basic protein (MBP) induced tolerance in EAE mice.[12] In this study, we have applied the CTB-CB-11 to tolerate chondritis induced by type II collagen. The CB-11 is a T-cell epitiope peptide from type II collagen. The goal for this study is to compare and differentiate the immune response to type II collagen in arthritis with that in ear diseases in mice.

MATERIALS AND METHODS

A total of 168 mice were obtained from the Jackson Laboratories (Bar Harbor, Maine) and bred and maintaind in the Veterans Administration Hospital or the University of Tennessee. Details follow: 125 DBA/1 mice consisting of 70 as the immunized group (*I*) and 55 as the control group (*C*); 43 B10.RIII mice (*I* = 35 and *C* = 8). The ages of the animals range from 6 weeks old to 10 weeks old. Twenty of the B10.RIII mice and two of the DBA/1 mice were female. We immunized mice with either bovine or chicken type II collagen or treated with a mixture of monoclonal antibodies against CB-8 in 5 DBA/1 mice, and monoclonal antibody against CB-11 in 3 DBA/1 mice; in the control group, we used normal murine IgG in 2 DBA/1 mice, and phosphate buffered saline (PBS) in 2 DBA/1 mice. The remaining mice were studied as the age-matched controls without any immunization.

Preparation of Type II Collagen and Immunization

Native type II collagens were obtained by limited pepsin digestion of fetal bovine cartilage or chick sternum. The purity of collagen was determind by amino-acid analysis and by sodium dodecyl sulphate polyacrylamide gel electrophoresis. These isolates are free from type I, IX, and XI collagens. Type II collagen was dissolved in 0.05-M acetic acid at a concentration of 4 mg/mL and emulsified in an equal volume. The mice were immunized subcutaneously at the base of tail with 100 μg of type II collagen 10 days later.

Producing Monoclonal Antibodies against CB-8 or CB-11 Fragment of Type II Collagen

Monoclonal antibodies were produced in mice by a hybridoma technique based on the principles described previously. Monoclonal antibodies were purified from clarified ascites fluid using a rec-Protein A Sepharose 4B column (Zymed Laboratories Inc., San Francisco). Each monoclonal antibody was tested for its ability to react with CB-8 or CB-11 fragment of type II collagen.

We injected intraperitoneally 400 μg of anti-CB-8 antibody derived from one B-cell clone (E9) and intravenously injected 10 mg of a mixture of anti-CB-11 antibodies derived from four B-cell clones (A2, D1, D2, and F10).

Observation of Auricular Chondritis

Four weeks after initial immunization with type II collagen, a hole 2 mm in diameter was punched at the base of both pinnae of the mice. The monoclonal antibody was injected when the holes were punched. The manifestations in the punched regions were followed and a biopsy sample was taken at the occurrence of ear diseases. The control mouse pinnae were treated identically without immunization or antibody and followed. The biopsied specimens were used for light-microscopic observation or immunohistochemistry for specific TCRs.

Myringotomy and Observation of its Sequelae

Four weeks after initial immunization with type II collagen or monoclonal antibody injection, the eardrum was incised throughout most of its width from the anterior to posterior part at the level below the malleus tip. This procedure was carried out under the microscope by a 30-gauge needle to avoid injuring the skin of the external auditory canal, the malleus, and the posterior wall of the middle-ear cavity. The animals were followed every month using operation-microscopic observation of the eardrum. This method was used for recognition of otitis media and retention of middle-ear effusion (unpublished data). Histologic studies were carried out under both a light and an electron microscope.

Light and Electron Microscopy

For transmission electron microscopy the specimens were fixed with Karnovsky's fixative (2.5% glutaraldehyde and 2% paraformaldehyde in 0.2 M of cacodylate buffer; pH, 7.4), postfixed in buffered 2% osmium tetroxide, dehydrated through graded concentrations of ethanol, and embedded in epoxy resin (Epon). Thin sections were stained with uranyl acetate and lead citrate. Observations were made with a transmission electron microscope (IEM-1200EX, Jeol, Tokyo, Japan). For light microscopy, the specimen was fixed with 10% formaldehyde or Bouin solution (a mixture of picric acid saturated solution, formaldehyde, and acetic acid in the relative amounts of 15:5.1), decalcified with 10% ethylenediaminetetraacetic acid (EDTA) in 0.1 mol/L of tris-HCl buffer (pH, 7.0) in the case of bony tissue, dehydrated, and embedded in paraffin or glycol methacrylate (JB-4, Polysciences, Warrington, Pennsylvania). Sections were stained with hematoxylin/eosin.

Immunohistochemistry for TCRs

The tissues (joints and pinnae of mice) were fixed with a periodate–lysine–paraformaldehyde solution for 16 h at 4°C. The joint tissue was decalcified with EDTA in a tris-HCl buffer for 2 to 3 weeks at 4°C. The specimen was rinsed with 0.01 M of PBS (pH, 7.2) for 36 h at 4°C, embedded in OCT compound (Miles Laboratories Inc., Elkhart, Indiana), and immediately frozen. Frozen sections 4 to 6 mm in thickness were obtained. After rehydration and rinsing in cold PBS, the sections were treated with 3% normal goat serum in PBS to reduce the nonspecific reaction, and then the endogenous peroxidase was blocked with absolute methanol containing 0.5% hydrogen peroxide for 20 min at room temperature. Biotin conjugated antimouse Vβ-8.1, Vβ-8.2 TCR, or antimouse Vβ-6 TCR monoclonal antibodies (Pharmingen, San Diego), diluted to 1:200 in PBS containing 1% bovine serum albumin, were applied to the sections, and incubated overnight at 4°C. After rinsing and treating with normal goat serum, the sections were incubated with a avidin–biotin–peroxidase complex (Vectastain Elite ABC Kit, Vector Lab., Inc., Burlingame, California) for 30 min at room temperature and rinsed sufficiently with PBS. The reaction product was developed with 0.02% 3,3′-diaminobenzidine in 0.05 M of tris-HCl buffer (pH 7.6) with 0.005% hydrogen peroxide for 7 min. The sections, with or without counterstaining, were dehydrated, cleared in xylene, and mounted.

Control staining for specificity of antibodies was studied with PBS instead of antibodies, while the reactivity of antibodies was examined with frozen sections of thymus, spleen, lymph nodes, and Peyer's patch. Although not shown in this communication, this reactivity was also compared with positive staining obtained by biotin-conjugated hamster antimouse TCR α/β receptor monoclonal antibody (Pharmingen). The positive staining of Vβ-8.1, Vβ-8.2, and Vβ-6 TCRs in spleen, lymph nodes, and Peyer's patch was confirmed to be inside the T-cell area indicated by TCR α/β staining.

In Vitro *T-cell Proliferation and Inhibition by CDR2 of TCR Vβ-8.2 Peptide*

CII was emulsified with equal volume of complete Freund's adjuvant (CFA, Difco Lab., Detroit, Michigan). A group of three DBA/1 lac mice were immunized with CII (100 μg per mouse) at the base of the tail. Ten days later the mice were again boosted with CII in incomplete Freund's adjuvant (ICFA, Difco Lab.). One week later, the draining lymph node cells were harvested from the inguinal, popliteal, and para-aortic lymph nodes. The lymph node cells (4×10^6 cells/mL) were cultured with antigen in Ventrex HL-1 serum-free medium (Hycon Biomedical Inc., Portland, Maine) in the presence of syngeneic irradiated spleen cells (2000 rad, 2×10^6 cells/mL). These T cells responded to P1 peptide (residue 121–147, *N′*-GPTGPLGPKGQTGEL-GIAGFKGEQGPK-*C′*) derived from a CII CB-11 fragment at a concentration ranging from 0 to 250 μM.[13] The CDR2 peptide derived from mouse Vβ-8.2 TCR (residue 54–77, *N′*-RQDTGHGLRLIHYSYVADSTEKGD-*C′*) was synthesized using the solid-phase technique on a Model 430A Applied Biosystem peptide synthesizer and purified through high-pressure liquid chromatography. In the inhibition study, the cells were incubated with 20 μM of CDR2 Vβ-8.2 peptide and a concentration of P1 peptide ranging from 0 to 200 μM. The control cells were incubated with various concentrations of P1 peptide without CDR2 Vβ-8.2 peptide. The incubation time was 96 h and 1 mCi of [^{3}H-methyl] thymidine was pulsed during the last 16 h of incubation. The tymidine incorporation was measured by liquid scintillation counting. Values were expressed in counts per minute (cpm). Each sample was run in triplicate.

Prevention of Arthritis by Monoclonal Antibodies against TCRs

Monoclonal antibody against Vβ-8.1, Vβ-8.2, and Vβ-8.3 TCRs was obtained from hydridoma F23.1. Briefly, the hybridoma was grown in complete medium (10^{-3} M of sodium pyruvate, 100 mg/mL of penicillin, 100 mg/mL of streptomycin, $2×10^{-5}$ of glutamine, $5×10^{-5}$ M of β-mercapthoethanol, $2×10^{-2}$ M of Hepes, and 1 X nonessential amino acids in RPMI 1640 medium). The supernatant was purified through a protein A column (Pierce, Rockford, Illinois), and the concentration was determined. Five DBA/1 mice (male) were immunized inraperitoneally with 100 μg of monoclonal antibody on the same day as immunization with bovine type II collagen, and a monoclonal antibody injection of the same dose was repeated every 7 days for as many as three times. The onset and severity of arthritis were compared with those seen in five immunized but untreated DBA/1 mice (male).

Determination of the Nucleotide Sequence of BII-specific Vβ and Jβ Beta Gene Segments in the Lesion

The mRNA was prepared from arthritic joints of B10.RIII mice as described. cDNA was generated by using Cβ beta-specific primer (5′-TGATGGCTCAAA-CAAGGAGAC-3′). The ds cDNA was ligated to a linker oligomer pair (PL4,5′-GATCGTGGTACCGCGGCCCGCATCGATGTCGAC; PL3,5′-CACCATGGCGC-CGGCGTAGCTACAGCTG-3′) and subjected to PCR amplification as described. Briefly, the PCR reaction containing 250 mM of dNTP, 100 pmole of primers (Cβ and PL4), 50 mM tris-Cl (pH 9.0), 50 mM NaCl, 2.5 mM MgCl$_2$, 0.5 mM DTT, and one unit of Taq polymerase (Cetus) in the final volume of 100 μL. Denaturing was performed at 92°C for 30 s, annealing at 55°C for 40 s, and elongation at 72°C for 1 min. DNA was amplified in Perkin-Elmer thermal cycler (Norwalk, Connecticut). The amplified DNA was purified and cloned into a modified M13mp18 bacteriophage vector for single-strand sequencing with sequenase (U.S. Biochemical).

RESULTS

Antibodies against Type II and IX Collagen in Patients with Inner-ear Disease

Collagen molecules are major extracellular matrix proteins involved in the development and support of delicate auditory sensory organs. Type II collagen is widely distributed within inner-ear tissues, while type IX is found only within the labyrinthine membrane and dense fibers of the tectorial membrane. Antibody-specific for type II collagen has been shown to be elevated in some patients with hearing loss due to several presumably autoimmune illnesses (including Ménière's disease, otosclerosis, chronic progressive sensorineural hearing loss, and relapsing polychondritis).

To further study this, purified human types II and IX collagen and an extract of human cochlear tissue were subjected to isolation by SDS-PAGE and transferred to nitrocellulose. The sera of 21 patients diagnosed as having inner-ear disease were examined for the presence of anticollagen and anticochlear antibodies; the sera were used to probe western blots of purified human collagens II, IX, and XI, and cochlear protein extract, with peroxidase conjugated goat antihuman polyvalent Ig as the second antibody.

Anti-type-II collagen antibodies were seen in 12/21 (57%) of patients, while 13/21 (62%) had anti-type-IX antibodies detectable by western blot. A previously unreported 30-kD (probably noncollagen) protein of human cochlear tissue extracts was found by SDS-PAGE in three patients, all with Ménière's disease, having antibody activity to this protein detected by western blot. Anti-type-II and -type-IX antibodies were found in a high percentage of patients with Ménière's disease, otosclerosis, and strial atrophy. Six patients (29%), and all control patients, had no detectable antibodies to these proteins by our assay.[3]

Type II Collagen-induced Autoimmune Ear Disease in Mice

In order to identify the epitope on the type II collagen molecule that induced autoimmune ear disease, electrophysiological and histological studies were carried out in DBA/1J mice immunized with native chick type II collagen (CIIn) and cyanogen bromide (CNBr) peptide 11 (CB-11 peptide), which was cleaved from chicken type II collagen with CNBr digestion. Four months after immunization, 3 out of 6 CIIn-immunized mice and 5 out of 6 CB-11 peptide-immunized mice developed moderate hearing loss. No control animals showed hearing loss. The pattern of hearing loss was characteristic of progressive deafness. Further, the immunized mice showed temporal lesions involving atrophy of the Corti organ and degeneration of the spiral ganglion, in proportion to the level of hearing loss. Since similar inner-ear lesions were induced by immunization with CIIn and CB-11 peptide, CB-11 peptide contains at least one epitope that induces autoimmune inner-ear disease in collagen-II-induced disease on the chick type II collagen molecule involved in pathogenesis of autoimmune ear disease. It was concluded that CB-11 peptides contain the epitope that induces autoimmune inner-ear disease in collagen-IIn-induced disease.[14]

T-cell Receptor with V β-8 and V β-6 Gene Segments Recognize Multiepitopes in CB-11 Peptide in Type II Collagen-induced Autoimmune Disease

We have found autoimmune peptide epitopes from the CB-11 peptide of type II collagen for TCR and examined the TCR V region usage and its Vß gene structures. In CIAD, the TCR from the original different H2 mice recognize multiepitopes of type II collagen. The TCR with H-2^q source recognizes peptide residues 121–147 of

CB-11, but not residues 211–247. The TCR with H-2^r source responds to residues 211–247 (P2 peptide) better than to residues 121–147 (P1 peptide). The lysine residues at position 129 and 141 in P1, the arginine residue at position 227, and glutamic acid at position 230 in P2 might play an important role in trimolecular interaction. In CIAD, the restrictive usage of the TCR Vß gene was found to be Vß-8, Vß-6, and Vß-1 by DNA sequencing of T-cell hybridomas in addition to PCR and FACS. This preferential use of Vß-8 and Vß-6 in CIAD implies that an immunotherapy may be possible to control this autoimmune disease.[15]

Hearing Loss Induced by Monoclonal Antibody Against CB11 Peptide.

Type II collagen fragment CB-11-specific monoclonal antibodies were infused directly into the guinea pig cochlea (a mixture of #6, #10, #21, and #D12G was used). The concentration of each antibody was 1 mg/mL on 5 guinea pigs. Brain-stem auditory-evoked potential (BAEP) study was performed on days 0 (immediately after surgery), 3, 7, 10, and 14. Two of five guinea pigs showed more than 30 dB increased hearing threshold on days 7 to 10. The other two guinea pigs showed 20 dB increased hearing threshold on day 7. The increase in hearing threshold continued until the end of this study. Seven guinea pigs of the control group received infusions with diluted normal mouse serum. This study is still in process. However, at present none of the guinea pigs shows increased hearing threshold.

Auricular Chondritis

Punching a hole in the pinna produced some degree of redness and swelling around the hole; this acute inflammation always disappeared in 7 to 10 days. There was no difference in the average severity of this initial inflammation between immunized and control groups. However, the remarkable finding in this experiment is that 6 of the 41 (14.6%) immunized mice (6 of 86 pinnae, 7.0%) had recurrent redness and swelling in the punched area later on, while no lesion recurred in any of the 34 control mice that were treated only by punching a hole in the pinna. Detailed observations follow: during the first month after immunization, immunized group (I) = 0/86 pinnae, control group (C) = 0/68; during the second month, I = 4/80, C = 0/68; during the third month, I = 1/73, C = 0/62; and during the fourth month, I = 1/64, C = 0/62. The pinnae indicated by the reduced number in each observation were used for histologic study. Beside those pinnae, specimens biopsied within one week after punching (12 pinnae from 8 immunized mice and 4 pinnae from 2 control mice) were also studied histologically. The histologic findings of this lesion were characterized by nodular proliferation of chondrocytes, inflammatory cells infiltrating the normal cartilaginous layer as well as around proliferated chondrocytes, and fibrosis; these manifestations resembled those seen in the rat auricular chondritis. Immunohistochemistry demonstrated positive staining for Vβ-6 TCRs. In contrast to with these findings, in the region where the hole was punched and no inflammatory sign recurred obviously, a small number of proliferative chondrocytes and a thin layer of collagen fibers, contiguous to the edge of lacerated cartilaginous layer and perichondrium layer, respectively, were the only changes seen histologically. This manifestation, lacking obvious cell infiltrates around those tissues, was thought to be normal healing at the punched pinna. In the specimen biopsied in the early phase (within 7 days after punching), no inflammatory signs were seen inside the cartilaginous layer, but infiltration of inflammatory cells and the proliferation of fibroblasts, located in subdermal connective tissue at the edge of the punched hole, was not thought to be a specific change produced by immunization, and indeed, no average difference in severity was found between the immunized and control groups. All of the mice that developed recurrent lesions on the pinna had developed arthritis. In an identically designed experiment with B10.RIII mice, no such recurrent lesions were found on 21 pinnae (5 pinnae observed during the first 2 months after immunization, 4 pinnae during the first 5 months, and 12 pinnae during the first 10 months).[16]

Producing Ear-lobe Lesion by Monoclonal Antibody

An attempt at producing auricular chondritis by injecting a mixture of murine type II collagen specific monoclonal antibodies demonstrated various manifestations in the punched region. Redness and swelling assessed macroscopically were more remarkable at days 7 and 8 in the immunized mice than those in the controls. Histologic study with biopsied specimens, taken from one pinna of each group mouse at day 9, supported this observation; there was more severe inflammation in the subdermal connective tissue; however, this lesion did not contain any sign of chondritis. After further observation of the remaining pinnae, redness and swelling disappeared by day 14 and no recurrence of inflammation was recognized for 4 months, at which time the mice were sacrificed. Arthritis was recognized by swelling and redness in only one finger in 2 of the 3 mice, but it disappeared after 2 weeks.[16]

Sequelae after Myringotomy

The incised eardrums always healed without any sign of middle-ear infection in the control mice that were checked with an operation microscope one month after incision, and appeared clear for the 12 months until the mice were sacrificed. This observation was based on 20 eardrums in DBA/1 mice and 6 eardrums in B1O.RIII mice. However, healing of the incised eardrum in the type II collagen immunized mice showed different manifestations that were characterized by a crustlike covering on the eardrum. This covering was seen in 10 of the 24 DBA/1 eardrums and in 7 of the 8 B1O.RIII eardrums even 6 to 9 months after incision. However, middle-ear infection was not seen in any of the cases when they were sacrificed. Although the number of experimental mice was small, 3 DBA/1 mice injected with the mixture of CB-ll monoclonal antibodies had a similar pattern that lasted only for about one month, while the two control mice injected with normal mouse IgG healed the incised eardrums without such a covering. The histologic finding of one such eardrum taken 15 days after incision from a DBA/1 mouse injected with the mixture of monoclonal antibodies in comparison, with that in a control mouse (IgG injected) show that the incised eardrum healed as seen in both cases, but was thicker and accompanied with crustlike material, which appears of cell infiltration, desquamated epithelium, and exudate in the immunized mouse. Electron-microscopic pictures from the specimen taken from a type-II-collagen immunized B10.RIII mouse 9 months after the eardrum incision shows that the intact eardrum consists of two layers of epithelium (the thinner one is the middle-ear side and another is the external-ear side) and two layers of a collagen fiber arrangement (radially and circularly arranged). On the other hand, in the immunized mouse, the eardrum partially winds and its thickness is 2 to 4 times normal. The arrangement of collagen fibers is irregular in both layers and contains fibroblasts, which are rarely found in the intact eardrum. The appearance of the covering over the eardrum varies. It appears to be partially a homogenous low density containing cholesterine-crystal appearing material, cell infiltration, and a spongy tissue consisting of cell debris.[16]

Oral Tolerance

The mice were divided into four groups: the first group was fed PBS buffer orally; the second group was fed orally with 20 μg of CB11 peptide; the third group was fed orally with 500 μg of CB11; and the last group was fed orally with 20 μg of CTB-CB11. All the mice received either PBS buffer or antigen 7 days before the immunization. All the mice had their ears punched (~2mm) at the auricle on day 12 postimmunization. The serums from all four groups of mice were collected before and every two weeks after immunization. The development of chondritis was observed daily. The clinical score of chondritis was graded as 0: mild erythema with little swelling due to the ear punch; 1: moderate erythema and swelling of portions of the ear; 2: severe-erythema and swelling of the entire ear.

The results suggest that 20 μg of orally fed CTB-CB-11 is sufficient to induce tolerance in chondritis. The secretion of antigen-specific IgG in the tolerant mice is higher than in the 20- or 500-μg CB-11 orally fed group of mice and lower than the nontolerant group. A more detailed analysis of IgG1, IgG2a, and IgG2b shows that distribution of the antigen-specific subclass IgG is not even among these groups.

DISCUSSION

Autoimmune response to the components of connective tissue, in particular type II collagen, were proposed by Yoo *et al.*[2] Connective tissues, forming the architectural framework of the vertebrate structure, consist of the cell components and the extracellular matrix served by cells, such as fibroblasts, chondrocytes and osteoblasts. The extracellular matrix is made up of two main classes of macromolecules: (1) polysaccharides (glycosaminoglycans), which are usually found covalently linked to protein in the form of proteoglycans; and (2) fibrous proteins that have either a mainly structural function (collagen and elastin) or a mainly adhesive function (fibronectin and laminin). Thus, the fundamental structure of connective tissue is common among different organs, but the amounts of connective tissue vary greatly. They are a major component in skin and bone, and minor constituents in brain and spinal cord. The extracellular matrix also varies in form, such as the calcified forms in the bone or teeth, the transparent form in the cornea, and the ropelike form in tendons. With regard to collagen molecules, at least 17 genetically distinct types have been found[17] and their type-specific distribution in various tissues is well established.[18] Type II collagen is known as the major component of cartilage but immunohistochemical studies of the ear tissue in rodents has revealed its distribution in the following regions: the enchondral layer and the globuli interossei of the otic capsule, osseous spiral lamina, spiral ligament, limbus, tectorial membrane, endolymphatic duct.[13,19,20]

Type-II-collagen-induced ear lesions in Lewis rats and guinea pigs were first reported by Yoo *et al.* in 1983 and 1984.[21–23] However, in 1986 Harris *et al.* could not observe these phenomena.[24] Soliman reexamined these controversial results in 1990 and demonstrated impaired hearing threshold morphologic changes, endolymphatic hydrops, slight vasculitis of the cochlear artery, and slight degeneration of the spiral ganglion cells.[25]

Huang *et al.*[26,27] reproduced type-II-collagen-induced bone resorption in the temporal bone and salphingitis in rats, in contrast to the negative report of Bretlau *et al.,*[28] and confirming our previous observation. Cruz *et al.* also reproduced spiral ganglion degeneration in guinea pig with type II collagen immunization.[29] These animals had an increase of latency in wave one. Tomoda *et al.* reproduced type-II-collagen-induced the animal model in guinea pig in separate experiments.[30,31] Obviously, further studies are necessary to clarify those contradicting observations.

Autoimmune response to type II collagen with animal models was originally described as the collagen-induced arthritis in rats and mice.[32,33] As is known, the onset of arthritis can be recognized by redness and swelling of the paws 4 to 6 weeks after immunization with type II collagen. Histologically, the hypertrophied synovial membrane, the massive infiltration of mononuclear cells, and the destruction and pannus formation in both cartilage and subchondral bone are remarkable findings in the early phase of the lesion. Then the lesion persists into a chronic phase, resulting in ankylosis of the joint. The mechanism of this lesion is known as the following: (1) anticollagen IgG in the serum, which binds to type II collagen present in the articular cartilage, activates the complement system, and then leads to the generation of C3a and C5a; (2) C3a can increase vascular permeability and allows for trafficking of sensitized lymphocytes into the joint space; (3) these sensitized lymphocytes can proliferate in the joint space and secrete lymphokines that may induce proliferation of synovial tissue; and (4) C5a induces migration of the inflammatory cells into the joint space and allows them to produce connective tissue-degrading enzymes, such as collagenase, elastase, and neutral and acid cathepsin. Thus, humoral immunity plays a critical role in initiating the lesion. Yet, cell-mediated immunity is believed to be required to sustain the lesion because arthritis can be transferred to recipients by the intravenous administration of immune sera, but it is transient and lacks a chronic phase.[34] Transfer of arthritis can also be achieved in recipients by intravenous administration of sensitized T cells, leading to a sustained response.[35] Here we are able to induce tympanic lesions by monoclonal antibody specific against type II collagen. Thus, ear lesions can be transferred either by T cells[15] or antibodies.

Some patients of rheumatoid arthritis have been reported to have the elevated antibody to type II collagen in the serum.[36,37] When the mechanism of this clinical observation is compared with the collagen arthritis model, the inner-ear lesions reported in this animal model also attract attention, because of similar reports of elevated serum titer to type II collagen in various human inner-ear diseases.[3,23] Auricular chondritis induced by immunization with type II collagen was reported previously in rats as an animal model for the relapsing polychondritis in humans.[38] In our mouse experiments, we used mechanical damage (the punctured pinnae) to facilitate the collagen-induced auricular chondritis. However, it has been reported that the H-2^q strain of BZH mice is susceptible only to bovine collagen (not to chick collagen) and develops an atypical joint disease and frequent auricular chondritis resembling relapsing polychondritis.[39] Thus, different background genes acting in concert with major class II histocompatibility complex genes, and immunogenic epitope differences on the type II collagen molecule appear to have a strong influence on the occurrence of the lesions in various sites. In the present study, the auricular lesions in mice had a lower incidence than arthritis. However, they were characterized by massive infiltration of mononuclear cells and destruction and proliferation of the cartilage, exactly as seen in the arthritic joint.

Immunohistochemical studies of type II collagen have previously revealed its localization in the lamina propria of the eardrum,[19] and tympanosclerotic change has been reported in guinea pigs immunized with type II collagen.[40] These remarkable findings include hyperplasia of the eardrum with calcium deposition, especially after myringotomy. In our mouse experiments, we have failed to observe such calcification, but persistent inflammation of the eardrum after myringotomy was demonstrated. In the longest case the inflammatory product covering the eardrum lasted for 9 months before the mouse was sacrificed. The ear lesions are clearly distinguished from arthritic lesions by their decreased incidence and severity. However, relapsing polychondritis is sometimes clinically seen in association with arthritis.[41] The patients with relapsing polychondritis have been reported to develop inner-ear disorders at an incidence of 30 to 40%,[41,42] and to demonstrate anticollagen antibodies and cell-mediated immunity to cartilage components.[39,43] Auricular chondritis has been observed to occur spontaneously in a strain of rats, as well as following immunization with type II collagen.[38,44] Only type II collagen, as well as 68- and 30-kD inner-ear proteins and type IX and XI collagen,[3,4] appear to be the major proteins implicated in the autoimmune mechanism of inner ear lesion at present, although other antigens have been implicated.[6] Therefore, further studies of their molecular level of 68- and 30-kD inner-ear proteins would be an important study. It is also shown that the bovine inner-ear antigen 68 kD is a hsp70 protein.[45] The implication of this finding in human ear disease is not clear at this point. Further study of molecular events leading to the induction of autoimmune ear diseases is urgently needed.

A trimolecular complex, formed when an α/β TCR on a CD4$^+$ lymphocyte binds to its specific peptide antigen–class II major histocompatibility complex molecule combination on an antigen-presenting cell, is thought to transmit a signal to the CD4$^+$ lymphocyte from an antigen presenting cell. This initiating process of the lesion has been the subject of intense investigation.[46] If a specific TCR V region expression can be shown to correlate with a specific autoimmune disease, treatment of the disease with monoclonal antibodies specific for the particular TCR might be possible. Indeed, this type of therapy has already been used successfully to prevent and cure experimental allergic encephalomyelitis, a T-cell-mediated autoimmune disease in mice.[47] The most remarkable evidence for the role of specific TCRs in a human autoimmune disease has been reported in rheumatoid arthritis, in which particular

TCR β chain rearrangements predominate in T cells cultured from the synovia of individuals with an advanced case of the disease.[48–54] In the present study in conjunction with our reports elsewhere,[15] we were able to show a similar fundamental phenomenon in collagen-induced ear disease. Our monoclonal antibody and peptide therapies, as well as some similar studies reported previously, suggest a possible role for TCR β chain immunomodulation in this animal model.[55,56] These results also highlight the possibility of curing or preventing autoimmune diseases by antibody or peptide therapies without affecting the whole immunity system.

Positive staining of TCR was demonstrated not only by Vβ-8.1 or Vβ-8.2 in the arthritic lesion, but also by Vβ-6, although the implication of this result is still unknown. This differential TCR Vβ expression could be a clue to differences in these two types of lesions. However, it could be due to the sampling process, and so needs further investigation. It is of interest to note that one of the collagen specific T-cell hybridoma clone prepared from the lymph nodes of diseased mice has identical to the TCR Vβ-8.1 gene sequence as prepared from the arthritic joints. The TCR Vβ-8.1 and TCRVβ-8.2 gene segments were 91% alike in nucleotide sequence and 90% at the protein level. These results demonstrate that circulating antigen specific T cells infiltrate the arthritic joints. However, a detailed mechanism of this T-cells infiltration to the lesions is not clear. An extensive study of this mechanism could produce a possible lead to cure these autoimmune diseases. The role of the autoimmune response to type II collagen in auricular chondritis as shown here is highly suggested by its histologic similarity to that in arthritis.

It was also found that in the CIA model of DBA/1J and B10RIII, the arthogenic and tolerogenic T-cell epitopes are residues: 245–270 and 181-210 (DBA/1J) 430–466 and 607–621 (B10.RIII),[57–62] which are needed for study in CIAED model. The preliminary data on oral tolerance suggests that it might be possible to induce tolerance by the CTB-CB-11 peptide in the CIAED model.

REFERENCES

1. McCabe, B. F. 1979. Autoimmune sensorineural hearing loss. Ann. Otol. Rhinol. Laryngol. **88:** 585–589.
2. Yoo, T. J., J. M. Stuart, A. H. Kang, A.S. Townes, K. Tomoda & S. Dixit. 1982. Type II collagen autoimmunity in otosclerosis and Ménière's disease. Science **217:** 1153–1155.
3. Joliat, T., J. Seyer, J. Bernstein, M. Krug, X. J. Ye, J. S. Cho, T. Fujiyoshi & T. J. Yoo. 1992. Antibodies against a 30 KD cochlear protein and type II and IX collagens in the serum of patients with inner ear diseases. Ann. Otol. Rhinol. Laryngol. **101:** 12, 1000–1006.
4. Harris, J. P., M. Gastka, J. Cevallos & A. F. Ryan. 1992. Screening an inner ear gene library for targets of autoimmunity. Molecular Biology of Hearing Deafness (abstract 97).
5. Moscicki, R. A., J. E. San Martin, C. H. Quintero, S. D. Rauch, J. B. Nadol & K. J. Bloch. Serum antibody to inner ear proteins in patients with progressive hearing loss. JAMA **272:** 611–616.
6. Harris, J. P. 1987. Experimental autoimmune sensorineural hearing loss. Laryngoscope **97:** 63–76.
7. Zaller, D. M., G. Osman, O. Kanagawa & L. Hood. 1990. Prevention and tratment of experimental allergic encephalomyelitis with T-cell receptor Vβ-specific antibodies. J. Exp. Med. **171:** 1943–1955.

8. THOMPSON, H. S. G. & N. A. STAINES. 1985. Gastric administration of type II collagen delay the onset and severity of collagen induced arthritis in rats. Clin. Exp. Immunol. **64:** 581.

9. NAGLER-ANDERSON, C., L. A. BOBER, M. E. ROBINSON, G. W. SISKIND & G. J. THORBECKE. 1986. Suppression of type II collagen-induced arthritis by intragastric administration of soluble type II collagen. PNAS **83:** 7443.

10. LIDER, O., L. M. B. SANTOS, C. S. Y. LEE, P. J. HIGGINS & H. L. HEINER. 1989. Suppression of experimental autoimmune encephalomyelitis by oral administration of myelin basic protein; II suppression of disease and in vitro immune responses is mediated by antigen-specific CD8+ T lymphocytes. J. Immunol. **142:** 748.

11. Miller, A., O. Lider & H. L. Weiner. 1991. Antigen driven bystander suppression after oral administration of antigens. J. Exp. Med. **174:** 791.

12. SUN, J. B., C. RASK, T. OLSSON, J. HOLMGREN & C. CZERKINSKY. 1996. Treatment of experimental autoimmune encephalomyelitis by feeding myelin basic protein conjugated to cochlear toxin B subunit. PNAS **93:** 7196–7201.

13. SLEPECKY, N. B., J. E. SAVAGE & T. J. YOO. 1992. Localization of type II, IX and V collagen in the inner ear. Acta Otolaryngol. (Stockholm) **112:** 611–617.

14. TAKEDA, T., N. SUDO, H. KITANO & T. J. YOO. 1996. Type II collagen induced autoimmune ear disease in mice. Am. J. Otology **17:** 69–75.

15. YOO, T. J., M. K. LEE, Y.S. MIN, H. J. CHIANG, K. WANG, T. FUJIYOSHI, T. WATANABE, M. S. KRUG, J. SEYER & K. C. CHENG. 1994. Epitope specificity and T-cell receptor usage in type II collagen induced autoimmune ear disease. Cell. Immunol. **157:** 249–262.

16. FUJIYOSHI, T., K. C. CHENG, M. S. KRUG & T. J. YOO. 1997. Molecular basis of type II collagen autoimmune diseases. ORL **59:** 215–229.

17. ALBERTS, B., D. BRAY, J. LEWIS, M. RAFF, K. ROBERT & J. D. WATSON. 1989. Molecular Biology of the Cell, 2nd ed.: 802–803. Garland Publishing. New York.

18. DARNELL, J., H. LODISH & D. BALTIMORE. 1990. Molecular Cell Biology, 2nd ed.: 906–915. Scientific American Books. New York.

19. YOO, T. J. & K. TOMODA. 1988. Type II collagen distribution in rodents. Laryngoscope **98:** 1255–1260.

20. SLEPECKY, N. B., L. K. CEFARATTI & T. J. YOO. 1992. Type II and type IX collagen from heterotypic fibers in the tectorial membrane of the inner ear. Marix **11:** 80–86.

21. YOO, T. J., K. TOMODA & A. HERNANDEZ. 1984. Type II collagen induced autoimmune inner ear lesions in guinea pigs. Am. Otol. Rhinol. Laryngol. **93**(Suppl. 113): 3–5.

22. YOO, T. J., K. TOMODA, J. M. STUART, M. A. CREMER, A. S. TOWNES & A. H. KANG. 1983. Type II collagen induced autoimmune sensorineural hearing loss and vestibular dysfunction in rats. Ann. Otol. Rhinol. Laryngol. **92:** 267–272.

23. YOO, T. J., Y. YAZAWA, K. TOMODA & R. A. FLOYD. 1983. Type II collagen induced autoimmune endolymphatic hydrops in guinea pig. Science **222:** 65–67.

24. HARRIS, J. P., N. K. WOOLF & A. RYAN. 1986. A reexamination of experimental type II collagen autoimmunity: Middle and inner ear morphology and function. Ann Otol. Rhinol. Laryngol. **95:** 176–181.

25. SOLIMAN, A. M. 1990. Type II collagen induced inner ear disease: Critical evaluation of the guinea pig model. Am. J. Otol. **11**(1): 27–32.

26. HUANG, C., D. SAPORTA & M. ABRAMSON. 1985. Immunologically induced salpingitis in rats. Am. J. Otolaryngol. **6:** 368–372.

27. HUANG, C. 1987. Bone resorption in experimental otosclerosis in rats. Am. J. Otolaryngol. **8:** 332–341.

28. BRETLAU, P., V. BALLE, J. B. CAUSSE, K. HORSTEV-PETERSEN, C. H. SORENSEN & M. SOLVS-TEEN. 1987. Is otosclerosis an autoimmune disease? Proc. 2nd Int. Acad. Conf. on Immunobiology, Histophysiology and Tumor Immunology in Otolaryngology: 201–206. Kugler. Amsterdam, The Netherlands.

29. CRUZ, O. L., A. MINITI, W. COSSERMELLI & R. M. OLIVEIRA. 1990. Autoimmune sensorineural hearing loss: A preliminary experimental study. Am. J. Otol. **11**(5): 342–346.

30. TOMODA, K., N. MAEDA, T. YAMAWAKI, T. YAMSHITA, T. KUMAZAWA & T. OHASHI. 1989. Immunologically induced experimental hydrops: Its mechanisms and pathology, 2nd Int. Symp. on Ménière's Disease, J. B. Nadal, Ed.: 165–172. Kugler & Ghedini. Amsterdam/Berkley/Milan.

31. TOMODA, K., T. YAMAWAKI, Y. SUZUKA, T. YAMASHITA & T. Kumazawa. Inner ear immunology and the changes of charge barrier. Ear Res. (Jpn.) **21**: 275–276.

32. TRENTHAM, D. E., A. S. TOWNES, & H. KANG. 1977. Autoimmunity to type II collagen: An experimental model of arthritis, J. Exp. Med, **146**: 857–868.

33. COURTENAY, J. S., M. J. DALLMAN, A. D. DAYAN, A. MARTIN & B. MOSEDALE. 1980. Immunization against heterologous type II collagen induced arthritis in mice. Nature (London) **283**: 666–668.

34. STUART, J. M., M. A. CREMER, A. S. TOWNES & H. KANG. 1982. Type II collagen-induced arthritis in rats. Passive transfer with serum and evidence that IgG anticollagen antibodies can cause arthritis. J. Exp. Med. **155**: 168–178.

35. TRENTHAM, D. E., R. A. DYNESIUS & J. R. DAVIS. 1978. Passive transfer by cells of type II collagen induced arthritis in rat. J. Clin. Invest. **62**: 359–366.

36. ANDRIOPOULOS, N. A., J. MESTECKY, E. J. MILLER & E. L. BRADLEY. 1976. Antibodies to native and denatured collagen in sera of patients with rheumatoid arthritis. Arthritis Rheum. **19**: 613–617.

37. TERATO, K., Y. SHIMOZURU, K. KATAYAMA, Y. TAKEMITSU, I. YAMASHITA, M. MIYATSU, K. FUJII, M. SAGARA, S. KOBAYASHI, M. GOTO, K. NISHIOKA, N. MIYASAKA & Y. NAGAI. 1990. Specificity antibodies to type II collagen in rheumatoid arthritis. Arthritis Rheum. **33**: 1493–1500.

38. CREMER, M. A., J. A. PITCOCK, J. M. STUART, A. H. KANG & A. S. TOWNES. 1981. Auricular chondritis in rats. An experimental model of relapsing polychondritis induced with type II collagen. J. Exp. Med. **154**: 535–540.

39. WOOLEY, P. H. 1988. Collagen induced arthritis in the mouse. Methods Enzymol. **162**: 361–373.

40. YAZAWA, Y., T. J. YOO, T. ISHIBE & K. TOMODA. 1985. Type II collagen induced tympanosclerosis model in guinea pigs. Auris Nasus Larynx (Tokyo) **12**(Suppl. I): S200–S202.

41. EBRINGER, R., G. ROOK & G. T. SWANA. 1981. Autoantibodies to cartilage in type II collagen in relapsing polychondritis and other rheumatic disease. Ann. Rheum. Dis. **40**: 473–479.

42. MCADAMS, L. P., M. A. O'HANLAN & R. BLEUSTONE. 1976. Relapsing polychondritis; Prospective study of 23 patients and a review of the literature. Medicine **55**: 193–215.

43. CODY, D. T. R. & D. A. SONES. 1971. Relapsing polychondritis; Audiovestibular manifestations. Laryngoscope **2**(81): 1208–1222.

44. PRIEUR, D. J., D. M. YOUNG & D. F. COUNTS. 1984. Auricular chondritis in Fawn-hooded rats. Am. J. Pathol. **116**: 69–76.

45. BILLINGS, P. B., E. M. KEITHLEY & J. P. HARRIS. 1995. Evidence linking the 68-kd antigen associated with progressive sensorineural hearing loss with the highly induciable hsp70. Association for Research in Otolaryngology Abst. 588.

46. GOVERMAN, J. & J. R. PARNES. 1991. The T-cell receptor. *In* Basic and Clinical Immunology, 7th ed., D. P. Stites and A. L. Terr, Eds.: 73–77. Appleton and Lange. Norwalk, Conn.

47. URBAN, J. L., V. KUMAR, D. H. KONO, C. GOMEZ, S. J. HORVATH, J. CLAYTON, D. G. ANDO, E. E. SERCARZ & L. HOOD. 1988. Restricted use of T-cell receptor V genes in murine autoimmune ecephalomyelitis raises possibilities for antibody therapy. Cell **54**: 577–592.

48. PALIARD, X., S. G. WEST, J. A. LAFFERTY, J. R. CLEMENTS, J. W. KAPPLER, P. MARRACK & B.

L. KOTZIN. 1991. Evidence for the effects of a superantigen in rheumatoid arthritis. Science **253**: 325–329.

49. COOPER, S. M. 1944. T-cell receptor use in human rheumatoid arthritis. N.Y. Acad. Sci. Symp. T-Cell Receptor Use in Human Autoimmune Diseases, April 17–20.

50. BRENNER, M. 1994. T-cell populations in rheumatoid arthritis. N.Y. Acad. Sci. Symp. T-Cell Receptor Use in Human Autoimmune Diseases (Abst.), April 17–20.

51. NATVIG, J. B. 1994. T-cell receptor use in rheumatoid arthritis. N.Y. Acad. Sci. Symp. T-Cell Receptor Use in Human Autoimmune Diseases (Abst.), April 17–20.

52. PADULA, S. 1994. T-cell receptor use in rheumatoid arthritis. N.Y. Acad. Sci. Symp. T-Cell Receptor Use in Human Autoimmune Diseases (Abst.), April 17–20.

53. JENKINS, R. N. 1994. T-cell receptor Vβ gene bias in rheumatoid arthritis. N.Y. Acad. Sci. Symp. T-Cell Receptor Use in Human Autoimmune Diseases (Abst.), April 17–20.

54. KATZIN, B. L. 1994. T-cell receptor use in human and murine inflammatory joint disease. N.Y. Acad. Sci. Symp. T-Cell Receptor Use in Human Autoimmune Diseases, April 17–20.

55. MODER, K. G., G. D. ANDERSON, H. S. LUTHRA & C. S. DAVIS. 1991. A significant reduction in the incidence of collagen induced arthritis in mice treated with anti-TCR Vβ antibodies in self reactivity and its regulation. 20th Annu. Meeting, Keystone Symp., Abst. C412.

56. CHIOCCHHIA, G., M. C. BOISSIER & C. FOURNIER. 1991. Therapy against murine collagen-induced arthritis with T-cell receptor Vβ specific antibodies. Eur. J. Immunol. (Germany) **21**: 2899–2905.

57. MIYAHARA, H., L. K. MYERS, E. F. ROSLONIEC, D. D. BRAND, J. M. SEYER, J. M. STUART & A. H. KANG. 1995. Identification and characterization of a major tolerogenic T-cell epitope of type II collagen that suppresses arthritis in B10.RIII mice. Immunology **86**: 110–115.

58. MYERS, L. K., H. MIYAHARA, K. TERATO, J. M. SEYER, J. M. STUART & A. H. KANG. 1995. Collagen-induced arthritis in B10.RIII mice (H-2ʳ) identification of an arthritogenic T-cell determinant. Immunology **84**: 509–513.

59. MYERS, L. K., S. W. COOPER, K. TERATO, J. M. SEYER, J. M. STUART & A. H. KANG. 1995. Identification and characterization of a tolerogenic T cell determinant within residues 181-209 of check type II collagen. Clin. Immun. Immunopath. **74**(1): 33–38.

60. MYERS, L. K., J. M. SEYER, J. M. STUART, K. TERATO, C. S. DAVID & A. H. KANG. 1993. T cell epitopes of type II collagen that regulate murine collagen-induced arthritis. J. Immun. **151**: 500–505.

61. MYERS, L. K., E. F. ROSLONIEC, J. M. SEYER, J. M. STUART & A. H. KANG. 1993. A synthetic peptide analogue of a determinant of type II collagen prevents the onset of collagen-induced arthritis. J. Immun. **150**: 4652–4658.

62. MYERS, L. K., K. TERATO, J. M. SEYER, J. M. STUART & A. H. KANG. 1992. Characterization of a tolerogenic T cell epitope of type II collagen and its relevance to collagen-induced arthritis. J. Immun. **149**: 1439–1443.

Lymphocyte Trafficking to the Inner Ear[a]

ALLEN F. RYAN, [b] BERTRAND GLODDEK AND JEFFREY P. HARRIS

Division of Otolaryngology
Department of Surgery
UCSD Medical School and VA Medical Center
9500 Gilman Drive
La Jolla, California 92093-0666

THE ORIGINS OF INNER EAR IMMUNITY

The concept that the inner ear serves as a site for the expression of immune responses has been accepted relatively recently. Because of the existence of the blood–labyrinthine barrier, similar in many respects to the blood–brain barrier, the labyrinth was long thought to be an immunoprivledged or protected site, sequestered from immunity because of the delicate nature of its tissues.[1]

In fact, the blood–labyrinthine barrier does serve to partially isolate the cochlea and vestibular labyrinth from systemic immunity. Antibody titers in perilymph are typically about 1/1000th of those in serum,[2] and under normal circumstances leukocytes are not present in the majority of the inner ear. However, this does not render the cochlea defenseless. Under the appropriate circumstances, immunity can be expressed at high levels in the inner ear. In some cases this immunity is protective, as when immunization protects the inner ear from viral infection.[3] In other circumstances, immunity can be a destructive force. Thus a primary viral infection of the labyrinth produces markedly less damage in immunosuppressed animals.[4] In addition, antigenic challenge of the inner ear in a systemically immunized animal can result in severe inflammatory damage.[5] During such cochlear immune responses, numerous lymphocytes and plasma cells can be found within the cochlea.

Because the cochlea lacks resident leukocytes, immune cells that appear in the ear must originate at other sites. While the normal cochlea lacks resident lymphocytes, immunocytes are present in small numbers in the normal endolymphatic sac.[6] However, lymphocytes can appear in large numbers quite rapidly in the cochlea, and they occur preferentially in scala tympani.[7] These observations suggest that migration of immmunocytes from the sac is not a likely source of these cells. However, another potential source of lymphocytes in the cochlea is the circulation. During a cochlear immune response, vessels in the cochlea develop morphological specializations that are associated with lymphocyte trafficking in other tissues.[8] Since extravasation of leukocytes plays an integral role in virtually all immune responses, it seems likely that it occurs in the cochlea as well.

[a]This research was supported by NIG/NIDCD Grants DC00129 and DC00189, by the Research Service of the Veterans Administration, and by the Duaei Hearing Research Fund.
[b]Author for correspondence. Phone: 619/534-4594; fax: 619/534-5319; e-mail: aryan@ucsd.edu

THE PROCESS OF LYMPHOCYTE EXTRAVASATION

Immunosurveilance and immune responses depend on the circulation of lymphocytes between immune organs and sites of antigen-induced inflammation. This circulation takes place primarily through the vasculature, and is mediated by sets of specific ligands on the surfaces of lymphocytes, which recognize receptors on the luminal surface of endothelial cells.

The process of extravasation for all leukocytes occurs in several well-documented steps.[9] The initial step is slowing of lymphocytes in the circulation, as they adhere weakly to the vessel wall and move along the surface of the endothelial cells, a process known as "rolling." The second step is tight adherence to a single location on the vessel wall, accompanied by flattening of the cell against the endothelium. Finally, the leukocyte penetrates the vessel wall through intraepithelial cell junctions. Each of these steps is mediated by cytokines and cytokine receptors, as well as cell surface molecules and specific receptors for these ligands.

Two groups of cytokines that play critical roles in leukocyte extravasation are proinflammatory interleukins and chemokines, both of which can be released by damaged tissues and leukocytes. A critical family of cell surface molecules involved in leukocyte recruitment is the selectins: L-selectin is expressed primarily on leukocytes, while E- and P-selectin are expressed primarily on endothelial cells. The binding between selectins and their cell surface ligands is relatively weak. Selectins are involved primarily in the initial capture of lymphocytes during the rolling process (see TABLE 1). A sec-

TABLE 1. Molecules Involved in Leukocyte Extravasation

	Site of Expression	Ligand	Role
Selectins			
P-selectin	Endothelial cells	Mucinlike molecules	Rolling on normal vessels
E-selectin	Inflamed venule endothelial cells	Fucosylated carbohydrates	Rolling on inflammed vessels
L-selectin	Leukocytes	Ig superfamily Mucinlike	Lymph node homing
Adhesion Molecules			
I-CAM1	Inflamed venule endothelial cells	$\alpha_L\beta_2$ Integrin $\alpha_M\beta_2$ Integrin	Activation, flattening, diapadesis
I-CAM2	Lymph node HEV endothelial cells	$\alpha_L\beta_2$ Integrin $\alpha_M\beta_2$ Integrin	Activation, flattening, diapadesis
V-CAM	Inflamed venule endothelial cells	$\alpha_4\beta_1$ Integrin $\alpha_4\beta_7$ Integrin	Activation, flattening, diapedesis
MAdCAM	Mucosal HEV endothelial cells	$\alpha_4\beta_7$ Integrin L-selectin	Activation, flattening
PECAM1	Leukocytes endothelial cells	PECAM1	Diapedesis

ond group of endothelial cell molecules, all members of the cell-adhesion molecule family, mediates tight adhesion of leukocytes and their flattening to the vessel wall (see TABLE 1).

MECHANISMS OF LYMPHOCYTE HOMING

The expression of unique combinations of vascular adhesion molecules is associated with different patterns of leukocyte and lymphocyte circulation. In the normal lymph node, constitutive expression of the ligands for L-selectin and of I-CAM2 on the cuboidal endothelial cells of specialized vessels called high endothelial venules, mediate the capture, flattening, and extravasation of circulating lymphocytes that express both L-selectin and I-CAM2 on their cell membranes.[9] This circulation mediates the spread of immunologic memory the peripheral lymph nodes.

A separate vascular adhesion system operates in mucosal lymphoid tissues. Mucosal lymphocytes express not only L-selectin, but also the $\alpha_4\beta_7$ integrin.[10] Both of these ligands recognize the mucosal addressin cell adhesion molecule (MAd-CAM).[11,12] MAdCAM mediates the capture and firm adhesion of mucosal lymphocytes to venules in the lamina propria of mucosae and in mucosa-associated lymphoid tissues. Circulation of mucosal lymphocytes mediates the spread of immunologic memory between these sites, especially in the system of gut-associated lymphoid tissue (GALT). It is possible that additional mucosal addressins exist, specific for other mucosal systems such as the bronchus-associated lymphoid tissue (BALT) or the immune organs of Waldeyer's ring.

During inflammation at peripheral sites, postcapillary venules express E-selectin, increased P-selectin, I-CAM1 and V-CAM in response to cytokines such as interleukin-1 (IL-1) and IL-8.[13] These surface molecules mediate capture, binding, and extravasation of leukocytes. In the inner ear, there is extensive evidence that the postcapillary venules of the cochlea, known as the spiral modiolar vein, are the primary site of recruitment for leukocytes of all types, including lymphocytes, into the inner ear.[14] The final step of extravasation through the vessel wall, diapedesis, involves platelet endothelial cell adhesion molecule 1 (PECAM1), and occurs in response to chemotactic signals released in the tissue. These chemotactic stimuli include a number of cytokines[13,15] as well as specific antigen.[16]

DEMONSTRATION OF LYMPHOCYTE RECRUITMENT
TO THE INNER EAR

The circulation of lymphocytes to the inner ear was evaluated using the passive transfer of radiolabeled lymphocytes.[17] Lymphocytes from several sources were employed to determine whether preferential recruitment of different types of lymphocytes might occur. Inbred guinea pigs were sensitized with antigen. Lymphocytes were harvested from the peripheral blood, lymph nodes in the neck and the spleens of these donors, and labeled with radioactive ^{51}Cr. Lymphocytes from unimmunized donors were also employed.

Additional inbred guinea pigs were sensitized with antigen, and later challenged

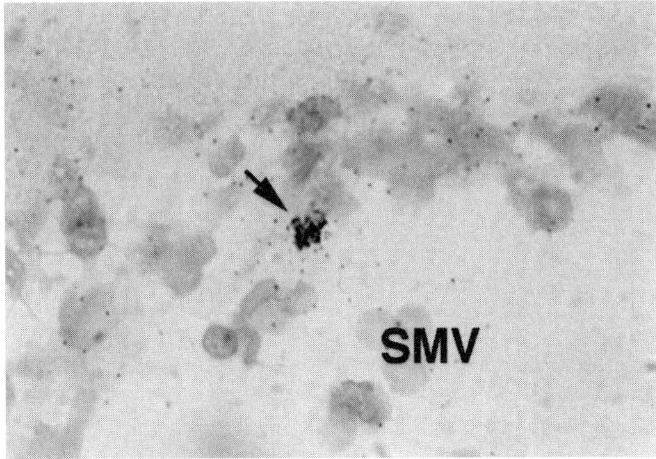

FIGURE 1. Radiolabeled lymphocyte (arrow) adjacent to the SMV of the guinea pig cochlea, following scala typani challenge of a sensitized animal with antigen.

in one cochlea with the same antigen, by direct injection into scala tympani. The opposite cochlea was injected with saline. These recipient animals were then injected with radiolabeled lymphocytes of one type. After 18 h, the inner ears and various immune organs were harvested for analysis by gamma counting and autoradiography.

Lymphoid tissues showed the expected patterns of lymphocyte trafficking. The spleen captured a large number of lymphocytes, and all three cell types were recruited with approximately equal efficiency. In contrast, lymph nodes preferentially recruited lymphocytes that were themselves harvested from lymph nodes. Also as expected, lymphocytes from sensitized animals showed higher rates of recruitment to all sites than those from naive animals.

In the inner ear, much higher levels of recruitment was observed in the inner ears challenged with antigen than in the saline-injected cochleas, suggesting that the vessels of the challenged inner ears express substantially more vascular adhesion molecules. Recruitment of peripheral blood and spleen lymphocytes occurred at higher levels than recruitment of lymphocytes harvested from neck nodes, suggesting that general adhesion molecules such as I-CAM1 and V-CAM, as opposed to I-CAM2, mediate lymphocyte capture in the cochlea. As at other sites, lymphocytes from sensitized animals showed higher rates of recruitment than those from nonsensitized animals. This presumably reflects the higher level of activation of lymphocytes from sensitized animals, with increased expression of integrins and other cell surface receptors that recognize endothelial cell adhesion molecules.

When cells were localized by autoradiography in the cochlea, lymphocytes were preferentially observed in the scala tympani of the challenged inner ears, although smaller numbers were also found in scala vestibuli and scala media. Other lymphocytes were observed in or near cochlear vessels. These cells were preferentially associated with the spiral modiolar vein. No cells were observed in the endolymphatic sac

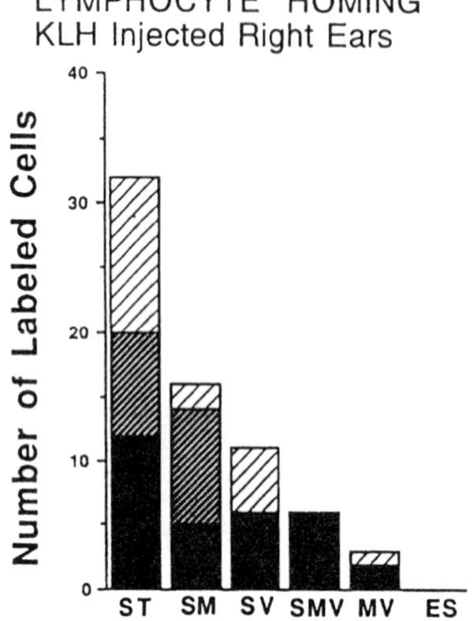

FIGURE 2. Amount and localization of labeled cells in the right (antigen-injected) and left (saline-injected) inner ears of systemically immunized, inner-ear-challenged guinea pigs. ST, scala tympani; SM, scala media; SV, scala vestibuli; SMV, spiral modiolar vein, MV, modiolar vein; ES, endolymphatic sac. (From Gloddek et al.[17] Reproduced by permission.)

of the antigenically challenged inner ears. These data are consistent with the spiral modiolar vein being the primary site of entry of lymphocytes into the cochlea.

Interestingly, the opposite inner ear showed lymphocytes within the spiral modiolar vein, but only in animals receiving lymphocytes from immunized animals. It seems likely that saline injection alone induced expression of endothelial cell adhesion molecules that were recognized by activated lymphocytes, causing the cells to slow and be captured on the endothelium. However, signals for the final step of lymphocyte extravasation were apparently absent. A few lymphocytes were also observed in the lumen of the control endolymphatic sac.

In a separate study, the expression of I-CAM1 was studied in the guinea pig inner ear, using immunocytochemistry.[18] Following antigenic challenge of previously sensitized animals, I-CAM1 immunoreactivity was observed in many cochlear cells, and most strongly in the endothelial cells of the spiral modiolar vein. Such expression provides a substrate for the capture of lymphocytes by cochlear vessels.

THE ORIGIN OF INNER-EAR LYMPHOCYTE RECRUITMENT SIGNALS

The response of the inner ear to antigen is dependent on the presence of an intact endolymphatic sac. Destruction of the sac prior to antigenic challenge dramatically reduces the immune response in the cochlea, including the appearance of lymphocytes.[19] Since lymphocyte trafficking during a cochlear immune response does not appear to directly involve the sac, this leaves an unanswered question as to the role of this structure in lymphocyte recruitment.

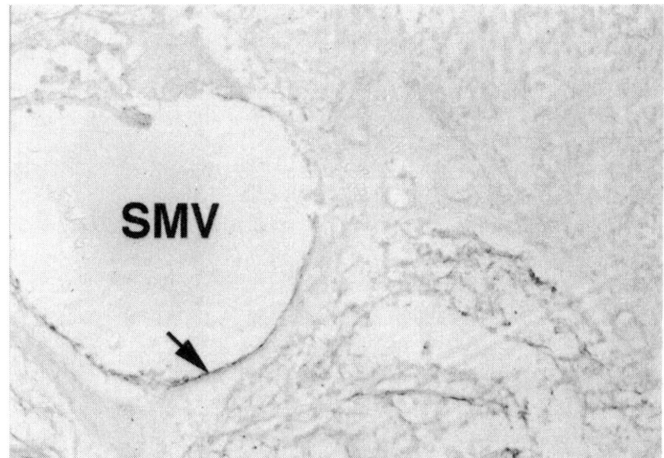

FIGURE 3. Immunolocalization of I-CAM in endothelial cells of the SMV in an immunologically challenged guinea pig inner ear. (From Suzuki and Harris.[18] Reproduced by permission.)

Evidence is provided by the fact that the sac is the only inner-ear site at which macrophages and lymphocytes normally reside.[6] It is therefore possible that antigen that enters the inner ear is transported to the sac, where it is initially processed by phagocytes and presented to resident lymphocytes. This could result in the production of inflammatory cytokines such as IL-1. Diffusion of IL-1 to the region of the spiral modiolar vein could stimulate the production of E-selectin, I-CAM, and V-CAM, leading to the recruitment of lymphocytes. A weakness of this hypothesis is that a similar response is not observed in vessels in the region of the sac itself. However, it is difficult to envision another mechanism by which the sac could exert such a powerful effect on cochlear immune responses.

Another possible relationship between lymphocyte trafficking and the endolymphatic sac involves the observation of IgA, IgA+ plasma cells, and the secretory component in the sac late in an immune response,[20,21] when they are rarely observed in the remainder of the inner ear. This raises the possibility that MAdCAM or perhaps another mucosal addressin is expressed in the sac under appropriate circumstances. Immunocytochemical evidence consistent with MAdCAM expression has been observed in the sac after antigenic challenge of the cochlea.[22] The sac may thus participate in mucosal immunity, by recruiting lymphocytes from other mucosal sites.

REFERENCES

1. HARRIS, J. P. & A. F. RYAN. 1995. Fundamental immune mechanisms of the brain and inner ear. Otolaryngol. Head Neck Surg. **112:** 639–653.
2. HARRIS, J. P. 1984. Immunology of the inner ear: Evidence of local antibody production. Ann. Otol. Rhinol. Laryngol. **93:** 157–162.

3. WOOLF, N., J. P. HARRIS, A. F. RYAN, D. M. BUTLER & D. D. RICHMAN. 1985. Hearing loss in experimental cytomegalovirus infection: Prevention by systemic immunity. Ann. Otol. Rhinol. Laryngol. **94:** 350–356.

4. DARMSTADT, G. L., E. M. KEITHLEY & J. P. HARRIS. 1990. Effects of cyclophosphamide on the pathogenesis of cytomegalovirus-induced labyrinthitis. Ann. Otol. Rhinol. Laryngol. **99:** 960–968.

5. WOOLF, N. K. & J. P. HARRIS. 1986. Cochlear pathophysiology associated with inner ear immune responses. Acta Otolaryngol. **102:** 353–364.

6. RASK-ANDERSON, A. & J. STAHLE. 1980. Immunodefense of the inner ear? Acta Otolaryngol. **89:** 283–294.

7. TAKAHASHI, M. & J. P. HARRIS. 1988. Analysis of immunocompetent cells following inner ear immunostimulation. Laryngoscope **98:** 1133–1138.

8. STEARNS, G. S., E. M. KEITHLEY & J. P. HARRIS. 1993. Development of high endothelial venule-like characteristics in the spiral modiolar vein induced by viral labrynthitis. Laryngoscope **103:** 890–898.

9. BUTCHER, E. C. & L. J. PICKER. 1996. Lymphocyte homing and homeostasis. Science **272:** 60–66.

10. BERLIN, C., E. L. BERG, M. J. BRISKIN, D. P. ANDREW, P. J. KILSHAW, B. HOLZMANN, I. L. WEISSMAN, A. HAMANN & E. C. BUTCHER. 1993. $\alpha_4\beta_7$ integrin mediates lymphocyte binding to the mucosal vascular addressin MAdCAM-1. Cell **74:** 185–185.

11. STREETER, P. R., E. BERG, B. ROUSE, R. BARGATZE & E. C. BUTCHER. 1988. A tissue-specific enduthelial cellmolecule involved in lymphocyte homing. Nature **331:** 41–46.

12. BRISKIN, M. J., L. M. McEVOY & E. C. BUTCHER. 1993. MAdCAM-1 has homology to immunoglobulin and mucin-like adhesion receptors and to IgA1. Nature **363:** 461–464.

13. ALBELDA, S., C. SMITH & P. WARD. 1994. Adhesion molecules and inflammatory injury. FASEB J. **8:** 504–512.

14. HARRIS, J. P, S. FUKUDA & E. M. KEITHLEY. 1990. Spiral modiolar vein: Its importance in inner ear inflammation. Acta Otolaryngol. **110:** 357–356.

15. WEBER, C., R. ALON, B. MOSER & T. A. SPRINGER. 1996. Sequential regulation of $\alpha_4\beta_1$ and $\alpha_5\beta_1$ integrin avidity by CC chemokines in monocytes: Implications for transendothelial chemotaxis. J. Cell Biol. **134:** 1063–1073.

16. ROWLEY, D. A., J. L. GOWANS, R. C. ATKINS, R. C. FORD & W. L. SMITH. 1972. The specific selection of recirculating lymphocytes by antigen in normal and pre-immunized rats. J. Exp. Med. **136:** 499–513.

17. GLODDEK, B., A. F. RYAN & J. P. HARRIS. 1991. Homing of lymphocytes to the inner ear. Acta Otolaryngol. **111:** 1051–1059.

18. SUZUKI, M. & J. P. HARRIS. 1995. Expression of intercellular adhesion molecule-1 in the inner ear during experimental labyrinthitis in rat. Ann. Otol. Rhinol. Laryngol. **104:** 69–75

19. TOMIYAMA, S. & J. P. HARRIS. 1987. The role of the endolymphatic sac in inner ear immunity. Acta Otolaryngol. **103:** 182–188.

20. TAKAHASHI, M. & J. P. HARRIS. 1988. Anatomic distribution and localization of immunocompetent cells in normal mouse endolymphatic sac. Acta Otolaryngol. **106:** 409–416.

21. TAKAHASHI, M. & J. P. HARRIS. 1993. Secretory component and IgA in the endolymphatic sac. Acta Otolaryngol. **113:** 615–619.

22. GLODDEK, B. & W. ARNOLD. 1995. Role of adhesion molecules in the immunological defense of the inner ear. Oto.-Rhino.-Laryngol. **57:** 10–14.

The Endolymphatic Sac as the Immunocompetent Organ of the Inner Ear

M. BARBARA,[a,c] G. ATTANASIO,[a] V. PETROZZA,[a] A. MODESTI,[b]
AND R. FILIPO[a]

[a]Institute of Otorhinolaryngology
Department of Experimental Medicine
University of Rome "La Sapienza"
Viale del Policlinico
00185 Rome, Italy

[b]Department of Pathology
University of Rome "Tor Vergata"
00185 Rome, Italy

INTRODUCTION

The existence of immune activity within the inner ear regulated by the endolymphatic sac (ES) is a relatively recent finding, demonstrated through several studies carried out in the last two decades. However, it would be incorrect to state that this issue had been left completely unrecognized until the 1980s. Some of the recently developed concepts were, in fact, already present in the specific literature of the beginning of the century. For example Guild's observed in 1927 that:[1,2]

1. The ES possesses morphological features that suggest it is the main structure for the absorption of endolymph, which flows longitudinally from the cochlear region;
2. Free-floating cells of different origin are recognizable in the ES lumen, including macrophages and white blood cells.

Both findings are important in terms of protection of the inner ear, however, this "protection" does not necessarily involve the activation of an immune activity. In fact, the major risk for the inner ear stems from the loss of its homeostatic balance, based on a stable water/electrolyte environment. Hearing and balance equilibrium are achieved in the inner ear by a morphofunctional unit called the blood–labyrinth barrier (BLB),[3] which functions to filter the foreign material carried with systemic circulation, thus impeding noxious, or potentially noxious agents entering the inner-ear fluid environment. Nonfenestrated capillaries and "tight" intercellular junctions represent the ultrastructural basis for this defense activity.

Although the topic of this review concerns the immunologic role of the ES, it is worth mentioning that other defense mechanisms have been attributed to this structure (FIG. 1).

[c]Author for correspondence.

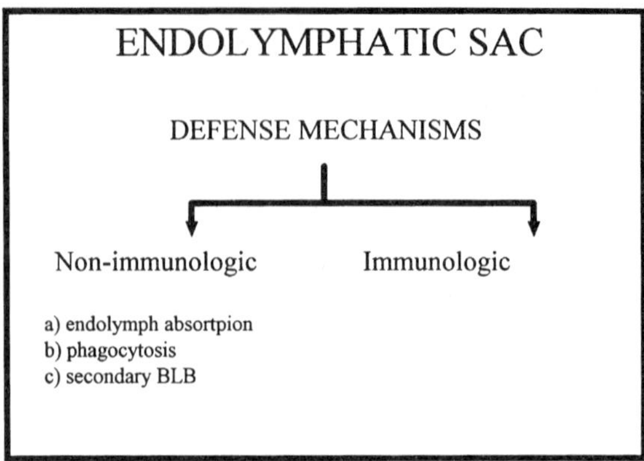

FIGURE 1.

Absorption of Endolymph

It is common knowledge that the ES actively participates in the dynamics of endolymph flow. With its absorptive function, the ES impedes fluid overloading and thus guarantees a physiologic function of the inner ear. Absorption of endolymph could possibly take place in specific areas of the endolymphatic duct and proximal ES, due to the presence of epithelial cells specifically equipped for a phagocytotic activity.[4] "Leaky" intercellular junctions and a large surface contact with the underlying areolar, plus loose subepithelial tissue particularly rich in fenestrated blood vessels represent further circumstantial evidence for an absorptive function.

Phagocytosis

Phagocytosis has been extensively described in detailed studies published in the late 1940s.[5–7] Successively, starting from Guild's observations, Lundquist[4] hypothesized that the ES dark cells might play such a role at the level of the intermediate portion where, once dispelled from the epithelial surface, they float freely in the luminal space, isolated or more often in clusters, with the task of engulfing and expelling the foreign material coming via the longitudinal endolymph flow, and also to digest the endolymph itself. The origin of phagocytes has long been debated: Rask-Andersen and Stahle[8] proposed a scheme based on previous coauthors and their own morphological observations, identifying a free cell turnover involving epithelial cell exfoliation, histiocytes coming from neighboring tissues, as well as blood elements from systemic circulation.

"Secondary" BLB

A few studies have raised the possibility that the ES could act as the "secondary" defensive route of the inner ear. Due to the presence of "leaky" intercellular junctions and fenestrated blood vessels immersed within a loose subepithelial tissue, aggressive substances or situations provoke temporary, rarely permanent ES ultrastructural changes that alert the inner-ear fluid environment. Yamane *et al.*[9] reported that Kanamicin was already detectable at the level of the ES one minute after a single-dose systemic injection, passing through the subepithelium toward the luminal space, where it is phagocytosed by free-floating cells, much before the described cochlear noxious effects take place, that is, 10 consecutive days of i.m. administration.[10] The remarkable subepithelial edema occurring in the gerbilline ES under a prolonged hyperosmotic situation obtained by depriving the animals of water for 12 days, without concomitant hearing changes, has also been interpreted as a compensatory tissutal fluid overloading which thus allows the inner-ear fluid to retain homeostasis.[11]

As far as the immunologic topic *sensu stricto* is concerned, it is again important to recall that Guild's description of white blood cells within the ES luminal space prompted the first speculation of a possible immunological activity taking place within the ES.[12]

Rask-Andersen and Stahle[13] deserve credit for having resurrected previous research, opening the door for the development of the era of inner-ear immunology. Through a detailed electronmicroscopical documentation, intimate contact between lymphocytes and macrophages within the guinea-pig ES luminal space was described and the hypothesis of possible functional cooperation in view of an immunologic defense of the inner ear was then raised. The importance of this contact resides in the fact that macrophages are capable of entrapping antigenic material and presenting it to immunospecific lymphocytes before the antigen response becomes evident.[14] Such a possibility was really a novelty, especially if one considers that the inner ear, like the brain, was thought to be an immunoprivileged site of the human body.

A new line in inner-ear research was then traced and begun to be followed by a few, very active research groups. Through serial studies, Harris investigated a possible inner-ear autonomous humoral immune response. After perfusion of the perilymphatic compartment with keyhole limpet hemocyanin (KLH), a T-dependent antigen, detection of relevant levels of antibodies (primary response) was reported.[15] Systemic immunization with KLH, with consequent high titers of circulating anti-KLH antibodies, demonstrated markedly increased anti-KLH perilymphatic titers (secondary response), once the perilymphatic space was perfused with KHL.[16] These experiments indicated that these antibodies were produced locally. Almost contemporarily, the presence of IgG and secretory IgA in the subepithelium as well as in the lumen of the human ES was reported.[17,18]

In order to verify whether immune processing takes place within the ES or in another compartment of the inner ear, the former experiment was reproduced, but with a group of animals with surgically obliterated ES, in which the immune activity was found to be significantly suppressed.[19] The central role of the ES for the immunologic activity within the inner ear was thus definitively confirmed.

The source of the immunocompetent cells found at the ES level, then, started to be analyzed. Since the first morphologic reports, lymphocytes and macrophages were seen to reside at the level of the ES subepithelial and endoluminal space under normal conditions as well as after heterogeneous stimulation (osmotic changes,[20] ototoxicity,[21] and noise exposure[22]). Whether such a finding represents a nonspecific observation or is, on the contrary, peculiar of an ongoing immunologic activity is difficult to say. Systemic circulation is the main pathway for the presence of blood cells, and the presence of a rich network of fenestrated vessels, venules, and lymphatics around the ES, especially in its distal and intermediate portion, is positively accounting for this assumption. In particular, lymphocytes passing through the capillary walls, that is, from the intra- to the extravasated location in the ES subepithelium, would indicate an active immunologic reaction. In synthesis, as in other regions of the human body, any particular stimulation of the inner ear may induce migration of the immune cells from systemic circulation through postcapillary venules into the surrounding stroma, after venule dilatation by released chemical mediators. The different classes of lymphocytes (helper, suppressor, activator, and killer) within the ES were also described in detail.[23]

The bone marrow adjacent to the ES represents the other source for immune-cell recruitment. Specific areas of the ES (distal portion) have been shown to have intimate contact with it.[24,25] Small bony channels between bone marrow and ES have been described as permitting the passage during experimental labyrinthitis of macrophages and polymorphonuclear neutrophils.[26]

During recent years, the concept of memory lymphocytes has also arisen and transferred within the rationale of the immune activity of the normal ES.[27] In the normal ES there were, in fact, identified memory lymphocytes, with homing receptors on their surface, that enable them to interact with target molecules of the high endothelial venules, that is, specialized postcapillary venules. Under normal conditions, this phenomenon was observed only at the ES level, while the same finding was seen at the level of the posterior spiral modiolar vein, port of entry for lymphocytes during an inflammatory reaction,[28] only when inflammation is evident. This finding led to inclusion of the ES within the mucosa-associated lymphoid tissue (MALT) system, which is composed of organs in which a constant recirculation of exchanging memory lymphocytes takes place.[29]

To summarize this short review, much progress has been made in the field of inner-ear immunology, but further efforts have to be made in order to make them applicable to human inner-ear diseases.

Our personal contribution to the topic regards a direct antigenic challenge of the inner ear, by using the direct inoculation of malignant cells into the cochlea through the round window membrane. The initial aim of this experiment was to establish whether or not the inner-ear sensory structures could develop any malignancy, since no description in this regard has ever been published in relation to this region of the body. For this purpose, the local, direct inoculation was chosen in order to avoid as much as possible the biasing effect of a systemic aggression, which could reach the inner ear once the BLB is overcome.

MATERIAL AND METHODS

Adult Mongolian gerbils (Meriones Unguiculatus) were used for this study. Under general anaesthesia, a ventro-lateral approach to the bulla was carried out and the round-window membrane region exposed. After creating a small hole in the round-window membrane, three microliters (1 million cells/mL) of a solution containing murine neuroblastoma cells (CH3/HEJ), courteously donated by Prof. G. Augusti Tocco from the Department of Cellular and Developmental Biology of the University of Rome "La Sapienza," were gently perfused into the perilymphatic space by a small needle operated by a mechanical micromanipulator. A small suction tube was concomitantly used in order to limit backflowing of the solution in the middle-ear space. The perforation of the round-window membrane was then sealed and the animals allowed to recover. Sacrifice was planned 24 hours, 7 days, and 30 days after surgery. The temporal bones of the operated side were immediately immersed either in a buffered 2% glutaraldehyde or in a buffered 4% paraformaldehyde solutions and kept for 24 and 6 h, respectively. The specimens were then decalcified for 10 days in 10% buffered EDTA and then processed either for routine light (LM) and transmission electron microscopy (TEM) or for immunochemical staining, in order to detect positivity of T- and B-lymphocytes. For this purpose the following human monoclonal antibodies were used: DAKO UCHL-1 (CD45RO) for detection of activated and resting T-lymphocytes and DAKO YCB117 (CD79a) for B-lymphocytes.

RESULTS

One Day

At the level of the *cochlea,* tumoral cells mixed with blood cells are found in the scala tympani, close to the lateral wall of the cochlea, at the level of the basal turn as well as at the apex, corresponding to the elicotrema. No tumoral cells can, however, be observed at the level of the scala media.

The lumen of the ES appears devoid of free-floating cells, and no relevant alteration affects the epithelial cell layer (FIG. 2).

In the bone-marrow region proximal to the ES, a few tumoral cells are recognizable (FIG. 2). White blood cells also appears to occupy the lumen of the bony channels along with the ES subepithelium. Lymphocyte-like cells are arranged in a rosette-like fashion around the neuroblastoma cells, identified as T-lymphocytes by immunochemistry (FIG. 3).

Seven Days

Neither tumoral nor red blood cells are found in the perilymphatic and endolymphatic spaces of the cochlea.

	

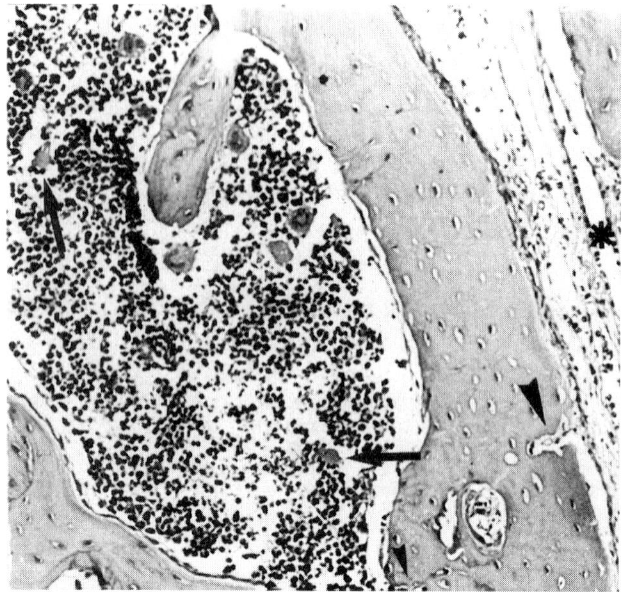

FIGURE 2. Hematoxylin-eosin stained light micrograph of the gerbilline temporal bone, *1 day* after antigenic challenge. The ES lumen (*asterisk*) appears devoid of cell corpuscles. The bone-marrow region of the petrous bone located anteriorly to the ES presents with a few cellular components surrounded by white blood cells arranged in a rosette-like fashion (*arrows*). Note portions of a bony channel located in between the ES region and the bone marrow (*arrowhead*).

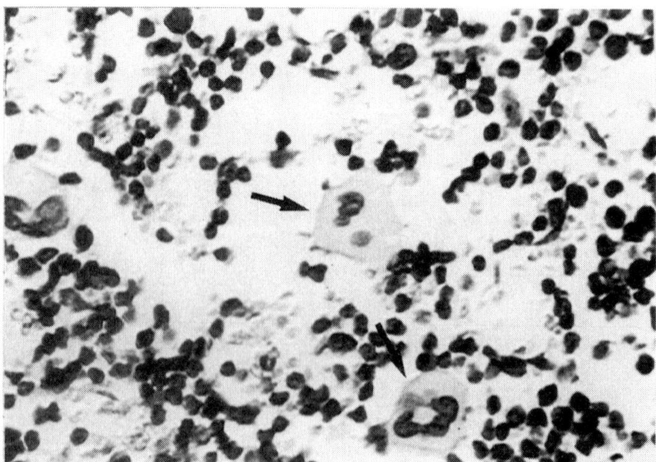

FIGURE 3. Light micrograph of the bone marrow close to the gerbilline ES after incubation with monoclonal antibody CD45RO (DAKO UCHL-1) for detection of activated and resting T-lymphocytes. Note the neuroblastoma cells (*arrow*) surrounded by positively stained lymphocytes.

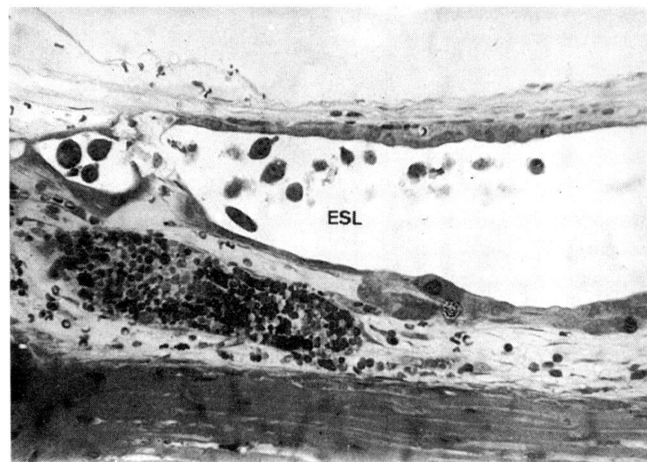

FIGURE 4. Blue-toluidine stained light micrograph of the gerbilline ES *7 days* after antigenic challenge. Several differently shaped cell corpuscles are seen to occupy the ES luminal space (*ESL*). The ES epithelial cell layer appears normal.

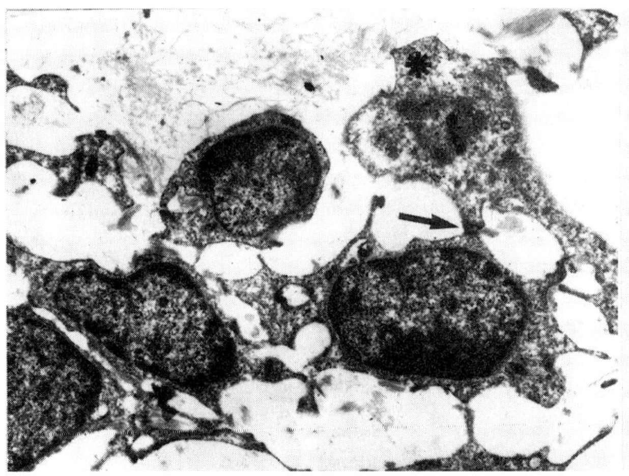

FIGURE 5. High-magnification of electronmicrograph of the gerbilline spiral ganglion region *30 days* after antigenic challenge. A cluster of neuroblastoma cells are recognizable through a large nucleus pushing a poorly represented cytoplasm that gives rise to external protrusions. A macrophage (*asterisk*) is seen in contiguity to a tumoral cell with a desmosome-like intercellular junction (*arrow*).

At the ES level, the endoluminal space appears with numerous, differently shaped corpuscles (FIG. 4), while the epithelial cell layer shows no significant alterations.

Thirty Days

At the level of the cochlea, despite the fast clearance of the heterogeneous cells from the turns of the cochlea, a few tumoral cells are seen at the level of the spiral ganglion of the middle turn (FIG. 5). These tumoral cells appear to be in proximity, sometimes in contact with polimorphonucleated cells and macrophages.

DISCUSSION

The direct antigenic challenge of the inner ear by using malignant cells was first reported by Harris (oral presentation, A.R.O. Meeting, 1989), who described the effects of inoculating human sarcoma cells into the cochlea, without any mention on the ES findings. Yamane and coworkers,[30] in 1994, challenged the guinea-pig inner ear with human chronic myelogenous leukemia cells. Also in this case, the ES was not explored, the study being focused on the cochlear region only.

The originality of our study consisted in:

1. The use of murine instead of human tumoral cultured cells;
2. In the typology of cells used, that is, neuroblastoma it is more likely to be related to the rationale of a malignancy in a sensorineural structure;
3. Finally, in also taking into analytic consideration the inner-ear structure mainly involved in the immune regulation, that is, the ES.

Even though from the results of our time-related study it is not possible to draw definitive conclusions concerning the finality of our experimental design, that is, whether or not the inner ear is protected from being involved by malignant tumors, a few, interesting observations are worth being stressed and discussed.

A few days after inoculation, the tumoral cells showed up in the ES luminal space. This finding means that these cells can pass from the perilymphatic (inoculation site) to the endolymphatic compartment, overcoming the perilymph/endolymph barrier through unknown membrane mechanisms. Moreover, this localization further confirms the presence of a longitudinal flow of endolymph. Their ES endoluminal presence was, however, observed at day 7 and not on day 1, which means that the tumoral cells do not passively flow with the endolymph bulk as previously described for red blood cells one hour after perilymphatic contamination.[31]

The presence of neuroblastoma cells at the level of the bone marrow closely proximal to the ES one day after perilymphatic inoculation is difficult to explain. In fact, such an involvement would be the expression of a systemic aggression, which cannot be ruled out even though the tumoral solution was carefully introduced into the scala tympani only. The consequence of the presence of neuroblastoma cells within the bone-marrow tissue is expected, with white blood cells, identified as T-lymphocytes, surrounding them. This finding further suggests that this organ, activated by the immune challenge, plays a significant role in recruiting the white blood cell components in immune reactions involving the inner ear. Positivity for T-lymphocytes indicates the presence of a cell-mediated immune response.

The more striking findings at the level of the inoculation site, that is, the cochlea, are observed only at day 30. A few neuroblastoma cells appeared locally at the spiral ganglion level in the modiolar region. This finding is of particular significance, considering that the posterior spiral modiolar vein resides at that anatomic level, where lymphocytes are known to enter the inner ear. Furthermore, it also seems to prove that the elimination of injected murine neuroblastoma cells from the inner-ear environment is not a fast process, as was also observed by Yamane and coworkers[31] nine days after inoculation of human tumoral cells, and presumably involves both known and unknown local immune mechanisms.

REFERENCES

1. GUILD, S. 1927. Observations upon the structure and normal contents of the ductus and saccus endolymphaticus in the guinea-pig (cavia cobaya). Am. J. Anat. **39**(1): 1–56.
2. GUILD, S. 1927. The circulation of the endolymph. Am. J. Anat. **39**(1): 57– .
3. JUHN, S., L. P. RYBAK & S. PRADO. 1981. Nature of blood–labyrinth barrier in experimental conditions. Ann. Otol. Rhinol. Laryngol. **90**: 135–141.
4. LUNDQUIST, P.-G. 1965. The endolymphatic duct and sac in the guinea-pig. An electron microscopic and experimental investigation. Acta Otolaryngol. (Stockholm) **201**(Suppl.): 1–108.
5. ANDERSEN, H. C. 1948. Passage of trypan blue into the endolymphatic system of the labyrinth. Acta Otolaryngol. (Stockholm) **36**: 273–283.
6. ENGSTROM, H. & S. HJORTH. 1950. On the distribution and localization of injected dyes in the labyrinth of the guinea-pig. Acta Otolaryngol. (Stockholm) **95**(Suppl.): 149–158.
7. ARNVIG, J. 1951. Lymph vessels in the wall of the endolymphatic sac. Arch. Otorhinolaryngol. **53**: 290–295.
8. RASK-ANDERSEN, H. & J. STAHLE. 1980. Immunodefence of the inner ear? Lymphocyte-macrophage interaction in the endolymphatic sac. Acta Otolaryngol. (Stockholm) **89**: 283–294.
9. YAMANE, H., Y. NAKAI, M. SUGIYAMA, K. KONISHI, K. TAKAHASHI & T. OKADA. 1987. Drug permeability of the endolymphatic sac. Ann. Otol. Rhinol. Laryngol. **96**: 411–414.
10. NAKAI, Y., K. ZUSHI, K. C. CHANG, H. YAGI & T. TOKIMOTO. 1981. Acta Otolaryngol. (Stockholm) **91**: 199–206.
11. BARBARA, M., D. BAGGER-SJOBACK, H. RASK-ANDERSEN & R. FILIPO. 1989. Does severe water deprivation affect the inner ear? An experimental study of the gerbilline endolymphatic sac. J. Laryngol. Otol. **103**: 22–29.
12. LIM, D. & P. SILVER. 1974. The endolymphatic duct system. A light and electron microscopic investigation. *In* Barany Society Meeting, J. Pulec, Ed.: 390. Los Angeles.
13. RASK-ANDERSEN, H. & J. STAHLE. 1979. Lymphocyte-macrophage activity in the endolymphatic sac. An ultrastructural investigation of the rugose endolymphatic sac in the guinea-pig. ORL **41**: 177–192.
14. HERSH, E. M. & J. E. HARRIS. 1968. Macrophage-lymphocyte interaction in the antigen-induced blastogenic response of human peripheral blood leukocytes.
15. HARRIS, J. P. 1983. Immunology of the inner ear: Response of the inner ear to antigenic challenge. Otolaryngol. Head Neck Surg. **91**: 17–23.

16. HARRIS J. P. 1984. Immunology of the inner ear: Evidence of local antibody production. Ann. Otol. Rhinol. Laryngol. **93:** 157–162.

17. ARNOLD, W., H.-J. ALTERMATT & J. O. GEBBERS. 1984. Demonstration of immunoglobulins (SIgA, IgG) in the human endolymphatic sac. Laryngol. Rhinol. Otol. **63:** 464–467.

18. YAMANE, H., Y. NAKAI, M. SUGIYAMA, K. KONISHI & K. TAKAHASHI. 1987. The occurrence of IgG in the endolymphatic sac of the guinea-pig. Arch. Otorhinolaryngol. **243:** 370–373.

19. TOMIYAMA, S. & J. P. HARRIS. 1986. The endolymphatic sac: Its importance in inner ear immune responses. Laryngoscope **96:** 685–691.

20. JANSSON, B. & H. RASK-ANDERSEN. 1992. Osmotically induced macrophage activity in the endolymphatic sac. ORL **54:** 191–197.

21. GRAY, R. F., R. A. SCHINDLER, K. Y. CHEN & Z. Z. WANG. 1982. Am. J. Otolaryngol. **3:** 254–261.

22. FREDELIUS, L., D. BAGGER-SJOBACK & H. RASK-ANDERSEN. 1987. Effects of high intensity pure tone stimulation on the endolymphatic sac correlations between cochlear morphology and endolymphatic sac response. Hear. Res. **29:** 139–146.

23. TAKAHASHI, M. & S.-I. TOMIYAMA. 1995. Cell proliferation in the endolymphatic sac in situ after inner ear immunostimulation. Acta Otolaryngol. (Stockholm) **115:** 396–399.

24. RASK-ANDERSEN, H. 1979. The vascular supply of the endolymphatic sac. Acta Otolaryngol. **89:** 283–294.

25. BARBARA, M. & M. HULTCRANTZ. 1990. Vascular supply of the endolymphatic sac. A gross and ultrastructural study in the mongolian gerbil under normal and experimental conditions. Acta Otolaryngol. (Stockholm) **111:** 728–737.

26. YAMANOBE, S., J. P. HARRIS & E. M. KEITHLEY. 1993. Evidence of direct communication of bone marrow cells with the endolymphatic sac in experimental autoimmune labyrinthitis. Acta Otolaryngol. (Stockholm) **113:** 166–170.

27. GLODDEK, B., A. F. RYAN & J. P. HARRIS. 1991. Homing of lymphocytes to the inner ear. Acta Otolaryngol. (Stockholm) **111:** 1051–1059.

28. HARRIS, J. P., S. FUKUDA & E. M. KEITHLEY. 1990. Spiral modiolar vein: Its importance in inner ear inflammation. Acta Otolaryngol. (Stockholm) **110:** 357–365.

29. GLODDEK, B. & W. ARNOLD. 1994. The endolymphatic sac as part of the organs of the mucosa-associated lymphatic system. *In* Immunobiology in Otorhinolaryngology—Progress of a Decade, G. Mogi, J. E. Veldman, and H. Kawauchi, Eds.: 205–207. Kugler. Amsterdam/New York.

30. YAMANE, Y., H. IGUCHI, Y. NAKAI, K. KONISHI, T. NAGAKAWA, M. TAKAYAMA & K. TAKAHASHI. 1994. The first defense of the inner ear. *In* Immunobiology in Otorhinolaryngology—Progress of a Decade, G. Mogi, J. E. Veldman, and H. Kawauchi, Eds.: 165–174. Kugler. Amsterdam/New York.

31. JANSSON, B. & H. RASK-ANDERSEN. 1996. Erythrocyte removal and blood clearance in the endolymphatic sac. An experimental and TEM study. Acta Otolaryngol. (Stockholm) **116:** 429–434.

Human Autoantibodies and Monoclonal Antibody KHRI-3 Bind to a Phylogenetically Conserved Inner-ear-supporting Cell Antigen[a]

MICHAEL J. DISHER,[c] ANNA RAMAKRISHNAN, THANKAM S. NAIR,
JOSEF M. MILLER, STEVEN A. TELIAN, H. ALEXANDER ARTS,
ROBERT T. SATALOFF,[d] RICHARD A. ALTSCHULER,
YEHOASH RAPHAEL, THOMAS E. CAREY[b]

Department of Otolaryngology/Head and Neck Surgery
The University of Michigan
Kresge Hearing Research Institute
1301 East Ann Street
Ann Arbor, Michigan 48109-0506

INTRODUCTION

Autoimmunity as a cause of sensorineural hearing loss[1-3] has yet to be completely confirmed or characterized. However, the evidence of antibody to inner-ear antigens in sera from patients with the clinical diagnosis of autoimmune sensorineural hearing loss (AISNHL) and experimental models strongly support this possibility.[4-21]

In 1987, Harris[6] demonstrated hearing loss and inner-ear lesions in guinea pigs immunized with bovine inner-ear extract. Subsequently, Orosco *et al.*[8] immunized mice and guinea pigs with chick and guinea pig inner-ear tissues and found that the animals developed transient hearing loss and serum antibodies to hair cell stereocilia. We followed these experiments with the development of monoclonal antibodies to inner-ear antigens by immunizing mice with chick and guinea pig inner-ear tissue.[22,23] We characterized two classes of monoclonal antibodies (MAb) to inner-ear antigens. One class (KHRI-5 and KHRI-6) stains stereocilia.[23] The other class is represented by MAb KHRI-3, which binds to inner ear supporting cells in a characteristic punctate "stacked wine glass" staining pattern.[22] It also identifies a 68-kD protein in Western blots of inner-ear extracts.[20]

In vivo studies showed that mice carrying the KHRI-3 hybridoma develop high-frequency hearing loss.[20] The hearing loss is associated with high circulating KHRI-3 antibody titers and loss of outer hair cells in the basal turn of the cochlea, the region that encodes high-frequency sounds. More recent studies using *in vivo* infusion

[a]This work was supported by the Lynn and Ruth Townsend Fund, Deafness Research Foundation, NIH P01-DC00078-27, NIH NIDCD R01-DC02272.

[b]Address for correspondence: Thomas E. Carey, Ph.D., Cell Biology and Immunology Lab, 6020 KHRI, 1301 East Ann Street, Ann Arbor, MI 48109-0506. Phone: 313/764-4371; fax 313/764-0014; e-mail: careyte@umich.edu

[c]Present address: Ear, Nose and Throat Associates, 347 West Berry Street, Fort Wayne, IN 46802.

[d]Present address: 1721 Pine Street, Philadelphia, PA 19103.

of KHRI-3 antibody directly into the guinea pig cochlea have shown that KHRI-3 binds to supporting cells *in vivo,* and that animals receiving this antibody, but not an isotype-matched IgG1 myeloma protein, develop hearing loss.[24] These experimental studies provide strong evidence for antibody-mediated disruption of hearing.

Support for antibody-mediated hearing loss in humans also has accumulated. Harris and his colleagues demonstrated that serum antibodies from patients with AISNHL bind to a 68-kD protein in bovine inner-ear tissue extracts.[7,16–18] In a recent report, the cumulative data were summarized.[16] Of 279 patients with rapidly progressive sensorineural hearing loss, 32% were positive for the 68-kD antigen on Western blots.[16] Hughes *et al.*[25] reported finding antibodies to a 68-kD antigen in 86% of patients with what they termed idiopathic, progressive, bilateral sensorineural hearing loss (IPBSNHL), whereas Moscicki *et al.*[18] found this type of antibody activity in 42 of 72 (58%) patients. These groups also found that the presence of antibody predicted a clinical response to treatment with steroids.

The reactivity of human autoantibodies with heterologous tissues is based on the assumption that the autoantibodies bind to phylogenetically conserved proteins in the inner ear. Thus, human autoantibodies to inner ear have been detected using bovine inner-ear substrates.[7,15–18,25] In support of this concept, Harris and Sharp[7] showed similar antibody binding on human, bovine, and guinea pig inner-ear substrates. Cao *et al.*[19,21] recently reported the use of guinea pig inner-ear extracts as a substrate for detecting autoantibodies from patients with AISNHL. This group found antibodies to proteins of 58 and 30 kD on Western blots, which differs from the more common finding of a 68-kD protein.

In the present study, we used guinea pig inner-ear tissue as the substrate for detection of inner-ear reactive antibodies in sera from patients with AISNHL. We show that roughly one-half of patients clinically assessed as having possible AISNHL have antibodies that bind to a 68–70-kD protein in guinea pig inner-ear extracts. The same sera also stain supporting cells in the organ of Corti with a pattern like that of the KHRI-3 monoclonal antibody. This is the first demonstration that sera from humans with sudden/rapidly progressive hearing loss have a reproducible binding pattern in the inner ear. In addition, we show that a 68–70-kD inner ear protein immunoprecipitated by KHRI-3 is also reactive with human autoantibodies. Furthermore, human inner-ear-tissue, but not blood cells from the same donor, absorbs the reactivity to guinea pig inner-ear substrate, indicating that the antibodies define a phylogenetically conserved protein expressed in human and guinea pig ears.

METHODS

Serum Samples

Patients with suspected autoimmune inner-ear disorders evaluated in the Department of Otolaryngology at the University of Michigan and in cooperating private otolaryngology practices in Pennsylvania, Michigan, and Indiana, were asked to participate in the study, which was approved by the University of Michigan Institutional Review Board. Serum samples and histories were obtained from patients giving written informed consent. Sera from 91 patients thought to have autoimmune hearing loss were analyzed, and the records of the patients were subsequently reviewed and categorized. Although the criteria for patients with AISNHL was to include only patients with sudden onset and rapidly progressive or fluctuating hearing loss, not all cases fit this criterion on review. Hearing loss was defined as greater than 30 dB at any frequency, or less than 85% speech discrimination in either one (unilateral) or both ears (bilateral). If the hearing loss developed within a 24-h period and did not progress subsequently, the patient was considered to have sudden hearing loss. Either unilateral or bilateral hearing loss with greater than 10-dB progression within three months was classified as rapidly progressive. Seventeen patients that did not fit in these categories were not included in the analysis. KHRI-3 monoclonal antibody batches were prepared from hybridoma supernatant, ascites fluid, or concentrated supernatant from hybridoma cells grown in a bioreactor.[20,22,24]

Western Blotting

All studies described in this report were approved by the University of Michigan Committee on Use and Care of Animals and NIH NIDCD P01 DC00078 and R01 DC02272. Veterinary care and housing were provided by the Unit for Laboratory Animal Medicine of the University of Michigan. Guinea pig inner-ear extracts were made as described previously.[20,22] The organ of Corti and vestibular tissues were collected on ice and immediately dissolved in lysis buffer (1% NP-40 in phosphate-buffered saline pH 7.2 (PBS) containing protease inhibitors, including 1 mM PMSF, leupeptin 1 μg/mL, antipain 2 μg/mL, benzamidine 10 μl/mL, aprotinin 10 ku/mL, chymostatin 1 μg/mL, pepstatin 1 μg/mL), and allowed to stand on ice for 30 min after homogenizing. The homogenates and the molecular-weight standards were prepared for polyacrylamide gel electrophoresis (PAGE) using sample buffer containing 0.0625 M tris-HCL pH 6.8, 2% SDS, 10% glycerol, and 0.005% bromophenol blue. For reducing conditions, the sample buffer contained 5% (v/v) 2-mercaptoethanol. The samples were boiled for 5 min and separated on 3% stacking and 7% separating gels.[26] For the 7 × 8-cm gels, 30-μg protein was loaded per lane and 100 μg of protein per lane was loaded in the 14 × 16-cm gel. Standards (200–14.3 kD) were from Amersham (Arlington Heights, Illinois). The gels were run at constant current of 25 mA/gel for 90 minutes for the minigels and at constant current of 35 mA/gel for 4 h for the larger gels. Electrophoretic transfer to nitrocellulose paper was performed at constant voltage of 35 V overnight.[27] The nitrocellulose paper was cut into strips, incubated with milk buffer (Blotto) (50 mM tris-HCL, pH 8.0, containing 5% nonfat dry milk, 2 mM $CaCl_2$, and 5% Tween 20) to block nonspecific binding. All subsequent incubations were done in this buffer. The strips were incubated for 2 h at room temperature with human serum diluted at 1:50, or KHRI-3 diluted to 10 μg/mL, washed three times for 10 min each, and incubated for 2 h in secondary antibody (goat antihuman IgG/IgM or antimouse IgG heavy and light chain-specific conjugated to horseradish peroxidase from Jackson ImmunoResearch Laboratories Inc., West Grove, Pennsylvania) diluted at 1:500. The blots were developed with 4-chloro-1-naphthol (0.5 mg/mL) in methanol-PBS, pH 7.6 (1:5) containing 0.05% H_2O_2.

Immunofluorescence

Guinea pigs were decapitated and the bullas were fixed locally with 4% paraformaldehyde for 2 h. The cochleae were dissected free of the surrounding bone, the spiral ligament and tectorial membrane were removed, and the central bony cochleae containing the organ of Corti were incubated in 3% normal goat serum for 1 h. The specimens were washed three times for five minutes in PBS, incubated in the primary antibody (serum diluted at 1:50 or KHRI-3 10 µg/mL) overnight at 4°C, washed three times for 5 min in PBS, and incubated for 45 min at room temperature in the secondary antibody (Lissamine Rhodamine LRSC anti-Human IgG/IgM heavy and light chain-specific from Jackson ImmunoResearch Laboratories Inc, West Grove, or rhodamine (TRITC) conjugated to goat antimouse anti-IgG, Accurate Chemicals, Old Westbury, New York), diluted 1:200 in PBS (pH 7.4). The cochleae were washed in PBS, and then the organ of Corti was carefully peeled off the modiolus and mounted in GVA mounting media (Zymed Labs, San Francisco, California).

Immunoprecipitation and Western Blotting

The KHRI-3 antigen was immunoprecipitated from guinea pig cochlea and vestibular tissue extracts using KHRI-3 antibody. For each lane in an experiment, cochlear and vestibular tissue from both ears of a guinea pig were homogenized in 25-µL lysis buffer with protease inhibitors as described earlier. The lysate (25-µL) was mixed with 50 µL of BSA and 150 µL of wash buffer containing 1% Nonidet P-40, 50 mM tris-Cl (pH 8), 150 mM NaCl, 0.1% sodium deoxycholate, 0.1% SDS, and 1 mM phenylmethylsulfonyl fluoride per sample. The samples were precleared twice with protein G-agarose for 30 minutes and incubated overnight at 4°C with 200 µL of the KHRI-3 antibody from hybridoma supernatant. Antibody–antigen complexes were precipitated by incubation with protein G-agarose for 2 hours at 4°C. The supernatant was removed after centrifugation at 5000 × g for 5 min. The precipitates were washed four times with wash buffer, centrifuged, resuspended in running buffer under reducing or nonreducing conditions, and separated by SDS-PAGE using a 7% gel.[22,23] The gel was electrophoresed at 25 mA of constant current. The proteins were transferred as described earlier and Western blotted with human sera or KHRI-3 antibody as described before.

Absorption

Two absorptions of human sera containing antibody reactive with the guinea pig inner ear were performed using part of the cochlea and labyrinth of two acoustic neuroma patients who were undergoing ablative surgery. The tissue was saved and transported to the lab together with an anticoagulated sample of each patient's whole blood. The patients gave prior written consent to use these tissues. The blood was centrifuged at 700 × g to pellet the buffy coat and red cells. The buffy coat was carefully removed and washed once in PBS. An aliquot of the red cell layer was also removed and washed in PBS. The inner-ear tissue was put into a microcentrifuge tube and washed once with PBS. The volume of the inner-ear tissue was estimated, and an equal volume of packed white cells and packed red cells were placed in similar tubes. Each sample was mixed with an equal volume of serum (diluted 1:50 in PBS) from an antibody-positive patient, UM-HL-37, incubated overnight at 4°C, then warmed to room temperature for 30 min. One aliquot of the same serum dilution was incubated identically without any absorbing tissue as a positive control. The tubes were centrifuged for 4 min, the sera was carefully pipetted out, and the absorbed and sham absorbed samples were incubated with segments of surface preparations of guinea pig organ of Corti prepared as described earlier for immunofluorescence staining. After three washes in PBS, the cochleae were incubated with lissamine rhodamine goat antihuman IgG/IgM from Jackson Immunochemicals at 1:200 for 1 h at room temperature. After four 5-min washes in PBS, the surface preparations were mounted with GVA mounting media from Zymed Labs (San Francisco).

RESULTS

Sera from 74 patients with rapidly progressive or sudden onset hearing loss were evaluated for reactivity with guinea pig inner-ear antigens using either Western blot (73 patients) or immunofluorescence (36 patients). The breakdown of the patients by type of hearing loss is shown in TABLE 1. Fifty-four patients had rapidly progressive hearing loss. Thirty-six of these had bilateral involvement, and 18 had unilateral involvement. Twenty patients had sudden hearing loss; of these, only two had bilateral effects. Of the 54 patients with rapidly progressive hearing loss, tested by Western blot, 28 (52%) stained a 68–70-kD protein. Similarly, one half of the of the sudden hearing loss patients 9/19 (47%) were positive. Of the patients with rapidly progressive hearing loss 50% (18/36) with bilateral involvement and a slightly higher proportion, 56% (10/18), of the patients with unilateral involvement were Western blot positive. Examples of the Western blots are shown in FIGURE 1.

To determine the location of the inner-ear antigen, we tested Western blot positive sera, negative sera, normal donor sera, and a sera from a few previously untested patients by immunofluorescence on surface preparations of guinea pig organ of Corti.

TABLE 1. Serological Results by Type of Hearing Loss

	Type of Hearing loss		
	Rapidly Progressive	Sudden	Total
Number of patients	54	20	74
Western blot			
Number positive/number tested	28/54	9/19	37/73
Percent positive	(52%)	(47%)	(51%)
Immunofluorescence			
Number positive/number tested	24/28	8/8	32/36
Percent positive	(86%)	(100%)	(89%)

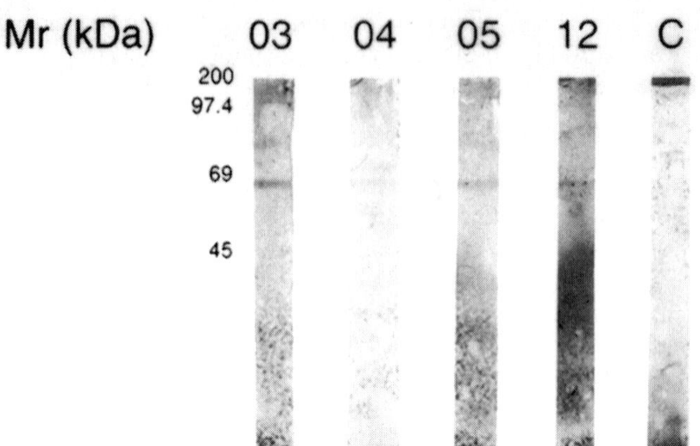

FIGURE 1. Western blot of human sera on guinea pig inner-ear extract. UM-HL indicates University of Michigan Hearing Loss patients 03 through 12. **Lane C** is serum from a normal donor.

Thus far, 32/36 (89%) of the patients' sera stained supporting cells in the organ of Corti. The staining was distributed in punctate clusters over the surfaces of the supporting cells, including the surface of the pillar cells and the phalangeal processes of the Deiters' cells. Most Western blot positive sera, 29/31 (94%), also were positive by IF (TABLE 2). Of the 36 cases that were tested by both assays, 29 sera were positive in both assays, three were negative in both, two were IF positive but Western blot negative, and two stained the 68-kD protein on Western blot but did not stain supporting cells in the organ of Corti. Examples of supporting cell staining by seven-patient sera and one normal control serum are illustrated in FIGURE 2. This pattern was of particular interest to us because the patient sera replicated the staining pattern observed with the monoclonal antibody KHRI-3.[20,22,24] Examples of staining by a patient's serum and the KHRI-3 antibody are compared in FIGURE 3.

TABLE 2. Results for Sera from Sudden and Rapidly Progressive Hearing-loss Patients Tested by Both Assays

		Immunofluorescence		
		+	−	Total
Western blot	+	29	2	31
	−	2	3	5
	Total	31	5	36

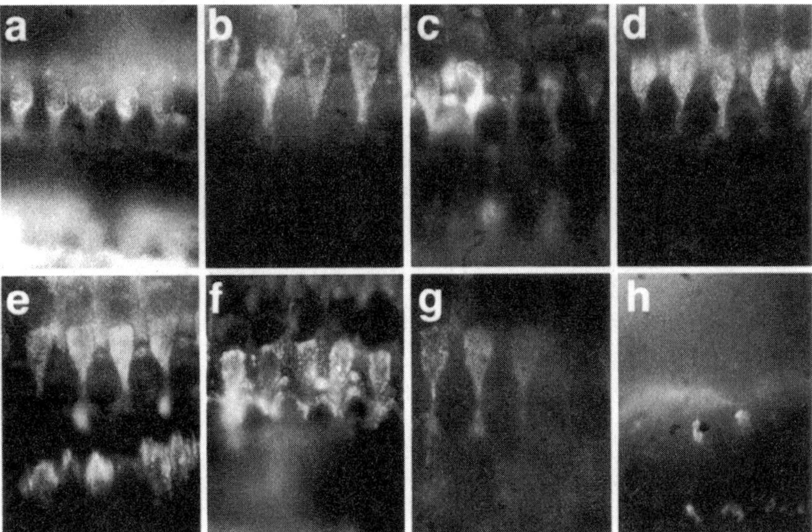

FIGURE 2. Immunofluorescence photomicrographs of surface preparations of guinea pig organ of Corti immunostained with human sera. Panels (**a**)–(**g**), sera from patients UM-HL-5, UM-HL-21, UM-HL-25, UM-HL-26, UM-HL-37, UM-HL-53, with sudden onset or rapidly progressive hearing loss; panel (**h**), serum from a normal donor. Note the punctate "wine glass" staining pattern of the supporting cells in each case incubated with the patients' sera. No such staining was observed with control sera, although the normal serum stained the stereocilia.

The similarity of staining and the prior observations that KHRI-3 can cause hearing loss[20,24] suggested that the human sera might bind to the same antigen as KHRI-3. To test this hypothesis, proteins precipitated from inner-ear extracts by KHRI-3 were subjected to SDS PAGE, Western blotted, and stained with patient sera. An example of this experiment is shown in FIGURE 4. Thus far, 4/4 patients' sera that were positive for the 68–70-kD band by Western blot also stained a 70-kD band in the ma-

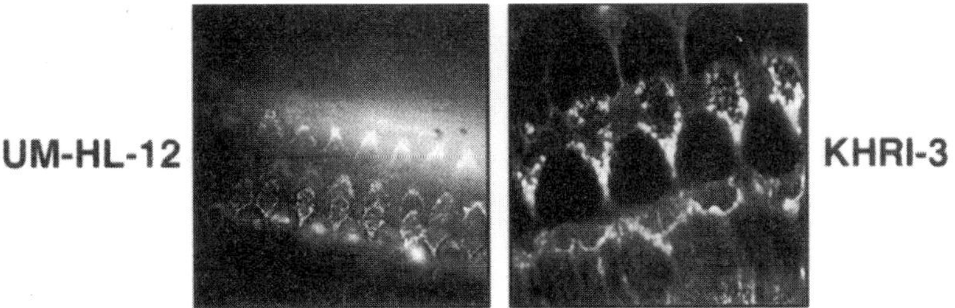

FIGURE 3. Confocal immunofluorescence photomicrographs of guinea pig organ of Corti surface preparations stained with serum from patient UM-HL-12 (**left panel**) and KHRI-3 monoclonal antibody (**right panel**). Note the similarity of the staining pattern on the supporting cells.

KHRI-3 Precipitates a 68 kDa Protein Identified by Human Autoantibody

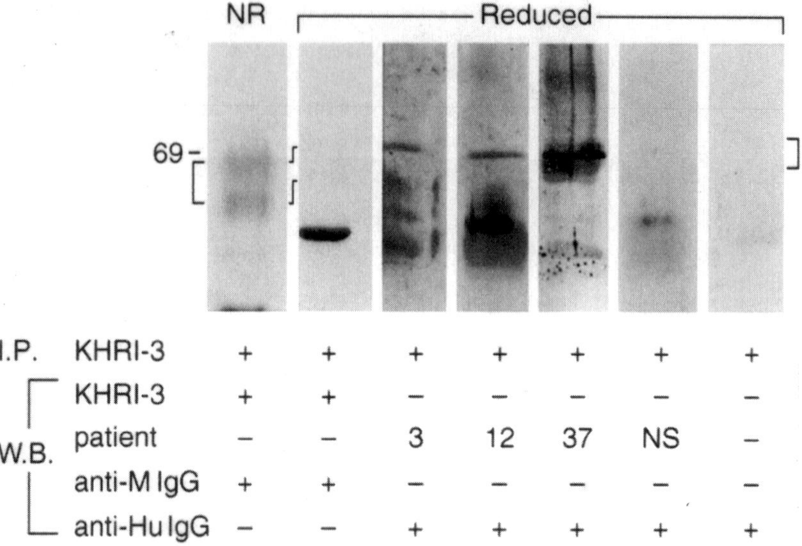

FIGURE 4. Immunoprecipitation and Western blot of guinea pig inner-ear tissue. Guinea pig inner-ear extracts were immunoprecipitated with the KHRI-3 mouse monoclonal antibody, and then the precipitated proteins were separated by electrophoresis under nonreducing conditions (NR, **lane 1**) or reducing conditions (reduced, **lanes 2–7**) and transferred to a nitrocellulose membrane. The left two lanes were then incubated with KHRI-3 antibody and developed with antimouse immunoglobulin. Lanes 3–6 were incubated with human sera from patients UM-HL-03, -12, and -37, or with a normal serum sample and developed with antihuman immunoglobulin. Lane 7 is the second antibody control. Note that the autoimmune human sera stain a 68–70-kD protein (*bracket* shows the region of the protein band) immunoprecipitated by KHRI-3 antibody. KHRI-3 antibody reacts best with nonreduced proteins, whereas the human sera react with the reduced proteins, indicating that the human sera bind to a different epitope than the murine antibody.

terial immunoprecipitated by KHRI-3. Normal sera controls were negative. The KHRI-3 antibody reacts best with nonreduced inner-ear proteins (FIG. 4, bracket on left). Under these conditions we can usually resolve a doublet of 65 and 67 kD. KHRI-3 reacts poorly with reduced proteins, but faint staining of the bands that shift to 68 and 70 kD under reducing conditions can be discerned in lane 2. The human sera appear to stain most strongly the upper band detected by KHRI-3 under reducing conditions (FIG. 4, bracket on right). The heavy band at 55 kD in lane 2 is the reduced Ig heavy chain of the KHRI-3 antibody used to precipitate the inner-ear proteins. In contrast to KHRI-3, the human sera react best with reduced proteins, indicating that the human antibodies and the murine antibody may identify different conformational epitopes on the same protein.

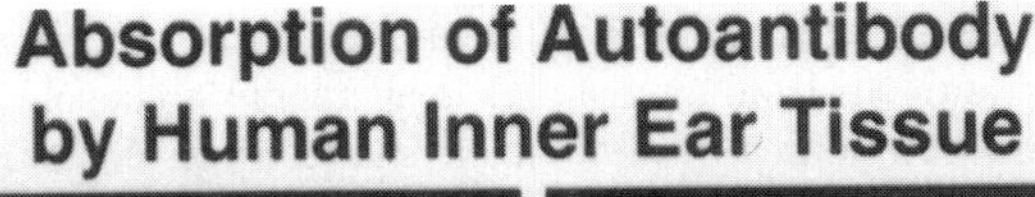

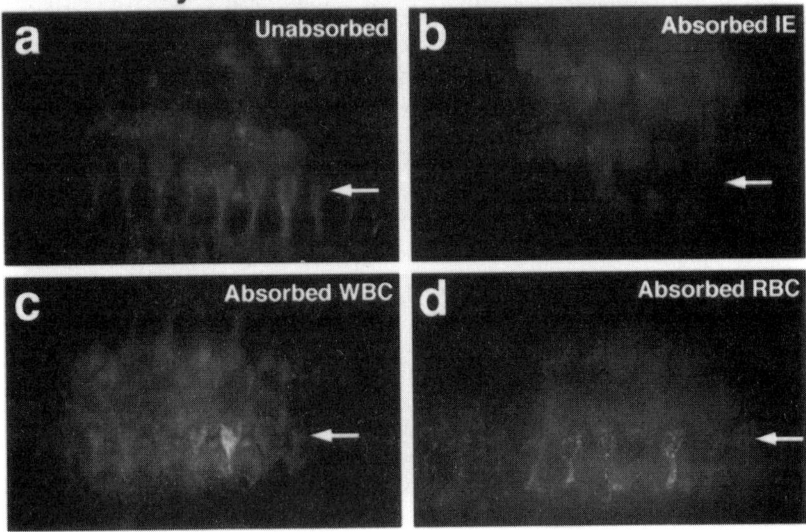

FIGURE 5. Immunofluorescence photomicrographs of guinea pig organ of Corti immunostained with an autoimmune hearing-loss serum showing the effects of absorption of the serum with: (**a**) no tissue; (**b**) human inner-ear tissue; (**c**) white blood cells from the inner-ear tissue donor; (**d**) red blood cells from the inner-ear tissue donor. *Arrows* indicate the location of the first row of supporting cells. Note that the staining of the supporting cells is eliminated after absorption with human inner ear, but not after absorption with blood cells from the same donor.

To determine if the antigen detected by patient sera in guinea pig inner-ear tissue is present in human inner ear, absorption analysis was performed. Inner-ear tissue removed from patients undergoing ablative inner-ear surgery was used as the source of inner-ear antigen, and white and red blood cells from the same donors were used as histocompatibility and blood group antigen controls. Equal volumes of either packed blood cells or inner-ear tissue were mixed with an aliquot of IF positive patient sera and then retested on guinea pig inner-ear substrate. As shown in FIGURE 5, absorption with inner ear but not blood cells removed the antibody reactivity to guinea pig inner ear. In a second experiment not shown, a similar but less complete absorption was obtained.

DISCUSSION

Although autoimmunity as one etiologic alternative for SNHL[1,2] has not been conclusively confirmed, there is mounting evidence to suggest that it is one of the causes of SNHL in patients who have rapidly progressive loss. Much of the experimental and clinical evidence has involved the use of bovine inner-ear antigens.[7,15–18] We used inner-ear antigens from guinea pigs in an attempt to develop a more readily available and consistent source of antigen for study.[22,23] In this study with human sera, the use of guinea pig tissue also allowed us to employ established immunohistochemistry techniques and a previously prepared monoclonal antibody.[22] Using Western blots, we have been able to demonstrate that 51% of patients with sudden onset and/or rapidly progressive hearing loss have antibody that reacts strongly with guinea pig inner-ear antigens. Our findings are similar to the observations of other investigators. The highest frequency of positive cases is reported by Hughes *et al.,*[25] who found antibodies to a 68-kD antigen in 86% of patients. Moscicki *et al.*[15] found that 58% of the 72 patients they tested with bilateral rapidly progressive hearing loss had antibody to a 68–72-kD protein in bovine inner-ear extracts. Likewise, Harris and Ryan[16] reported 32% of their large series of presumptive autoimmune hearing-loss cases were positive for antibody to a 68-kD protein in bovine inner-ear extract. Veldman *et al.*[28] found 65–73% of patients with sudden onset or rapidly progressing hearing loss, respectively, had antibody to multiple bands in Western blots including 27, 45, 50, and 68 kD. Cao *et al.*[19,21] used guinea pig inner-ear extracts similar to ours to detect human autoantibodies. These investigators did not observe a 68–70-kD band; instead, they reported bands of 58 and 30 kD. We also noted that some patients sera stain multiple bands at 200, 85, and 55 kD, but for the purposes of this study we scored as positive only those sera staining a 68–70-kD protein. The 68–70-kD band was the most consistent and usually the most strongly stained band. As we reported previously, the inner-ear extracts are very sensitive to proteolytic breakdown.[23] If stringent extraction conditions using quick processing, rapid chilling on ice, and protease inhibitors are not used, then high molecular-weight bands may disappear and lower molecular-weight bands may appear in their place. However, Cao *et al.*[19,21] used protease inhibitors, so the reasons for the absence of the 68–70-kD protein in their results is not clear.

There have been a number of reports of human sera staining inner-ear tissue and human temporal bone specimens[29] as summarized by Soliman.[30] However, to our knowledge there have been no previous reports of consistent staining of the supporting cells in the organ of Corti such as we observed. This may be because many of the other investigators used cross sections rather than surface preparations. In cross section, supporting cell staining, unless it is very intense,[22,31] is less apparent than it is when viewed from the surface. The "wine-glass" staining pattern we observed with the human autoimmune sera on the phalangeal processes of the outer pillar cells and Deiters' cells is like that which we previously reported with the KHRI-3 monoclonal antibody.[20,22,24] Furthermore, there was a strong concordance between staining of the 68-kD protein and the wine-glass staining pattern on organ of Corti supporting cells, since >90% of sera that had antibody to the 68-kD band also stained supporting cells. This is consistent with the notion that the 68-kD protein is expressed on the supporting cells. Since the KHRI-3 antibody has been linked to hearing loss and damage to the organ of Corti in both mice[20] and guinea pigs,[24] we found this pattern of staining to be quite interesting. It suggested to us that the human autoantibodies might bind to the same protein as the KHRI-3 antibody and that both antibodies might have a common mechanism of inducing hearing loss. To further investigate this possibility, we immunoprecipitated inner-ear proteins using the KHRI-3 antibody and then tested if the human antibodies would stain those immunoprecipitated proteins. As shown in FIGURE 4, this is the case. Our results support the concept that the human antibodies detected with guinea pig inner-ear tissue could be pathogenic in humans. However, until now there has been no evidence that antigens detected by human sera in guinea pig or bovine inner ear are also expressed in the human inner ear. Our last experiment shown in this paper demonstrates that the antigen we detect in guinea pig inner ear using human sera is also expressed specifically in human inner-ear tissue. Human inner-ear tissue but not lymphocytes or red blood cells from two tissue donors was capable of absorbing the antibodies that bind to the guinea pig supporting cells. If the human inner ear did not contain the same antigen as the guinea pig inner ear, then the absorption would not have removed the antibody. This is compelling evidence that antibodies to inner-ear antigens that are present in the sera of a high proportion of sudden onset, rapidly progressive hearing loss patients do bind to human inner-ear antigens and may well have pathogenic effects themselves as suggested by their similarity to the pathogenic KHRI-3 antibody.

The nature of the target antigen of human autoimmune sera has been suggested to be heat shock protein, specifically HSP-70.[17] We don't know if this is correct or not, but we strongly suspect that HSP-70 is not the target of KHRI-3, because when proteins are precipitated from inner-ear extracts by KHRI-3 and Western blotted, nothing in the immunoprecipitate reacts with anti-HSP-70 antibodies. Thus, if KHRI-3 and human autoantibodies define the same antigen, then it seems unlikely that HSP-70 is the primary target of the human antibodies that stain proteins precipitated by KHRI-3. This is an area of investigation in our and other laboratories and requires more work before any conclusions can be drawn.

The findings of this study support the hypothesis that autoimmune sensorineural hearing loss occurs in humans, and that its presence can be established by laboratory testing in at least some patients. Such test results may correlate with therapeutic response.[15] In light of the clinical importance of accurately and rapidly diagnosing treatable, potentially reversible causes of sensorineural hearing loss, and considering the complications associated with the use of cytotoxic medications and corticosteroids, there is clearly a need for a readily available test to diagnose this condition.

SUMMARY

Autoimmunity is thought to be one cause of sensorineural hearing loss (SNHL). Sera from patients with rapidly progressive hearing loss have been shown to contain antibodies to a 68-kD protein in heterologous inner-ear tissue. Using guinea pig inner-ear tissue as the antigenic substrate and either Western blot or immunofluorescence (IF) or both, we tested sera from 74 patients suspected to have autoimmune hearing loss for inner-ear antibodies. Sera from 73 patients were tested by Western blot, and sera from 36 were tested by IF. Thirty-seven of 73 (51%) had antibody to a 68–70-kD protein by Western blot. Sera positive by IF stained supporting cells with a staining pattern like that previously observed with the KHRI-3 monoclonal antibody. There was concordance between Western blot and IF assays. Of 36 patients tested by both assays, 29/31 (94%) that were positive in Western blot were also positive by IF, three were negative by both tests, and two each were positive by one assay but negative by the other. Absorption of patient sera with human inner-ear tissue removed antibody reactivity to the guinea pig supporting cells, indicating that the antigen detected by the autoantibody is also present in the human inner ear. Absorption with an equal volume of white or red blood cells from the tissue donor did not remove the antibody reactivity to inner ear, showing that the absorption by inner-ear tissue is specific. Sera from three patients positive in both assays also stained a 68–70-kD inner-ear protein immunoprecipitated by the KHRI-3 monoclonal antibody, indicating that the monoclonal and human antibodies recognize the same antigen. The results support the hypothesis that patients with autoimmune sensorineural hearing loss produce autoantibodies to an inner-ear supporting cell antigen that is phylogenetically conserved and defined by the murine monoclonal antibody KHRI-3. Since KHRI-3 can induce hearing loss after infusion into the inner ear, it is likely that autoantibodies with the same antigenic target are also pathogenic in humans.

REFERENCES

1. LEHNHARDT, E. 1958. Plotzliche Horstorungen, auf beiden Selten gleichzeitig oder nacheinander aufgetreten. Z. Laryngol. Rhinol. Otol. **37:** 1.
2. McCABE, B. F. 1979. Autoimmune sensorineural hearing loss. Ann. Otol. **88:** 585–859.
3. YOO, T. J., J. M. STUART, A. H. KANG, A. S. TOWNES, K. TOMODA & S. DIXIT. 1982. Type II collagen autoimmunity in otosclerosis and Meniere's disease. Science **217:** 1153–1155.
4. HARRIS, J. P. 1983. Immunology of the inner ear: Response of the inner ear to antigen challenge. Otolaryngol. Head Neck Surg. **91:** 18–23.
5. YOO, T. J., R. A. FLOYD, N. SUDO, T. ISHIBE, T. TAKEDA, K. TOMODA, Y. YAZAWA, J. STUART, I. S. CHOE & S. C. HA. 1983. Factors influencing collagen-induced autoimmune ear disease. Am. J. Otolaryngol. **6:** 209–216.
6. HARRIS, J. P. 1987. Experimental autoimmune sensorineural hearing loss. Laryngoscope **97:** 63–76.
7. HARRIS, J. P. & P. A. SHARP. 1990. Inner ear autoantibodies in patients with rapidly progressive sensorineural hearing loss. Laryngoscope **100:** 516–524.
8. OROZCO, C. R., J. K. NIPARKO, B. C. RICHARDSON, D. F. DOLAN, M. U. PTOK & R. A. ALTSCHULER. 1990. Experimental model of immune-mediated hearing loss using cross-species immunization. Laryngoscope **100:** 941–947.
9. CRUZ, O. L. M., A. MINITI, W. COSSERMELLI & R. M. OLIVEIRA. 1990. Autoimmune sensorineural hearing loss: A preliminary experimental study. Am. J. Otol. **11:** 342–346.
10. McCABE, B. F. 1991. Autoimmune inner ear disease: Results of therapy. Adv. Otorhinolaryngol. **46:** 78–81.
11. KUSAKARI, C., K. HOZAWA, S. KOIKE, M. KYOGUKU & T. TAKASAKA. 1992. MLR/MP-lpr/lpr mouse as a model of immune-induced sensorineural hearing loss. Ann. Otol. Rhinol. Laryngol. **101:** 82–86.
12. TAGO, C. & N. YANGITA. 1992. Cochlear and renal pathology in the autoimmune strain mouse. Ann. Otol. Rhinol. Laryngol. **157**(Suppl.): 87–91.
13. WONG, M. L., J. S. YOUNG, G. NILAVER, J. I. MORTON & D. R. TRUNE. 1992. Cochlear IgG in the C3H/lpr autoimmune strain mouse. Hear. Res. **59:** 93–100.
14. SONE, M., H. NARIUCHI, K. SAITO & N. YANAGITA. 1994. A substrain of NZB mouse as an animal model of autoimmune inner ear disease. Hear. Res. **83:** 26–36.
15. MOSCICKI, R. A., J. E. SAN MARTIN, C. H. QUINTERO, S. D. RAUCH, J. B. NADOL & K. B. BLOCH. 1994. Serum antibody to inner ear proteins in patients with progressive hearing loss: Correlation with disease activity and response to corticosteroid treatment. JAMA **272:** 611–616.

16. HARRIS, J. P. & A. F. RYAN. 1995. Fundamental immune mechanisms of the brain and inner ear. Otolaryngol. Head Neck Surg. **112:** 639–653.

17. BILLINGS, P. B., E. M. KEITHLEY & J. P. HARRIS. 1995. Evidence linking the 68 kilodalton antigen identified in progressive sensorineural hearing loss patient sera with heat shock protein 70. Ann. Otolol. Rhinol. Laryngol. **104:** 181–188.

18. GOTTSCHLICH, S., P. B. BILLINGS, E. M. KEITHLEY, M. H. WEISMAN & J. P. HARRIS. 1995. Assessment of serum antibodies in patients with rapidly progressive sensorineural hearing loss and Meniere's disease. Laryngoscope **105:** 1347–1352.

19. CAO, M.-Y., M. GERSDORFF, N. DEGGOUJ, M. WARNY & J.-P. TOMASI. 1995. Detection of inner ear disease autoantibodies by immunoblotting. Mol. Cell Biochem. **146:** 157–163.

20. NAIR, T. S., Y. RAPHAEL, D. F DOLAN, T. J. PARRETT, L. S. PERLMAN, V. R. BRAHMBHATT, Y. WANG, X. HOU, G. GHOLIZADEH, A. L. NUTTALL, R. A. ALTSCHULER & T. E. CAREY. 1995. Monoclonal antibody induced hearing loss. Hear. Res. **83:** 101–113.

21. CAO, M. Y., N. DEGGOUJ, M. GERSDORFF & J.-P. TOMASI. 1996. Guinea pig inner ear antigens: Extraction and application to the study of human autoimmune inner ear disease. Laryngoscope **106:** 207–212.

22. ZAJIC, G., T. S. NAIR, M. PTOK, C. VAN WAES, R. A. ALTSCHULER, J. SCHACHT & T. E. CAREY. 1991. Monoclonal antibodies to inner ear antigens: I. Antigens expressed by supporting cells in guinea pig cochlea. Hear. Res. **52:** 59–72.

23. PTOK, M., T. S. NAIR, R. A. ALTSCHULER, J. SCHACHT & T. E. CAREY. 1991. Monoclonal antibodies to inner ear antigens: II. Antigens expressed in sensory cell stereocilia. Hear. Res. **57:** 79–90.

24. NAIR, T. S., D. M. PRIESKORN, J. M. MILLER, A. MORI, J. GRAY & T. E. CAREY. 1997. In vivo binding and hearing loss after intracochlear infusion of KHRI-3 antibody. Hear. Res. **107:** 93–101.

25. HUGHES, G. B., R. MOSCICKI, B. P. BARNA & J. E. SAN MARTIN. 1994. Laboratory diagnosis of immune inner ear disease. Am. J. Otology. **15:** 198–202.

26. LAEMMLI, U. K. 1970. Cleavage of structural proteins during the assembly of the head of bacteriophage T4. Nature **277:** 680–685.

27. TOWBIN, H., T. STAEHLIN & J. GORDON. 1979. Electrophoretic transfer of proteins from polyacrylamide gels to nitrocellulose sheets. Procedure and some applications. Proc. Natl. Acad. Sci. USA **73:** 2599–2604.

28. VELDMAN, J. E., T. HANADA & F. MEEUWSEN. 1993. Diagnostic and therapeutic dilemmas in rapidly progressive sensorineural hearing loss and sudden hearing loss. A reappraisal of immune reactivity in inner ear disorders. Acta Otolaryngol. (Stockholm) **113:** 303–306.

29. ARNOLD, W. & C. R. PFALTZ. 1987. Critical evaluation of the immunofluorescence microscopic tests for identification of serum antibodies against human inner ear tissue. Acta Otolaryngol. (Stockholm) **103:** 371–378.

30. SOLIMAN, A. M. 1992. Immune mediated inner ear disease. Am. J. Otol. **13:** 575–579.

31. CHEN, H., I. THALMANN, J. C. ADAMS, K. B. AVRAHAM, N. G. COPELAND, N. A. JENKINS, D. R. BEIER, D. P. COREY, R. THALMANN & G. M. DUYK. 1995. cDNA cloning, tissue distribution, and chromosomal localization of Ocp2, a gene encoding a putative transcription-associated factor predominantly expressed in the auditory organs. Genomics **27:** 389–398.

Induction of an Inner-ear-specific Autoreactive T-Cell Line for the Diagnostic Evaluation of an Autoimmune Disease of the Inner Ear

BERTRAND GLODDEK,[a,c] JUTTA GLODDEK,[b]
AND WOLFGANG ARNOLD,[a]

*aDepartment of Otolaryngology/Head & Neck Surgery
Klinikum rechts der Isar der Technischen Universität München
Ismaninger Strasse 22
81675 München, Germany*

*bDepartment of Endocrinology
Max-Planck-Institute for Psychiatry
München, Germany*

INTRODUCTION

Otolaryngologists have long sought to identify causes of sensorineural hearing loss that might be reversed by medical treatment. One such entity that has been postulated is autoimmune inner-ear disease.[1–3] The potential improvement in auditory function in these patients following immunosuppressive therapy supports this hypothesis.[4] Because of the lack of well-defined detection methods to identify autoimmune processes within the inner ear and the fact that the human inner ear is one of the few organs of the body not amenable to diagnostic biopsy there has been great interest in developing animal models. Previous studies gave evidence that this entity might be cellular mediated.[5,6]

However, there is still the need to identify the cochlear autoantigen, which could induce an autoimmune inner-ear disease. The aim of this study was to establish an inner-ear-specific autoreactive T-celline that could be used as a tool to define the causing autoantigen.

MATERIAL AND METHODS

Animals

Inbread Lewis rats weighing 250–280 g (Charles River Wiga GmbH) were used for all experiments. Animals were checked otoscopically and excluded if they showed any sign of middle-ear infection. For all procedures the animals were anesthetized with ether.

[c]Author for correspondence. Phone: 49-89-41-40-23-70; fax: 49-89-41-40-48-53.

Antigen

Cochleas from swine collected in the slaugtherhouse were used to prepare antigen. After removal from the skull the temporal bones were immediately frozen in liquid nitrogen. The cochlea was microscopically dissected and tissue from the membraneous labyrinth and modiolus taken separately in sterile phosphate buffered saline (pH=7.4). A quantitative protein estimation according to the Lowry method was performed.

Immunization History

Donor animals were divided into three groups and immunized in the hind footpads with a mixture containing 100 µg of the respective antigen dissolved in 50 µL PBS and emulsified in an equal volume of complete Freund's adjuvant (CFA). Group A was immunized with modiolus antigen, group B was immunized with membraneous labyrinth antigen, and a control group C was immunized only with CFA (FIG. 1).

Primary Cell Culture

Ten days following injection the draining lymph nodes of the animals were removed and stored in sterile Eagles Hepes (EH) medium. The tissue was homogenized

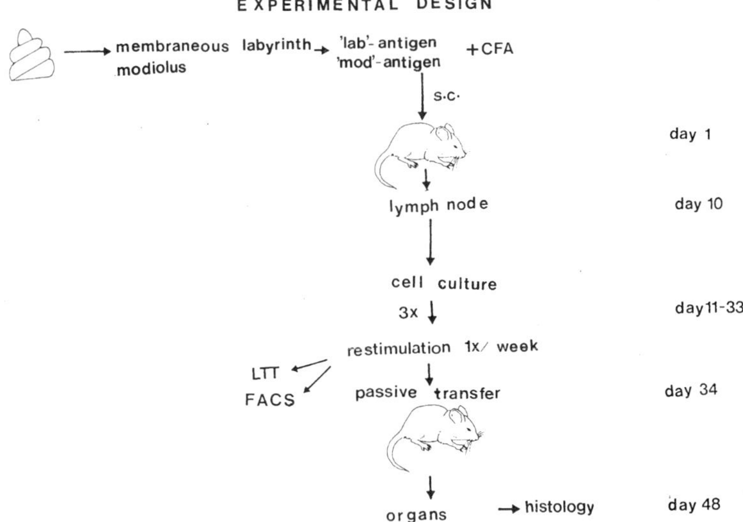

FIGURE 1. Experimental design.

with a Glasshomogeniser (Belco, New York) in a volume of 40 mL EH. The cells were centrifugated (1200 rpm/4°C/10 min), washed twice with EH, and their viability assessed by trypan blue exclusion. These cells were cultured for three days in bulks with a concentration of 10^7 cells per mL restimulation medium together with 20 μg/mL of the respective antigen. The cells were incubated at 37°C in a humidified incubator (5% CO_2/95% air). After three days the cells were centrifugated, washed with EH, and cultured in a concentration of 2.5×10^8 cells in 20-mL T-cell growth-factor medium (TCGF medium).

Restimulation

Peptide-specific T-cell lines were derived from bulk cultures of the lymph node cells as previously described.[7] Antigen-specific T-cell lines were selected by repeated cycles of propagation in T-cell growth factor containing medium, followed by antigen-specific restimulation using irradiated, syngenic thymocytes as antigen-presenting cells. This procedure was repeated every eight days for three times.

Lymphocyte Transformation Test

The successful antigen-specific stimulation of cells could be demonstrated by a lymphocyte transformation test (LTT). (^{3}H) Thymidine (1 μCi/well) was added to the culture for the last 16 h of a 72-h culture. (^{3}H) Thymidine incorporation was determined on filter mats using a Packard Matrix 96 Direct Beta counter. For this test a single-cell suspension was prepared from cell culture and the cells cultured at a concentration of 10^6/mL in 200 μL DMEM-medium supplemented with glutamine, penicillin/streptomycin, sodium pyruvate, essential amino acids, and 1% rat serum in flat-bottom 96-well tissue culture plates.

Aditional positive and negative tests were performed with 20 μL concavalin A (Con A) and 20 μL tuberculin purified protein derivative (PPD). The lymphocytes were incubated at 37°C in a humidified environment with 5% CO_2 for 72 h. This test was repeated every time parallel to the restimulation processes (FIG. 1).

Fluorescein-activated Cell Sorter

Before passive transfer of the proliferating blasts, a cell typing of the lymphocyte subtypes was performed with a fluorescein-activated cell sorter (FACScan). Then cell-surface markers were tested with their specific first antibodies: W3/25 (CD4), OX8 (CD8), OX22 (CD45), OX52 (Pan T-cell), G4.18 (G4.18), and R73 (constant region of TCR-alpha/beta). The T-cell blasts were used after the third restimulation and diluted in FACS buffer at a concentration of 2×10^6 cells/mL buffer. The absorption was measured at 495 nm.

Passive Cell Transfer

Following the third restimulation with their specific antigen, the cells were aspirated by gently pipetting and washed twice. Viability was determined by trypan blue exclusion. Cells were suspended in EH at 10^7–10^8 viable cells/mL and injected into the tail vein (FIG. 1). Recipient animals were naive Lewis rats without immunization. Ten to fourteen day's following the cell transfer, the animals were anesthetized with ether and perfused intracardially with 4% paraformaldehyd before the cochleas and control kidney, liver, and brain tissues were removed.

Histology

The cochleas were decalcified in 10% EDTA at room temperature for two weeks while the control organs were fixed and stored in 4% paraformaldehyde. The cochleas were paraffin embedded and sectioned with a microtome. One part of the slides was used for H&E staining, and the other part for immunohistochemistry, using the peroxidase technique. Therefore specific antibodies against cell-surface antigens were employed to identify and classify lymphocytes in the cochlea and control tissue.

The following antibodies were used:

W 3/25 (1:10) = CD 4 (T-helper cells);
ED 1 (1:20) = monocytes and macrophages;
W 3/13 (1:20) = pan T cells and granulocytes;
MRC OX-33 (1:20) = CD 45 RA present on B-lymphocytes.

After deparaffinization endogeneous peroxidase on the slides was blocked with 0.6% H_2O_2/methanol for 20 min. Every section was incubated with 50 μL of the diluted first antibody at 4°C in a humid-box overnight. The following day slides were washed twice with PBS and incubated with the second antibody (coupled goat anti-mouse IgG peroxidase) at 37°C for 30 min. After washing twice with PBS, sections were stained with 1 μL H_2O_2/1 mL amino-ethyl-carbazole (1:75) and slightly counterstained with Meyer's hematoxilin.

RESULTS

Lymphocyte Transformation Test

The results first of all demonstrate the successful selection and stimulation of lymphocytes with the respective inner-ear antigen as shown with lymphocyte transformation test. The increasing antigen specificity after repeated restimulation is evident by increasing stimulation index. This observation is true for the membraneous labyrinth-celline and modiolus-celline (FIGS. 2 and 3). Additionally, the cross-reactivity of the modiolus cell population with the guinea pig brain antigen is striking.

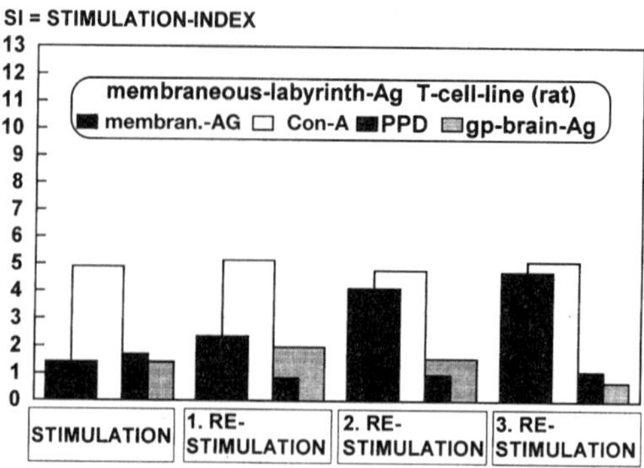

FIGURE 2. Results of lymphocyte transformation test (LTT) for membraneous labyrinth cell-line after repeated stimulation.

FACS-analysis of the Transferred Cells

The FACS-analysis shows that approximately 95% of transferred cells were T-cells and belong to the T-helper cell population (FIG. 4). Only a small part consisted of T supressor or B cells. Almost all cells expressed the alpha/beta T-cell receptor (FIG. 5).

Histology/Immunohistochemistry

In the animal group receiving lymphocytes raised against modiolus antigen the modiolar vessels showed a perivascular lymphocyte conglomeration in contrast to the control group (FIG. 6). In the modiolus itself, and especially at the area of the internal

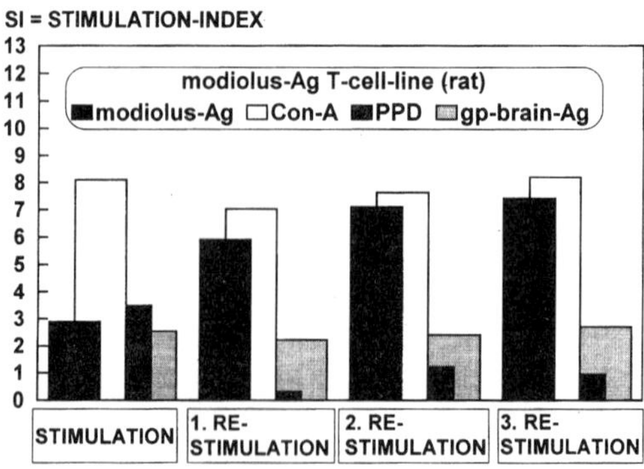

FIGURE 3. Results of LTT for the modiolus cell-line after repeated stimulation.

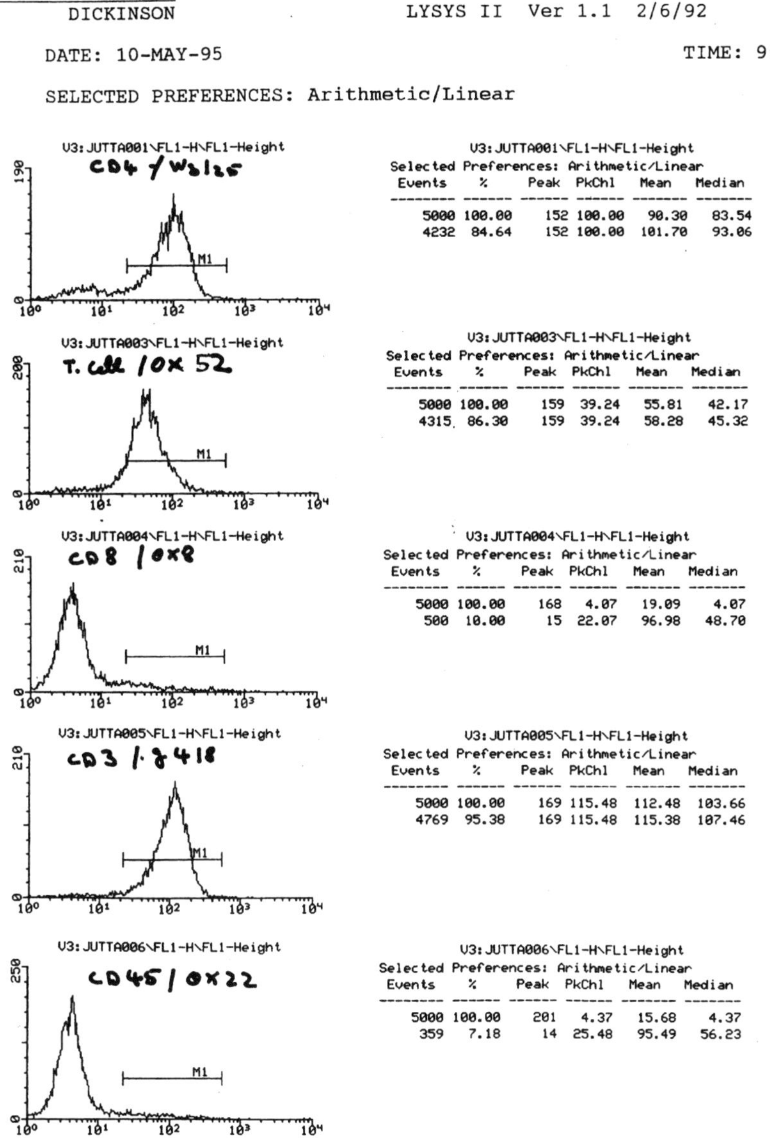

FIGURE 4. FACS results of the transferred cell line to identify the lymphocyte subpopulation.

BECTON
DICKINSON LYSYS II Ver 1.1 2/6/92

DATE: 10-MAY-95 TIME: 9:52:35

SELECTED PREFERENCES: Arithmetic/Linear

V3: JUTTA007\FL1-H\FL1-Height

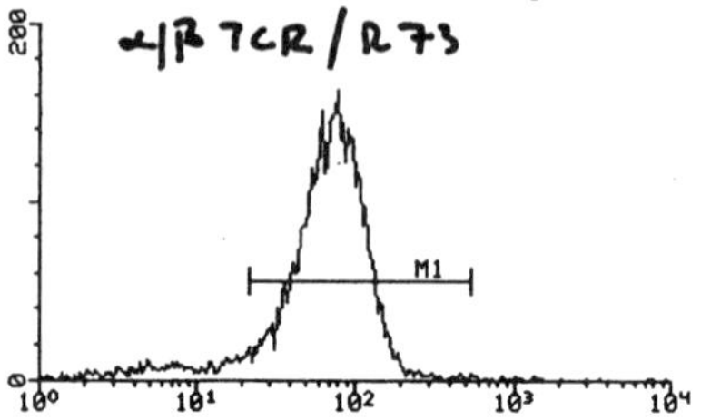

V3: JUTTA007\FL1-H\FL1-Height
Selected Preferences: Arithmetic/Linear

Events	%	Peak	PkChl	Mean	Median
5000	100.00	163	77.74	85.44	69.78
4523	90.46	163	77.74	80.20	72.34

V3: JUTTA008\FL1-H\FL1-Height

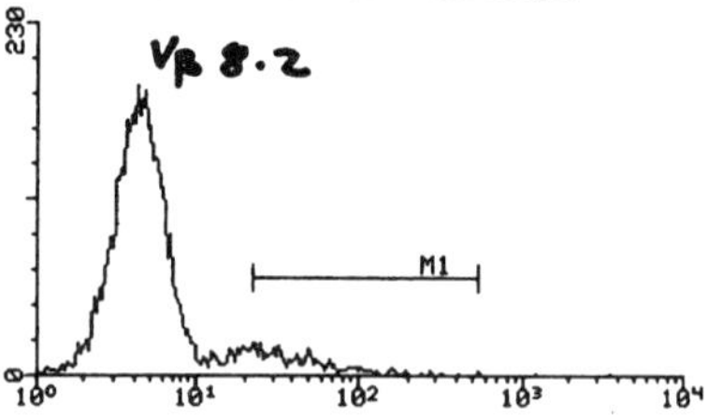

V3: JUTTA008\FL1-H\FL1-Height
Selected Preferences: Arithmetic/Linear

Events	%	Peak	PkChl	Mean	Median
5000	100.00	188	4.22	10.44	4.53
429	8.58	21	24.58	55.16	37.86

V3: JUTTA009\FL1-H\FL1-Height

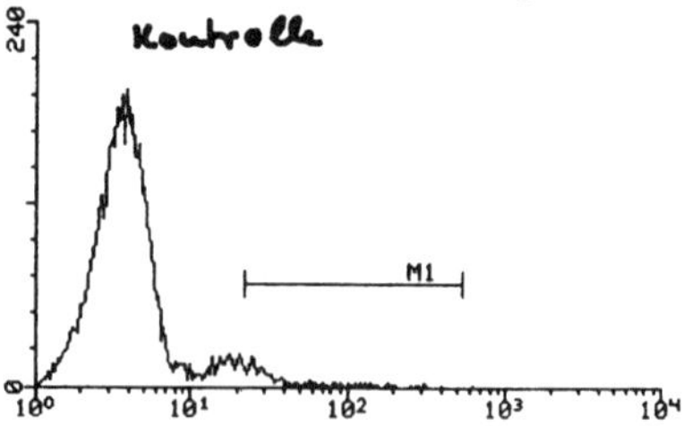

V3: JUTTA009\FL1-H\FL1-Height
Selected Preferences: Arithmetic/Linear

Events	%	Peak	PkChl	Mean	Median
5000	100.00	195	3.79	6.66	3.65
214	4.28	19	24.58	53.46	29.97

V3: JUTTA010\FL1-H\FL1-Height

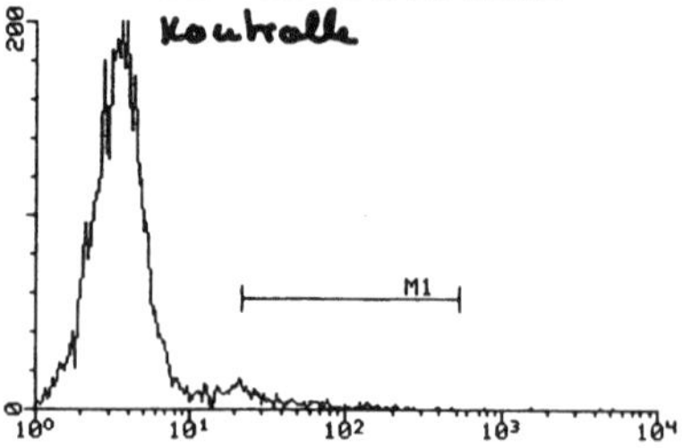

V3: JUTTA010\FL1-H\FL1-Height
Selected Preferences: Arithmetic/Linear

Events	%	Peak	PkChl	Mean	Median
5000	100.00	213	3.52	8.49	3.52
183	3.66	11	22.07	61.09	36.52

FIGURE 5. FACS results of the transfered cell-line to identify the lymphocyte subpopulation.

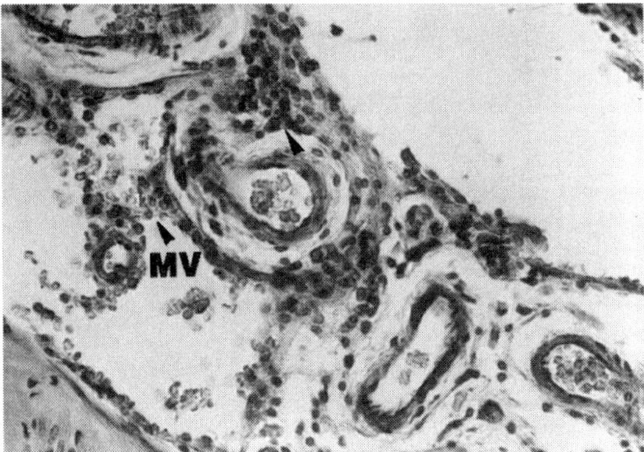

FIGURE 6. Perivasculitis of modiolar vessels (MV) in the cochlea of the "modiolus group," indicated by *arrows.*

auditory canal, a severe lymphocyte infiltration was evident with edema and bleeding of the nerve. Predominantly T-helper cells could be detected immunohistochemically (FIG. 7).

In the group with membraneous labyrinth as antigen, a cellular infiltration of lymphocytes was observed in the perilymph compartements, especially in the scala vestibuli was observed (FIG. 8). The main lymphocyte subtype was also T-helper cells (FIG. 9).

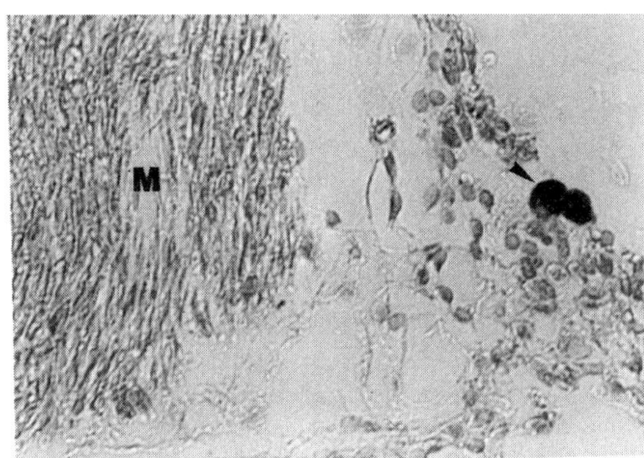

FIGURE 7. Immunohistochemical identification of T-helper cells (*arrow*) close to the modiolus (M) in the "modiolus group."

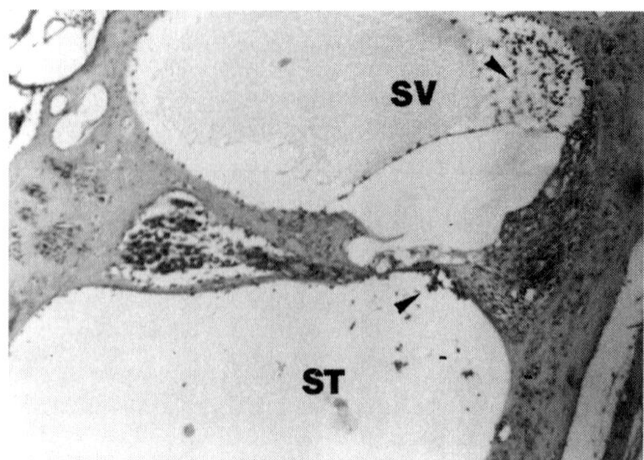

FIGURE 8. Cellular infiltration of perilymph compartments (*arrows*) in the cochlea of "membraneous labyrinth" group. ST = scala tympani, SV = scala vestibuli.

DISCUSSION

The aim of this study was to establish an animal model for an autoimmune disease of the inner ear. In order to clasify a disease as autoimmunological mediated, it is mandatory to prove that the immune system reacts against an endogeneous protein.[8] The proteins of the inner ear are normally behind the blood–labyrinth barrier, but could come into contact with the systemic circulation by trauma, operation, or infection and then be recognized as foreign.[3,9] Previous studies gave evidence that this process might be cellular mediated.[5,6]

It is general immunological knowledge that autoreactive B-lymphocytes cause systemic nonorgan-specific autoimmune diseases, while autoreactive T cells induce

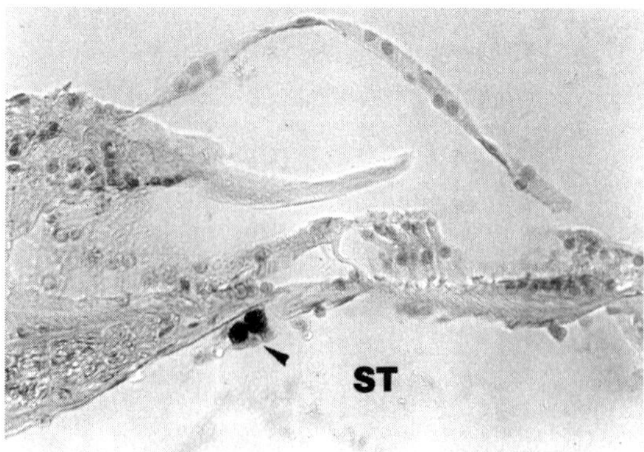

FIGURE 9. Immunohistochemical identification of T-helper cells (*arrow*) in the cochlea of "membraneous labyrinth group." ST = sala tympani.

an organ-specific process.[10] Clinical observation of patients with hypothesized autoimmunologically mediated inner-ear dysfunction indicate that other organs are not involved.[11,12] This puts emphasis on a T-lymphocyte mediated process.

In this study two inner-ear-specific T-cell lines were developed using heterologeous immunization of Lewis rats. The transfer of these mainly T-helper cells (CD_4+) induced two different histopathological pictures: a perivasculitis and neuritis in the "modiolus group," and a labyrinthitis in the group with membraneous labyrinth as antigen. The first cells invading the inner ear were T-helper cells, as demonstrated immunohistologically. These cells probably contain the autoantigenic determinant.

The experimental design of the study can serve as an animal model for a cellular-mediated autoimmune disease of the inner ear. With the establishment of a T-cell line, an *in vitro* control of the possible causes of cochlea-protein seems possible employing the lymphocyte transformation test. So further studies have to split the cochlea proteins and to identify the protein with the strongest autoimmunological potency. After biotechnical production of this protein, a sufficient clinical test should be possible to diagnose an autoimmune disease of the inner ear in man.

SUMMARY

Different patterns of sensorineural hearing loss with a potential improvement in auditory function following immunosuppressive therapy might be caused by an isolated autoimmune disease of the inner ear. Because of the lack of well-defined detection methods to identify autoimmune processes within the inner ear and the fact that the human inner ear is one of the few organs of the body not amenable to diagnostic biopsy, there has been great interest in developing animal models.

Previous studies found evidence that this entity might be cellular mediated.

By heterologeous immunization of inbred Lewis rats with inner-ear tissue, an autoreactive inner-ear-specific T-cell line was established. After passive transfer of these cells, a labyrinthitis was induced in recipient animals. The experimental design can serve as an animal model for a cellular-mediated autoimmune disease of the inner ear. Further studies have to split the cochlear proteins and to identify the protein with the strongest autoimmunological potency. After biotechnical production of this protein, a clinical test to diagnose an autoimmune disease of the inner ear in man should be possible.

REFERENCES

1. McCabe, B. F. 1979. Autoimmune sensorineural hearing loss. Ann. Otol. Rhinol. Laryngol. **88:** 585–589.
2. Harris, J. P. 1987. Experimental autoimmune hearing loss. Laryngoscope **87:** 63–76.
3. Gloddek, B., W. Arnold & M. Conrad. 1993. Sudden sensorineural hearing loss in the last hearing ear. *In* 3rd Int. Symp. on Meniere's Disease, R. Filipo *et al.*, Eds.: 121–123. Kugler. Amsterdam.
4. Vischer M. & W. Arnold. 1991. Kortisonsensible Innenohrschwerhörigkeit. ORL Nova **1:** 75–79.

5. HUGHES G. B., B. P. BARNA & S. E. KINNEY. 1988. Clinical diagnosis of immune inner ear disease. Laryngoscope **98:** 251–253.
6. GLODDEK, B., M. ROGOWSKI & W. ARNOLD. 1994. Adoptive transfer of an autoimmunological labyrinthitis in the guinea pig. Animal model for a sympathetic cochleolabyrinthitis. Clin. Exp. Immunol. **97:** 133–137.
7. LINNINGTON, C., T. BERGER, L. PERRY, S. WERTH, D. HINZE- SELCH, Y. ZHANG, H. LU, H. LASSMANN & H. WEKERLE. 1993. Eur. J. Immunol. **23:** 1364–1369.
8. ROSE N. R. & C. BONA. 1993. Defining criteria for autoimmune diseases (Witebsky's postulates revisted). Immunol. Today **14:** 426–430.
9. HARRIS J. P., N. C. LOW & W. F. HOUSE. 1985. Contralateral hearing loss following inner ear injury: Sympathetic cochleo-labyrinthitis? Am. J. Otol. **23:** 371–377.
10. ABBAS, A. K., A. H. LICHTMAN & J. S. POBER. 1994. Cellular and Molecular Immunology, 2nd ed., Saunders. Philadelphia.
11. HUGHES, G. B., S. E. KINNEY, B. P. BARNA & L. H. CALABRESE. 1984. Practical versus theretical management of autoimmune inner ear disease. Laryngoscope **94:** 758–767.
12. HARRIS, J. & P., P. A. SHARP. 1990. Inner ear autoantibodoes in patients with rapidly progressive sensorineural hearing loss. Laryngoscope **100:** 516–524.

Auditory Findings in Subjects with Immunomediated Sensorineural Hearing Loss

ANTONIO QUARANTA,[a] ANGELO SCARINGI, PAOLA PORTALATINI, AND DONATELLA VANTAGGIATO

Audiology and Otology Center
ENT Department
University of Bari
Policlinico
Piazza Giulio Cesare, 11
70124, Bari, Italy

INTRODUCTION

In 1979 McCabe[1] described that first series of patients with progressive bilateral sensorineural hearing loss (SNHL) who were responsive to immunosuppressive therapy. Subsequently, he[2] and others[3,4] have reported that in immunomediated inner-ear disease hearing loss can begin at any age, with unilateral or bilateral sudden onset, with fluctuating or progressive symptoms, with or without dizziness. Patients may have vestibular symptoms mimicking Ménière's disease. The audiometric curve may be upsloping as well as downsloping. Discrimination scores may be either disproportionately good or disproportionately poor as compared to pure tone thresholds. Audiovestibular testing suggests that the cochlea is the target organ, although retrocochlear involvement has also been reported.

The present study was undertaken in order to explore the performance of subjects with inner-ear disorder, with suspected immunomediated pathogenesis, in advanced tests that assess primary cochlear functions (temporal integration, frequency selectivity, cochlear mechanics).

MATERIALS AND METHODS

Subjects

Six subjects were selected according to the following criteria: SNHL and laboratory tests encompassing autoimmunity (circulating immune complexes or CICs, elevated immunoglobulins, autoantibodies); SNHL nonresponding to conventional therapy that were responsive to immunosuppressive drugs; no history of middle-ear disease, noise exposure, trauma, use of ototoxic drugs, or any drugs that affect the central nervous system, and no obvious pathological factors involving the brain or the

[a]Author for correspondence. Phone: 0039 80 5478850; fax: 0039 80 5562171; e-mail: audiolog@cimedoc.UNIBA.it

central nervous system; clinically normal tympanic membranes and type-A tympanograms.

Equipment

The apparatus used for the present study consisted of a two-channel clinical audiometer (ANSI 3.6; ISO 389); two electroacoustic bridges equipped with graphic registration for tympanometry and acoustic stapedius reflex measurements; a hearing science laboratory EM40; an otodynamics standard IL092; a clinical averaging system (Amplaid MK7) for stimulation and recording of auditory brain-stem responses.

Procedure

In each patient the following were preliminarily evaluated: standard tonal audiometry (frequencies from 0.25 to 8 kHz; pure thresholds average, or PTA of about 0.5, 1, and 2 kHz); speech discrimination scores; stapedius reflex (SR) thresholds (0.5, 1, and 2 kHz; contralateral stimulation), and tone decay (1 kHz; 10 dB SL); auditory brain-stem responses (ABRs; 2048 wideband clicks, each lasting 0.1 ms, sent through headphones with alternating polarity, at a repetition rate of 11 and 47 pps, and at an intensity level of 114 dB SPL p.e.); electronystagmography (ENG; caloric test). Primary cochlear functions were only studied in ears with PTA $\leq$ 40 dB HL.

Temporal Integration

Temporal integration refers to the change in the sensitivity of a signal as a function of signal duration. As the duration of a signal decreases, its threshold increases. This function is attributed to outer hair cell (OHC) activity.[5] Clinical studies utilizing brief tone audiometry (BTA) have shown that the temporal integration can be reduced by a temporary or chronic dysfunction of the enzymometabolic processes of the inner ear.[6] The slope of temporal integration functions have been recorded unilaterally at 1 kHz, studying pulsed tones of 20 and 200 ms with a rise/fall time of 10 ms and with a 2-s interval between stimuli. The BTA factor recorded in normal subjects ranged from 6 dB to 15 dB.

Frequency Selectivity

Frequency selectivity refers to the ability of the auditory system to detect one signal in the presence of another.[7] This analytic ability was attributed to the filter process both of the basilar membrane and of the organ of Corti, particularly the OHCs.[8] Clinical data have revealed that frequency selectivity is abnormal in ears with cochlear pathology.[9] This important function was measured utilizing both the critical ratio (CR)[10] and the Q 10 dB of the psychoacoustical tuning curves (PTCs).[11]

CR was recorded ipsilaterally for 1-kHz pulsed tones (500-ms duration, 25-ms rise/fall time, 50% duty cycle);[12] the masking stimulus was a continuous wideband noise ranging from 98 Hz to 6 kHz, delivered at an overall level of 81 dB SPL, so it had a spectrum level of 42.8 dB.

PTCs were measured for 1 kHz using simultaneously continuous masking tones and pulsed probe tones (250 ms duration, 20 ms rise/fall time, 50% duty cycle). Q 10 was calculated as the ratio between the test frequency and the bandwidth of the PTC when the masked tone intensity was 10 dB above the tip. Normal subjects show CRs between 18 and 26 dB, and Q values from 3.3 to 4.4.

Cochlear Mechanics

Cochlear mechanics refer to the active mechanical process in the cochlea due to OHCs activity and to basilar membrane motion. Cochlear mechanics were evaluated recording spontaneous (SOAEs) and evoked otoacoustic emissions (EOAEs) and measuring nonlinear distortion products. Outer hair cells are capable of producing a rapid force generating length change in response to electrical stimulation. This electromotility is thought to be responsible for the generation of otoacoustic emissions.[13,14] In ears with SNHL, the recording of OAEs helps in differentiating "pure" cochlear impairment from retrocochlear involvement[15] and gives early information of functional changes occurring in OHCs.[16]

SOAEs were recorded with a frequency resolution of 12.3 Hz in the range 0.012 kHz to 6.25 kHz. The measurements were made in dB SPL and the SOAEs were considered present for at least a 10 dB ratio against background noise.

EOAEs were recorded for click (CEOAEs) and 1-kHz tone-burst stimulation (TBEOAEs). Clicks were constituted by very short pulses (< 50 μs) with a wideband spectrum generated in the ILO88 standard nonlinear mode at an effective 0.3-Pa sound pressure in the ear canal. The noise-rejection level was set at 4.6 mPa corresponding to 47.3 dB SPL. The spectrum analyzer was triggered at 4 ms after stimulus presentation to avoid acoustic ringing of the input stimuli, and the temporal window was set at about 20 ms. The average was set for 260 averages. The tone bursts were constituted by 1-kHz brief stimuli of four complete cycles. The other setting parameters were the same as click stimuli. In the averaged spectra (0.012–6.25 kHz) EOAEs were considered present for at least a 10-dB ratio against background noise.

Nonlinear distortion products were studied by recording 2f1/f2 evoked emission (DPOAEs) and measuring remote masking (RM) effect.

The DPOAEs were recorded using two pure tones (f1 and f2 of 100-ms duration) at the same intensity with a f2/f1=1.22 frequency range. Three different stimulations were performed with f2=2, 4, and 6 kHz. The probe-fitting check and the two tone adjustments were performed before each stimulation session. Each registration consisted of an input/output function, of a growth-rate test for 2f1/f2 distortion products in which the two probe tones were delivered at an intensity ranging from 25 to 75 dB SPL (5-dB step) in the downward direction. The noise rejection level was 5 mPa, and the final graph for each test was drawn using at least 128 valid averages collected in a subgroup of 16. DPOAEs were considered present for a ratio > 10 dB against background noise.

The RM consists of a threshold increase for low-frequency tones when the ear is exposed to high-frequency noise band delivered at an overall noise level of 80 dB SPL or more. This phenomenon has been attributed to mechanical nonlinear distortion of the vibrating structure within the inner ear,[17] and has been proposed as a test of cochlear partition elasticity.[18,19] RM values were recorded ipsilaterally for pulsed tones (250-ms duration, 25-ms rise/fall time, 50% duty cycle) at 0.25 kHz using a continuous narrowband noise masker centered at 3 kHz with a bandwidth of 305 Hz, and delivered at an overall level of 98 dB SPL. In normal subjects RM values range from 13 dB to 45 dB.

All measurements were recorded in a silent room using Telephonics ear phones (TDH-39).

RESULTS

Case Analyses

CASE 1. A 24-year-old girl was referred in September 1996 for a sudden hearing loss with high-pitched tinnitus on the left and spells of incapacitating vertigo lasting three days. Five months before being referred, the patient had a sudden drop in hearing in the right ear with continuous tinnitus and one spell of vertigo. She was hospitalized for a 10-day course of diuretics, cortisone, and vasodilators without benefit for hearing and tinnitus. A few days into the treatment the vertiginous spells ceased. At the time of admission her audiogram (FIG. 1(a)) revealed, from 125 Hz to 2 kHz, an upsloping SNLH with a PTA of 47 dB HL and 80% speech discrimination score on the left, and a flat SNHL with a PTA of 70 dB HL and 0% speech discrimination on the right; in both ears, there was a downsloping SNHL at frequencies > 2 kHz. SR was not elicited on the right and had thresholds $\geq$ 90 dB HL and normal tone decay on the left. ABRs were normal on both ears. ENGs showed normal caloric responses on the left and none on the right. MRI showed no cerebellopontine angle pathology. The clinical immunology work-up showed normal values except for the presence of antinuclear and antimitochondrial autoantibodies and for increased circulating immunocomplexes (CICs). After two days of therapy with oral prednisone (60 mg/day), PTA in the left ear had improved 15 dB HL (FIG. 1(b)). On that side, the BTA value was 4 dB, CR 34 dB, PTC Q value 2.8, and RM 12 dB; SOAEs, EOAEs, and DPOAEs were absent. One week (FIG. 1(c)) later her PTA was 5 dB HL with a high frequency (> 3 kHz) SNHL; BTA was 6 dB, CR 29, PTC Q value 6.7, and RM 28 dB; SOAEs, EOAEs, and DPOAEs were present. The hearing in the right ear demonstrated no response whatsoever to treatment. Therapy still continues.

Of note is that in this patient temporal integration, frequency selectivity, and products of cochlear mechanics were affected two days after admission, when PTA was 32 dB HL; cochlear functions improved after 10 days of therapy when PTA normalized.

CASE 2. A 9-year-old boy was referred in March 1996 for continuous high-pitched tinnitus in the right ear lasting two months. His parents stated that over the last few months his hearing had worsened. He did not have audiometry prior to referral. At the time of admission his audiogram (FIG. 2a) showed an upsloping SNLH with a PTA of 43 dB HL on the right and a profound downsloping SNLH on the left. His speech-discrimination score was 100% in the right ear; there was no speech discrim-

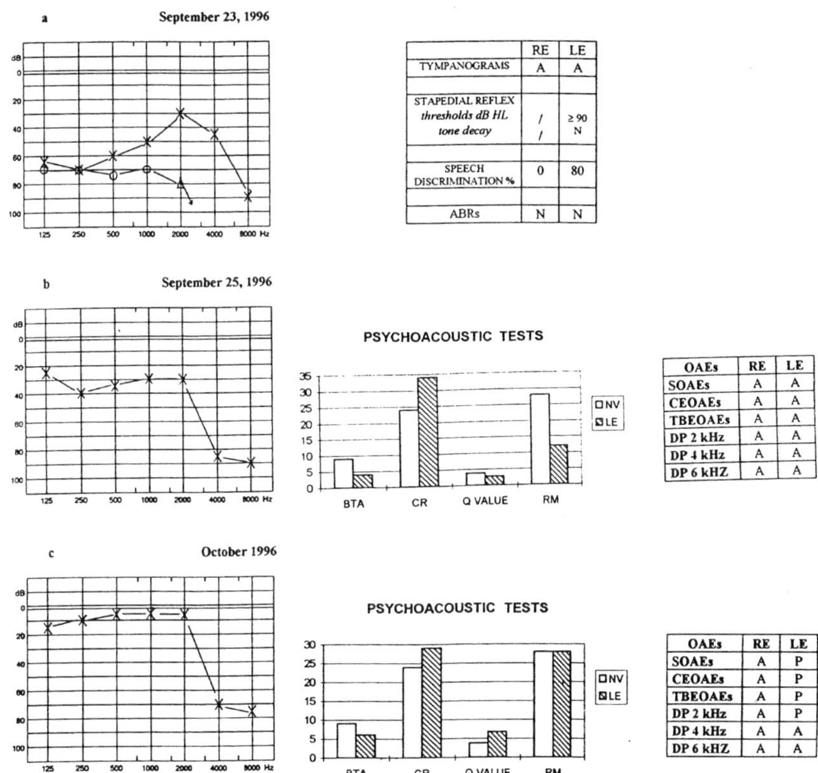

FIGURE 1. Auditory findings of Case 1 (24-year-old woman) prior to therapy (a), after two days (b), and nine days (c) of therapy. RE= right ear; LE= left ear; N= normal; NV= normal value; OAEs A= absent, P= present.

ination on the left side. SR was not elicited on the left, and had thresholds $\geq$ 100 dB HL on the right. ABRs were absent in the left ear and normal in the right. ENGs showed a normal caloric response on both sides. MRI showed no cerebellopontine angle pathology. Clinical immunology work-up showed normal values. Within a week (FIG. 2(b)), prednisone therapy (30 mg/day) gave a PTA improved by 20 dB on the right; in that ear BTA value was 7 dB, CR 32 dB and PTC Q value 1.6, RM value 25 dB; SOAEs, EOAEs, and DPOAEs were present. After two weeks prednisone was reduced to 20 mg/day. Twelve days later, the patient's audiogram showed a 15-dB loss at low frequencies on the right. Prednisone dosage was then increased (30 mg/day), and within two weeks low frequencies improved by 20 dB. Audiograms were made periodically during follow-up, and they showed a fluctuating SNHL related to prednisone dosage. These fluctuations of hearing still continue. The hearing in the left ear demonstrated no response to treatment. In September 1996 (FIG. 2(c)), the right ear showed a downsloping SNHL with a PTA of 15 dB HL; BTA value was 7 dB, CR 25

CASE 2

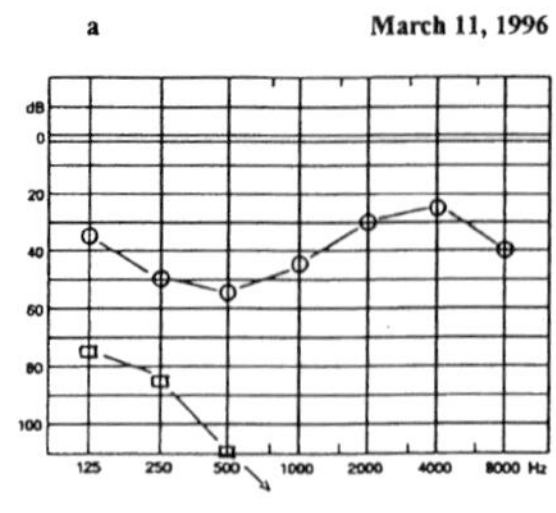

a March 11, 1996

	RE	LE
TYMPANOGRAMS	A	A
STAPEDIAL REFLEX *thresholds dB HL tone decay*	≥100 N	/ /
SPEECH DISCRIMINATION %	100	0
ABRs	N	A

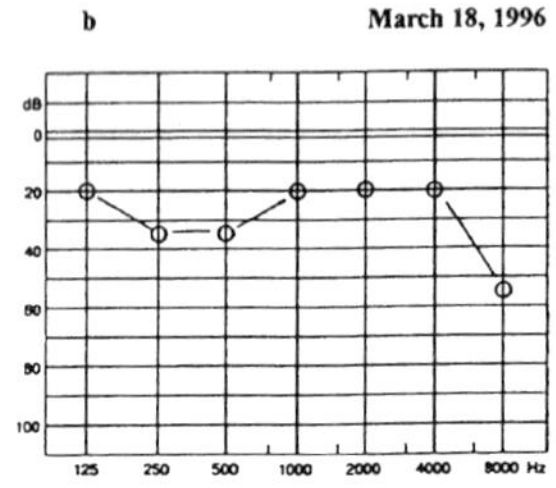

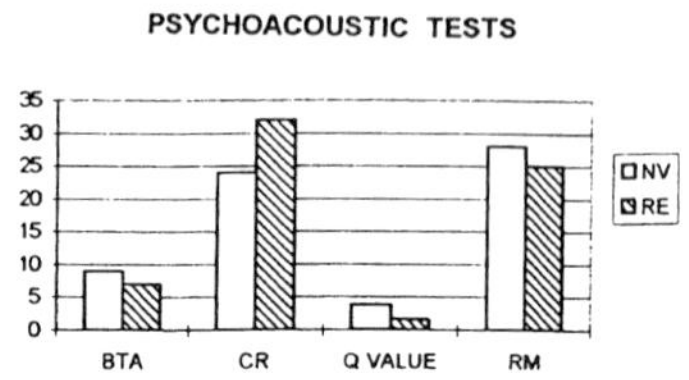

b March 18, 1996

PSYCHOACOUSTIC TESTS

□ NV ☒ RE

OAEs	RE	LE
SOAEs	P	A
CEOAEs	P	A
TBEOAEs	P	A
DP 2 kHz	P	A
DP 4 kHz	P	A
DP 6 kHZ	P	A

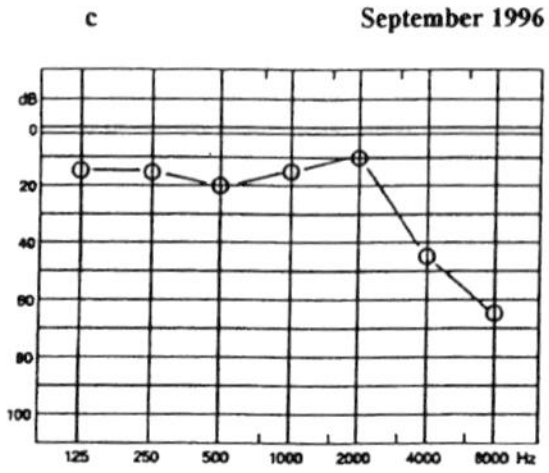

c September 1996

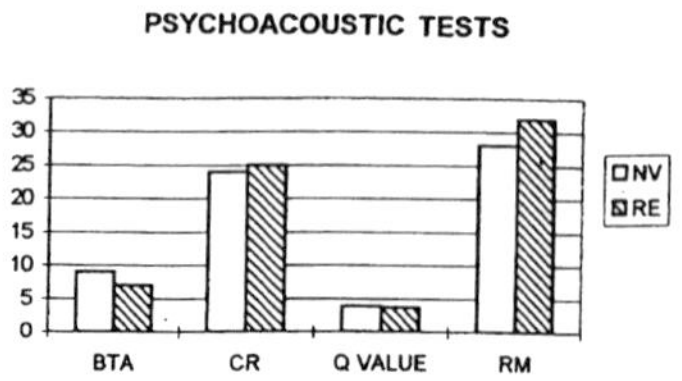

PSYCHOACOUSTIC TESTS

□ NV ☒ RE

OAEs	RE	LE
SOAEs	P	A
CEOAEs	P	A
TBEOAEs	P	A
DP 2 kHz	P	A
DP 4 kHz	P	A
DP 6 kHZ	P	A

FIGURE 2. Auditory findings of Case 2 (9-year-old boy) prior to therapy (a), after a week (b), and six months (c) of therapy. RE = right ear; LE = left ear; N = normal; NV = normal value; OAEs A = absent, P = present.

dB, PTC Q value 3.6, and RM 32 dB; SOAEs, EOAEs, and DPOAEs were present.

In this case, after a week of therapy, when the PTA was 25 dB HL, primary cochlear functions were normal, except for frequency selectivity; six months later, when PTA returned to normal, frequency selectivity function showed normal.

CASE 3. A 21-year-old woman with a history of slowly progressive hearing loss and a low pitched tinnitus in the right ear for twelve months. She had noticed recurrent spells of incapacitating vertigo over the last three months. At the time of admission, in March 1996, her audiogram (FIG. 3(a)) revealed a flat SNHL with a PTA of 70 dB HL and a 70% speech discrimination score in the right ear. The hearing was normal on the left. SRs and ABRs showed no abnormalities. ENGs showed a normal caloric response on both sides. MRI showed no cerebellopontine angle pathology.

CASE 3

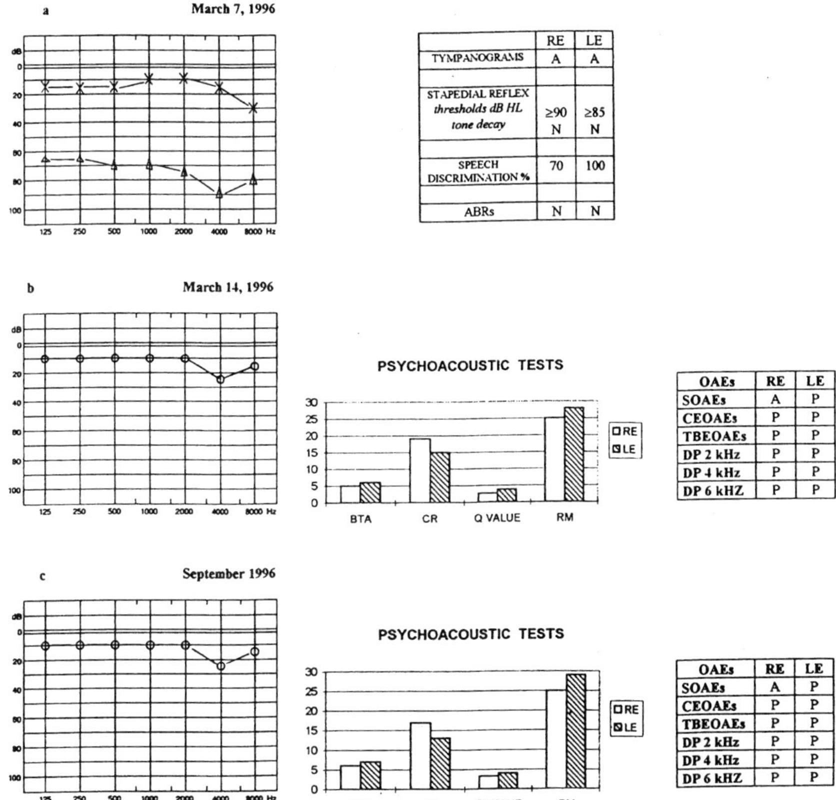

FIGURE 3. Auditory findings of Case 3 (21-year-old woman) prior to therapy (a), after seven days of therapy (b), and after six months off treatment (c). RE = right ear; LE = left ear; N = normal: OAEs A = absent, P = present.

Her nonspecific inflammation indexes were normal. Dosage of the immunoglobulin fractions showed increased IgG and normal IgA and IgM. Antigen-nonspecific immunological tests were normal except for the presence of antinuclear and antimitochondrial autoantibodies and for the increase of CICs. The patient received prednisone (60 mg/day) for 15 days. Within seven days of therapy a complete recovery of her hearing was observed (FIG. 3(b)); BTA factor was 5 dB, RC 19 dB, PTC Q 2.7, RM 25 dB; SOAEs were absent, EOAEs and DPOAEs present. Her tinnitus and vertigo also disappeared. Hearing remained normal over the following six months without therapy. In September 1996, CICs were in the normal range; the right ear (FIG. 3(c)) had a PTA of 10 dB HL; BTA value was 6 dB, CR 17 dB; PTC *Q* value 3.2, RM 25 dB; EOAEs and DPOAEs were present. No SOAEs were recordable.

It is notable that after 10 days of corticosteroid therapy, when the hearing had returned to normal, temporal integration and frequency selectivity were slightly depressed; after five months these functions were normal.

CASE 4. A man aged 39 with a sudden drop in hearing in the left ear recovered, in a few days without therapy, five months prior to referral. In February 1993 he was referred for evaluation of a new hearing loss in the left ear with a feeling of aural pressure. Five days after the event the patient noticed intermittent high-pitched tinnitus in the left ear; then an increase of tinnitus preceded a violent episode of objective rotatory vertigo with neurovegetative symptoms that suggested admission to the Clinic.

CASE 4

a   February 1993

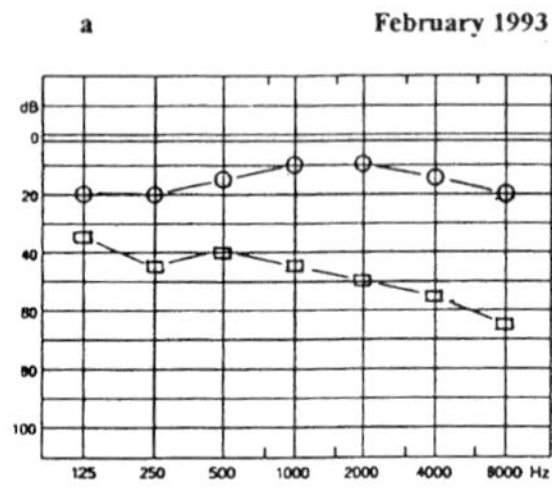

	RE	LE
TYMPANOGRAMS	A	A
STAPEDIAL REFLEX *thresholds dB HL* *tone decay*	≥80 N	≥90 P
SPEECH DISCRIMINATION %	100	70
ABRs	N	N*

b   November 6, 1993

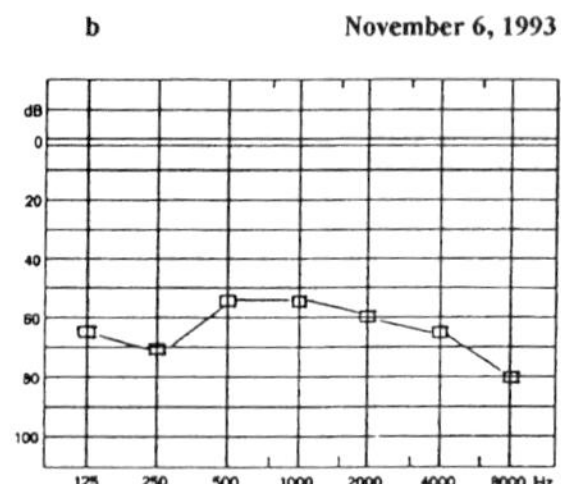

	RE	LE
TYMPANOGRAMS	A	A
STAPEDIAL REFLEX *thresholds dB HL* *tone decay*	≥85 N	≥95 N
SPEECH DISCRIMINATION %	100	70
ABRs	N	N

c   November 10, 1993 - September 1996

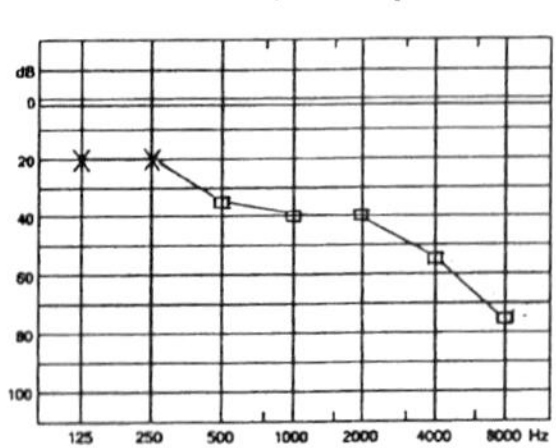

OAEs	RE	LE
SOAEs	A	A
CEOAEs	P	A
TBEOAEs	P	A
DP 2 kHz	P	A
DP 4 kHz	P	A
DP 6 kHZ	P	A

FIGURE 4. Auditory findings of Case 4 (39-year-old man) prior to therapy (a), upon relapse (b), and after four days of therapy (c). Hearing and primary cochlear functions remained stable off treatment over three years. RE = right ear; LE = left ear; N = normal; tone decay P = pathological; * = slight increase of latency; OAEs A = absent, P = present.

His head, neck, and neurootologic examinations were normal, but an audiogram (FIG. 4(a)) revealed a unilateral flat SNHL with a PTA of 45 dB HL in the left ear. A 70% speech discrimination score was obtained from that side. SRs showed no abnormalities except for a pathological tone decay in the left ear. ABRs were normal on the right, while on the left the waves showed a moderate increase of latency. ENGs showed normal caloric responses on both sides. MRI showed no cerebellopontine angle pathology. Clinical immunology work-up showed normal value except for an increase in CICs. The patient received prednisone (60 mg/day) and amiloride+idrocloro-tiazide (5mg+50mg/day), both orally, for two weeks. On the twelfth day of treatment pure tone thresholds had improved by 10 dB over all frequencies. Within two months (April 1993) his CICs and hearing had completely returned to normal. Seven months later (November 1993) the hearing in the left ear suddenly fell to a PTA of 60 dB HL (FIG. 4(b)); the audiometric curve was flat; his speech-discrimination score was 70%; impedance and SRs showed no abnormalities; ABRs still showed a slight increase in latency. CICs were again increased. After four days of prednisone therapy (60 mg/day), his audiogram (FIG. 4(c)) showed a downsloping SNHL with PTA of 38 dB HL. BTA was 3 dB, CR 26 dB, PTC Q value 2.8, RM 18 dB; SOAEs, EOAEs, and DPOAEs were absent. Prednisone therapy continued for five months (25 mg/day). Over the following three years, his hearing and primary cochlear functions have remained stable off treatment. The last follow-up was in September 1996.

Of note is that in this patient temporal integration, frequency selectivity, and products of cochlear mechanics were affected nine months from the beginning of therapy, when PTA stabilized at 40 dB HL; over the following three years, hearing and cochlear functions remained unchanged off treatment.

CASE 5. A 12-year-old girl was referred in September 1993 for evaluation of sudden hearing loss in the left ear. She reported intermittent low-pitched tinnitus in both ears and no vertigo. She had previously noticed a sudden bilateral drop of hearing at the age of 9; after corticosteroid therapy, her hearing completely recovered to normal thresholds on the left and stabilized flat SNHL with PTA of 55 dB HL on the right. These were documented by serial audiograms. At the time of admission, her audiogram (FIG. 5(a)) revealed a bilateral downsloping SNHL with PTA of 93 dB HL in the right ear and 48 dB HL in the left. Speech discrimination score was 0% on the right and 50% on the left. SR was not elicited on the right and had thresholds ≥ 105 dB HL on the left. ABRs waveforms didn't show any significant response in the right ear and showed a moderate increase of latency of all waves on the left. ENGs showed a bilateral reduced caloric response. The MRI showed no cerebellopontine-angle pathology. The clinical immunology work-up showed normal values except for a complement (C4) activation and a circulating immune complex increase. Within a week, prednisone therapy (50 mg/day) gave an improvement of 30 dB at frequencies > 2 kHz in the left ear. The hearing in the right ear demonstrated no response whatsoever to treatment. Twenty days later, the corticosteroid dosage was reduced to 15 mg/day and she developed a new sudden SNHL in the left ear. She was admitted once again and given 20 mg/day prednisone. After a week her hearing returned to pretreatment levels, so cyclosporine (150 mg/day) was added to prednisone. Within two days, pure tone thresholds improved by 20 dB over all frequencies on the left. Circu-

CASE 5

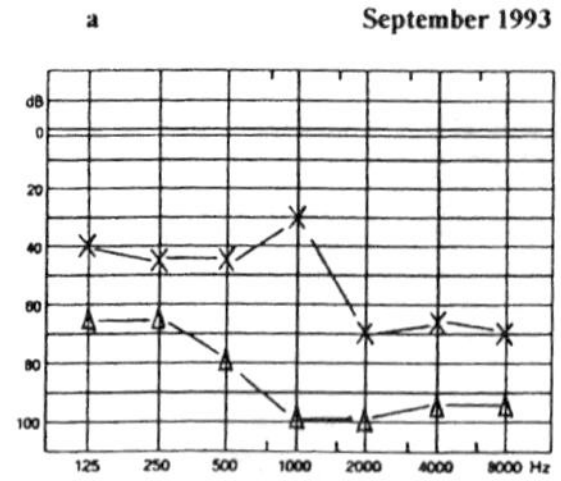

	RE	LE
TYMPANOGRAMS	A	A
STAPEDIAL REFLEX thresholds dB HL tone decay	/ /	≥105 /
SPEECH DISCRIMINATION %	0	50
ABRs	A	N*

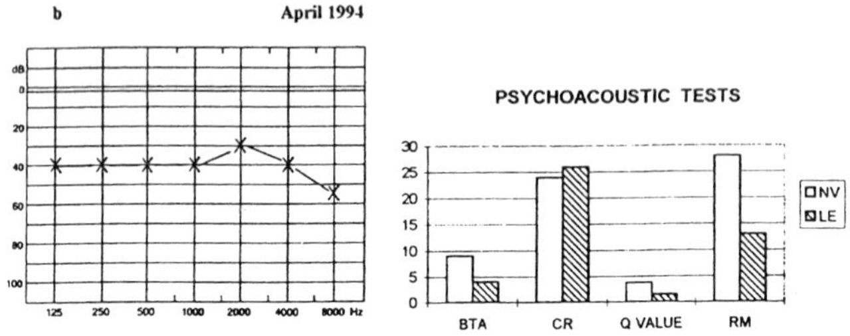

OAEs	RE	LE
SOAEs	A	A
CEOAEs	A	A
TBEOAEs	A	A
DP 2 kHz	A	A
DP 4 kHz	A	A
DP 6 kHZ	A	A

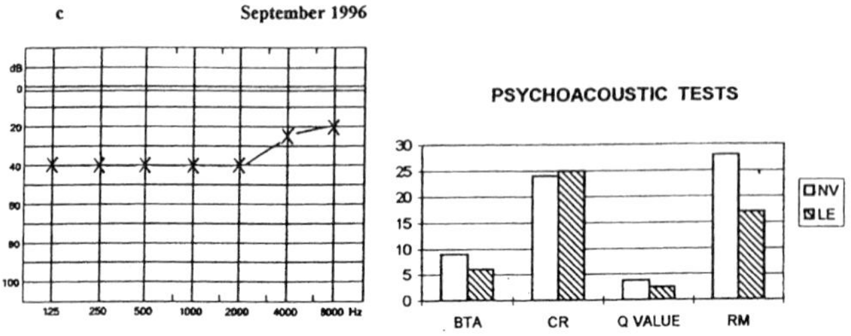

OAEs	RE	LE
SOAEs	A	A
CEOAEs	A	P
TBEOAEs	A	A
DP 2 kHz	A	A
DP 4 kHz	A	P
DP 6 kHZ	A	P

FIGURE 5. Auditory findings of Case 5 (12-year-old girl) prior to therapy (a), after eight months of therapy (b), and after two years off treatment (c); RE = right ear; LE = left ear; N = normal; NV = normal value; OAEs A = absent, P = present.

lating immunocomplexes disappeared within a few weeks. Repeated audiograms (twice weekly) showed a fluctuating SNHL related to the dosage of medication, if successful. These fluctuations lasted for eight months, then the hearing stabilized with prednisone at 10 mg/day and cyclosporine at 100 mg on even days and 50 mg on odd days. In April 1994 (FIG. 5(b)) her audiogram showed a flat SNHL in the left ear, with a PTA of 37 dB HL; BTA value was 4 dB, CR 25 dB, PTC Q value 1.5, RM effect 13 dB; SEOAEs, EOAEs, and DPOAEs were absent. In July 1994 therapy was stopped. Her hearing remained stable for the following months. In September 1996 (FIG. 5(c)), the patient's CICs were in the normal range; her audiogram revealed downsloping SNHL with PTA of 93 dB HL on the right and upsloping SNHL with a

PTA of 40 dB HL on the left. At the same side, her BTA was 6 dB, CR 25 dB and PTC Q value 2.5, RM 17 dB; SOAEs and EOAEs by tone bursts were absent, EOAEs by clicks were present, DPOAEs were absent at 2 kHz and present at 4 and 6 kHz.

In this patient, temporal integration, frequency selectivity, and products of resulting cochlear mechanics were affected after eight months of therapy when the hearing stabilized with a flat SNHL with PTA of 37 dB HL; a further two years of therapy improved cochlear functions without any change of PTA.

CASE 6. A 14-year-old girl presented a 4-year history of slowly progressive SNHL in the left ear and fluctuations in hearing, with continuous low-pitched tinnitus in the right (these fluctuations were documented by serial audiograms). She did not complain of spells of vertigo or unsteadiness. Clinical immunology showed normal values except for complement (C4) activation and CICs increase. Antinuclear and antimitochondrial autoantibodies were present. She was treated with prednisone (30 mg/day) and cyclosporine (100 mg/day), both orally, for 14 months, and her hearing has remained steady over the last two years without therapy. At the time of referral, in July 1996, she had (FIG. 6) a flat SNHL with a PTA of 80 dB HL and a speech-discrimination score of 0% on the left and a borderline low-frequency SNHL with a PTA of 15 dB HL and speech discrimination score of 100% on the right. SR thresholds were ≥ 100 dB HL on the left and ≥ 90 dB on the right. Tone decay was normal in the right ear and pathologic in the left. In the right ear, BTA values were 8 dB, CR 25 dB, PTC Q value 2.5, RM effect 31 dB; SOAEs were absent and EOAEs and

CASE 6

July 1996

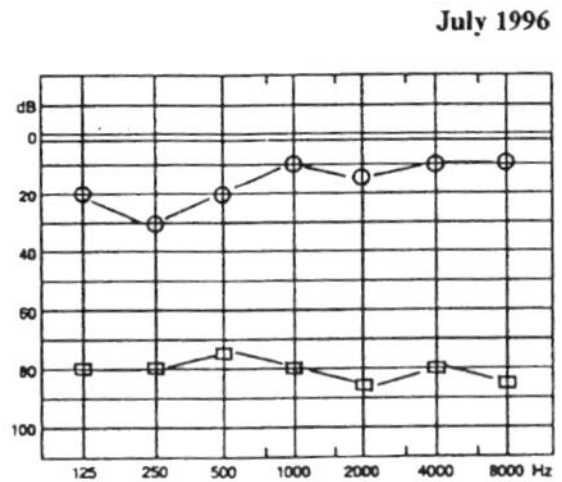

	RE	LE
TYMPANOGRAMS	A	A
STAPEDIAL REFLEX *thresholds dB HL* *tone decay*	≥90 / N	≥100 / P
SPEECH DISCRIMINATION %	100	0
ABRs	N	P

PSYCHOACOUSTIC TESTS

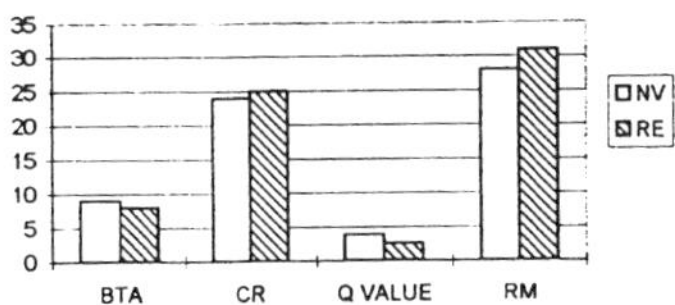

OAEs	RE	LE
SOAEs	A	A
CEOAEs	P	A
TBEOAEs	P	A
DP 2 kHz	P	A
DP 4 kHz	P	A
DP 6 kHZ	P	A

FIGURE 6. Auditory findings of Case 6 (14-year-old girl) four years after beginning of disease with two years off treatment. RE = right ear; LE = left ear; N = normal; tone decay P = pathological; * = slight increase of latency; NV = normal value; OAEs A =absent, P = present.

DPOAEs present. ABRs were normal on the right, while on the left the lone V wave was detected and showed an increased latency; IT5 was abnormally increased. ENGs showed normal vestibular responses on both sides. The MRI showed no cerebellopontine angle pathology. The clinical immunology work-up showed CICs in the normal range.

It is notable that in this patient, four years from the beginning of therapy, frequency selectivity was slightly alterated in the presence of a borderline low-frequency SNHL.

DISCUSSION

The six case reports discussed in the present paper emphasize, first of all, the variability in the clinical course of the immunomediated SNHL syndromes. The disease began in middle age in three patients and during childhood in the other three; the hearing loss was sudden in onset in three patients and slowly progressive in three; bilateral although asymmetric in four cases and unilateral in two; three patients had vestibular symptoms, which in one mimicked Ménière's syndrome. At the time of admission, three of the ten ears with SNHL had downsloping audiometric curves, three upsloping, and four were flat. Discrimination scores were ≥ 80% in three ears, between 50 and 80% in three, and < 50% in four; in three ears they were disproportionately poor and in two disproportionately good as compared to PTA. SR audiometry and/or ABRs, when evaluable, indicated a retrocochlear involvement in three ears. Vestibular functions were involved in both ears of one patient and in one ear of another. Steroid treatment resulted in a dramatic positive response in two ears, while two ears showed fluctuating hearing losses related to the dosage of drug. Two cases didn't respond to cortisone alone, but were treated successfully using combinations of steroid with immunosuppressive medication (cyclosporine). Only one subject had a relapse after a first course of therapy. After treatment six ears improved and their hearing stabilized with a PTA of 10–15 dB HL in the four ears and of 40 dB in two; therapy didn't restore any function in four ears with longlasting and severe SNHL.

Concerning primary cochlear functions, the present study has shown that in immunomediated SNHL, temporal integration, frequency selectivity, and products of cochlear mechanics are affected during the hearing loss and tend to normalize after therapy when hearing returns to normal. This finding would seem to confirm that the cochlea is the target organ in such cases. Experimental and clinical evidence suggest CICs are important as one of the pathogenetic mechanisms of autoimmune SNHL.[20] It appears that CIC deposits in the blood vessel of the stria vascularis damage the capillary endothelium, increase the vascular permeability, and secondarily result in endolymphatic hydrops. The histopathological features observed in the patients[21–27] and in animal models[28] with immunomediated inner-ear disorders support this vascular pathogenesis. In fact, temporal bone studies have shown that in such cases the most common findings were vasculitis in the internal auditory artery and capillary damage within the stria vascularis, followed by spiral ganglion cell degeneration, atrophy of the organ of Corti, collapse of Reissner's membrane, distortion of the tectoral membrane, and endolymphatic hydrops with atrophy of the surface epithelium of the endolymphatic duct. These findings, experimentally producible by sudden interruption of cochlear blood flow,[29,30] could explain the auditory dysfunctions observed in the six cases reported in the present paper. It is noteworthy that all patients except one had elevated levels of CICs at the outset of hearing loss. Moreover, the outcome of the tests that we used to assess primary cochlear function led us to assume that the immunomediated inner-ear disease results, in the first stages, in the development of endolymphatic hydrops, which increases the stiffness of the vibrating structures within the inner ear and causes dysfunctions of the OHCs. The auditory findings in this stage are upsloping or flat SNHL, absence of EOAEs and DPOAEs, and abnormal results for RM, BTA, CR, and PTC Q10. After treatment, if successful, hydrops recovers and hearing subsequently returns to normal, the audiometric curve becomes flat at low-middle frequencies, RM values tend to normalize, EOAEs and DPOAEs reappear; in some ears, a subclinical dysfunction of the OHCs, which is evident only in an abnormal temporal integration and/or frequency selectivity, could persist for a certain time. Finally, when the disease has caused irreversible anatomofunctional changes within the cochlea, hearing and primary cochlear functions remain persistently altered. The present study seems to support the usefulness of testing primary cochlear functions to monitor the clinical course of immunomediated inner-ear disorders.

ACKNOWLEDGMENTS

The authors gratefully acknowledge the assistance of Drs. Olga Defidio and Eileen Mulligan.

REFERENCES

1. McCabe, B. F. 1979. Autoimmune sensorineural hearing loss. Ann. Otol. Rhino. Laryngol. **88:** 585–589.
2. McCabe, B. F. 1987. Autoimmune inner ear disease: Clinical varieties of presentation. *In* Otoimmunology, Chap. 15, J. E. Veldman and B. F. McCabe, Eds.: 143–148. Kugler. Amsterdam.
3. Hughes, G. B., S. E. Kinney, P. A. Barna, *et al.* 1987. Autoimmune inner ear disease. Laboratory tests and audio-vestibular treatment reponses. *In* Otoimmunology, Chap. 16, J. E. Veldman and B. F. McCabe, Eds.: 149–155. Kugler. Amsterdam.
4. Veldman, J. E. 1987. Immune-mediated inner ear disorders. New syndromes and their etiopathogenesis. *In* Otoimmunology, Chap. 14, J. E. Veldman and B. F. McCabe, Eds.: 125–141. Kugler. Amsterdam.
5. Pedersen, C. B. 1973. Brief-tone audiometry in patients with acoustic trauma. Acta Otolaryngol. **75:** 332–333.
6. Pedersen, C. B. 1974. Brief-tone audiometry in persons treated with salicylate. Audiology **13:** 311–319.
7. Scharf, B. 1978. Comparison of normal and impaired hearing. II. Frequency analysis, speech perception. *In* Sensorineural Hearing Impairment and Hearing Aids, C. Ludvigsen and J. Barfod, Eds.: 81–106. Scand. Audiol. (Suppl. 6).
8. Evans, E. F. 1982. Recent advances in cochlear physiology. *In* Otology, A. Gibb and M. F. W. Smith, Eds.: 105–131. Butterworth. London.

9. TYLER, R. S. 1986. Frequency resolution in hearing-impaired listeners. *In* Frequency Selectivity in Hearing, B. C. J. Moore, Ed.: 309–371. Academic Press. London.
10. FLETCHER, H. 1940. Auditory patterns. Rev. Mod. Phys. **12:** 47–85.
11. ZWICKER, E. 1974. On a psychoacoustical equivalent of tuning curves. *In* Facts and Models in Hearing, E. Zwicker and E. Terhardt, Eds.: 132–140. Springer-Verlag. Heidelberg.
12. VANDEN ABEELE, D., P. H. VAN DE HEYNING, W. CRETEN, A. GRAFF & J. F. E. MARQUET. 1992. Psychoacoustical tuning curves. Normative data for clinical use. Scand. Audiol. **21:** 3–8.
13. BROWNELL, W. E., C. R. BADER, D. BERTRAND & Y. DE RIBAUPIERRE. 1985. Evoked mechanical responses of isolated cochlear outer hair cells. Science. **227:** 194–198.
14. BROWNELL, W. E. 1990. Outer hair cell electromotility and otoacoustic emissions. Ear Hear. **11:** 82–92.
15. BONFILS, P., A. UZIEL & R. PUJOL. 1988. Evoked otoacoustic emissions: A fundamental and clinical survey. ORL **50:** 212–218.
16. LONG, G. R. & A. TUBIS. 1988. Modification of spontaneous and evoked otoacoustic emissions and associated psychoacoustic microstructure by aspirin consumption. J. Acoust. Soc. Am. **84:** 1343–1353.
17. DEATHERAGE, B. H., R. C. BILGER & D. H. ELDREDGE. 1957. Remote masking in selected frequency regions. J. Acoust. Soc. Am. **29:** 512–514.
18. CERVELLERA, G., A. QUARANTA & P. CASSANO. 1978. Le "remote masking": Un test de surdité de transmission cochléaire. Audiology **17:** 317–323.
19. CERVELLERA, G., A. QUARANTA & C. AMOROSO. 1980. Clinical experience with remote masking. Audiology **19:** 404–410.
20. HARADA, T., M. SANO, M. SAKAGAMI, S. OGINO & T. MATSUNAGA. 1992. Mechanisms of immune complex-mediated inner ear diseases. Ann. Otol. Rhinol. Laryngol. **101:** 72–77.
21. GUSSEN, R. 1977. Polyarteritis nodosa and deafness: A human temporal bone study. Arch. Otorhinolaryngol. **217:** 263–271.
22. JENKINS, H. A., A. M. POLLAK & U. FISCH. 1981. Polyarteritis nodosa as a cause of sudden deafness: A human temporal bone study. Am. J. Otolaryngol. **2:** 99–107.
23. YANAGITA, N., *et al.* 1987. Acute bilateral deafness with nephritis: A human temporal bone study. Laryngoscope **97:** 345–352.
24. FISHER, E. R. & H. R. HELLSTROM, 1961. Cogan's syndrome and systemic vascular disease. Analysis of pathologic features with reference to its relationship to thromboangiitis obliterans (Buerger). Arch. Pathol. 72:572–592.
25. WOLFF, D., *et al.* 1965. The pathology of Cogan's syndrome causing profound deafness. Ann. Otol. Rhinol. Laryngol. **74:** 507–520.
26. ZECHNER, G. 1980. Zum Cogan-Syndrom. Acta Otolaryngol. (Stockholm) **89:** 310–316.
27. SCHUKNECHT, H. F. 1991. Ear pathology in otoimmune disease. *In* Bearing of Basic Research on Clinical Otolaryngology, Vol. 46, C.R. Pfaltz, W. Arnold, and O. Kleinsasser, Eds.: 50–70. Adv. Otorhinolaryngol. Karger. Basel.
28. YOO, T. J., *et al.* 1983. Type II collagen-induced autoimmune sensorineural hearing loss and vestibular dysfunction in rats. Ann. Otol. Rhinol. Laryngol. **92:** 267–271.
29. ALFORD, B. R., *et al.* 1965. Physiologic and histopathologic effects of microembolism of the internal auditory artery. Ann. Otol. Rhinol. Laryngol. **74:** 728–748.
30. KIMURA, R. & H. B. PERLMAN. 1958. Arterial obstruction of the labyrinth: I. Cochlear changes; II. Vestibular changes. Ann. Otol. Rhinol. Laryngol. **67:** 5–24.

Measles, Mumps, and Sensorineural Hearing Loss[a]

MICHAEL J. McKENNA[b]

Department of Otolaryngology
Massachusetts Eye and Ear Infirmary
243 Charles Street
Boston, Massachusetts 02114-3096

INTRODUCTION

On the basis of both clinical and histopathologic investigations, there is a well established association between viral infection and sensorineural hearing loss. Several viruses with varying classifications have been implicated, including measles, mumps, influenza, rubella, cytomegalovirus, and herpes. Since humans are known to be the host of over a hundred different viruses, it is reasonable to speculate that many other viral agents may also result in inner-ear pathology. Despite the well established association between certain specific viruses and corresponding characteristic cochlear and vestibular pathology, the mechanisms by which some of these viruses result in end organ pathology has not been determined. Specifically, it is not known whether the damage that occurs within the cochlea and vestibular labyrinth is the result of viral infection of specific target cells or the sequela of a reactive inflammatory response to viral infection or the presence of viral antigens or some combination of both. Recent studies on inner-ear immune reactivity suggest that the immune response to inner-ear antigenic challenge may be a critical determinant of the resultant pathology and sensory impairment.[1,2] Furthermore, these studies indicate that secondary exposures may result in a more robust amnestic immune response with potentially greater effects than that which occurred as the result of the initial infection or exposure.[3] These findings provide a rational mechanistic explanation for the pathologic basis of viral related inner-ear dysfunction and potentially related conditions, including Ménière's disease, sudden hearing loss, delayed hydrops, and some immune-mediated inner-ear disorders.

Review of the inner-ear histopathology in selected cases of well-established specific viral-related otopathology may serve to illuminate some of the mechanisms of cochlear and vestibular injury, especially when viewed in the context of the established mechanism of infection, systemic manifestations, and secondary immune response. The pathophysiology and the basic mechanism of systemic viral infection, replication, and host immune response has been described for several viruses. This review and discussion focuses on the otopathology, characteristics of systemic infec-

[a]This work was support by Grant KO8 DC00065 from the National Institute on Deafness and Other Communication Disorders.
[b]Phone: 617/573-3672; fax: 617/573-3914.

tion, and immune response of measles and mumps infection, which may serve as a model for other related viruses.

MEASLES

Measles is among the most contagious viruses known to infect man. Its portal of entry is through the respiratory tract. The incubation period varies from 10 to 14 days, which is followed by a prodromal stage with predominately respiratory tract manifestations including laryngitis, tracheobronchitis, bronchiolitis, and some degree of interstitial pneumonitis. As these symptoms begin to increase in severity, increasing fever develops, which is followed shortly by the development of the pathognomonic Koplik's spots in the buccal and labial mucosa. This is followed by an exanthematous rash that begins on the head and neck and within three days progresses to involve the upper extremities, trunk, and lower extremities. Once the rash reaches the lower extremities, the fever recedes. In some cases, a secondary bacterial infection of the upper respiratory tract occurs which has been attributed to measles-virus-induced immunosuppression. The degree of immunosuppression from measles infection may last for months, as can be demonstrated by the loss of delayed hypersensitivity to tuberculin injection. Patients with active tuberculosis often experience a severe exacerbation during this period. The severity of measles infection has been related to the age, nutritional status, and immune competence of the infected individual. Viremia occurs in association with the early upper respiratory tract symptoms, and its spread occurs hematogenously via infected lymphocytes.

Among the most dreaded complications of measles virus infection is an associated measles encephalitis which occurs in approximately 1 in 1000 cases. Usually, this occurs three to four days following the acute illness and is clinically characterized by seizures, obtundation, and coma. The mortality rate of central nervous system involvement is approximately 25%. Half of those who survive have permanent sequelae, including mental retardation, seizures, motor abnormalities, and deafness. Despite the relatively low incidence of CNS clinical manifestations, it is estimated that more than half of individuals infected with measles have some degree of CNS involvement, as evidenced by the presence of pleocytosis in CSF of uncomplicated cases and transient EEG abnormalities.[4,5] A rare and usually late CNS sequela of measles infection is the development of subacute sclerosing panencephalitis (SSPE). SSPE occurs months to years following infection of measles virus and in some cases the administration of the live attenuated vaccine. The clinical course is characterized by the initial manifestation of subtle cognitive and behavioral dysfunction which slowly progresses with the ultimate development of severe neurologic symptoms and death. The presence of a slowly progressive persistent measles virus infection has been established.[6]

Widespread vaccination against measles virus began in the United States in 1966. The vaccine is a live attenuated measles virus that has been passed through other animal hosts to decrease its pathogenicity in man. The vaccine results in the development of both cellular and humoral immunity. Since measles remains a ubiquitous virus, most individuals continue to experience repeat infection throughout life, as is evidenced by periodic elevations of measles antibody titers. Multiple reports of secondary clinical measles infection after vaccination exist. There are also reports of measles infection with CNS complications that have occurred in association with vaccination, suggesting that in some individuals, the attenuated virus is pathogenic. The live attenuated vaccine is contraindicated in immunocompromised individuals.

The incidence of measles-related sensorineural hearing loss has been studied by several investigators. It is estimated that measles infections accounted for 5–10% of all cases of profound bilateral sensorineural hearing loss prior to the advent of the live measles vaccine.[7–12] Although evidence suggests that the incidence of measles-related sensorineural hearing loss has declined since the introduction of the vaccine, the magnitude of the impact has yet to be established.[13] It is also not clear whether or not the vaccine has altered the clinical course of sensorineural hearing loss from profound bilateral deafness to some intermediate degree of stable or progressive impairment. Cases of unilateral and bilateral profound sudden deafness have been reported with the administration of the vaccine.[14] However, since the current form of the vaccine is administered in combination with mumps and rubella (MMR), the role of the live attenuated measles virus in the etiology of this condition has been difficult to establish. Some data suggest that the live attenuated mumps virus may be the more likely cause.

Histopathologic studies of temporal bones from individuals with sensorineural hearing loss following measles virus infection have been reported. A comprehensive review of the histopathologic temporal bone findings of both measles and mumps infection can be found in Schuknecht's *Pathology of the Ear*.[15] Bilateral involvement is most common with severe cochlear and vestibular pathology. Diffuse cochlear pathology with destruction or degeneration of the organ of Corti, stria, and cochlear neurons is typical. The most severe changes are usually found in the basal turn. Although endolymphatic hydrops may be seen in some specimens, it is not a typical feature of measles infection. Of particular significance is the presence of fibrous tissue in the scala of the basal turns, which is suggestive of an associated inflammatory process (FIG. 1). Some specimens demonstrate new bone growth in the vestibular labyrinth, which is also consistent with an associated inflammatory process. No obvious abnormalities of the endolymphatic duct or sac are present.

Of particular interest is a case of an infant who died shortly following the development of measles leukoencephalitis. The temporal bones reveal the presence of an inflammatory process within the cochlea that appears to be a direct extension from the subarachnoid space that contains a dense small-cell inflammatory infiltrate. The scala tympani contains both small cells and polymorphonuclear leukocytes . There is early severe degeneration of the cochlear neurons, which is most pronounced in the basal turn. The cochlea reveals severe degeneration of the organ of Corti and stria (FIG. 2). In contradistinction to the other cases of measles infection that were studied years following the acute insult, the vestibular labyrinth is well preserved without evidence of sensory epithelial degeneration.

MUMPS

Like measles, mumps is a paramyxo virus whose portal of entry is through the upper respiratory tract. The incubation period between exposure and the development

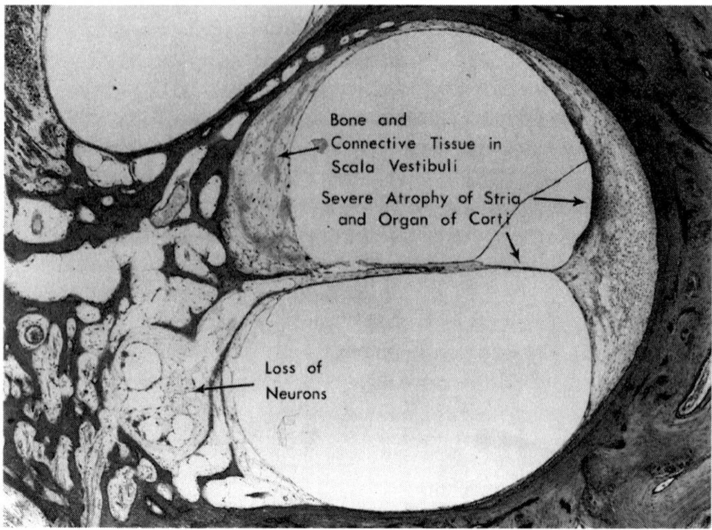

FIGURE 1. Case of profound bilateral hearing loss at age four in association with measles. Patient died of a myocardial infarction at age 53. Pathologic changes are similar in both ears. Predominant histopathologic features include atrophy of the organ of Corti and stria vascularis with degeneration of cochlear neurons.

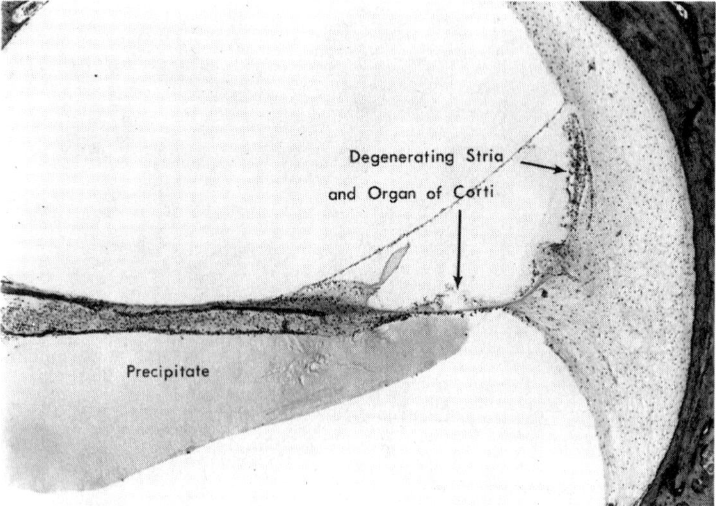

FIGURE 2. Case of an infant who died at age one and one-half years from measles leukoencephalitis approximately 10 days after developing routine measles infection. Predominant histopathologic features include proteinaceous precipitate and round cell infiltrate in scala tympani with degeneration of stria and organ of Corti. Vestibular end-organ (not seen) is well preserved.

of clinical symptoms is between 14 and 21 days. Viremia occurs shortly following exposure. The specific tissues in which viral replication occurs, other than the respiratory epithelium and parotid gland, has not been well established. Infectious virus is secreted in the saliva. The most common clinical manifestations of infection include parotidis, pancreatitis, and inflammation of the testes and meninges. Other organs known to be affected include the thyroid, heart, ovaries, and kidneys. CNS involvement is common and is estimated to occur in approximately 65% of cases based on the presence of pleocytosis and the development of mild meningeal signs that are common and are attributed to aseptic meningitis. Much less common is the development of mumps postinfectious encephalitis, which occurs in approximately 2.5/1000 patients with an onset that is usually 7–10 days later than the common aseptic meningitis. The clinical course is initially similar to measles encephalitis with seizures, obtundation, and coma. Survival is more common than with measles encephalitis and recovery is more often complete. A common sequela of mumps postinfectious encephalitis is the development of hydrocephalous and inflammatory stenosis of the sylvian aqueduct. Evidence of viral infection has been seen in the ependymal cells, and in the cells of the choroid plexus.

The live attenuated mumps vaccine was licensed in 1968 and is now commonly administered to infants in the United States in combination with measles and rubella (MMR). Subsequent infection following vaccination is known to occur, and complications following vaccination, including typical mumps infection, encephalitis, and sudden unilateral and bilateral hearing loss, have been reported. As is the case with measles, the vaccine has not eliminated the mumps virus from the general population, and amnestic immune responses with periodic elevation of antibody titers are known to occur.

Deafness following mumps infection is believed to be more often unilateral than bilateral, although the data to support this are not conclusive. Because of the presumed unilaterality of the disease, children are frequently not diagnosed until they reach school, making the direct association between past infection and sensorineural loss far from certain. As such, it is difficult to establish the causal relationship and frequency of associated hearing loss. Several lines of indirect evidence support the association of unilateral sudden hearing loss and mumps infection. These include the association of sudden unilateral deafness in adults with established mumps infection,[16] and the common finding of rising titer of antibody to mumps in individuals with sudden unilateral hearing loss.[17] The histopathology of a case of sudden bilateral sensorineural deafness shortly following mumps infection was reported by Lindsay *et al.,* whose findings are identical to cases of reported unilateral loss.[18] Also, animal models of mumps labyrinthitis are consistent with the human pathology in cases of presumed mumps labyrinthitis.[19] Although there appears to be no association between mumps aseptic meningitis and postinfectious encephalitis and the development of acute profound hearing loss, recent audiometric and neurotologic assessment of patients with mild and severe CNS involvement reveal that transient sensorineural hearing loss is common.[20]

The histopathology of temporal bones from patients with presumed mumps-related unilateral deafness reveal severe atrophy of the organ of Corti and stria vascularis with good preservation of the utricle, saccule, and crista of the semicircular canals. Endolymphatic hydrops is common, as is obstruction and obliteration of the endolymphatic duct and increased fibrosis of the endolymphatic sac. Unlike with measles, fibrous tissue formation and new bone formation within the cochlea and vestibule are uncommon. Schuknecht *et al.* have reported a case of delayed contralateral hydrops in a patient with presumed unilateral profound deafness from mumps.[21] A common finding in both ears is the presence of hydrops, and obliteration of the endolymphatic duct approximately 2 mm from the vestibule is suggestive of past ductal inflammation (FIG. 3).

DISCUSSION

The association between sensorineural hearing loss and measles infection is well established, and the histopathology of cases of bilateral profound sensorineural hearing loss resulting from measles infection has been described. However, because measles infection is known to result in profound bilateral loss in some cases that produces impairment that is immediately obvious to parents and physicians, the evidence to support that measles results in solely or predominately bilateral loss is lacking, and is speculative at best. Cases of unilateral profound loss in childhood with histologic evidence of both cochlear and vestibular pathologic changes have been reported and may well be the result of measles infection. It is also conceivable that less

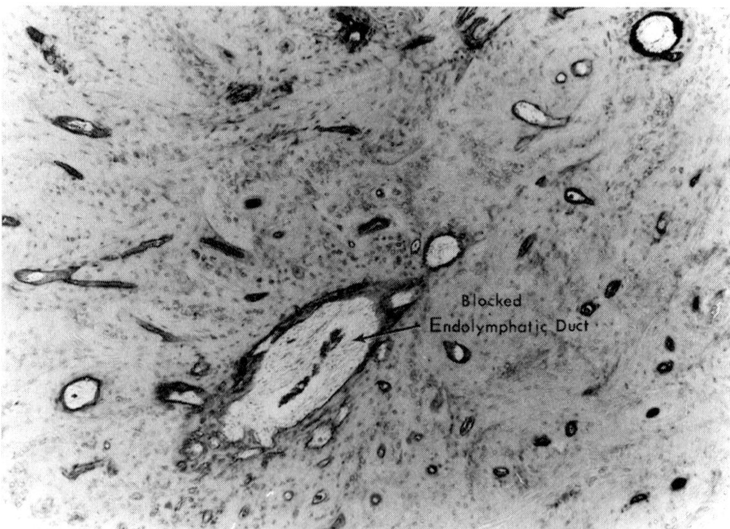

FIGURE 3. Case of delayed contralateral hydrops from a patient with profound unilateral sensorineural hearing loss in early childhood from presumed mumps infection. At age 31 he developed symptoms of Ménière's disease in the opposite ear. He died at age 35 from aspiration of emesis during an attack of vertigo. Both ears revealed hydrops with obstruction of the endolymphatic ducts. (Reprinted with permission from the Annals Publishing Company.[21])

extensive pathology may occur in cases of measles infection with the preservation of some residual auditory and vestibular function, and that this may be both bilateral and unilateral. The case presented earlier from a child with measles leukoencephalitis and early degeneration of cochlear and cochlear neuronal structures with preservation of the vestibular elements would support this concept. The formation of cochlear and vestibular fibrous tissue and new bone formation would suggest that the accompanying inflammatory reaction that occurs in association with acute measles infection or possibly as the result of secondary systemic exposure with an amnestic inflammatory response is a significant component of the underlying pathology and perhaps critical to the resultant auditory and vestibular dysfunction.

Although the association between unilateral profound sensorineural hearing loss and mumps infection has not been rigorously established, the histopathology of reported cases with involvement of the endolymphatic duct and sac, the report of delayed contralateral hydrops in a case of presumed unilateral deafness from mumps, and the association between mumps antibodies and sudden hearing loss raise speculation regarding the role of this virus in the development of other forms of inner-ear pathology.

A feature common to both measles and mumps infection that may be relevant to the resultant otopathology is that both viruses result in a high incidence of clinical and subclinical central nervous system involvement. Since it is well established that CSF and perilymph freely communicate with one another, this portal of entry may represent one mechanism by which the virus gains entry to the inner ear. If the virus is then processed by established inner-ear immune mechanisms, with or without labyrinthine infection, the inner ear would then be poised to respond to future challenges with the potential for delayed cochlear and vestibular manifestations. Whether or not secondary systemic challenges with viruses that have been previously processed by inner-ear immune mechanism are capable of resulting in an amnestic response with resultant inner-ear dysfunction and pathology has yet to be determined. If so, this may prove to be a valuable model in understanding the pathogenesis of Ménière's disease, sudden hearing loss, and some forms of immune-mediated inner-ear disorders.

REFERENCES

1. KEITHLEY, E. M. & J. P. HARRIS. 1996. Late sequelae of cochlear infection. Laryngoscope **106:** 341–345.
2. HARRIS, J. P., J. T. FAN & E. M. KEITHLEY. 1990. Immunologic responses in experimental cytomegalovirus labyrinthitis. Am. J. Otolaryngol. **11:** 304–308.
3. WOOLF, N. K. & J. P. HARRIS. 1986. Cochlear pathophysiology associated with inner ear immune responses. Acta Otolaryngol. (Stockholm) **102:** 353–364.
4. OJALA, A. 1947. On changes in the cerebrospinal fluid in measles. Ann. Med. Intern. Fenn. **35:** 321–331.
5. GIBBS, F. A., E. L. GIBBS, P. L. CARPENTER & H. W. SPIES. 1959. Electroencephalographic abnormalities in "uncomplicated" childhood diseases. JAMA **71:** 1050–1055.
6. HORTA-BARBOSA, L., D. A. FUCCILLO, W. T. LONDON, J. T. JABOUR, W. ZEMAN & J. L. SEVER. 1969. Isolation of measles virus from brain cell cultures of two patients with subacute sclerosing panencephalitis. Proc. Soc. Exp. Biol. Med. **132:** 272–277.

7. SHAMBAUGH, G. E., E. W. HAGENS, J. W. HOLDERMAN & R. W. WATKINS. 1928. Statistical studies of children in the public schools for the deaf. Arch. Otolaryngol. **7:** 424–513.

8. YEARSLEY, M. 1935. An analysis of over four thousand cases of educational deafness studied during the past twenty-five years. Br. J. Child. Dis. **31:** 177–192.

9. GOODMAN, A. I. 1949. Residual capacity to hear of pupils in schools for the deaf. J. Laryngol. Otol. **63:** 551–579.

10. SIMPSON, R. R. 1949. The causes of perceptive deafness. Proc. Roy. Soc. Med. **42:** 536–539.

11. BORDLEY, J. E. 1952. The problem of the preschool deaf child. (Diagnostic methods and the otologist's role in his rehabilitation.) Laryngoscope **62:** 514–520.

12. KINNEY, C. E. 1953. Hearing impairments in children. Laryngoscope **63:** 220–226.

13. WRIGHT, D. O. & B. LEIGH. 1995. The impact of the expanded programme on immunisation on measles-induced sensorineural hearing loss in the western area of Sierra Leone. West. Afr. J. Med. **14:** 205–209.

14. STEWART, B. J. & P. U. PRABHU. 1993. Reports of sensorineural deafness after measles, mumps and rubella immunisation. Arch. Dis. Child. **69:** 153–154.

15. SCHUKNECHT, H. F. 1993. Pathology of the Ear, 2nd ed. Lea & Febiger. Philadelphia.

16. VAN DISHOECK, H. A. E. & T. A. BIERMAN. 1957. Sudden perceptive deafness and viral infection. Ann. Otol. Rhinol. Laryngol. **66:** 963–980.

17. SAUNDERS, W. H. & W. H. LIPPY. 1959. Sudden deafness and Bell's palsy: A common cause. Ann. Otol. Rhinol. Laryngol. **68:** 830–837.

18. LINDSAY, J. R., P. R. DAVEY & P. H. WARD. 1960. Inner ear pathology in deafness due to mumps. Ann. Otol. Rhinol. Laryngol. **69:** 918–935

19. TANAKA, K., S. FUKUDA, T. SUENAGA & Y. TERAYAMA. 1988. Experimental mumps virus induced labyrinthitis. Immunohistochemical and ultrastructural studies. Acta Otolaryngol. (Stockholm) **456**(Suppl.): 98–105.

20. YAMAMOTO, M., Y. WATANABE & K. MIZUKOSHI. 1993. Neurotological findings in patients with acute mumps deafness. Acta Otolaryngol (Stockholm) **504**(Suppl.): 94–97.

21. SCHUKNECHT, H. F., Y. SUZUKA & C. ZIMMERMANN. 1990. Delayed endolymphatic hydrops and its relationship to Ménière's disease. Ann. Otol. Rhinol. Laryngol. **99:** 843–853.

Ménière's Disease and Autoimmunity

ROBERTO FILIPO, PATRIZIA MANCINI,[a] AND GABRIELE NOSTRO

Otolaryngology Department
University "La Sapienza"
Viale del Policlinico
00185 Rome, Italy

INTRODUCTION

Identifying the etiopathogenesis of Ménière's disease (MD) has been the object of several studies since Prosper Ménière first described the main symptoms of this disease in 1861: fluctuating hearing loss, vertigo, and tinnitus. Endolymphatic hydrops is considered the main pathological finding associated with MD and a good deal of research has been directed toward the identification and understanding of its underlying mechanisms. Because the sensory neural elements of the inner ear cannot be visualized in their diseased state *in vivo,* diagnosis of MD has been based mainly on the evaluation of the clinical symptoms and results of audiological tests. Since Rask-Andersen and Stahle[1] first recognized the inner ear as having an immunological function, several authors have added their support to the idea of a multifactorial origin by hypothesizing a possible role of the immunological system in MD pathogenesis. In fact, in 1983 Shea described the possible role of autoimmune mechanisms in patients with typical MD who responded favorably to steroid treatment or plasmapheresis.[2] Immunohistochemical studies also revealed the presence of an immunological reaction within the inner-ear tissues, such as stria vascularis, supporting connective tissues and blood vessels, in only a small number of patients investigated.[3–5] Although these studies are certainly affected by technical problems mainly linked to tissue preservation and processing, they are still suggestive of the idea that certain types of MD are caused by immunological factors of the inner ear. Immune inner-ear disease is a comparatively new area of clinical research, and over time different immunological reactions have been recognized and this has led to the introduction of several laboratory tests in the clinical evaluation of these patients.

The pathogenetic mechanisms underlying inner-ear disorders seem to be mainly due to either type 2 cytotoxic interaction of autoantibodies with tissue-bond antigen or a type-3 IgG- and IgM-mediated reaction that creates circulating immune complexes. The generic mechanism inducing tissue damage is a specific T-cell clonal expansion, specific autoantibody formation, complement cascade activation with inflammatory cell recruitment. Inner-ear damage and the resultant symptoms could depend upon the type of antigen and tissues as well as the anatomical site involved in the inflammatory reaction, which could be critical in determining endolymphatic hydrops. One of the main issues is the factor that triggers a T- and B-lymphocytes reaction and the production of autoantibodies against inner-ear structure in patients with

[a]Author for correspondence: Phone: 39-6-445-4607; fax: 39-6-445-4864.

idiopathic MD. One possibility is the modification or increased exposure of inner-ear protein induced by aging processes or by infectious agents and inflammatory processes, or molecular mimicry with antigens expressed by infectious agents similar to those found in the normal human inner ear.[6] However, the identification of the specific antigen or antigens responsible for MD pathogenesis is still controversial.

Autoimmune diseases affecting the inner ear might be the result of an organ-specific reaction or be one of the targets in a systemic disorder. To establish an organ-specific disorder, a cell-mediated or humoral response against the tissue-specific antigen must be proved. In 1955 Witebsky *et al.*, after their studies on chronic thyroiditis, wrote:

> ... certain criteria ideally should be fulfilled in order to prove the role of an autoantibody in the pathogenesis of a particular disease, namely, (1) the direct demonstration of free, circulating antibodies that are active at body temperature or of cell-bound antibodies by indirect means; (2) the recognition of the specific antigen against which this antibody is directed; (3) the production of antibodies against the same antigen in experimental animals; (4) the appearance of pathological changes in the corresponding tissues of an actively sensitized experimental animal that are basically similar to those in the human disease.[7]

Witebsky *et al.*'s original concept was recently reevaluated on the basis of molecular and cellular biology findings on immune responses and autoimmunity. The revised criteria for autoimmune disease (AD) were published by Rose and Bona,[8] who proposed three types of evidence to establish that a human disease is actually autoimmune in origin: (1) direct proof; (2) indirect evidence; (3) circumstantial evidence. The direct proof is the most straightforward evidence for autoimmune etiology of a human disease, and is the ability to reproduce the disease in a normal animal model by direct transfer of autoantibody or autoantigen-specific T cells. Direct evidence of MD autoimmune etiology has not been found. Nevertheless some indirect evidence has been investigated by creating animal models of autoimmunity against eterologous and homologous inner-ear antigen.

A reliable animal model has not yet been established although many attempts have been made since the first animal model was developed by Yoo and coauthors using bovine type II collagen to induce endolymphatic hydrops. Although these authors report several inner-ear changes coinciding with progressive sensorineural hearing loss, only 50% of the animals showed endolymphatic hydrops.[9,10] The validity of this model was questioned by Harris and coauthors, who were unable to reproduce Yoo *et al.*'s results.[11] In later studies systemic and endolymphatic administration of autologous inner-ear antigen and keyhole limpet hemocyanin[12–14] were used to induce sensorineural hearing loss (SNHL) and endolymphatic hydrops. As in previous studies, these results strongly suggest that the inner ear is able to produce an immune response to either systemic or local antigenic challenge. Nevertheless, all animal models have an insufficient correlation between histopathological findings and antibody titers, and even if a wide range of histopathological correlates has been found, endolymphatic hydrops is an inconsistent finding, and many significant inner-ear structures (i.e., organ of Corti) remained unaffected.

Most of our knowledge of possible autoimmune etiology of MD comes from circumstantial evidence and clinical observations such as: (1) association with other AD in the same individual or the same family; (2) infiltration of target organ by lymphocytes; (3) statistical association with a particular MHC haplotype or aberrant expression of MHC class II antigens on the affected organ; (4) favorable response to immunosuppressive therapy.[8] Clinical evidence of autoimmune inner-ear disease was researched over time by many authors using laboratory tests available at the time of the investigations, such as evaluation of circulating immune complexes, IgE titer for type I allergies, lymphocyte transformation test, and Western blot immunoassay.

Circulating immune complexes (CIC) occur when a circulating or local antigen binds to its specific antibody. Although large-size complexes are rapidly removed, small-size complexes remain in circulation for a long time, which results in deposits in many tissues, thus inducing complement fixation, inflammatory process activation, and tissue damage. As in the case of kidney glomeruli in the systemic circulation, the stria vascularis and the endolymphatic sac are the main site of investigation for CIC deposits within the inner ear,[15] and are mainly due to similarities existing between the stria and glomerular capillaries in ultrastructure and physiology function. Elevated levels of CIC have been reported in MD patients, ranging from 32% to more than 50%,[16,17] and its level is higher in MD patients compared to normal controls.[18] A type 1 reaction has also been investigated because of the frequently referred association between food intake and allergy to inhalant allergens by MD patients that seems to increase or trigger their symptoms. Results obtained on total serum IgE titer, skin tests, and subcutaneous food test showed that there is no significant statistical association between type 1 reaction and MD symptoms, leading to the conclusion that type 1 reaction might play a secondary role in MD, by releasing inflammatory mediators into the blood stream.[17,19,20]

Expression of specific HLA genes is a characteristic, which together with positive family history and a tendency to acquire other autoimmune systemic disorders, is considered to be common in many autoimmune disorders. When expression of HLA antigens has been evaluated in MD patients, a correlation with the CW7 antigen was found in 65 to 75% of patients with MD,[21,22] while in a study carried out in the Japanese population, a higher expression of CW4 and DR2 antigen has been found.[23] Although data obtained from the peripheral immune status are highly suggestive of immune reaction against the inner ear, they still might not reflect the local situation since the inner ear is capable of local immune regulation,[1] and we might be in the presence of an organ-specific reaction. More information on local immune status come from laboratory tests that employ inner-ear antigen as a substrate to evaluate both lymphocyte T and B activation. Lymphocyte migration and transformation tests were used by Hughes and coauthors[24–26] to diagnose MD of autoimmune origin in which they first used as a substrate fresh human inner-ear antigen obtained from labyrinthine surgery as a screening for autoimmune reaction in the inner ear. The authors published several reports claiming that a positive test had a predictive value of approximately 70%, although the main criterion for evaluation is the patient's response to immunosuppressive therapy.

The most recent and widely used laboratory test to investigate autoimmune inner-ear diseases is Western blot immunoassay, in an attempt to show evidence of specific antibodies against homologous and eterologous proteins of the inner ear identified by molecular-weight determination. Since Yoo *et al.*[27] first pointed out that the levels of Ab to type II collagen were significantly higher in a population of patients with MD and otosclerosis, Western blot immunoassay has been carried out on serum of patients with MD and other forms of SNHL. Using fresh homologous inner-ear proteins, antibodies against type II and also type IX collagen were found positive in 50–60% of patients, together with a nonidentified 30-kDa inner-ear protein.[28] Harris and coauthors were the first to use fresh bovine inner-ear antigen to determine the reactivity of patients suffering from MD and other forms of SNHL.[29,30] In their results, 30% of MD patients showed a band in the region of 68-kDa molecular weight, while 22% had a protein band in the region of 33–35-kDa molecular weight. Their results were confirmed by Rauch *et al.*[31] who found 46.7% of MD patients positive with a 68–70-kDa band. Although a greater prevalence of bilateral MD was found, they could identify no characteristics of the hearing loss or vestibular symptoms that correlated with serologic status.[31] By using guinea pig antigen, Cao and coauthors identified 50% of MD patients with bands ranging from 30 to 58 kDa.[32,33] Distribution of the inner-ear protein bands was different in the various regions of the inner ear, although MD patients showed a prevalent distribution in the 30-kDa molecular-weight range. Veldman and coauthors, by employing swine inner-ear antigen, did not confirm previous findings, and reported the presence of antibodies reactive against several antigens ranging from 27 to 80 kDa.[34]

We have established a research protocol for the study of autoimmune mechanisms in patients with MD, involving the use of Western blot immunoassay and the study of patients' response to immunosuppressive therapy.

MATERIALS AND METHOD

Twenty-five patients (18 female and 7 male, average age 45 yr) were diagnosed as having Ménière's disease according to the criteria of the 1995 AAO-HNS, and were included in our study protocol. Diagnosis was based on clinical manifestation and audiometric data. All patients had unilateral or bilateral HL, and had experienced fluctuation of hearing, although this was not necessarily present at the time they were included in the protocol. Transtympanic electrochochleografy test (ECochG) was carried out to investigate the presence of endolymphatic hydrops, using Click stimuli to study the AP/SP ratio. The AP/SP ratio was considered to be positive when equal or greater than 0.51% (3 standard deviation from the average). All patients were treated with steroid therapy consisting in 1 mg/kg prednisone daily for 30 days and then decreased to a maintenance therapy of 10 mg given every other day.[26] The audiometric pure tone average (500–1000–2000) was compared pre- and posttreatment, and a difference greater than 10 dB was considered to be significant. Western blot immunoassay on patients' serum was carried out to investigate the presence of autoantibodies against inner-ear proteins. Vestibular tissue dissected during labyrinthine surgery was fresh frozen and treated for standard electrophoresis in 10% SDS polyacrylamide gel and transferred to nitrocellulose paper and followed standard immunoblotting with a primary reaction against patient serum followed by goat antihuman IgG (G-specific) alkaline phosphatase conjugate secondary antibody and color reaction. Patients' serum was run together with a wide range of multicolor standard to evaluate band weight.

RESULTS AND DISCUSSION

Only 15 (60%) of the patients who underwent this study responded to steroid therapy. Twenty (80%) of them showed positive ECochG findings, but response to treatment was also found in those patients not showing endolymphatic hydrops. The Western blot immunoassay was positive in only five (20%), three of whom showed positive ECochG findings. Analysis of western blot results revealed a predominance of low kDa bands of 32 and 46 kDa in four patients, whereas only one patient showed a band ranging from 60 kDa to 70 kDa. Our results seem to differ from those obtained by Harris and coauthors,[29,30] for the low incidence of the 68-kDa band found in the serum of our MD patients. On the contrary, a higher incidence of low molecular weight ranging from 30 kDa to 35 kDa has already been described in studies where human inner-ear antigen was used.[28] Although eterologous antigen has been proved to yield results comparable with homologous antigen,[35] still not all inner-ear proteins are preserved across species, and a simple aminoacid change in antigen epitope might affect antibody recognition. The variability of results could therefore depend upon both tissue processing and protein extraction, and on multiple sources of inner-ear antigen used by different authors. In general, allogenic human inner-ear tissues should be a more suitable source of antigen. Limitation in its use derives from the scarce sources of fresh antigen, often exclusive of vestibular tissues. In fact, fresh human antigen is usually obtained from translabyrinthine surgery, consisting of neural and vestibular tissues lacking in cochlear components. Differences in Western blot results might therefore depend upon the lack of cochlear protein, and therefore the 68–70-kDa protein might reflect a more specific cochlear damage. In our opinion it is unclear whether the 68 kDa along with other proteins detected by Western blot analysis are a cause of organ specific damage or simply an epiphenomenon of inner-ear injury. Hence , further trials will need to be carried out in order to identify these proteins, to confirm the validity of Western blot assay procedures as test for the identification of autoimmune etiology in MD and other forms of SNHL.

REFERENCES

1. Rask-Andersen, H. & J. Stahle. 1980. Immunodeficence of the inner ear?: Lymphocyte-macrophage interaction in the endolymphatic sac. Acta Otolayrgol. (Stockholm) **89:** 283–294.
2. Shea, J. J. 1983. Autoimmune sensorineural hearing loss as aggravating factor in Ménière's disease: A preliminary report. Laryngoscope **93:** 410–7.
3. Wei, N. R., J. Helms & W. Giebel. 1990. Immunochemical findings in the vestibular ganglion from patient with Ménière's disease. Eur. Arch. Otolaryngol. **247:** 340–34.
4. Yazawa, Y. & M. Kitahara. 1989. Immunofluorescent study of the endolymphatic sac in Ménière's disease. Acta Otolaryngol. (Stockholm) **468**(Suppl.): 71–76.
5. Arnold, W., R. Pfaltz & H. J. Altermatt. 1985. Evidence of serum antibodies against in-

ner ear tissues in the blood of patients with certain sensorineural hearing disorders. Acta Otolaryngol. (Stockholm) **99**: 437–444.

6. RUCKENSTAIN, M. J. & R. V. HARRISON. 1991. Autoimmune inner ear disease: A review of basic mechanisms and clinical correlates. J. Otolaryngol. **20**: 196–202.

7. WITEBSKY, E., N. R. ROSE & S. SHULMAN. 1955. Studies on organ specificity: I Serological specificity of thyroid extracts. J. Immunol. **75**: 269–281.

8. ROSE, N. R. & C. BONA. 1993. Defining criteria for autoimmune diseases (Witebsky's postulates revisited). Immunol. Today **9**: 426–429.

9. YOO, T. J., Y. YAZAWA, K. TOMODA & R. FLOYD. 1983. Type II collagen-induced autoimmune endolymphatic hydrops in guinea pig. Science **222**: 65–67.

10. YOO, T. J., K. TOMODA, J. M. STUART , M. A. CREMER, A. S. TOWNES & A. H. KANG. 1983. Type II collagen-induced autoimmune sensorineural hearing loss and vestibular dysfunction in rats. Ann. Otol. Rhinol. Laryngol. **92**: 267–71.

11. HARRIS, J. P., N. K. WOOLF & A. F. RYAN. 1986. A reexamination of experimental type II collagen autoimmunity: Middle and inner ear morphology and function. Ann. Otol. Rhinol. Laryngol. **95**: 176–180.

12. HARRIS, J. P. 1983. Immunology of the inner ear: Response of the inner ear to antigenic challenge. Otolaryngol. Head Neck Surg. **91**: 18–23.

13. HARRIS, J. P., N. K. WOOLF & A. F. RYAN. 1985. Elaboration of systemic immunity following inner ear immunization. Am. J. Otolaryngol. **6**: 148–152.

14. TOMIYAMA, S. 1992. Endolymphatic hydrops induced by immune response of the endolymphatic sac: Relation to perilymph antibody levels. Ann. Otol. Rhinol. Laryngol. **101**: 48–53.

15. HARADA, T., T. MATSUNAGA, K. HONG & K. INOUE. 1984. Endolymphatic hydrops and type III allergic reaction. Acta Otolaryngol. (Stockholm) **97**: 450–459.

16. BROOKES, G. B. 1986. Circulating immune complexes in Ménière's disease. Arch. Otolaryngol. **112**: 536–540.

17. HSU, L., X. N. ZHU & Y. S. ZHAO. 1990. Immunoglobulin and circulating immune complexes in endolymphatic hydrops. Ann. Otol. Laryngol. **99**: 535–538.

18. YOSHINO, K., T. OHASHI, T. URUSHIBATA, M. KENMOCHI & M. AKAGI. 1996. Antibodies to type II collagen and immune complexes in Ménière's disease. Acta Otolaryngol. (Stockholm) **522**(Suppl.): 79–85.

19. DEREBERY, M. J. & S. VALENZUELA. 1992 Ménière's syndrome and allergy. Otolarygol. Clin. North Am. **25**(1):213–224.

20. STAHLE, J., H. DEUSCHL & S. G. JOANSSON. 1974. Ménière's disease and allergy, with special reference to immunoglobuline E and IgE antibody in serum. Int. J. Equil. Res. **4**: 22–27.

21. EVANS, K. L., D. L. BALDWIN, D. BAINBRIDGE & A. W. MORRISON. 1988. Immune status in patients with Ménière's disease. Arch. Otolaryngol. **245**: 287–292.

22. XENELLIS J., A. W. MORRISON, D. MCCLOWSKEY, H. FESTENSTEÍN & F. R. C. PATH. 1986. HLA antigens in pathogenesis of Ménière's disease. J. Laryngol. Otol. **100**: 21–24.

23. KOYAMA, S., Y. MITSUISHI, P. I. TERASAKI & I. WATANABE. 1993. HLA in patients with Ménière's disease. *In* Ménière's Disease: Perspectives in the 90's, Proc. 3rd Int. Symp. on Ménière's Disease, Vol. 1, R. Filipo and M. Barbara, Eds.: 85–87. Kugler. Amsterdam/New York.

24. HUGHES, G. B., B. P. BARNA, S. E. KINNEY & L. H. CALABRESE. 1983. Autoimmune reactivity in Ménière's disease: A preliminary report. Laryngoscope **93**: 410–417.

25. HUGHES, G. B., B. P. BARNA, S. E. KINNEY, L. H. CALABRESE & N. J. NALEPA. 1988. Clinical diagnosis of immune inner ear disease. Laryngoscope **98**: 251–253.

26. HUGHES, G. B., R. L. FAIRCHILD & P. BARNA. 1994. Laboratory diagnosis of immune inner ear disease. Immunobiology in Otorhinolaryngology—Progress of a Decade. Proc. 4th

Int. Academic Conf. Vol. 1, G. Mogi, J. E. Veldman, and H. Kawauchi, Eds.: 231–235. Kugler. Amsterdam/New York.

27. Yoo, T. J., J. M. Stuart, A. H. Kang, A. S. Townes, K. Tomoda & S. Dixit. 1982. Type II collagen autoimmunity in otosclerosis and Ménière's disease. Science **217:** 1153–1155.

28. Joliat, T., J. Seyer, J. Bernstain, M. Krug, X. J. Ye, J. S. Cho, T. Fujiyoshi & T. J. Yoo. 1992. Antibodies against a 30 kilodalton cochlear protein and type II and IX collagens in the serum of patients with inner ear diseases. Ann. Otol. Rhinol. Laryngol. **101:** 1000–1006.

29. Harris, J. P. & P. A. Sharp. 1990. Inner ear autoantibodies in patients with rapidly progressive sensorineural hearing loss. Laryngoscope **100:** 516–524.

30. Gottschlich, S., P. B. Billings, E. M. Keithley, M. H. Weisman & J. P. Harris. 1995. Assessment of serum antibodies in patients with rapidly progressive sensorineural hearing loss and Ménière's disease. Laryngoscope **105:** 1347–1352.

31. Rauch, S. D., J. E. san Martin, R. A. Moscicki & K. J. Bloch. 1995. Serum antibodies against heat shock protein 70 in Meniere's disease. Am. J. Otol. **16:** 648–652.

32. Cao, M. Y., N. Deggouj, M. Gersdorff & J. P. Tomasi. 1996. Guinea pig inner ear antigens: Extraction and application to the study of human autoimmune inner ear disease. Laryngoscope **106:** 207–212.

33. Cao, M. Y., J. P. Tomasi, M. Gersdorff & N. Deggouj. 1994. Detection of guinea pig inner ear antigens by sera from patients with inner ear disease. Immunobiology in Otorhinolaryngology—Progress of a Decade. Proc. 4th Int. Academic Conf., G. Mogi, J. E. Veldman, and H. Kawauchi, Eds.: 263–268. Kugler. Amsterdam/New York.

34. Veldman , J. E., T. Hanada & F. Meeuwsen. 1993. Diagnostic and therapeutic dilemmas in rapidly progressive hearing loss. Acta Otolaryngol. **113:** 303–306.

35. Yamanobe S. & J. P. Harris. 1993. Extraction of inner ear antigens for studies in inner ear autoimmunity. Ann. Otol. Rhinol. Laryngol. **102:** 22–27.

Viral Theory for Ménière's Disease and Endolymphatic Hydrops: Overview and New Therapeutic Options for Viral Labyrinthitis

I. KAUFMAN ARENBERG,[a,d] CHRISTINE LEMKE,[b]
AND GEORGE E. SHAMBAUGH, JR.[c]

[a]International Meniere's Disease Research Institute
300 East Hampden Avenue, Suite 400
Englewood, Colorado 80110

[b]Hanover, Germany

[c]Hinsdale, IL

In six cases of Meniere's disease, the sac wall was definitely fibrotic and ischemic and the epithelium either absent or markedly altered. There was partial or complete obliteration of the lumen in every case. In cases where the duct was not seen by polytomography, the epithelium was usually absent in the sac. Since none of these patients had a history of suppurative otitis media or mastoiditis, the most likely etiology for the changes observed is an old viral labyrinthitis affecting especially or perhaps primarily the duct and sac, destroying or markedly impairing the normal resorption of endolymph.

—GEORGE E. SHAMBAUGH AND I. KAUFMAN ARENBERG

OVERVIEW OF MÉNIÈRE'S DISEASE AND ANY INNER-EAR DYSFUNCTION

Ménière's disease is not one disease, but the clinical manifestation to various degrees of everything that can go wrong with the inner-ear hearing and balance mechanism. It is, in its classic form, a progressive end stage inner-ear disease. If we think of the inner ear "black box" as a little kidney, Ménière's disease would be analogous to end-stage renal disease, which requires dialysis and/or transplantation. Ménière's disease and endolymphatic hydrops are also analogous to glaucoma and increased intraocular pressure. Control and regulation of the fluid hydrodynamics and the pres-

[d]Address for correspondence: 7995 East Prentice Ave., Suite 110, Greenwood Village, CO 80111. Phone: 303/850-0670; fax: 303/850-0671; e-mail: 76513.2007@compuserve.com

sure within these two exquisitely sensitive neuroepithelial peripheral sense organs is critical to normal function.

We will review in detail and update the Shambaugh–Arenberg theory of the viral etiopathogenesis of Ménière's disease first presented in 1969[1] and based on clinical experience and light microscopic histopathologic analysis of endolymphatic sac biopsies taken from patients at acoustic neuroma surgery or for perilymph fistula[2] and compared to normal ELS.[3]

BASIC CLINICAL CONCEPT OF SHAMBAUGH–ARENBERG VIRAL THEORY OF MÉNIÈRE'S DISEASE

Viral labyrinthitis or viral inner-ear infection is probably the most common and often made clinical diagnosis for the first episodes of apparent inner-ear dysfunction either auditory or vestibular or both. This diagnosis of viral labyrinthitis is very often used not only by the ENT doctor, but also by the emergency room doctor, the family physician, and the internist. It would be extremely rare today for this diagnosis to be made rigorously to confirm the likely clinical suspicion of a viral labyrinthitis and associated inflammatory-immune response by serology, cultures, immuno-histopathology, or ultrastructural means in order to fulfill Koch's postulates. This approach has not been practical, and until recently, there were no specific drug treatments for viral diseases.

The basic theory is that a virus or its immunologic equivalent, ototropic in nature, gets into the inner ear most likely either across the round-window membrane or hematogenously. This can occur concurrently with an upper-respiratory-type infection, with a middle-ear effusion, which would be the direct method to the inner ear by the round-window membrane. However, and probably more likely, the virus gets into the inner ear hematogenously without an apparent direct relationship to an obvious viral illness. In terms of clinical onset, there is probably an inoculation time interval to clinical manifestation of inner-ear symptoms of days to weeks or months. Thus the associated low-grade fever, malaise, and other nonspecific viral "flulike" symptoms that didn't materialize clinically is often forgotten and not connected to the temporally separate onset of the inner-ear symptoms. Thus, the inner-ear symptoms appear to have come out of nowhere. No obvious explanation. Once the virus gets into the inner ear, each different virus can attack and pathologically damage different areas or components of the inner ear with variable clinical manifestations and variable documented audiovestibular test abnormalities. These variations in clinical response can be related to the inoculating dose, the host immune status at the time, whether there is a concurrent viral or bacterial infection, and so forth. It also would make a difference if it was hematogenous and both inner ears were exposed, and differentially effected. (This could explain the long-term high incidence of Ménière's disease in the contralateral ear.) If it was from a middle-ear effusion across the round-window membrane, it may more likely be unilateral. These variations may help explain the very variable spectrum of clinical presentation of inner-ear disorders from unknown causes or presumed viral labyrinthitis. There are distinct advantages for just reporting exactly the clinical stages of involvements for each ear for hearing, tinnitus, pressure, vertigo, imbalance, and disability. This allows the clinician to go back to basics and clinical descriptive medicine. This is accomplished by reporting exactly what is seen clinically without a specific diagnosis.

The original theory suggested that the first episodes of vertigo and hearing loss were directly from the virus and its inflammatory-immune and microvascular effects on the inner ear. That is why, often, the first so-called attack of Ménière's disease is the worst and that subsequent attacks rarely equal the first attacks in severity and the fear the attacks provoke. Subsequent attacks are not due to active, persistent viruses (although recurrent reactivated virus is possible, particularly with HSV), but due to the damage to various structures such as the stria vascularis, dark cells within the vestibular labyrinth, and most likely the endolymphatic sac and endolymphatic duct, which are the primary filters for the inner-ear debris from the viral immune and inflammatory processes. Thus, the first episode of so-called "Ménière's disease," or "Ménière's Syndrome," or "Ménière's Symptom Complex" (in some undetermined percent of cases) was due to, and the clinical manifestations of, a viral labyrinthitis. The subsequent episodes and characteristic attacks of vertigo, and the progressive, fluctuating but often deteriorating sensorineural hearing loss is due to the actual histopathologic damage to various components of the inner-ear labyrinth and particularly the immunodefense system of the inner ear, primarily the endolymphatic sac and duct. This paper focuses on the endolymphatic sac as the immunodefense system of the inner ear and the ultrastructural pathologic evidence of viral immune inflammatory disease at various stages. The entire spectrum of these observed pathologic processes will be presented to further elucidate and support the original theory, which was based on only histopathologic data. There has been much progress in supporting the Shambaugh–Arenberg viral theory of Ménière's disease since 1969.

MRI IMAGING EVIDENCE

MRI imaging studies with gadolinium have shown focal enhancement of the labyrinth, either vestibular, auditory, or both.[4] This enhancement strongly suggests a focal or localized inflammatory vascular response. This has been correlated in some cases with the clinical diagnosis of viral labyrinthitis.[5–7] Alternatively, there are MRI studies that show enhancement of only the eighth nerve or its components.[8] Thus radiologically you can clinically diagnose vestibular neuronitis (involving the eighth nerve). This would have direct clinical treatment algorhythm implications. Direct drug delivery of steroids to round-window membrane/inner ear would be expected to be efficacious if only the cochlear and/or vestibular labyrinth shows enhancement.

There may be no direct benefit to the eighth nerve from direct drug delivery to the inner ear when only the eighth nerve involvement is demonstrated on enhanced imaging studies., If there is a combined disorder of the labyrinth and the eighth nerve, enhanced MRI would also show this as well the status of the opposite ear. Without MRI, it would be otherwise clinically difficult if not impossible to localize specifically the site of viral immune inflammatory vascular response as current audiovestibular differential site specific testing, for specificity or sensitivity cannot approach the reliability of a positive MRI finding. We should focus attention on the time correlation and frequency of MRI findings and changes, present or not, with onset of symptoms, viral history, low-grade fever, malaise, and so on, as well as inner-ear symptoms. This should be correlated with serial audiovestibular tests, and specifically with electrocochleography (ECoG) to determine the presence or absence of endolymphatic hydrops as demonstrated by enhanced summating potential and basilar membrane distortion. This will help to pinpoint the clinical symptoms with the MRI findings (positive or negative) and the the time course of clinical change and evolution of the audiovestibular and electrophysiologic changes. If there is a combined inner-ear and eighth-nerve inflammation, as seen on MRI in some cases, this might explain the increased success of direct drug delivery to the inner ear combined with systemic steroids. MRI information on site, and the presence or abscence or evolution of enhancement, can help tailor the treatment to the specific pathologic site and confirm generally the underlying pathology.

EPIDEMIOLOGIC EVIDENCE

This concept of a virus being the otopathologic agent in inner-ear disorder as a direct result of an ototropic virus, although not new, received a major boost when the Centers for Disease Control and Prevention (CDC) sent two Epidemic Intelligence Service (EIS) agents to analyze an epidemic outbreak of vertigo in Thermaopolis, Wyoming, in 1992.[9] Although the actual numbers were small, if the outbreak in Thermopolis was extrapolated to the U.S. population for the same six-month period, about 2.5 million Americans would have clinically developed epidemic vertigo, and other associated inner-ear problems. The CDC authors and consultants concluded from their studies that the cause was most likely an enterovirus that was ototropic, after they ruled out all other explanations for the epidemic of vertigo. This was the first study using accepted epidemiologic and statistical methods to prospectively demonstrate a specific viral etiology for viral labyrinthitis using concurrent case-control group analysis. This patient group is now being followed prospectively and longitudinally to determine the incidence and scope of any future inner-ear symptoms and/or the development of clinical Ménière's disease.

PATHOLOGY

There is temporal bone histopathology confirmation of ototropic virus attacking the labyrinth as well as the eighth nerve or both the labyrinth and the eighth nerve. There is serologic and viral culture evidence for a host of ototropic viruses, particularly in fetus and newborn material for CMV, HSV, as well as rubella, and so on. The endolymphatic sac as the main immune defense component of the inner ear is now well accepted. The pathology of the ELS in humans with Ménière's disease, at the light and ultrastructural level, is not as well appreciated. The reader is referred to the original studies and illustrations at the light microscopic level,[1–3] as well as the ultrastructural level.[10–12] The entire spectrum of the pathology from almost normal ELS to end-stage inner-ear disease suggests a role for a virus as the causative factor in some of the cases.[13] The demonstrated spectrum ranges from patients with a congenitally/developmentally small ELS without notable fibrosis or evidence of epithelial damage to end-stage inner-ear disease in which there is no recognizable or functional epithelium. There is also an extensive disarray of perisaccular fibrosis and almost complete abscence of a microvascular system.[10] A summary of the evidence of a viral etiology or possible cause for the observed ultrastructural changes, including thickened basement membrane, loss of epithelial integrity, presence of nuclear bodies, as well as possible viruslike particles has been elaborated.[10]

Evidence of a viral genome within the ELS of patients with ELH and Ménière's disease is an important missing link in this viral theory for Ménière's disease. Recently we investigated the occurrence of human cytomegalovirus (CMV) by polymerase chain reaction (PCR) in the endolymphatic sac (ELS) tissues of patients with inner-ear disorders, Ménière's disease, and endolymphatic hydrops (ELH) compared to a control group of ELS from patients with acoustic neuroma. ELS biopsies obtained from patients during surgery were analyzed for the presence of CMV genome by PCR utilizing primers specific for human CMV-DNA. ELS tissues were obtained from nine Ménière's disease/syndrome patients. All patients with this diagnosis had abnormal ECoG consistent with the diagnosis of ELH. All nine inner-ear disease patients were seropositive for CMV antibodies. ELS tissue samples were positive for CMV deoxyribonucleic acid (DNA) by PCR in seven of the nine ELH patients (77.8%). All of the controls with only primary eighth-nerve pathology were negative by PCR amplification for CMV-DNA. The clinical significance of the presence of CMV in the ELS of patients with various subgroups of Ménière's disease and ELH and not in the control group is not yet known. However, these data indicate that a significant number of Ménière's disease patients may harbor CMV in a latent but persistently infected state within the ELS. The CMV infection may promote the development of ELH and subsequently Ménière's disease. However, the role of CMV or other ototropic viruses, possibly interacting with inner-ear immune system, remains intriguing, but speculative.

TREATMENT OPTIONS FOR VIRAL LABYRINTHITIS

Currently, end-stage Ménière's disease and endolymphatic hydrops is treated many years after its onset with expensive, destructive surgery such as vestibular nerve section (VNS) (roughly $20,000–$40,000) or labyrinthectomy (roughly $7000–$20,000). Nondestructive inner-ear surgery, such as any one of many variations of endolymphatic sac surgery with or without intraoperative ECoG monitoring is still expensive (roughly $7000–$20,000) and is rarely performed early in the course of the disease. Rather, it is performed primarily for end-stage inner-ear disorders. Most recently, a destructive vestibular chemical labyrinthectomy with aminoglycosides has started to gain favor internationally. It is the least expensive (roughly $1000–$4000) and minimally invasive therapeutic option available. It is also done for end-stage inner-ear disease, but has an unacceptably high incidence of drug/dose-related hearing loss. Recently, Nedzelski reported a rate of hearing loss, as high as 42–52%, depending on whether the patient had serviceable or nonserviceable hearing at the onset of treatment.[13]

Direct drug delivery to the round-window membrane by transtympanic injection needle, with or without a vent tube, was first developed and used for aminoglycoside chemical labyrinthectomy perfusion of the inner ear (CPT code 68601). This is a very positive improvement in this, developing cost-effective management of minimally invasive therapeutic interventions for inner ear disease. The direct drug delivery of steroids to the round window membrane is nondestructive and therefore a significant improvement. Steroids are being used to treat Ménière's disease somewhat earlier in the course of the disease with good preliminary results.[14] It is also being used to treat sudden hearing loss, presumably of viral-immune etiology, as well as tinnitus and other manifestations of viral labyrinthitis. This application in the ongoing treatment of autoimmune inner-ear disease should be notable as well.[15] The advantages of direct application of steroids to the inner ear by the round-window membrane (RWM) to treat a variety of inner-ear clinical manifestations are obvious, since you essentially eliminate the significant side effects and complications of systemic steroids. Thus, you can intervene early, quickly, and maintain a high concentration of steroids in the inner-ear fluids. This opens the therapeutic window widely to intervene and treat, minimally invasively and cost effectively, a variety of inner-ear disorders that specifically respond to steroids. Many of the otherwise unexplained etiopathogenic mechanisms for inner-ear dysfunction are thought to be viral-immune in nature. Therein lies the future therapeutic goals and direction of almost all aspects and various pathologies of the inner ear.

In the acute phase, steroids are often given in short bursts, but an exact treatment regimen has not been established. In a recent study using Acyclovir, patients with a clinical diagnosis of acute disease (less than eight weeks since clinical onset) were treated with large doses. The patients were segregated into groups with a clinical history or manifestation of HSV infection. Preliminary, unpublished data suggest that these patients have a milder course and more rapid recovery with less sequelae. Valacyclovir and other new generation antivirals may be more specific. Concurrent treatment with a nerve growth factor (NGF) and steroids may better help protect neural components from the damaging effects of viral-immune and inflammatory insults before irreversible damage occurs. This type of direct drug delivery can occur via the transtympanic (shotgun) route with or without a vent tube in place. A new IV-like (bull's-eye) targeted system to the inner ear via the round-window membrane is now being used in animal studies, and may become a viable alternative. In the future, it will be important to be able to deliver drugs in a controlled microdosing protocol. It may be clinically beneficial to treat viral labyrinthitis with antiviral drugs like acyclovir on an individual basis. Additionally, diuretics such as atrial naturetic peptide (ANP) and urodilatin can be used to treat the resultant endolymphatic hydrops. Nerve growth factors could be given to protect hair cells and neurons, and to stimulate their regeneration.

Late-stage (after eight weeks) treatment could be similar but be less effective if irreversible inner-ear pathology and scarring have already occurred. It may be a better therapeutic plan to intervene early in the course of the disease to prevent damage as much as possible. Thus a minimally invasive, cost-effective, bull's-eye-targeted delivery of drugs direct to the inner ear early in the course of the inflammatory process may have a very beneficial effect. It could prevent irreversible damage to vital inner-ear structures and prevent long-term sequelae, such as full-blown Ménière's disease and endolymphatic hydrops. The damage may be mitigated and future reoccurrences minimized. It would be the same concept as treating strep throat and rheumatic fever early in the course of the disease with antibiotics to prevent the child from developing rheumatic fever. If the infection, inflammation-immune response is not treated early and adequately, irreversible pathologic changes occur in the heart valves, but may not show up clinically for many years. In the same way, a viral labyrinthitis untreated or inadequately treated can cause varying degrees of irreversible pathologic damage to certain key structures in the inner ear, as best assessed by changes in the endolymphatic sac and duct. The endolymphatic sac and duct are thought to show the most damage at the ultrastructural level because almost all viral inflammatory debris from an inner-ear infection is longitudinaly moved by the ELS/ELD for immunologic processing and phagocytosis. When the concentration of the inner-ear debris exceeds the ELS/ELD capacity for effective cleanup and damage control, then damage to the ELS epithelium and subepithelial connective-tissue matrix and microvascular systems occur; this results in loss or decreased ability of ELS to regulate inner-ear fluid hydrodynamics, volume, pressure, and distention. When untreated, these pathologic processes result in endolymphatic hydrops within the inner ear and clinically result in Ménière's disease many months or years later because of direct damage to the ELS, as speculated by Shambaugh and Arenberg in 1969.[1]

We think this is a common occurrence and that most cases of idiopathic Ménière's disease and endolymphatic hydrops are the result of untreated viral labyrinthitis. These idiopathic cases of Ménière's disease and endolymphatic hydrops, which can be presumed to be viral-immune mediated, can have a significant impact on healthcare dollars as well as cost to society in terms of lost productivity, wages, and so forth. The human cost to the quality of life of the individual patient can be huge. We advocate an open-minded, aggressive, proactive approach to treating all inner-ear disease early with drugs, specific for the underlying, etiopathogenetic mechanisms, such as viral labyrinthitis.

REFERENCES

1. SHAMBAUGH, G. E. & I. K. ARENBERG. 1969. The endolymphatic sac in Ménière's disease. *In* Proc. Centennial Symp. Manhattan Eye, Ear and Throat Hospital. Otolaryngology, Vol. 2, Sec. IV, Chap. 13, W. F. Robbett, Ed.: 105–119. Mosby. St. Louis.
2. SHAMBAUGH, G. E., J. D. CLEMIS & I. K. ARENBERG. 1969. Endolymphatic duct and sac in Ménière's disease: I. Surgical and histopathologic observations. Arch. Otolaryngol. **89:** 116–125.
3. ARENBERG, I. K., W. F. MAROVITZ & G. E. SHAMBAUGH. 1970. The role of the endolymphatic sac in the pathogenesis of the endolymphatic hydrops in man. Acta Otolaryngol. **275**(Suppl.): 1–49.
4. FITZGERALD, D. C. & A. S. MARK. 1996. Endolymphatic duct/sac enhancement on gadolinium magnetic resonance imaging of the inner ear: Preliminary observations and case reports. Am. J. Otol. **17:** 603–606.
5. SLETZER, S. & A. S. MARK. 1991. Constrast enhancement of the labyrinth on MR scans in patients with sudden hearing loss and vertigo: Evidence of labyrinthine disease. ANJR **12:** 13–16.
6. MARK, A. S., S. SELTZER & H. R. HARNSBERGER. 1993. Sensorineural hearing loss: More than meets the eye. ANJR **14:** 37–45.
7. WILSON, D. F., J. M. TALBOT & R. S. HODGSON. 1994. Magnetic resonance imaging-enhancing lesions of the labyrinth and facial nerve. Arch. Otolaryngol. Head Neck Surg. **120:** 560–564.

8. SELESNICK, S. H., R. K. JACKLER & L. W. PITTS. 1993. The changing clinical presentation of acoustic tumors in the MRI era. Laryngoscope **103:** 431–436.

9. SIMONSEN, L., A. S. KHAN, H. E. GARY, *et al.* 1996. Outbreak of vertigo in Wyoming: Possible role of an enterovirus infection. Epidemiol. Infect. **117:** 149–157.

10. ARENBERG, I. K., D. W. WALKER & G. E. SHAMBAUGH. 1991. The role of the endolymphatic sac and viruses in the pathogenisis of endolymphatic hydrops: An ultrastructural analysis of endolymphatic sac biopsies. *In* Surgery of the Ear, I. K. Arenberg, Ed.: 31–52. Kugler. Amsterdam.

11. ARENBERG, I. K., D. H. NORBACK & G. E. SHAMBAUGH. 1982. Ultrastrucural analysis of endolymphatic sac biopsies: I. The biopsy technique and identification of the endolymphatic sac. Arch. Otolaryngol. **108:** 292–298.

12. ARENBERG, I. K., D. H. NORBACK & G. E. SHAMBAUGH. 1985. Distribution and density of subepithelial collagen in the endolymphatic sac in patients with Ménière's disease. Am. J. Otol. **6:** 449–454.

13. NEDZELSKI, J. 1996. Remarks on gentamycin perfusion of the labyrinth in Ménière's disease at the American Neurootologic Society, Washington, D.C., Sept. 28.

14. SILVERSTEIN, H., D. CHOO, S. I. ROSENBERG, *et al.* 1969. Intratympanic steroid treatment of inner ear disease and tinnitus (Preliminary Rep.). Ear, Nose & Throat J. **75**(8):468–488.

15. McCABE, B. F. 1979. Autoimmune sensory neural hearing loss. Ann. Otol. Rhinol. Laryngol. **88:** 585–589.

Cytomegalovirus Antibodies in Endolymphatic Sac Biopsies of Patients with Endolymphatic Hydrops and Ménière's Disease

I. KAUFMAN ARENBERG,[a,d] GARY CABRIAC,[b] STEFAN MARKS,[a]
JULIE G. ARENBERG,[a] PETER R. PFEIFFER,[a]
AND RONALD S. MURRAY[c]

[a]International Ménière's Disease Research Institute
300 East Hampden Avenue, Suite 400
Englewood, Colorado 80110

[b]Rocky Mountain Multiple Sclerosis Center

[c]National Jewish Center for Immunology and Respiratory Disease
The Colorado Neurological Institute
Denver, Colorado

INTRODUCTION

Numerous viruses have been implicated as ototropic and as a contributing or initiating factor in inner-ear disorders. These ototropic viruses (mumps, CMV, herpes simplex virus, varicella-zoster, and the coxsackie virus) can cause damage or death to various hair cells, resulting in hearing loss and balance disorders.

CMV infections are classified as two major types: the first is clinically seen at birth and is systemic in nature, and the second is not clinically apparent at birth and is termed asymptomatic or subclinical. Importantly, both types of CMV infections have reported otologic sequelae and involvement with the property of neurotropism.[1,2] Thirty to fifty percent of patients with symptomatic CMV have reported hearing loss,[3–6] whereas a substantially lower number (7–13%) of patients who are asymptomatic have reported hearing loss,[4,5,7] presumably related to the CMV infection. Recent speculations suggest that CMV infections may not be solely associated with congenital infections, but also with the reactivation of latent virus or with primary infections later in life, or as a primary or secondary trigger mechanism.

However, definitive evidence of a viral etiology of Ménière's disease is lacking. Ménière's disease may be secondary to dysfunction of the ELS. The main function of the ELS is to act as a resorptive site for endolymph and is the main defensive mechanism for the inner ear. It is an important site for endolymph absorption,[8] regulation of the inner ear pressure,[9–12] and inner-ear fluid dynamics.[13,14]

Recent evidence indicates that dysfunction of the ELS and its inability to resorb endolymph resulting in ELH, may be a contributing factor, but not the only factor in the development of Ménière's disease. Studies involving immunohistochemical

[d]Address for correspondence: 7995 East Prentice Ave., Suite 110, Greenwood Village, CO 80111. Phone: 303/850-0670; fax: 303/850-0671; e-mail: 76513.2007@compuserve.com

analysis of the ELS in the normal and immunologically stimulated condition have demonstrated that each of the cell populations required for immune processing exist in the normal ELS and expand following immunological stimulation.[15–17] The ELS has been suggested as the primary site of host defense of the inner ear and the center of its immunological occurrence. The ELS is the only part of the inner ear that contains a macrophage system and has interplay with the systemic vascular and lymphatic systems. The capillaries in the ELS have been shown to be fenestrated as compared to the cochlea.[18] Fenestrated vessels, which are often found in organs involved with fluid absorption, are more permeable and subject to immune complex deposition.

Virus or viral products have yet to be isolated consistently from Ménière's disease inner-ear tissues. However, CMV has been isolated from inner-ear fluid and tissue in patients with congenital CMV and from AIDS patients.[19] Additionally, CMV in the guinea pig model produces pathologic ELH and similar changes, as seen in human Ménière's disease. As CMV is an ubiquitous pathogen with ototropic propensity, we hypothesized a relationship between CMV infection and inner-ear disorders, specifically Ménière's disease. We propose either CMV as a direct cause of the pathologic changes in ELS epithelium's decreased capacity to transport endolymph with resultant ELH, or a secondary or cointeractive factor such as a trigger mechanism for viral immune reaction. These pathologic changes in the ELS adversely affect the inner-ear fluid hydrodynamics and result in ELH, which is clinically manifested as Ménière's disease.

MATERIALS AND METHODS

ELS tissue was obtained from nine patients with inner-ear disorders. Six of the patients had Ménière's disease and ELH, while the remaining three had idiopathic vestibular ELH, idiopathic SNHL, or posttraumatic inner-ear dysfunction with ELH. Ménière's disease was diagnosed in accordance with the AAOO criteria (1985).

All patients had serological analysis for antiviral antibody titres against CMV, routine biochemical surveys, and transtympanic electrocochleography (ECoG). ECoG was considered abnormal if the summating potential/action potential (SP/AP) ratio was greater than 33% with a click stimulus. All serological testing was performed at commercial laboratories. The reference range for CMV AB [IgG] includes: negative [unexposed], 0.8–1.0 equivocal, 1.1–2.6 low positive, 2.7–6.3 midpositive, 6.4 or more high positive.

Pathologic ELS tissue was obtained from a double-wall ELS biopsy from all of the Ménière's disease patients at the time of valve implant–sac surgery, and "normal" ELS in a control group of acoustic neurinoma patients undergoing transtemporal surgery extirpation. All ELS samples were stored in sterile isotonic saline at 4°C for a maximum of 4 h before processing as described below.

Each ELS was removed from the saline and stored at −70°C in 1.5-mL Eppendorf tubes until nucleic acids were extracted by the following procedure. Samples were removed from storage at −70°C and 100 μL of 50 mM tris (pH 8.0), so mM EDTA, 0.5% SDS, and 500-μg/mL proteinase K was immediately added to each. Tissues were macerated using plastic microcentrifuge pestles and digested for approximately 16 h at 37°C. Samples were then extracted once with buffer equilibrated phenol, once with phenol:chloroform (1:1), and once with chloroform. Nucleic acids were precipitated by the addition of sodium acetate to a final concentration of 0.25 M and two sample volumes of 100% ethanol, followed by overnight storage at 4°C. Nucleic acid was collected by centrifugation, washed once with cold 70% ethanol, dried under vacuum, and dissolved in 10 μL of 0.1× TE (1 mM tris, pH 8.0, 0.1 mM EDTA). Extreme precautions were taken during nucleic acid purification to minimize the possibility of sample contamination with exogenous sources of DNA.

PCR Analysis

Nucleic acid extracted from the ELS samples was assayed for CMV genomic DNA by PCR. To increase sensitivity, nested pairs of CMV-specific primers were used. The external primers used were MIE4 and MIE5,[20] and the internal primers were MIEN1 and MIEN2; these primers amplify a region of the major immediate early gene of CMV. The sequences for MIEN1 and MIEN2 are 5′-CACTGGCTCA-GACTTGACAGACACT and 5′-GATCCTCTGAGAGTCTGCTCTCCT, respectively. The primers MIE4/5 and MIEN1/2 produce amplified products of 435 bp and 288 bp, respectively. PCR amplification reactions were performed using conditions previously described.[20,21] For amplification with the MIEN1 and 2 primers, 5 μL was removed from the MIE4/5 reaction, diluted with 95 μL of water, then 10 μL of this dilution was used for the amplification reaction with the MIEN1 and 2 primers. PCR reaction products were analyzed by agarose gel electrophoresis and Southern blot hybridization.[20,22] The oligonucleotide MIE[23] was 5′ radiolabeled with ^{32}P for use as the hybridization probe. The specificity of the PCR primers and probe was evaluated by using tissue culture samples of low passage clinical isolates of CMV harvested seven days postinfection. Precautions were taken at all times to avoid contamination of the patient samples or reagents with exogenous CMV-DNA, and the proper negative controls were included at all steps to detect any such contamination.

RESULTS

Autoradiography showed PCR detection of CMV-DNA in ELS samples. Patient sample DNAs were PCR amplified with CMV-specific primers as described. Reaction products were separated by agarose gel electrophoresis, transferred to membranes, and hybridized with a radiolabeled oligonucleotide probe. The autoradiogram shows that patient samples 1–3 and 5–8 contain amplified CMV product, while samples 4 and 9 are negative (+ indicates positive control lane). Different exposure times were used for different samples.

In the Ménière's disease patients with ELH, seven out of the nine ELS tissue samples were positive for CMV by PCR. Five of these were from classic Ménière's disease patients, and the remaining two had idiopathic endolymphatic hydrops and SNHL. All nine patients revealed anti-CMV antibodies in their sera. None of the nine ELS biopsy "controls" (0/9) were positive for CMV by PCR. The occurrence of CMV in patients with ELH and Ménière's disease was statistically significant ($p < 0.001$).

DISCUSSION

The occurrence of CMV genome in ELS tissues (obtained during inner-ear valve/shunt sac surgery) of patients with ELH and Ménière's disease ($n = 9$) were compared to that found in a control group ($n = 9$) of acoustic neurinoma patients with primary eighth-nerve pathology (obtained during transtemporal surgery). Using the highly sensitive polymerase chain reaction (PCR) technique,[24] we were able to detect CMV in nucleic acid extracted from the ELS tissues in 7 out of 9 (77.8%) of Ménière's disease patients and 0 out of 9 (0%) in the control group. This is a statistically significant difference.

The presence of CMV in a high percentage of patients with ELH and Ménière's (77.8%) and its statistically significant ($p < 0.001$) absence of CMV in ELS in a control group suggests that this ototropic virus with a known propensity for a pathologic correlation of inner-ear changes[6] with ELH, may have directly or indirectly caused the pathologic damages demonstrated to the ELS subunits. This ELS damage can result in ELH pathologically and Ménière's disease clinically. If it is not a direct pathologic insult to the ELS cellular component, tissues, and microvasculature, then a secondary interactive triggerlike mechanism for CMV is speculated in the etiopathogenesis of ELH either with other interactive viruses or immune reactions. Thus, the clinical significance of the presence of CMV in the ELS of patients with various clinical subgroups of Ménière's disease and not the control group is not yet known. However, these data do indicate that a significant number of patients with various clinical variations of Ménière's disease may harbor CMV in a latent, but persistently infected state within the ELS. Thus CMV infection may promote the development of ELH and subsequently Ménière's disease. However, the role of CMV infections or other ototropic viruses, possibly interacting with the inner-ear immune system leading to clinically apparent inner-ear disease, requires further study.

REFERENCES

1. WILLIAMSON, W. D., M. M. DESMOND, N. LaFEVERS, *et al.* 1982. Symptomatic cytomegalovirus. Am. J. Dis. Child. **136:** 902–905.
2. STAGNO, S., D. W. REYNOLDS, C. S. AMOS, *et al.* 1977. Auditory and visual defects resulting from symptomatic and subclinical congenital cytomegalovirus and toxoplasma infection. Pediatrics **59:** 669–678.
3. PASS, R. F., S. STAGNO, G. J. MEYERS, *et al.* 1980. Outcome of symptomatic congenital cytomegalovirus infection: Results of long term longitudingal follow-up. Pediatrics **66:** 758–762.
4. STAGNO, S., R. F. PASS, M. E. DWORSKY, *et al.* 1983. Congenital and perinatal cytomegalovirus infection. Semin. Perinatol. **7:** 31–42.
5. SAIGAL, S., O. LUNYK, R. P. B. LARKE, *et al.* 1982. The outcome in children with congenital cytomegalovirus infection. Am. J. Dis. Child. **136:** 896–901.
6. STRAUSS, M. 1990. Human cytomegalovirus labyrinthitis. Am. J. Otolaryngol. **11:** 292–298.
7. WILLIAMSON, W. D., A. K. PERCY, M. D. YOW, *et al.* 1990. Asymptomatic congenital cytomegalovirus infection. Am. J. Dis. Child. **144:** 1365–1368.
8. LUNQUIST, P. G. 1976. Aspects of endolymphatic sac morphology and function. Arch. Otorhinolaryngol. **212:** 231–240.

9. McCABE, B. F. & D. WOLSK. 1961. Experimental inner ear pressure changes: Functional effects. Ann. Otol. Rhinol. Laryngol. **70:** 541–555.

10. LONG, C. H. & T. MORIZONO. 1984. Hydrostatis pressure measurements of endolymph in a guinea pig model of endolymphatic hydrops. Otolaryngol. Head Neck Surg. **96:** 83–95.

11. ITO, S., U. FISCH, N. DILLIER & A. POLLAK. 1987. Endolymphatic pressure in experimental hydrops. Arch. Otolaryngol. **113:** 833–835.

12. BOHMER, A., J. C. ANDREWS & N. DILLIER. 1989. Inner ear pressure and cochlear function in experimental endolymphatic hydrops. *In* Ménière's Disease, J. B. Nadol, Ed.: 221–224. Kugler & Ghedini. Amsterdam.

13. KIMURA, R. S. 1967. Experimental blockade of the endolymphatic sac and duct and its effect in the inner ear of the guinea pig. A study of endolymphatic hydrops. Ann. Otol. Rhinol. Laryngol. **76:** 664–685.

14. SCHUKNECHT, H. F. & R. A. McNEIL. 1966. Light microscopic observation on the pathology of endolymph. J. Laryngol. Otol. **80:** 1–10.

15. ARNOLD, W. & C. R. PFALZ. 1987. Critical evaluation of the immunofluorescence microscopic test for identification of serum antibodies against human inner ear tissue. Acta Otolaryngol. (Stockholm) **103:** 373–378.

16. HARRIS, J. P., S. TOMIYAMA, S. FUKUDA, *et al.* 1988. The endolymphatic sac: Its importance as a site of inner ear host defense and immunity. 2nd Int. Symp. on Ménière's Disease, Cambridge, Mass., pp. 125–132.

17. RASK-ANDERSEN, H. & J. STAHLE. 1979. Lymphocyte-macrophage activity in the endolymphatic sac. Oto. Rhino. Laryngol. **41:** 177–192.

18. LEONE, C. A., J. G. GEGHALI & F. H. LINTHICUM, JR. 1984. Endolymphatic sac: Possible role in autoimmune sensorineural hearing loss. Ann. Otol. Rhinol. Laryngol. **93:** 208–209.

19. DAVIS, L. E., B. L. HJELLE, N. E. MILLER, *et al.* 1992. Early viral brain invasion in latrogenic human immunodeficiency virus infection. Neurology **42:** 1736–1739.

20. ALEXANDER, R. C., G. F. CABRIAC, T. LOWENKOPF, M. CASANOVA, J. KLEINMAN, R. J. WYATT & D. G. KIRCH. 1992. Search for evidence of herpes simplex virus type I or varicella-zoster virus infection in postmortem brain tissue from schizophrenic patients. Acta Psychiatr. Scand. **86:** 418–420.

21. MURRAY, R. S., G.-Y. CAI, K. HOEL, J.-Y. ZHANG, K. F. SOIKE & G. F. CABRIAC. 1992. Coronavirus infects and causes demyelination in primates. Virology **188:** 274–284.

22. CABRIAC, G. F., J. J. MULLOY, D. S. STRAYER, S. SELL & J. L. LEIBOWITZ. 1986. Transcriptional mapping of early RNA from regions of the shape fibroma and malignant rabbit ribroma virus genomes. Virology **153:** 53–69.

23. DEMMLER, G. J., G. J. BUFFONE, C. M. SCHIMBOR & R. A. MAY. 1988. Detection of cytomegalovirus in urine from newborns by using polymerase chain reaction DNA amplification. J. Infect. Dis. **158:** 1177–1184.

24. SAIKI, R. K., S. SCHARF, F. FALOONA, K. B. MULLIS, G. T. HORN, H. A. ERLICH & N. ARNHEIM. 1985. Enzymatic amplification of beta-globin genomic sequences and restriction site analysis for diagnosis of sickle cell anemia. Science **230:** 1350–1354.

Sudden Hearing Loss in Childhood Consequent to Hepatitis B Vaccination: A Case Report

M. P. ORLANDO,[a] S. MASIERI, M. A. PASCARELLA,
A. CIOFALO, AND F. FILIACI

*ENT Clinic
University "La Sapienza"
Viale del Policlinico
Rome, 00185, Italy*

INTRODUCTION

The adoption of a policy of vaccination against the hepatitis B virus (HBV) for the entire population has been suggested on the basis of several studies carried out in the United States. Subjects at risk for hepatitis B are babies born to women positive for HBsAg, homosexuals, medical doctors, and nurses. Twenty-one percent of babies born to women positive for HBsAg presented with HBsAg at the age of 2, 16% of homosexuals,[1] and 18% of sanitary personnel.[2] In Italy, HBV vaccination is obligatory for children under 12 years of age and workers at risk for HBV, such as medical doctors and nurses. In newborns, three doses of the vaccine against HBV are administered, the first at the age of 3 months, the second one month later, and the third six months later. Unfortunately the vaccination against HBV is not without the risk of complications;[3–5] for example, the boy in the following Case Report who developed monaurol sudden deafness in connection with HBV vaccine administration.

CASE REPORT

The boy, aged 11, was taken by his parents to the ENT Clinic of the University of Rome, complaining of unilateral hearing loss. The parents reported that he had undergone surgery for hernioplasty at the age of 20 months and had been affected by epidemic parotitis and chickenpox by the age of 3 years. He developed edema due to a food allergy at the age of 7 years. The boy was given the second vaccine against HBV (Engerix B) at a public medical office. After 48 hours, he complained of tinnitus and sudden left deafness associated with vertigo and nausea. Because the symptoms persisted, the parents took the boy to an ENT Clinic 24 hours later. No pathological finding was observed during the clinical examination. Impedenzometry showed Jerger's A curve (normal tympanic compliance) bilaterally; the acoustic reflex was evoked on the right side, while it was absent on the left. At pure tone audiometry, the boy presented marked neurosensorial hearing loss on the left side and

[a]Author for correspondence. Phone: 39-6-445-4607; fax: 39-6-818-5865.

normal threshold on the right side. No identifiable ABR waveforms were observed, even at maximum levels (120 dB SPL) of stimulus presentations on the left side. However, ABR on the right side was within normal limits. No pathological findings were observed by MRI, particularly no demyelinated areas were present. Routine blood chemical and hematological tests were normal apart from the presence of a slight lymphocytosis. Further blood exams were sent for PRIST, antibodies against DNA and mitochondria, CD3, CD4, CD8, C3, C4, T3, T4, TSH, antibodies against toxoplasma, cytomegalovirus, herpes virus, chickenpox, and HBsAg; all the tests were normal. Blood was also analyzed for mercury level, since Engerix B vaccine contains this metal (thiomersal).[6]

Therapy with corticosteroids (methylprednisolone 20 mg im BID) and carbogen (5% of carbogen in oxygen, 2 1/min, 20 min. every 2 h) was immediately instituted and given for five days. Further therapy with vitamine B12 was given for two months. The hearing loss improved only slightly. After two years, a marked neurosensorial left hypoacusia is still present.

DISCUSSION

This case was characterized by the absence of any pathological finding at the anamnesis and blood tests, but a temporal connection with the administration of the vaccine against HBsAg given 48 hours before the sudden appearance of unilateral hearing loss.

The mechanism by which the vaccine could act is not clear.[7,8] However, it could theoretically reveal a latent autoimmune disease not necessarily related to the HLA B7 antigen but possibly related to other phenotypes and allotypes. Both aluminum and mercury salts are present in Engerix B vaccine.[9] Mercury is known to exert a toxic action on central and peripheral nervous system, but the relation between dosage and toxicity has not yet been clearly established.[10–12]

REFERENCES

1. HADLER, S. C., D. P. FRANCIS, J. E. MAYNARD, S. E. THOMPSON, F. N. JUDSON, D. F. ECHENBERG, D. G. OSTROW, P. M. O'MALLEY, K. A. PENLEY, N. L. ALTMAN, *et al.* 1986. Long-term immunogenecity and efficacy of hepatitis B vaccine in homosexual men. New Eng. J. Med. **315:** 209–214.
2. FOLLETT, E. A., I. S. SYMINGTON & M. G. CAMERON. 1987. Experience with hepatitis B vaccination in nurses in a hospital for the mentally handicapped. Lancet **2:** 728–731.
3. HERROLEN, L., J. DEKEYSER & G. EBINGHER. 1991. Central nervous system demyelination after immunization with recombinant hepatitis B vaccine. Lancet **338:** 1174–1175.
4. BREZIN, M. LAUTER-FRAU, M. HAMEDANI & O. ROGEAUX. 1994. Perdita di verus ed eosinofilia dopo vaccino ricombinante antiepatite B. Lancet (ediz. Ital.) **2:**
5. EL-HIFNAWI, H. 1984. Sudden deafness in gastrointestinal infections: Microbial genesis or autoimmune reaction? Laryngol. Rhinol. Otol. **63:** 445–447.
6. ABERE, W. 1992. Vaccination despite thiomersal sensitivity. Excerpta medica.
7. NAIR, T. S., Y. RAPHAEL, D. F. DOLAN, T. J. PARRET, L. S. PERLMAN, V. R. BRANHMBHATT, Y. WANG, X. HOU, G. GANJEI, A. L. NUTTAL, R. A. ALTSCHULER & T. E. CAREY. 1995. Monoclonal antibody induced hearing loss. Hear. Res. **83:** 101–113.

8. KOSAKA, K., S. YAMANOBE, S.-I. TOMIYAMA & T. YAGI. 1995. Inner ear autoantibodies in patients with sensorineural hearing loss. Acta Otolaryngol. **S519:** 176–177.

9. SBRANA, I., A. DISIIBIO, A. LOMI & V. SCARCELLI. 1993. C. mitosis and numerical chromosome aberration analyses in human lymphocytes: 10 known or suspected spindle poisons. Mutat. Res. **287:** 57–70.

10. MILLER, B. M. & I. D. ADLER. 1992. Aneuploid induction in mouse spermatocytes mutagenesis: Mutagenesis **7:** 69–76.

11. GUDI, R., J. XU & A. THAILAGER. 1992. Assessment of the in vivo aneuployd/micronucleus assay in mouse bone marrow cells with 16 chemicals. Environ. Mol. Mutagen. **20:** 106–116.

12. FAWCETT, H., *et al.* 1994. Injection site granuloma due to aluminum. Arch. Dermatol. **120:** 1318.

Screening Patients Affected by Common Variable Immunodeficiency

S. MASIERI, M. P. ORLANDO,[a] A. CIOFALO, G. LUZI,
C. ZAMBETTI, AND F. FILIACI

ENT Clinic
University "La Sapienza"
Viale del Policlinico
Rome, 00185, Italy

INTRODUCTION

Common variable immunodeficiency (CVI) is characterized by primitive impairment of antibody production.[1–5] A few immunological deficits have been observed in these patients; they include decreased B lymphocytes and hypogammaglobulinemia involving both IgG (usually less than 500 mg/dL), IgA, and IgM (decreased or absent in blood). CVI is a hereditary disease; relatives of CVI patients frequently present low IgA blood levels and higher incidence of autoimmune diseases and malignant neoplasms in comparison with the general population. These families are characterized by a high incidence of HLA-DR3 associated with polymorphic class III antigens of histocompatibility with rare alleles and gene deletions on chromosome 6 (C4A, 21-OH hydrossilase A, HSP 70, TNF-α). T Lymphocytes can be normal in number or exhibit an inversion of the CD4/CD8 ratio.

The incidence of CVI ranges between 1:50000 and 1:200000 and is unaffected by sex. Clinical symptoms may appear in early childhood, but more often arise at the age of 20–30. CVI patients are usually affected by recurrent pulmonary infections that result in bronchiectasis and respiratory failure. Otitis, rhinitis, sinusitis, and meningitis, as well as digestive and urinary tract infections, are frequently observed. Autoimmune diseases are observed in about 25% of females affected by CVI. An increased incidence of neoplasma, particularly lymphomas and gastroenteric carcinomas, has been reported after the age of 40.

The periodic IV administration of immunoglobulins has been utilized in CVI patients for over 40 years and has had a positive effect on the course of the disease. Monthly IV administration of 400 mg/kg of immunoglobulins proved to be effective against chronic bronchial and pulmonary infections. To date the effectiveness of this therapy on upper airways has not been studied; therefore, in this study a group of CVI patients treated with chronic immunoglobulin therapy underwent an ENT screening to evaluate the incidence of ear and upper-airway disorders.

---

[a]Author for correspondence. Phone: 39-6-445-4607; fax: 39-6-818-5865.

TABLE 1. Symptoms

Pharynx		
Pain dysphagia	20	91%
Nose		
Obstruction, hypersecretion, pain	17	77%
Ear		
Otodinia, hypoacusia, tinnitus	12	57%
Larynx		
Pain, dysphonia	3	13%

MATERIALS AND METHODS

Twenty-two patients aged 13–70 (mean 39.2), 11 males and 11 females, affected by CVI were included in this study. They had been treated with chronic IV administration of immunoglobulins, 350–500 mg/kg/month, for a minimum of 2 years. ENT anamnesis was obtained and symptoms were classified as light, moderate, or serious; only moderate and serious cases were taken into this study. All patients underwent ENT physical examination, nasal endoscopy by fiberoptics, mucociliary transport test (MTT) by a colored indicator,[6] anterior rhinorheomanometry (RRM), specific nasal provocation test with cold (2–4°C) water (ANPT), audiometry and impedentiometry, olfactory evaluation by a Fortunato–Nicolini device, and paranasal sinus X rays. ANPT was considered positive if an increase or decrease of nasal resistance greater than 30% of basal value was registered.[7] TTM, RRM, and TPNA results are reported as means and standard deviations, and were compared by t-test and chi-square with values gathered from a control group including 15 healthy subjects.

RESULTS

ENT symptoms reported by the patients and classified as moderate or serious are shown in TABLE 1. Dysphagia occurred in 91% of the patients, nasal secretion and obstruction in 77%, and hypoacusia, tinnitus, and otodinia in 57%. The results of the physical examinations are shown in TABLE 2. Rhinitis and pharyngitis were observed in 86% of the patients, serous middle-ear effusion in 50%. Maxillary sinusitis confirmed by X rays was observed in five patients. Hyposmia was observed in 50% of the patients. MTT was significantly longer in the patients than in the controls (18.0 ± 10.5 vs. 11.2 ± 2.4 min; $p < .05$). Nasal resistance was lower in patients than in controls (0.46 ± 0.32 vs. 1.11 ± 0.22 Pa/L·s^{-1}; $p < .001$). Following ANPT, nasal resistance increased in controls (from 1.11 ± 0.22 to 1.31 ± 0.43 Pa/L·s^{-1}; $p < .05$); on the contrary, mean nasal resistance did not increase in patients (from 0.46 ± 0.32 to 0.47 ± 0.47 Pa/L·s^{-1}). Nevertheless, the test was positive in 9 patients out of 25 versus 1 control out of 15 ($p < .05$). Finally, seven patients were affected by transmissive hypoacusia and one patient by neurosensorial hypoacusia.

TABLE 2. Physical Examination

Rhinopharyngitis		
Hyperemia, hypersecretion, edema	19	86%
Serous middle-ear effusion		
Otoscopy, impedentiometry	11	50%
Turbinatus hypertrophy		
Mechanical obstruction	8	36. 3%
Sinusitis		
Positive X rays	5	22. 7%
Tympanic membrane perforation	3	22%
Laryngitis		
Hyperemia, dysphonia	2	9%
Tonsil hypertrophy	1	4. 5%

DISCUSSION

Our results point out that most CVI patients complain of ENT symptoms in spite of chronic immunoglobulin administration. In these patients, the decrease or absence of immunoglobulins, particularly IgA, impairs local defenses against infectious microorganisms in the nose and pharynx, and makes bacterial colonization easier, which in turn causes secretion, stagnation, and chronic phlogosis.[8,9] On the one hand, bacterial growth makes the secretion thicker, impairing mucociliary clearance in the nose, pharynx, paranasal sinuses, eustachian tube, and middle ear.[10] On the other hand, it attracts neutrophils, basophils, and mast cells toward the mucosa, so that chemical mediators, particularly histamine, are released and nasal hyperreactivity takes place. Such hyperreactivity has been pointed out by the high incidence of positive ANPT. Chronic mast edema and congestion of turbinatus superior explains why smell is impaired in most patients; analogously, the mechanical obstruction of the eustachian tube by chronic edema and mucociliary impairment through the tube causes the high incidence of middle-ear effusion. We conclude that although chronic immunoglobulin administration protects CVI patients from lower airway and pulmonary infections, it seems to be ineffective against ENT disorders, probably because of the important role played by nasal hyperreactivity. Hence, we suggest frequent ENT examination and early treatment of ENT disorders in order to prevent chronic disease.

SUMMARY

Chronic immunoglobulin administration decreases the incidence of bronchial and pulmonary infections in patients affected by chronic variable immunodeficiency (CVI). In this study, an ENT screening was carried out in 22 patients affected by chronic variable immunodeficiency and treated with chronic immunoglobulin administration. All the patients underwent ENT physical examination, nasal endoscopy by fiberoptics, mucociliary transport test (MTT), anterior rhinorheomanometry

(RRM), nasal provocation test with cold water (ANPT), audiometry and impedentiometry, olfactory evaluation, and paranasal sinus X rays. Dysphagia was present in 91% of the patients, nasal secretion and obstruction in 77%, and hypoacusia, tinnitus, and otodinia in 57%. Rhinitis and pharyngitis were observed in 86% of the patients, and serous middle ear effusion in 50%. Confirmed maxillary sinusitis was observed in five patients. Hyposmia was observed in 50% of the patients. MTT was significantly longer in the patients than in the controls (18.0 ± 10.5 vs. 11.2 ± 2.4 min; $p < .05$). Nasal resistance was lower in patients than in controls (0.46 ± 0.32 vs. 1.11 ± 0.22 Pa/L·s^{-1}; $p < .001$). ANPT was positive in 9 patients out of 25 versus 1 control out of 15 ($p < .05$). Finally, seven patients were affected by transmissive hypoacusia, and one patient by neurosensorial hypoacusia. Our results suggest that chronic immunoglobulin administration in CVI patients is not effective against ENT disorders, probably because of the important role played by nasal hyperreactivity. Frequent ENT examination and early treatment of ENT disorders are therefore suggested in order to prevent chronic disease.

REFERENCES

1. ROSEN, F. S., M. D. COOPER & R. J. P. WEDGWOOD. 1984. The primary immunodeficiencies. New Eng. J. Med. **311:** 235–242.
2. OCHS, H. D. & R. J. P. WEDGWOOD. 1987. IgG subclass deficiencies. Ann. Rev. Med. **38:** 325–340.
3. PAGANELLI, R., I. QUINTI, E. SCALA, E. FANALES-BELASIO, D. CARMINI, G. SPADARO & G. MARONE. 1991. Nuovi aspetti diagnostici e patogenetici dei difetti primitivi dell-immunita umorale. Giorn. It. Allergol. Immunol. Clin. **1:** 49–61.
4. GUPTA, S. & C. GRISCELLI. 1993. New concepts in immunodeficiency diseases. Wiley. Chichester, England.
5. REPORT OF A WHO SCIENTIFIC GROUP. 1994. Primary immunodeficiency diseases. NIH Conf. on New Insight into Common Variable Immunodeficiency. Ann. Intern. Med. **118:** 720–730.
6. FILIACI, F., N. LUCARELLI & M. ROSSI. 1981. Valutazione del TMC della mucosa nasale umana. Med. Mod. **31:** 3–7.
7. CRIFO, S., F. FILIACI, S. CITTADINI & E. DE SETA. 1975. RRM nasal provocation test. Rhinology **13:** 135–139.
8. MYGIND, N. & B. WINTHER. 1978. Immunological barriers in the nose and paranasal sinuses. Acta Otolaryngol. (Stockholm) **103:** 363–368.
9. BRANDTZAEG, P. 1988. Immunobarriers of the mucosa of the upper respiratory and digestive pathways. Acta Otolaryngol. (Stockholm) **105:** 172–180.
10. WILSON, R., D. A. SYKES, D. CURRIE & P. J. COLE. 1986. Beat frequency of cilia from sites of purulent infection. Thorax **41:** 453–458.

Summary: Progress in Inner-ear Immunology[a]

ALLEN F. RYAN[b]

Division of Otolaryngology,
Department of Surgery
UCSD Medical School and VA Medical Center
La Jolla, California 92093

INTRODUCTION

Numerous significant scientific advances in the immunobiology of the inner ear have recently been documented. This progress has occurred on both the basic science and clinical fronts, and is a testament to the high level of interest in immunity at this site. Part of this interest stems from basic science considerations regarding the operation of immunity in the unique environment of the labyrinth. As in the brain, the protective nature of immunity must be balanced in the inner ear against the destructive effects of inflammation on delicate tissues. Perhaps because of this, immunocytes have been excluded from the normal labyrinth, except for the physically remote endolymphatic sac.

It can be argued that even greater interest in inner-ear immunology has been stimulated by growing evidence of clinical manifestations of immune response within the inner ear, an organ that was once thought to be immunopriviledged. Hearing loss and vestibular dysfunction of suspected immune or inflammatory origin is unique among labyrinthine disorders, in that many symptoms can be reversed by treatment with anti-inflammatory steroids or immunosuppressive agents.

IMMUNITY IN THE INNER EAR

Our knowledge regarding the occurrence and nature of immune responses that occur in the inner ear continues to increase. For several years, it has been clear that the inner ear possesses efficient communication with systemic immunity. Sensitization of systemic immunity following introduction of antigen into the labyrinth is brisk, and the response to antigen introduced into the inner ear of sensitized individuals can be dramatic. The biological basis for these responses is emerging. Interaction of antigen and antibody in the inner-ear fluids, and/or interaction of antigen with sensitized lymphocytes in the endolymphatic sac, presumably produces an initial inflammatory response. This in turn induces the formation of endothelial cell receptors, including

[a]This work was supported by NIH/NIDCD Grants DC00129 and DC00193, and by the Research Service of the Veterans Administration.

[b]Address for correspondence: Allen F. Ryan, Ph.D., Division of Otolaryngology, 0666, UCSD School of Medicine, 9500 Gilman Drive, La Jolla, CA 92093. Phone: 619/534-4594; fax: 619/534-5319; e-mail: aryan@ucsd.edu

I-CAM, at specialized vessels such as the spiral modiolar vein. These receptors mediate the capture of activated leukocytes, including sensitized B and T lymphocytes, from the circulating peripheral pool, leading to interaction of immunocytes with antigen and triggering a cascade of immune and inflammatory events.[1–3] This can result in significant tissue remodeling in the inner ear, with negative impacts on labyrinthine function.

A unique role of the endolymphatic sac in inner-ear immunity continues to be clear. The sac contains the only resident lymphocytes in the labyrinth, and ablation of the sac or duct substantially reduces the response to inner-ear antigenic challenge.[1] The lymphocytes in the sac appear to originate both from the peripheral blood, suggesting the possibility of the circulation of immunologic memory through the inner ear, and from the adjacent bone marrow.

AUTOIMMUNE DAMAGE TO THE COCHLEA

It is now abundantly clear that autoimmunity can lead to damage to the delicate tissues of the inner ear. Several systemic autoimmune disorders, and especially those involving vasculatis or deposition of immune complexes, have been shown to include hearing loss or vestibular disorders as a component.[5] Type II collagen autoimmunity may also result in inner-ear disorders.[6,7] Viral infection has been implicated in several forms of hearing loss, including otosclerosis, Ménière's disease, and sudden hearing loss.[8–12] In such cases, inner-ear damage is most probably due to bystander injury, secondary to immune response against the infecting agent.

More specific is the suggestion that immune responses directed against antigens within the inner ear can lead to organ-specific autoimmune inner-ear diseases, and evidence steadily accumulates to support this view. Experimental studies have shown that high levels of circulating antibodies directed against a protein in the supporting cells of the organ of Corti can lead to sensorineural hearing loss in animals.[13] A number of studies have examined the prevalence and prognostic significance of antibodies against inner-ear proteins in patients exhibiting several forms of hearing loss. Western blotting of patient sera has revealed significant correlations between idiopathic, slowly progressive SNHL and positive Western blots against cochlear antigens.[1,14–16] To a lesser extent, this may also be true in Ménière's disease. The most commonly observed antigen has an apparent molecular weight of about 68 kDa. This antigen may be related to a heat-shock protein,[1,16] although an unidentified supporting cell protein[13] has also been implicated. These data lend credence to the concept of organ-specific autoimmune inner-ear disease.

To date, the Western blot assay against cochlear antigens appears to be the most specific and accurate diagnostic test for autoimmune inner-ear disease.[1,14–16] In most cases, Western blot positivity is correlated with responsiveness to steroid therapy. However, other tests such as the CH50 (total hemolytic activity) assay may be predictive of hearing recovery.

Management of autoimmune inner-ear disease typically involves immunosuppression. Burst and taper steroid therapy is often the initial treatment of choice.[1,16] For cases refractory to steroids or as an adjunct, more aggressive immunosuppressive agents such as cyclosporin A can be effective. Recovery of function following immunosuppression includes pure tone thresholds as well as several other measures of auditory acuity in the frequency and intensity domains.[17]

CONCLUSIONS AND FUTURE DIRECTIONS

The inner ear has now been firmly established as a site of immune response and immune-mediated disease. We have amassed a significant body of data regarding the manner in which immunity operates in the ear. Uniform diagnostic criteria have been developed for autoimmune inner-ear disease, and are gaining wide acceptance. Steroid treatment often leads to improved inner-ear function. However, many unanswered questions remain.

On the basic science front, the role of the endolymphatic sac in initiating inner-ear immune responses needs to be explored. How and whether the lymphocytes within the sac communicate with the remainder of the inner ear is unknown. The identities of antigens that are potential targets of autoimmunity in the cochlea remain uncertain. While evidence for the existence of organ-specific autoimmune inner-ear disease is mounting, convincing proof would be offered by positive identification of antigenic targets within the labyrinth, a documented etiology of hearing loss, and more robust animal models. Such evidence would lead to wider recognition of this condition, both within and especially outside of our field. Diagnostic tests for autoimmune inner-ear disease are imperfect. Available treatments need to be improved, and to be validated by controlled clinical trials. The role of genetics in autoimmune inner-ear disease[18] should be explored.

REFERENCES

1. HARRIS, J. P., J. HEYDT, E. M. KEITHLEY & M.-C. CHEN. 1997. Immunopathology of the inner ear: An update. This issue.
2. RYAN, A. F., B. GLODDEK & J. P. HARRIS. 1997. Lymphocyte trafficking in the inner ear. This issue.
3. GLODDEK, B., J. GLODDEK & W. ARNOLD. 1997. Induction of an inner-ear-specific autoreactive T-cell line for the diagnostic evaluation of an autoimmune disease of the inner ear. This issue.
4. BARBARA, M., G. ATTANASIO, V. PETROZZA, A. MODESTI & R. FILIPO. 1997. The endolymphatic sac as the immunocompetent organ of the inner ear. This issue.
5. ARNOLD, W. 1997. Systemic autoimmune diseases associated with hearing loss. This issue.
6. SUZUKI, M., K.-C. CHENG, H. MATSUOKA, M. KRUG, J. BERNSTEIN & T.-J. YOO. 1997. The cochlear protein antigens 28 kd and 30 kd, and their antibodies in Ménière's disease. This issue.
7. YOO, T. J., T. FUJIYOSHI, K.-C. CHENG, M. S. KRUG, N. S. KIM, K. M. LEE, T. SHEN & H. MATSUOKA. 1997. Molecular basis of type II collagen autoimmune ear diseases. This issue.
8. MCKENNA, M. J. 1997. Measles, mumps, and sensorineural hearing loss. This issue.
9. ARENBERG, I. K., C. LEMKE & G. E. SHAMBAUGH, JR. 1997. Viral theory for Ménière's disease and endolymphatic hydrops: Overview and new therapeutic options for viral labyrinthitis. This issue.

10. ARENBERG, I. K., G. CABRIAC, S. MARKS, J. G. ARENBERG, P. R. PFEIFFER & R. S. MURRAY. 1997. Cytomegalovirus antibodies in endolymphatic sac biopsies of patients with endolymphatic hydrops and Ménière's disease. This issue.

11. ORLANDO, M. P., S. MASIERI, M. A. PASCARELLA, A. CIOFALO & F. FILIACI. 1997. Sudden hearing loss in childhood consequent to hepatitis B vaccination: A case report. This issue.

12. MASIERI, S., M. P. ORLANDO, A. CIOFALO, G. LUZI, C. ZAMBETTI & F. FILIACI. 1997. Screening patients affected by common variable immunodeficiency. This issue.

13. DISHER, M. J., A. RAMAKRISHNAN, T. S. NAIR, J. M. MILLER, S. A. TELIAN, H. A. ARTS, R. T. SATALOFF, R. A. ALTSCHULER, Y. RAPHAEL & T. E. CAREY. 1997. Human autoantibodies and monoclonal antibody KHRI-3 bind to a phylogenetically conserved inner-ear-supporting cell antigen. This issue.

14. VELDMAN, J. E. 1997. Immune-mediated sensorineural hearing loss with or without endolymphatic hydrops. This issue.

15. FILIPO, R. & P. MANCINI. 1997. Ménière's disease and autoimmunity. This issue.

16. RAUCH, S. D. 1997. Clinical management of immune-mediated inner-ear disease. This issue.

17. QUARANTA, A., A. SCARINGI, P. PORTALATINI & D. VANTAGGIATO. 1997. Auditory findings in subjects with immunomediated sensorineural hearing loss. This issue.

18. MARTINI, A., M. MAZZOLI & W. KIMBERLING. 1997. An introduction to the genetics of normal and defective hearing. This issue.

Vaccination Against Middle-ear Bacterial and Viral Pathogens

G. SCOTT GIEBINK[a]

Otitis Media Research Center
Department of Pediatrics and Otolaryngology
University of Minnesota School of Medicine
Minneapolis, Minnesota 55455

INTRODUCTION

The enormous childhood morbidity and health care costs of otitis media (OM), together with the increasing prevalence of antibiotic-resistant middle-ear bacterial pathogens, create an imperative to develop effective immunoprophylactic interventions for this disease. Teele *et al.*[1] found that over 80% of children have symptomatic OM by their third birthday, and about one-third have three or more episodes. Direct costs of treating OM in the United States are estimated at $2 billion annually, and indirect costs are much higher.[2] OM leads to chronic otitis media with effusion (OME) in about 10% of children, and chronic OME is associated with hearing loss[3] and delayed speech and language development.[4,5]

Studies of OM epidemiology provide evidence that middle-ear infection elicits protection against reinfection with the homologous organism. Austrian *et al.* found that *Streptococcus pneumoniae* middle-ear isolates in recurrent acute OM were rarely the same type.[6] Barenkamp *et al.* also showed that recurrent nontypable *Haemophilus influenzae* (NTHi) acute OM episodes are caused by new strains.[7] Children with OM due to NTHi lack bactericidal antibody before infection and develop strain-specific bactericidal antibody after middle-ear infection.

We observed in the chinchilla OM model that susceptibility to pneumococcal OM was reduced from 88% after ipsilateral initial middle-ear inoculation to 38% when both ears were reinoculated; moreover, only 46% of previously uninoculated left ears became infected.[8] Thus, previous unilateral infection provided both ipsilateral and contralateral middle-ear protection, suggesting that unilateral pneumococcal OM induced systemic immune defenses.

Middle-ear infection induces both serum and local antibodies against the invading pathogen. Higher middle-ear fluid antibody concentrations against pneumococcal capsular polysaccharides (PCP) have been associated with more rapid clearing of infection in children and in the chinchilla model.[9,10]

Childhood pneumococcal vaccine trials in Massachusetts, Alabama, and Finland were reported in the late 1970s.[11–13] Children who received a vaccine composed of eight purified PCPs from types frequently causing acute OM experienced fewer

[a]Address for correspondence: G. Scott Giebink, M.D., Box 296 Mayo, 420 Delaware Street S.E., Minneapolis, MN 55455. Phone: 612/624-6159; fax: 612-624-8927; e-mail: giebi001@maroon.tc.umn.edu

episodes of acute OM due to pneumococcal types in the vaccine than children who received a control vaccine. Among 7- to 24-month-old Finnish children, vaccine prevented 67% of vaccine-type pneumococcal otitis media episodes after excluding infections caused by type 6, which was poorly immunogenic.[13] However, few of the vaccine antigens stimulated a protective antibody response, and the overall clinical experience of active and control vaccine recipients in these three trials was not significantly different.

In the chinchilla pneumococcal OM model, animals that experienced at least a twofold serum antibody increase after subcutaneous administration of purified PCP showed an 87% reduction in vaccine-type pneumococcal OM, compared to only a 28% reduction in vaccinated chinchillas lacking a systemic antibody response.[14] Moreover, prophylactic administration to OM-prone children of hyperimmune human immune globulin that contained antibodies to pneumococcal polysaccharides significantly decreased the incidence of pneumococcal OM.[15]

Potential OM vaccines include *S. pneumoniae* capsular polysaccharides and common protein antigens, NTHi outer-membrane proteins (OMP), fimbriae and pili, *Moraxella catarrhalis* outer membrane proteins, and attenuated viral vaccines (respiratory syncytial virus, influenza A virus, parainfluenza virus, adenovirus). The ideal OM vaccine will, of course, need to include the immunogenic antigen(s) that elicit protective antibody against relevant pathogen(s). These antigens must be conserved among bacterial and viral strains, and antibodies elicited by the vaccine must be preserved for sufficient time to protect the ear throughout the period of greatest risk— the first three years of life. While several other factors, such as eustachian tube dysfunction, respiratory viral infection, and immune function, contribute to OM pathogenesis, it is likely that bacterial vaccines against *S. pneumoniae* and NTHi will "tip the balance" against the occurrence of OM.

PNEUMOCOCCAL VACCINES

Elegant studies by Gray *et al.* demonstrated that children acquire their first pneumococcus in the nasopharynx by age 6 months.[16] Duration of carriage decreases with successive types, and types are reacquired during the first two years. Pneumococcal acquisition peaks in the winter months. About 15% of all pneumococcal acquisitions result in disease, and disease generally occurs within one month of the acquisition. In the cohort of children followed by Gray *et al.*,[16] 29% had a pneumococcal infection by age 2 years.

Pneumococcal capsular polysaccharides are the protective antigens for *S. pneumoniae*. While there are 90 different capsular types, only nine account for 90% of childhood disease. A 23-valent capsular polysaccharide vaccine is currently available and covers 87% of bacteremic pneumococcal infections in the United States; adult protection for invasive disease is estimated to be 61%. The vaccine is recommended for use in children over the age of 2 years who are at risk for pneumococcal infection, in adults over the age of 65, and in various high-risk groups. This vaccine is not generally effective below age 2 years due to low polysaccharide immunogenicity.

Bacterial polysaccharides do not stimulate T-cell help, but most can stimulate mature B cells; that is, they are T-independent antigens. These antigens stimulate mature

B cells directly, do not require the helper function of T cells, and induce variable amounts of antibody. They produce large amounts of IgM antibodies. They do not demonstrate a booster response; that is, they do not induce immunological memory; hence, they provide a short-lived immune response. Antibodies against complex bacterial polysaccharides demonstrate poor antibody affinity and do not induce affinity maturation.

Conjugate Vaccines

Development of vaccines effective against Hib encountered the same immunologic obstacles as *S. pneumoniae.* Polysaccharides from both bacteria are not very immunogenic in young infants. Glycoconjugate chemistry, a strategy pioneered by Avery and Goebel over 60 years ago that covalently links carbohydrate antigens and haptens to protein carriers, has overcome this problem.[17] We now know that proteins associate with cell-surface major histocompatibility complex (MHC) molecules, which trigger T-helper cells to promote effective B-cell antibody responses. Polysaccharides acquire new antigenic properties typical of "T-dependent" protein antigens when coupled to protein carriers.[18,19] Experimental animal studies have shown that these conjugates stimulate a T-cell response, generating stronger "booster" responses on revaccination.[20]

Conjugate vaccine technology has proven highly successful in *H. influenzae* type b (Hib) disease prevention. Polyribosylribitol phosphate, the capsular polysaccharide of Hib, linked to protein carriers is processed by T-lymphocytes, yielding significant antibody responses in infants as young as 4 months of age, longer lasting protective antibodies, and the characteristic T-dependent response to booster vaccine doses. Building on this technology, conjugate pneumococcal vaccines are being developed.

Eight pneumococcal conjugate vaccines are currently being developed (TABLE 1).[21] Schneerson *et al.*[22] first reported the immunogenicity of PCP-protein conjugate vaccines; this tetanus toxoid conjugate of type 6A PCP raised both 6A and tetanus antibodies in adults. Anderson and Betts[23] studied in adult volunteers the immunogenicity of types 6A, 14, 18C, 19F, and 23F saccharides of varying length and composition coupled by reductive amination to diphtheria toxoid. Immunogenicity of the type 6A conjugate was associated with higher overall saccharide content rather than chain length. Parallel changes in total anticapsular and IgG-specific antibodies were noted. Eleven of 19 subjects who demonstrated significant antibody responses to one of the several conjugate preparations also had a significant rise in type-specific opsonic activity, and eight subjects did not.

Vaccine Efficacy in an Animal Model

The chinchilla model has been useful in studying middle-ear protection against pneumococci after systemic immunization. We studied the immunogenicity and efficacy of PCP conjugates composed of hydrolyzed PCP conjugated to outer-membrane protein complex (OMPC) from *Neisseria meningitidis* group B bacteria in the chinchilla model.[24] Type 6B monovalent, type 23F monovalent, type 6B+23F bivalent,

TABLE 1. Pneumococcal Conjugate Vaccines Currently Developed in Various Phases of Clinical Testing

Organization	Polysaccharide Types	Saccharide Length	Protein Carrier	Linker
Pasteur-Merieux-Connaught	3, 4, 6, 9, 14, 18, 19, 23 3, 4, 6, 9, 14, 18, 19, 23	— —	Tetanus toxoid, Diphtheria toxoid	Short (new technology)
Wyeth Lederle Vaccines	4, 6, 9, 14, 18, 19, 23 1, 5, 6, 14, 18, 19, 23	Short Short	CRM[197] CRM[197]	Short + amine Short + amine
Merck	4, 6, 9, 14, 18, 19, 23	Long	OMPC-meningococcus B	Thioether
University of Rochester	6, 14, 19, 23	Short	CRM[197], tetanus toxoid	Amine
NICHD	6, 12	Long	Tetanus toxoid	Short
Dutch-Nordic Consortium	6, 14, 19, 23	Variable	Tetanus toxoid	Thioether

Source: From D. L. Klein.[21]

and type 6B+14+19F+23F tetravalent PCP-OMPC conjugate vaccines were very immunogenic in chinchillas, producing 100 to 1000 times more anti-PCP antibody in serum than plain PCP vaccines. These serum responses are relevant since both an earlier study[9] and this study showed strong relationships between serum antibody and middle-ear protection. IgG, IgM, and some IgA type-6B antibodies were produced, and animals boosted 28 days after priming showed an anamnestic increase in IgG antibodies. Shorter intervals between priming and booster (7 and 14 days) did not accelerate type 6B antibody responses as has been observed in mice (P. Vella, unpublished observation).

Interactions between PCP antigens in the vaccines were examined in chinchillas using monovalent, bivalent, and tetravalent preparations.[24] There was no interference of types 6B, 14, or 19F PCP on the antibody response to type 23F PCP, nor was there interference of type 23F PCP on the antibody response to type 6B PCP. However, the type 6B anti-PCP antibody response to a booster dose of tetravalent vaccine was lower than the response to a booster dose of monovalent type 6B vaccine. Whether this represents antigen interference will require additional study. Such interference has not been observed with the tetravalent vaccine in infant Rhesus monkeys (P. Vella, unpublished observation). To our knowledge, this issue has not been addressed in previous publications of multivalent plain PCP vaccines.

Collectively, the three type 6B containing conjugate vaccines prevented or greatly attenuated pneumococcal acute OM in 63% of immunized animals.[24] Middle-ear protection tended to be better in animals given one or two vaccine doses and challenged after 42 to 56 days. Protection was not significantly different among animals given one or two doses of monovalent vaccine, one dose of bivalent vaccine, or two doses of tetravalent vaccine, although the 28-day challenge protocol yielded significantly greater protection with bivalent than monovalent vaccine.

Type 19F conjugate in the tetravalent mixture elicited a highly protective middle-ear response, but type 14 conjugate in the same mixture failed to protect.[24] Since type 14 conjugate elicited a slightly higher total mean serum antibody concentration before challenge (2.07 mg/mL) than either type 19F conjugate (1.85 mg/mL) or type 6B conjugate (0.82 mg/mL), differences in middle-ear outcome among the three PCP types could be explained by a different isotype antibody response to type 14 conjugate or by an enhanced host inflammatory response to type 14 pneumococci.

Serum Antibody Correlates of Middle-ear Protection

The concentrations of serum antibodies against 6B-PCP and 19F-PCP measured by RIA immediately before challenge were strongly associated with protection in the chinchilla model.[24] Correlation coefficients for the regression analysis of log10 antibody concentration versus OM severity area under the curve were 0.59 ($P < 0.001$) for type 6B and 0.76 ($P < 0.001$) for type 19F. Type 6B pneumococcal OM developed in 72% of animals with anti-6B-PCP serum antibody concentrations of less than 1.0 mg/mL, and in only 13% with higher antibody concentrations ($P < 0.001$). Type 19F pneumococcal OM developed in 75% of animals with anti-19F-PCP serum antibody concentrations of less than 1.0 mg/mL, and in none of seven with higher antibody concentrations ($P < 0.001$).

Cross-protection Between PCP Subtypes

Types 6B and 23F monovalent vaccines did not elicit heterologous antibodies (i.e., anti-23F and anti-6B, respectively), and immunization with type 23F vaccine did not protect against type 6B infection.[24] Cross-protection among subtypes was also studied.[25] Chinchillas were given two doses of a tetravalent vaccine composed of four pneumococcal PCP types (6B, 14, 19F, 23F) conjugated to OMPC. Vaccination induced at least a twofold anti-PCP IgG serum antibody rise against types 6A, 6B, 19A, and 19F PCP in 71, 89, 94, and 96% of chinchillas, respectively. Geometric mean week 8 antibody titers tended to be higher for PCP subtypes contained in the vaccine (6B, 19F) than for related subtypes (6A, 19A).

Middle-ear outcomes of the vaccinated groups challenged with types 6B, 6A, and 19F, but not 19A, were significantly better than the respective placebo vaccine groups. Middle-ear outcomes were not significantly different in ears of vaccinated chinchillas challenged with types 6B and 6A strains, demonstrating cross-protection within group 6. The vaccine was significantly more protective for type 19F OM than type 19A disease, demonstrating lack of cross-protection within group 19. Postchallenge OM severity for individual chinchillas was inversely correlated with serum anti-PCP IgG antibody concentration at the time of challenge. Therefore, types 6B and 19F PCP-OMPC elicited type-specific and heterologous antibody within serogroups, but middle-ear protection was variable for heterologous types.

Vaccine Polyvalency

Clinically effective pneumococcal vaccines must be able to protect against several pneumococcal types. Vaccine polyvalency may be a concern with PCP conjugate vaccines, since the conjugated protein antigens could adversely interact to reduce vaccine immunogenicity and efficacy. We studied this interaction in the chinchilla model using monovalent (types 6B and 14), tetravalent (types 6B, 14, 19F, 23F), and heptavalent (types 4, 6B, 9V, 14, 18C, 19F, 23F) PCP-OMPC conjugate vaccines.[26] Type 6B and 14 IgG antibody distributions in serum were not significantly different in the respective monovalent and polyvalent vaccine groups; type 19F IgG antibody distributions were similar in the two polyvalent vaccine groups.

Vaccine efficacy was tested by injecting both middle ears of immunized and control chinchillas with type 6B, 14, or 19F pneumococci. Middle-ear outcomes after types 6B and 19F challenge were significantly better for immunized chinchillas than controls. Disease was not modified in the tetravalent vaccine group challenged with type 14 pneumococci, perhaps due to lower type 14 antibody concentrations prechallenge than in the 6B and 19F vaccine groups. Monovalent, tetravalent, and heptavalent preparations of 6B-OMPC vaccine yielded similar efficacy, as did tetravalent and heptavalent preparations of 19F-OMPC vaccine. Thus, 6B and 19F PCP-OMPC monovalent and polyvalent vaccine mixtures have similar immunogenicity and OM efficacy.

Vaccine Efficacy during Influenza Infection

Direct middle-ear inoculation of pneumococci is an extremely vigorous test of vaccine efficacy. It bypasses the natural nasopharyngeal acquisition of pneumococci, their adherence to nasopharyngeal epithelium, and ascent to the middle ear via the eustachian tube. Mucosal defense mechanisms are therefore, less likely to contribute to middle-ear protection in the direct middle-ear challenge model than in nasopharyngeal colonization. While a conservative test of vaccine efficacy is an important step in the evaluation of a new vaccine, conditions associated with the natural history of an illness should also be tested to measure true vaccine effectiveness in the target population of children.

We tested the efficacy of monovalent type 6B and type 14 PCP-OMPC conjugate vaccines by injecting the anterior nares of chinchillas with wild influenza A (H3N2) virus, and four days later injected the vaccine-type pneumococcal strain intranasally.[27] Both vaccines administered intramuscularly in two doses produced significant serum IgG anti-PCP antibody responses. Prechallenge serum anti-PCP IgG antibody titers were 0.5 μg/mL or greater in 93% of chinchillas given type 6B conjugate vaccine and in 88% given type 14 conjugate vaccine; this serum titer was previously demonstrated to predict vaccine-type middle-ear protection in the chinchilla model.[25]

After intranasal challenge with influenza A virus followed four days later by intranasal vaccine-type pneumococcus, type 6B pneumococcal OM (POM) developed in 45% and type 14 POM developed in 75% of unvaccinated control chinchillas. Compared with controls, type 6B vaccine efficacy was 72% against pneumococcal OM and 55% against any OM. Compared with controls, type 14 vaccine efficacy was

29% against pneumococcal OM and 33% against any OM. Previously reported efficacy rates using direct middle-ear pneumococcal challenge without influenza virus infection were 64% and 17% for type 6B and type 14 conjugate vaccines, respectively.[24,25] Thus, conjugate vaccine efficacy for type 14 pneumococcal OM was demonstrated more clearly after intranasal challenge with pneumococci and influenza A virus than after direct middle-ear challenge with pneumococci alone. Efficacy of type 6B conjugate vaccine was similar using both challenge protocols. Greater virulence of type 14 than type 6B pneumococci in the chinchilla model probably accounted for lower vaccine efficacy with type 14 conjugate vaccine in both challenge models.

Pneumococcal Conjugate Vaccine in Human Clinical Trials

Clinical trials are in progress with several of the pneumococcal conjugate vaccines. All conjugates tested to date have induced dose-dependent T-cell-dependent responses, predominantly IgG1, and certain types (e.g., 6B) elicited a weaker response. Antibody responses have been greater after two and three injections at two-month intervals than after a single injection. A seven-valent vaccine OM clinical efficacy trial sponsored by Merck Research Laboratories began in 1993, and a Finnish comparative vaccine trial for OM efficacy began late 1995.

The Merck PCP-OMPC vaccines are immunogenic in human infants. We reported that one dose of type 6B-OMPC conjugate vaccine elicited a significant IgG anti-6B PCP antibody response in infants four to six months of age, and two doses elicited significant IgG responses in infants two to four months of age.[28] Primary antibody responses to larger doses of 6B-OMPC and 14-OMPC vaccines (2.5 and 5.0 mg) were greater than to lower doses (0.5 and 1.0 mg), but similar antibody responses were observed after a booster dose was given in the second year irrespective of primary dose size.[29,30] Tetravalent PCP-OMPC vaccine containing types 6B, 14, 19F, and 23F antigens was given to infants at two, four, and six months of age; and significant antibody responses to all four types were observed after the second and third dose[31] Three doses of a seven-valent PCP-OMPC vaccine (types 4, 6B, 9V, 14, 19F, 18C, 23F) were given to over 100 infants at two, four, and six months of age.[32] Serum antibody responses to 4, 9V, 19F, and 23F were better than responses to types 6B, 18C, and 19F, but 63% to 100% of infants had serum antibody concentrations greater than 1.0-mg type-specific IgG/mL after the third dose (age seven months). This serum antibody concentration is protective in the chinchilla model.[24]

Wyeth Lederle Vaccines and Pediatrics have linked pneumococcal capsular oligosaccharides to the same diphtheria toxin mutant (CRM[197]) used in their Hib oligosaccharide conjugate vaccine. Saccharides of varying length and composition have been tested with this conjugate. Greater immunogenicity of a type 6A-CRM[197] conjugate vaccine in adults was associated with higher overall saccharide content rather than chain length.[23] In animal studies, short-chain oligosaccharides were significantly better immunogens than long-chain homologous oligosaccharides after coupling to a carrier protein.[33] The IgG immune response specific for the carbohydrate chain of a glycoconjugate appeared to be restricted to the linking area of the glycoconjugate and confined to a few monosaccharide residues of the carbohydrate structure.[33] However, a recent report demonstrated that both oligo- and polysaccharide-CRM[197] conjugate vaccines given to two- to six-month old infants primed for 6- to 19-fold anamnestic antibody increases after administration of plain 23-valent PS vaccine at age 18 months; saccharide chain length and dose were not significant in priming.[34]

A single dose of a pentavalent (types 6B, 14, 18C, 19F, 23F) CRM[197]-conjugate vaccine given to Finnish two-year-old children produced significant serum IgG antibody responses to each of the five PCPs, as well as PCP-specific responses in peripheral blood IgA antibody secreting cells.[35] These latter results suggest that pneumococcal conjugate vaccines may provide local IgA antibodies in addition to systemic IgG antibodies, a conclusion consistent with the observation that Hib conjugate vaccines reduce the nasopharyngeal carriage of Hib.[36]

In addition to the OMPC and CRM[197] carrier molecules, Schneerson *et al.* have linked type 6A PCP to tetanus toxoid and demonstrated immunogenicity in adults.[22]

Pneumococcal capsular polysaccharides have been coupled to both diphtheria and tetanus toxoids by Pasteur-Merieux-Connaught. Serum antibody responses to tetravalent PS-T vaccine given at two to six months were somewhat greater than responses to PS-D vaccine, but a booster response at 12 months to plain PS vaccine was demonstrated in both vaccine groups.[37] Octavalent preparations of PS-D and PS-T given at two to six months also significantly reduced the nasopharyngeal carriage of vaccine types in infants between 7 and 13 months of age, but immunization had no effect on carriage of nonvaccine types.[38] Vaccines that reduce infant colonization are likely to produce a immunoprophylactic effect in unvaccinated susceptible children. Neither PCP-T nor PCP-D vaccines given to infants interfered with the antibody response to concurrent Hib conjugate (PRP-T) vaccine response.[39]

Further development of pneumococcal conjugate vaccines is now a high national and international priority due not only to the high incidence of pneumococcal OM but also to the rapid emergence of pneumococci with high-level resistance to multiple antibiotics. Although the new conjugate vaccines offer great promise, a few obstacles remain. Because types causing human disease are not consistent among countries surveyed to date, PCP-type composition of polyvalent conjugate vaccines may need to be different in various regions of the world. Continuous PCP-type surveillance will need to be developed in a many countries to determine if vaccine introduction and widespread use alters PCP-type prevalence. Such an observation was made 15 years ago by Maxwell Finland, who showed that PCP types prevalent in Boston changed significantly during a period of five decades.[40]

In the United States, Canada, Belgium, Finland, Sweden, Ireland, Spain, and Denmark, types 6A/6B, 14F, 18C, 19F, and 23F are most frequent,[41,42] although types 1 and 5 are becoming more prevalent in Denmark (J. Henrickson, personal communication). A Finnish study of 365 invasive pneumococcal infections demonstrated that types 6A/6B, 14, 18C, 19F, and 23F covered 68% of infections; adding types 4, 7F, and 9N increased coverage to 90%.[43] In Israel, Egypt, Nigeria, and New Guinea, however, types 1 and 5 make up 35% of all pneumococcal infections.[44] The number of different capsular polysaccharide types included in a polyvalent vaccine may lead to antigenic competition.

The nature of the protein carrier may be a critical determinant in the polyvalent limitations of conjugate vaccines. The type and amount of carrier protein may induce immune tolerance to itself if used in large quantities, or against other vaccine antigens that might be given simultaneously. Preexisting immunity to the carrier protein or saccharide may enhance or limit the immune response. The method used to covalently couple protein and saccharide molecules, the physical nature of the saccharides, the saccharide-to-protein ratio, and presence of free polysaccharide all contribute to vaccine immunogenicity. Biochemical considerations may preclude physical or chemical combinations of multiple polysaccharide antigens linked to protein carriers in these vaccines. Since an ultimate goal is to combine all vaccines given by injection to infants in single syringes, pneumococcal conjugates will have to perform well when mixed with Hib and *N. meningitides* conjugates, diphtheria and tetanus toxoids, pertussis antigens, and hepatitis B virus recombinant antigens.

Adjuvants such as aluminum hydroxide may be necessary. Additional factors include the frequency of immunization, age and immunocompetency of the host, and coadministration with other vaccines. Keyserling *et al.* recently showed that two adjuvants, monophosphoryl lipid A and QS-21, significantly enhanced the immunogenicity of heptavalent PCP-CRP[197] in infant rhesus monkeys.[45]

Pneumococcal conjugate vaccines must also be studied in high risk conditions such as human immunodeficiency virus (HIV) infection, organ and bone marrow transplant, functional and anatomic asplenia, nephrotic syndrome, renal failure, and the elderly. A recent report demonstrated that HIV infected and uninfected healthy children 6–23 months had similar antibody responses to a high-dose pentavalent oligosaccharide-CRM[197] vaccine; the two groups had similar rates of antibody decline one to eight months after vaccine dose 3.[46] A preliminary report suggests that the serum antibody response of patients who recovered from Hodgkin's disease to PCP-OMPC conjugate vaccine is lower than their response to polyvalent plain PCP vaccine.[47]

Vaccine antigen epitope suppression due to overuse of functional protein carriers used in most licensed and investigational polysaccharide–protein conjugate vaccines is a potential concern in conjugate vaccine development.[48] Novel carrier peptides could obviate this concern and might permit enhanced expression of multiple polysaccharide antigens from different pathogens including *S. pneumoniae.*[49]

It may be advantageous to use pneumococcal surface proteins known to play a role in pneumococcal disease pathogenesis for use as vaccine targets.[21] Several surface proteins—pneumolysin, surface protein A, surface adhesin A—and pneumococcal neuraminidase have been proposed as possible vaccine candidates or carriers for future conjugate vaccines.[50–52] Virolainen *et al.* recently showed that very young infants can produce PspA IgG antibodies after invasive pneumococcal disease, suggesting that this common protein antigen may be a reasonable vaccine antigen in young infants.[53] Efficacy of two pneumolysin-PCP conjugates has been demonstrated in a murine model of pneumococcal sepsis.[54,55] Surface protein vaccines can be produced inexpensively in bacterial cultures and thus may be more affordable in developing countries.[21] The potential ability of pneumococcal protein antigens to neutralize pneumococcal toxins, such as pneumolysin, adds a broader application to the use of these vaccines. Pneumolysin, for example, appears to play a critical role in the early pathogenesis of alveolar injury and tissue invasion during pneumococcal pneumonia and bacteremia.[56] A similar role for pneumolysin, however, was not demonstrated in experimental pneumococcal OM.[57]

NONTYPABLE *HAEMOPHILUS INFLUENZAE* VACCINES

H. influenzae isolated from infected middle ears are almost always nontypable. Results of biotyping, assays of metabolic enzymes, and OMP and lipooligosaccharide (LOS) analyses have revealed considerable diversity among the nontypable *H. influenzae* strains causing OM. The observation that chinchilla antiserum raised to formaldehyde-fixed NTHi conferred passive protection against OM in other chinchillas suggests that one or more surface antigens hold promise as an OM vaccine.[58] Their success as vaccine antigens will be based on their conservation among nontypable strains, their accessibility to the host's immune system, their immunogenicity in infants, and their requirement as a virulence factors for the organism.

Potential vaccine antigens for NTHi include outer membrane proteins (OMP), high-molecular-weight (HMW) proteins, pili, and fimbriae (TABLE 2). Several candidate OMP antigens have been identified. Protein-2 (P2) is a 36–41 kDa molecule that makes up about 50% of the OMP content, is the target of human bactericidal antibody, is protective in the infant rat Hib model, but shows antigen heterogeneity among strains.[59] P6 has a molecular weight of 16.6 kDa, makes up 1 to 5% of the OMP, elicits bactericidal antibody, and is highly conserved among strains.[59] Two other OMPs, P1 and P4, have elicited homologous and heterologous Hib protection in the infant rat model.[60] Further work is necessary to characterize the extent of homology of the antibody-accessible regions of these molecules. A recent report suggests that traces of reagents used during protein purification may play an important role in determining the success of *in vivo* and *in vitro* studies with OMPs.[61]

Bactericidal antibody response and protection from infection in animal models

TABLE 2. *H. influenzae* Potential Vaccine Antigens Including Outer Membrane Proteins, High-molecular-weight Proteins, Pili, and Fimbriae

Surface Antigen	Molecular Weight (kDa)	Surface Conservation Among Strains	Antibody is Bactericidal	Protection in Animal Model	Mediate Adherence
OMP P1[73,106]	45	?	?	+	?
OMP P2[59]	36–41	—	+	+	?
OMP P4[60]	45	?	?	+	?
OMP P6[67,70,72,109]	16.6	+	+	+	?
OMP PCP[68]	15	+	+	?	?
Protein D	?	+	?	?	?
HMW proteins[78,110]	100–150	?	?	?	+
Fimbriae / Pili[77,111,112]	23–27	?	?	?	+

Source: From Ogra *et al.*[113]

has been used to identify protective NTHi antigens. Indirect evidence suggests that serum bactericidal antibody is associated with protection from infection.[62,63] Therefore, an antigen that generates bactericidal antibodies holds promise as being capable of generating a protective immune response. The chinchilla OM model has been employed to study protection from infection by NTHi.[58,64–66] Green *et al.* have cautioned, however, that the immune response in chinchillas to *H. influenzae* antigens is different from that of other species.[65]

Immunization of animals with purified P6, P4, and PCP has generated bactericidal antibodies.[67–69] Murphy *et al.* have shown that immunopurified human antibodies to P6 are bactericidal.[70] Moreover, otitis-prone children have lower responses to P6 than healthy children, suggesting that antibody against P6 is important in protecting the middle ear from NTHi infection.[71] Antibodies to P1 and P6 of Hib are protective in the infant rat model of bacteremia.[72,73] Mucosal immunization with P6 in a rat model was most effective when Peyer's patch immunization was accompanied by an intratracheal boost; P6-specific antibodies in serum and bronchoalveolar lavage fluid were cross-reactive among strains with enhanced bacterial clearance of homologous and heterologous bacteria in the lungs.[74] Thus, P6, P4, and PCP are reasonable antigens to use in phase I studies in humans after appropriate purity and safety criteria are met.

Protein D is a surface-exposed immunoglobulin D-binding membrane protein of *H. influenzae,* and the gene encoding the lipoprotein (hpd) has been cloned.[75,76] Restriction fragment length polymorphism of the hpd region in 100 different NTHi strains showed a high degree of homology, suggesting that protein D is a possible vaccine candidate.[76]

Blocking attachment of NTHi to respiratory tract mucosa is another approach to preventing OM by vaccination. HMW proteins and pili mediate attachment of *H. influenzae* to human respiratory tract cells *in vitro.*[77–79] Four *H. influenzae* pili types have been identified. Brinton *et al.* determined that a 12-valent pilus vaccine would cover 69% of the NTHi otitis media strains, and a 20-valent vaccine would cover 80 to 90% of strains.[80] Strain-specific protection with a pilus vaccine has been demonstrated in the chinchilla model, although results were confounded by a small amount of lipooligosaccharide (LOS) in the vaccine that induced some agglutinating antibody.[81] Immunization of chinchillas with purified HMW1 and HMW2 adherence proteins modified the course of experimental NTHi OM and down-regulated the expression of HMW proteins in bacteria that caused infection in immunized animals.[82]

H. influenzae express morphologically and functionally distinct types of fimbriae, of which the LKP fimbriae mediate hemagglutination and adherence to human epithelial cells but hamper mucosal invasion. Therefore, fimbrial phase variation may contribute to the pathogenesis of NTHi infection.[83] The existence of greater than 14 LKP serotypes hampers vaccine development based on fimbriae, since a monovalent fimbria vaccine confers protection against only the homologous strain.[66]

Lipooligosaccharide is another major surface-exposed antigen on NTHi and is a potential target of human bactericidal antibodies. A detoxified LOS-protein conjugate has been prepared as a vaccine and is being characterized. However, NTHi LOS's are antigenically heterogeneous; thus, a multivalent conjugate will be needed to cover all the disease-producing strains.

TABLE 3. *Moraxella catarrhalis* Outer Membrane Antigens with Vaccine Potential

Surface Antigen	Molecular Weight (kDa)	Proposed Function	Other Observations
HMW-OMP[114,115]	350–700	Unknown	Oligomer. Antibodies enhance clearance in mice
OMP B1[116,117]	84	Iron acquisition	Major target of human antibody
OMP B2 (Cop B)[87,88]	80	Iron acquisition	Antibodies enhance clearance in mice
OMP CD[85,118,119]	46	Porin	Highly conserved. Homology with *Pseudomonas* OprF
OMP E[120,121]	50	Porin	Highly conserved

Source: From Ogra *et al.*[113]

MORAXELLA CATARRHALIS VACCINES

M. catarrhalis, previously called *Branhamella catarrhalis* and *Neisseria catarrhalis,* has been recognized as an important OM pathogen only in the recent past. Several OMP and HMW antigens have vaccine potential (TABLE 3).

Surface antigens of *M. catarrhalis* that are potential vaccine candidates include OMPs, LOS, and fimbriae.[84,85] OMPs from 50 strains obtained from diverse body sites and geographic locations showed a high degree of similarity of OMP patterns.[85] LOS is an important virulence factor that contributes to pathogenicity of nonenteric gram-negative bacteria. Murphy found evidence that *M. catarrhalis* LOS is relatively conserved among strains, raising the feasibility of using a portion of the LOS molecule in a vaccine.[84] Murphy also found that *M. catarrhalis* are fimbriated, suggesting that antibodies to fimbriae might block attachment of *M. catarrhalis* to mucosal surfaces.[84]

Unfortunately, no functional correlates of protection have been identified, and there is no clear evidence that antibody to *M. catarrhalis* is associated with OM protection. The chinchilla model has been disappointing for studying *M. catarrhalis* infection. Although a murine model has been developed, animals clear the organism from their respiratory tract without developing disease.[86–88] Because *M. catarrhalis* is exclusively a human pathogen, evaluating vaccine candidates in animal models may not reflect the antigenicity or efficacy of these antigens in humans.

RESPIRATORY VIRAL VACCINES

Attenuated viral vaccines also hold promise of preventing childhood OM, since viruses contribute to the pathogenesis of OM. Impaired eustachian tube opening and the resulting negative middle-ear pressure is a consequence of upper respiratory viral infection and often leads to OM.[89] Respiratory syncytial virus (RSV), adenovirus, and influenza viruses are strongly associated with symptomatic OM in children; OM was no more common after rhinovirus infection than in children without a viral infection.[90] Increased nasopharyngeal carriage of pneumococci has been documented after the onset of common colds, and it has been estimated that three common colds occur for each acquisition of a pneumococcus.[91,92] Viral vaccines are therefore an important consideration in OM control.

Two clinical trials with killed influenza vaccines have shown a significant reduction in OM among vaccine recipients compared to control children during periods of high influenza disease activity in the community. In a Finnish trial, the incidence of acute OM associated with influenza A virus was reduced 83% in one- to three-year-old children who received two doses of a trivalent subvirion influenza virus vaccine (Fluzone, Connaught Laboratories Inc, Swiftwater, PA) prior to the 1988–1989 influenza epidemic compared to unvaccinated control children.[93] There was a 36% reduction in the total number of children with acute OM in the vaccine group compared to controls.

Attenuated intranasal influenza vaccines are immunogenic in children, eliciting a secretory IgA antibody response. These vaccines have not been tested for OM efficacy, but theoretically would be as or more effective than killed vaccines. Attenuated RSV vaccines are also being evaluated for acute bronchiolitis efficacy in infants. Since RSV is highly associated with acute OM, these vaccines may also contribute to middle-ear protection, but these studies have not been performed. Similarly, parainfluenza virus and adenovirus vaccines may be effective.

In the chinchilla animal model, combined nasopharyngeal inoculation with wild-type influenza A virus and pneumococcus led to a high incidence of pneumococcal otitis media, whereas either pathogen inoculated alone infrequently caused OM.[94] Influenza A virus strains, however, differed in chinchillas as in humans in their capacity to enhance the development of pneumococcal OM.[95] These experiments suggested that immunoprophylaxis of bacterial OM may be addressed by identifying respiratory virus species with OM pathogenicity.

Influenza Vaccine Efficacy

We reported that a cold-tolerant, attenuated influenza A virus vaccine was more effective than an inactivated influenza A vaccine in blocking colonization with the wild-type influenza virus and pneumococcus, and in reducing the attack rate of OM in the chinchilla model.[96] Seroconversion rates in the attenuated and inactivated influenza vaccine groups were similar (62% and 57%, respectively). The attenuated viral vaccine but not the inactivated vaccine significantly reduced nasal titers of both the challenge wild virus strain and pneumococci. The incidence of OM was significantly lower in the attenuated vaccine group (18%) than in controls (41%), but was not lower in the inactivated vaccine group (39%). Thus, attenuated influenza virus immunization administered intranasally may be an effective pneumococcal OM prophylaxis strategy in children.

Adenovirus vaccine, containing attenuated live virus of immunotypes 4 and 7, has been used in military populations but is not licensed for general use. This vaccine, given in an oral enteric-coated capsule, has an adult efficacy exceeding 90%.[97] Efforts to develop effective RSV and parainfluenza vaccines are currently in progress.

PASSIVE IMMUNOPROPHYLAXIS

Passive immunoprophylaxis also has potential for preventing OM. Human bacterial polysaccharide immune globulin, prepared from the pooled plasma of donors immunized with polyvalent pneumococcal, meningococcal, and *H. influenzae* type b vaccines, was protective for pneumococcal OM in children and in the chinchilla model. High-dose respiratory syncytial virus-enriched immunoglobulin reduced the incidence and severity of RSV lower respiratory tract infection in high-risk children. Passive immunoprophylaxis may also be effective in children with specific immune deficiencies, such as IgG2 deficiency, and patients who fail to respond to future vaccines.

The rationale for systemic immunization in preventing OM comes from passive immunoprophylaxis studies. Intraperitoneal administration of a human bacterial polysaccharide immune globulin (BPIG), which contained high levels of anti-PCP immunoglobulin G from immunized human adult donors, protected chinchillas from pneumococcal OM.[98] Similarly, passive administration of antibody prevented experimental middle-ear infection caused by nontypable *H. influenzae,* and administration of serum IgG antibody against the capsular polysaccharide of *H. influenzae* type b (Hib) enhanced bacterial clearance in the murine lower respiratory tract.[58,64,99]

Shurin *et al.* gave BPIG intramuscularly to children 1 to 24 months of age with 1 to 3 prior episodes of acute OM, and saline placebo to a control group.[15] Although the incidence of acute OM during the four-month study was similar in BPIG and placebo recipients, pneumococcal acute OM was 50% less frequent, and time spent free of acute OM was significantly longer in BPIG recipients than controls. These animal and human studies show that circulating antibody, without stimulation of specific local immunity, can prevent middle-ear infection.

Two other recently published studies found no acute OM protection in children given pooled human immune globulin by the intramuscular route or intravenous route.[100,101] These studies, however, differed in the following respects from the BPIG trial reported by Shurin *et al.*:[15] (1) the immune globulin product used was not enriched in anti-PCP antibodies, as was the BPIG preparation, (2) middle-ear cultures of acute OM fluid were not performed to document bacteriologic efficacy, and (3) time free of acute OM was not measured. Since standard intravenously administered immune globulin preparations contain lower and more variable lot-to-lot levels of antibodies against PCPs,[102] these preparations should not be used for acute OM prophylaxis without further standardization and testing.

Shahid *et al.* recently reported an alternate method of passively delivering anti-PCP antibodies to infants.[103] Healthy Bangladesh women were given Pneumovax-

$23^®$ at approximately 7½ months gestation without adverse events. Mothers had good antibody responses to types 6B and 14 PCPs. Cord blood antibody levels were about 45% of maternal levels, and fourfold higher than those in infants of unimmunized control mothers. Thus, maternal immunization may provide a method to protect very young children against OM.

OTITIS MEDIA VACCINE IMPACT

Because OM is a disease of infancy with a predilection for recurrent OM established as young as two months of age, OM vaccines will be most effective if they are administered at two months of age and are fully effective by four to six months of age.[1,104,105] In one study, 61% of pneumococcal OM episodes occurred during the first year of life, 18% in the second, and 7% in the third year.[6] Children with specific risk factors for recurrent disease should have priority for immunization. Known risk factors include onset of bilateral disease early in life, siblings with recurrent OM, day care exposure, and absence of breast feeding.[106]

Vaccines effective in preventing acute OM in infancy and early childhood will most likely have a large impact on the entire spectrum of middle-ear disease, including OM with effusion and chronic OM, since these entities arise from early acute OM. Moreover, since sinusitis and pneumonia are caused by the same bacteria and viruses that infect the middle ear, OM vaccines will most likely be effective in preventing these diseases as well.

Will parents accept OM vaccines that are not fully protective? A recent report described parents' surprisingly high acceptability of low-efficacy vaccines for OM in five hypothetical scenarios.[107] About half of the 601 parents questioned would accept an intranasal or single-injection vaccine preventing three or more OM infections in six months. One-third would accept a vaccine preventing one OM episode in the next six months. Parents may choose to use such vaccines if they perceive that benefits outweigh the discomfort of vaccination. Their acceptance of a vaccine would most likely be enhanced if their other children had experienced recurrent OM.

SUMMARY

Considerable evidence suggests that otitis media (OM) can be prevented by systemic immunization. Building on the highly effective *H. influenzae* type b (Hib) conjugate vaccine technology, pneumococcal conjugate vaccines are being developed to circumvent T-independence of these antigens and provide durable immunity at a very young age. Several pneumococcal conjugate vaccines are currently in clinical testing. Potential vaccine antigens of nontypable *H. influenzae* (NTHi) include OMP, HMW, pili, and fimbriae. Several OMPs show extensive homology among strains, but surface determinants of others are highly variable so that antibodies to surface epitopes of one strain will not bind to surface epitopes of another. Several *M. catarrhalis* OMP and HMW antigens have vaccine potential, but no functional correlates of protection have been identified, and there is no clear evidence that antibody to *M. catarrhalis* is associated with OM protection. Attenuated viral vaccines also hold promise of preventing childhood OM. Two clinical trials with killed influenza vaccines have shown a significant reduction in OM among vaccine recipients compared to control children during periods of high influenza disease activity in the community. Passive immunoprophylaxis also has potential for preventing OM. Human bacterial polysaccharide immune globulin was protective for pneumococcal OM in children and in the chinchilla OM model. High-dose respiratory syncytial virus-enriched immunoglobulin reduced the incidence and severity of RSV lower respiratory tract infection in high-risk children. Passive immunoprophylaxis may also be effective in children with specific immune deficiencies, such as IgG2 deficiency, and patients who fail to respond to vaccines.

REFERENCES

1. TEELE, D. W., J. O. KLEIN, B. A. ROSNER, *et al.* 1989. Epidemiology of otitis media during the first seven years of life in children in Greater Boston: A prospective, cohort study. J. Infect. Dis. **160:** 83–94.
2. STOOL, S. E. & M. J. FIELD. 1989. The impact of otitis media. Pediatr. Infect. Dis. J. **8:** S11–S14, 1989.
3. FRIA, T. J., E. I. CANTEKIN & J. A. EICHLER. 1985. Hearing acuity of children with otitis media with effusion. Arch. Otolaryngol. **111:** 10–16.
4. ROBERTS, J. E., M. R. RUCHINAL, L. P. MEDLEY, S. A. ZEIAEL, M. MUNDY, J. ROUSH, S. HOOPER, D. BRYANT & F. W. HENDERSON. 1995. Otitis media, hearing sensitivity, and maternal responsiveness in relation to language during infancy. J. Pediatr. **126:** 481–489.
5. FRIEL-PATTI, S. & T. FINITZO. 1990. Language learning in a prospective study of otitis media with effusion in the first two years of life. J. Speech Hearing Res. **33:** 188–194.
6. AUSTRIAN, R., V. M. HOWIE & J. H. PLOUSSARD. 1977. The bacteriology of pneumococcal otitis media. Johns Hopkins Med. J. **141:** 104–111.
7. BARENKAMP, S. J., P. A. SHURIN, C. D. MARCHANT, R. B. KARASIC, *et al.* 1984. Do children with recurrent *H. influenzae* otitis media become infected with a new organism or reacquire the original strain? J. Pediatr. **105:** 533–537.
8. KARJALAINEN, H. K., M. K. QUARTEY, S. K. JUHN & G. S. GIEBINK. 1993. Pneumococcal otitis media treatment timing and susceptibility to homologous reinfection in the chinchilla model. Association for Research in Otolaryngology Ann. Meet., St. Petersburg, Fla.
9. GIEBINK, G. S. 1981. The pathogenesis of pneumococcal otitis media in chinchillas and the efficacy of vaccination in prophylaxis. Rev. Infect. Dis. 3(Suppl 2):42–52.
10. SLOYER, J. L., V. M. HOWIE, J. H. PLOUSSARD, G. SCHIFFMAN & R. B. JOHNSTON, JR. 1976. Immune response to acute otitis media: Association between middle ear fluid antibody and the clearing of clinical infection. J. Clin. Microbiol. **4:** 306–308.
11. TEELE, D. W., J. O. KLEIN & THE GREATER BOSTON COLLABORATIVE OTITIS MEDIA STUDY GROUP. 1981. Use of pneumococcal vaccine for prevention of recurrent acute otitis media in infants in Boston. Rev. Infect. Dis. **3:** S113–S118.
12. HOWIE, V. M., J. PLOUSSARD, J. L. SLOYER & J. C. HILL. 1984. Use of pneumococcal polysaccharide vaccine in preventing otitis media in infants: Different results between racial groups. Pediatrics **73:** 79–81.
13. MÄKELÄ, P. H., M. SIBAKOV, E. HERVA & J. HENRICKSEN. 1980. Pneumococcal vaccine and otitis media. Lancet **2:** 547–551.
14. GIEBINK, G. S., I. K. BERZINS, G. SCHIFFMAN & P. G. QUIE. 1979. Experimental otitis me-

dia following nasal colonization with type 7F *Streptococcus pneumoniae:* Prevention after vaccination with pneumococcal capsular polysaccharide. J. Infect. Dis. **140:** 716–723.

15. SHURIN, P. A., J. M. REHMUS, C. E. JOHNSON, C. D. MERCHANT, S. A. CARLIN, D. M. SU-PER, G. F. VAN HARE, P. K. JONES, D. M. AMBROSINO & G. R. SIBER. 1993. Bacterial polysaccharide immune globulin for prophylaxis of acute otitis media in high-risk children. J. Pediatr. **123:** 801–810.

16. GRAY, B. M., G. M. CONVERSE III & H. C. DILLON, JR. 1980. Epidemiologic studies of *Streptococcus pneumoniae* in infants: Acquisition, carriage, and infection during the first 24 months of life. J. Infect. Dis. **142:** 923–933.

17. AVERY, O. T. & W. F. GOEBEL. 1929. Chemoimmunological studies on conjugated carbohydrate proteins. II. Immunological specificity of synthetic sugar-protein antigens. J. Exp. Med. **50:** 533–550.

18. BEUVERY, E. C., F. VAN ROSSUM & J. NAGLE. 1982. Comparison of the induction of immunoglobulin M and G antibodies in mice with purified pneumococcal type 3 and meningogoccal group C polysaccharides and their protein conjugates. Infect. Immun. **37:** 15–22.

19. CHU, C., R. SCHNEERSON, J. B. ROBBINS & S. C. RASTOGI. 1983. Further studies on the immunogenicity of *Haemophilus influenzae* type b and pneumococcal type 6A polysaccharide-protein conjugates. Infect. Immun. **40:** 245–256.

20. GORDON, L. K. 1984. Characterization of a hapten-carrier conjugate vaccine: *H. influenzae*-diphtheria conjugate vaccine. *In* Modern Approaches to Vaccines, R. M. Chanock and R. A. Lerner, Eds.: 393–396. Cold Spring Harbor Laboratory Press. Cold Spring Harbor, N.Y.

21. KLEIN, D. L. 1995. Pneumococcal conjugate vaccines: Review and update. Microbl. Drug Resist. **1:** 49–58.

22. SCHNEERSON, R., J. B. ROBBINS, J. C. PARKE, JR., *et al.* 1986. Quantitative and qualitative analyses of serum antibodies elicited in adults by *Haemophilus influenzae* type b and pneumococcus type 6A capsular polysaccharide-tetanus toxoid conjugates. Infect. Immun. **52:** 519–528.

23. ANDERSON, P. & R. BETTS. 1989. Human adult immunogenicity of protein-coupled pneumococcal capsular antigens of serotypes prevalent in otitis media. Pediatr. Infect. Dis. J. **8:** S50–S53.

24. GIEBINK, G. S., M. KOSKELA, P. P. VELLA, M. HARRIS & C. LE. 1993. Pneumococcal capsular polysaccharide-meningococcal outer membrane protein complex conjugate vaccines: Immunogenicity and efficacy in experimental pneumococcal otitis media. J. Infect. Dis. **167:** 347–355.

25. GIEBINK, G. S., J. D. MEIER, M. K. QUARTEY, C. L. LIEBELER & C. T. LE. 1996. Immunogenicity and efficacy of *Streptococcus pneumoniae* polysaccharide-protein conjugate vaccines against homologous and heterologous serotypes in the chinchilla otitis media model. J. Infect. Dis. **173:** 119–127.

26. GIEBINK, G. S., J. D. MEIER & M. K. QUARTEY. 1996. Comparative immunogenicity and efficacy of monovalent and polyvalent pneumococcal conjugate vaccines.

27. GIEBINK, G. S., J. D. MEIER & M. K. QUARTEY. 1996. Pneumococcal capsular polysaccharide-protein conjugate vaccine efficacy in preventing pneumococcal otitis media during experimental influenza A virus infection in chinchillas.

28. GIEBINK, G. S., C. T. ALWARD, A. A. RZEPKA, *et al.* 1993. Isotype antibody responses to type 6B pneumococcal polysaccharide conjugate vaccine in infants [Abstr.]. Pediatr. Res. **33:** 168A.

29. MENDELMAN, P. M., E. ANDERSON, T. MARTIN, G. S. GIEBINK, C. RUSK, L. LUKACS, C. SHADLE, M. STALLWORTH, D. LOY, M. CHUNG, H. MATTHEWS, L. FEELEY & J. DONNELLY.

1994. A dose ranging study in young infants of a type 6B monovalent pneumococcal conjugate vaccine [Abst.]. Pediatr. Res. **35:** 187A.

30. KEYSERLING, H., C. BOSLEY, S. STARR, B. WATSON, D. LAUFER, E. ANDERSON, E. SHAPIRO, P. MENDELMAN, C. RUSK, J. DONNELLY, D. LOY, C. SHADLE, L. FEELEY & H. MATTHEWS. 1994. Immunogenicity of pneumococcal type 14 conjugate vaccine in infants [Abst.]. Pediatr. Res. **35:** 184A.

31. KEYSERLING, H. L., E. L. ANDERSON & J. T. MARTIN. 1993. Immunogenicity of a tetravalent (types 6B, 14, 19F, 23F) pneumococcal conjugate vaccine in infants [Abstract]. Pediatr. Res. **33:** 172A.

32. MENDELMAN, P. M., S. BLOCK, J. HEDRICK, E. ANDERSON, H. KEYSERLING, R. YOGEV, D. GREENBERG, C. RUSK, C. SHADLE, D. LOV, M. CHUNG, M. STALLWORTH, G. CALANDRA, H. MATTHEWS, J. WARD, L. FEELEY, J. DONNELLY, M. LIU, R. ELLIS & J. L. RYAN. 1994. Immunogenicity of a 7 valent pneumococcal conjugate vaccine in 2 month old infants [Abst.]. Pediatr. Res. **35:** 187A.

33. ARNDT, B. & M. PORRO. 1991. Strategies for type-specific glyconconjugate vaccines of *Streptococcus pneumoniae*. *In* Immunology of Proteins and Peptides VI, M. Z. Atassi, Ed.: 129–148. Plenum Press. New York.

34. STEINHOFF, M., K. REISINGER, H. KEYSERLING, S. BLOCK, F. MALINOSKI & R. S. DAUM. 1996. Immunologic priming of infants by *S. pneumoniae* oligo- and polysaccharide-CRM^{197} conjugate vaccines. Am. Soc. Microbiol. 36th ICAAC Abstr. **G43:** 151.

35. KÄYHTY, H., T. NIEMINEN, H. ÅHMAN, F. J. MALINOSKI & J. ESKOLA. 1994. Immunogenicity of pentavalent pneumococcal conjugate vaccine in Finnish 2-year-old children [Abstr.]. Pediatr. Res. **35:** 183A.

36. TAKALA, A. K., J. ESKOLA, M. LEINONEN, H. KÄYHTY, A. NISSINEN, E. PEKKANEN & P. H. MÄKELÄ. 1991. Reduction of oropharyngeal carriage of *Haemophilus influenzae* type b (Hib) in children immunized with an Hib conjugate vaccine. J. Infect. Dis. **164:** 982–985.

37. DAGAN, R., O. ZAMIR, R. MELAMED & O. LEROY. 1996. Immunogenicity of two tetravalent pneumococcal vaccines conjugated to either tetanus toxoid or diphtheria toxoid in young infants and their boosterability by native polysaccharide antigens. Am. Soc. Microbiol. 36th ICAAC Abstr. **G44:** 151.

38. DAGAN, R., M. MUALLEM, R. MELAMED, O. LEROY & P. YAGUPSKY. 1996. Reduction of pneumococcal nasopharyngeal carriage after immunization with tetravalent pneumococcal vaccines conjugated to either tetanus toxoid or diphtheria toxoid in early infancy. Am. Soc. Microbiol. 36th ICAAC Abstr. **G39:** 150.

39. AHMAN, H., H. KAYHTY, O. LEROY, J. FROESCHLE & J. ESKOLA. 1996. Immunogenicity of octavalent pneumococcal conjugate vaccines in Finnish infants. Am. Soc. Microbiol. 36th ICAAC Abstr. **G40:** 150.

40. FINLAND, M. & M. W. BARNES. 1977. Changes in occurrence of capsular serotypes of Streptococcus pneumoniae at Boston City Hospital during selected years between 1935 and 1974. J. Clin. Microbiol. **5:** 154–166.

41. KLEIN, J. O. 1981. The epidemiology of pneumococcal disease in infants and children. Rev. Inf. Dis. **3:** 246–253.

42. ORANGE, M. & B. M. GRAY. 1993. Pneumococcal serotypes causing disease in children in Alabama. Ped. Infect. Dis. **12:** 244–246.

43. ESKOLA, J., A. K. TAKALA, E. KELA, E. PEKKANEN, R. KALLIOKOSKI & M. LEINONEN. 1992. Epidemiology of invasive pneumococcal infections in children in Finland. JAMA **268:** 3323–3327.

44. DAGAN, R., D. ENGELHARD, E. PICCARD & D. ENGLEHARD. 1994. Epidemiology of invasive childhood pneumococcal infections in Israel (The Israeli Pediatric Bacteremia and Meningitis Group). JAMA **268:** 3328–3332.

45. KEYSERLING, H., B. KWAN, S. ROMERO-STEINER, L. PAIS, H. MCCLUR & G. CARLONE. 1996. Immunogenicity of a pneumococcal polysaccharide-protein conjugate vaccine with adjuvants in infant rhesus monkeys. Am. Soc. Microbiol. 36th ICAAC Abstr. **G36:** 149.

46. KING, J., P. VINK, J. FARLEY, I. CHANG & A. KIMURA. 1996. Duration of antibody levels after 3 doses of pneumococcal conjugate vaccine in HIV positive and HIV negative children less than 2 years of age. Am. Soc. Microbiol. 36th ICAAC Abstr. **G42:**150.

47. MOLRINE, D., S. GEORGE, N. TARBELL, P. MAUCH, L. DILLER, D. NEUBERG, R. SHAMBERGER, E. ANDERSON, N. PHILLIPS, K. KINSELLA & D. AMBROSINO. 1994. Antibody response to polysaccharide-conjugate vaccine following treatment for Hodgkin's disease [Abstr.]. Pediatr. Res. **35:** 189A.

48. SCHUTZE, M. P., C. LECLERC, M. JOLIVET, F. AUDIBERT & L. CHEDID. 1985. Carrier-induced epitope suppression, a major issue for synthetic vaccines. J. Immunol. **135:** 2319–2322.

49. TAM, J. P. 1988. Synthetic peptide vaccine design: Synthesis and properties of a high-density multiple antigenic peptide system. Proc. Natl. Acad. Sci. USA **85:** 5409–5413.

50. MCDANIEL, L. S., G. SCOTT, J. F. KEARNEY & D. E. BRILES. 1984. Monoclonal antibodies against protease sensitive pneumococcal antigens can protect mice from fatal infection with Streptococcus pneumoniae. J. Exp. Med. **160:** 386–397.

51. MCDANIEL, L. S., J. S. SHEFFIELD, P. DELUCCHI & D. BRILES. 1991. PspA, a surface protein of Streptococcus pneumoniae, is capable of eliciting protection against pneumococci of more than one capsular type. Infect. Immun. **59:** 222–228.

52. PATON, J. C., R. A. LOCK & D. J. HANSMAN. 1983. Effect of immunization with pneumolysin on survival time of mice challenged with Streptococcus pneumoniae. Infect. Immun. **40:** 548–552.

53. VIROLAINEN, A., W. RUSSELL, S. RAPOLA, D. BRILES & H. KAYHTY. 1996. Human antibodies to pneumococcal surface protein A. Am. Soc. Microbiol. 36th ICAAC Abstr. **G38:** 150.

54. PATON, J. C., R. A. LOCK & D. J. HANSMAN. 1983. Effect of immunization with pneumolysin on survival time of mice challenged with *Streptococcus pneumoniae.* Infect. Immun. **40:** 548–552.

55. KUO, J., M. DOUGLAS, H. K. REE & A. A. LINDBERG. 1995. Characterization of a recombinant pneumolysin and its use as a protein carrier for pneumococcal type 18C conjugate vaccines. Infect. Immun. **63:** 2706–2713.

56. RUBINS, J. B., P. G. DUANE, D. CHARBONEAU & E. N. JANOFF. 1992. Toxicity of pneumolysis to pulmonary endothelial cells in vitro. Infect. Immun. **60:** 1740–1746.

57. SATO, K., M. K. QUARTEY, C. L. LIEBELER, C. T. LE & G. S. GIEBINK. 1996. Roles of autolysin and pneumolysin in middle ear inflammation caused by a type 3 *Streptococcus pneumoniae* strain in the chinchilla otitis media model. Infect. Immun. **64:** 1140–1145.

58. BARENKAMP, S. J. 1986. Protection by serum antibodies in experimental nontypable *Haemophilus influenzae* otitis media. Infect. Immun. **52:** 572–578.

59. MURPHY, T. F., A. A. CAMPAGNARI, B. NELSON & M. A. APICELLA. 1989. Somatic antigens of *Haemophilus influenzae* as vaccine components. Pediatr. Infect. Dis. J. **8:** S66–S68.

60. LOEB, M. R. & E. PHILLIPS. 1989. Evaluating vaccine candidates for the prevention of otitis media. Pediatr. Infect. Dis. J. **8:** S48–S50.

61. KYD, J. M., D. TAYLOR & A. W. CRIPPS. 1995. Conservation of immune responses to proteins isolated by preparative polyacrylamide gel electrophoresis from the outer membrane of nontypeable *Haemophilus influenzae.* Infect. Immun. **62:** 5652–5658.

62. FADEN, H., J. BERNSTEIN, L. BRODSKY, J. STANIEVICH, D. KRYSTOFIK, C. SHUFF, J. J. HONG & P. L. OGRA. 1989. Otitis media in children. The systemic immune response to nontypable *Haemophilus influenzae.* J. Infect. Dis. **160:** 999–1004.

63. SHURIN, P. A., S. E. PELTON, I. B. TAZER & D. L. KASPER. 1980. Bactericidal antibody and susceptibility to otitis media caused by nontypeable strains of *Haemophilus influenzae*. J. Pediatr. **97:** 364–369.

64. KARASIC, R. B., C. E. TRUMPP, H. GNEHM, P. A. RICE & S. I. PELTON. 1985. Modification of otitis media in chinchillas rechallenged with nontypable *Haemophilus influenzae* and serological response to outer membrane antigens. J. Infect. Dis. **151:** 273–279.

65. GREEN, B. A., M. E. VAZQUEZ, G. W. ZLOTNICK, G. QUIGLEY-REAPE, J. D. SWARTS, I. GREEN, J. L. COWELL, C. D. BLUESTONE & W. J. DOYLE. 1993. Evaluation or mixtures of purified *Haemophilus influenzae* outer membrane proteins in protection against challenge with nontypeable *H. influenza* in the chinchilla otitis media model. Infect. Immun. **61:** 1950–1957.

66. SIRAKOVA, T., P. E. KOLATTUKUDY, D. MURWIN, J. BILLY, E. LEAKE, D. LIM, T. DeMARIA & L. BAKALETZ. 1994. Role of fimbriae expressed by nontypeable *Haemophilus influenzae* in pathogenesis of and protection against otitis media and relatedness of the fimbrin subunit to outer membrane protein A. Infect. Immun. **62:** 2002–2020.

67. GREEN, B. A., B. J. METCALF, T. QUINN-DEY, D. H. KIRKLEY, S. A. QUATAERT & R. A. DEICH. 1990. A recombinant non-fatty acylated form of the IE-PAL (P6) protein of *Haemophilus influenzae* elicits biologically active antibody against both nontypeable and type b *H. influenzae*. Infect. Immunol. **58:** 3272–3278.

68. DEICH, R. A., A. ANILIONIS, J. FULGINITI, B. M. METCALF, S. QUATAERT, T. QUINN-DEY, G. W. ZIOTNICK & B. A. GREEN. 1990. Antigenic conservation of the 15,000-dalton outer membrane lipoprotein PCP of *Haemophilus influenzae* and biologic activity of anti-PCP antisera. Infect. Immunol. **58:** 3388–3393.

69. GREEN, B. A., J. E. FARLEY, T. QUINN-DEY, R. A. DEICH & G. W. ZLOTNICK. 1991. The e (P4) outer membrane protein of *Haemophilus influenzae*: Biologic activity of anti-e serum and cloning and sequencing of the structural gene. Infect. Immun. **59:** 3191–3198.

70. MURPHY, T. F., L. C. BARTOS, P. A. RICE, M. B. NELSON, K. C. DUDAS & M. A. APICELLA. 1986. Identification of a 16,600-dalton outer membrane protein on nontypable *Haemophilus influenzae* as a target for human serum bactericidal antibody. J. Clin. Invest. **78:** 1020–1027.

71. YAMANAKA, N. & H. FADEN. 1993. Antibody response to outer membrane protein of nontypeable Haemophilus influenzae in otitis-prone children. J. Pediatr. **122:** 212–218.

72. MUNSON, R. S., JR. & D. M. GRANOFF. 1985. Purification and partial characterization of outer membrane proteins P5 and P6 from *Haemophilus influenzae* type b. Infect. Immunol. **49:** 544–549.

73. LOEB, M. R. 1987. Protection of infant rats from *Haemophilus influenzae* type b infection by antiserum to purified outer membrane protein 2. Infect. Immunol. **55:** 2612–2618.

74. KYD, J. M., M. L. DUNKLEY & A. W. CRIPPS. 1995. Enhanced respiratory clearance of nontypeable *Haemophilus influenzae* following mucosal immunization with P6 in a rat model. Infect. Immun. **63:** 2931–2940.

75. JANSON, H., L. O. HEDEN & A. FORSGREN. 1992. Protein D, the immunoglobulin D-binding protein of *Haemophilus influenzae*, is a lipoprotein. Infect. Immun. **60:** 1336–1342.

76. JANSON, H., M. RUAN & A. FORSGREN. 1994. Limited diversity of the protein D gene (hpd) among encapsulated and nonencapsulated *Haemophilus influenzae* strains. Infect. Immun. **61:** 4546–4552.

77. VANALPHEN, L., N. VAN DEN BERGHE & L. GEELEN-VAN DEN BROEK. 1988. Interaction of *Haemophilus influenzae* with human erythrocytes and oropharyngeal epithelial cells is mediated by a common fimbrial epitope. Infect. Immunol. **56:** 1800–1806.

78. ST. GEME, J. W., III, S. FALKOW & S. J. BARENKAMP. 1993. High-molecular weight proteins

of nontypeable *Haemophilus influenzae* mediate attachment to human epithelial cells. Proc. Natl. Acad. Sci. USA **90:** 2875–2879.

79. READ, R. C., R. WILSON, A. RUTMAN, V. LUND, H. C. TODD, A. P. R. BRAIN, P. K. JEFFERY & P. J. COLE. 1991. Interaction of nontypable *Haemophilus influenzae* with human respiratory mucosa in vitro. J. Infect. Dis. **163:** 549–558.

80. BRINTON, C. C., M. J. CARTER, D. B. DERBER, *et al.* 1989. Design and development of pilus vaccines for *Haemophilus influenzae* diseases. Pediatr. Infect. Dis. J. **8:** S54–S61.

81. KARASIC, R. B., D. J. BESTE, S. C.-M. TO, *et al.* 1989. Evaluation of pilus vaccines for prevention of experimental otitis media caused by nontypable *Haemophilus influenzae*. Pediatr. Infect. Dis. J. **8:** S62–S65.

82. BARENKAMP, S. J. 1996. Immunization with high-molecular-weight adhesion proteins of nontypeable *Haemophilus influenzae* modifies experimental otitis media in chinchillas. Infect. Immun. **64:** 1246–1251.

83. VAN HAM, S. M., L. VAN ALPHEN & F. R. MOOI. 1992. Fimbria-mediated adherence and hemagglutination of *Haemophilus influenzae*. J. Infect. Dis. **165** (Suppl 1):S97–S99.

84. MURPHY, T. 1989. The surface of *Branhamella catarrhalis*: A systematic approach to the surface antigens of an emerging pathogen. Pediatr. Infect. Dis. J. **8:** S75–S77.

85. BARTOS, L. C. & T. F. MURPHY. 1988. Comparison of the outer membrane proteins of 50 strains of *Branhamella catarrhalis*. J. Infect. Dis. **158:** 761–765.

86. HELMINEN, M. E., I. MACIVER, M. PARIS, J. L. LATIMER, S. L. LUMBLEY, L. D. COPE, G. H. MCCRACKEN, JR. & E. J. HANSEN. 1993. A mutation affecting expression of a major outer membrane protein of *Moraxella catarrhalis* alters serum resistance and survival in vivo. J. Infect. Dis. **168:** 1194–1201.

87. MACIVER, I., M. UNHANAND, G. H. MCCRACKEN, JR. & E. J. HANSEN. 1993. Effect of immunization on pulmonary clearance of *Moraxella catarrhalis* in an animal model. J. Infect. Dis. **168:** 469–472.

88. HELMINEN, M. E., I. MACIVER, J. L. LATIMER, L. D. COPE, G. H. MCCRACKEN, JR. & E. J. HANSEN. 1993. A major outer membrane protein of *Moraxella catarrhalis* is a target for antibodies that enhance pulmonary clearance of the pathogen in an animal model. Infect. Immunol. **61:** 2003–2010.

89. SANYAL, M. A., F. W. HENDERSON, E. C. STEMPEL, *et al.* 1980. Effect of upper respiratory tract infections on eustachian tube ventilatory function in the preschool child. J. Pediatr. **97:** 11–15.

90. HENDERSON, F. W., A. M. COLLIER, M. A. SANYAL, *et al.* 1982. A longitudinal study of respiratory viruses and bacteria in the etiology of acute otitis media with effusion. N. Eng. J. Med. **306:** 1377–1383.

91. STRAKER, E., A. B. HILL & R. LOVELL. 1939. A study of the nasopharyngeal flora of different groups of persons observed in London and South-east England during the years 1930 to 1937: 7–51. His Majesty's Stationery Office. London.

92. GWALTNEY, J. M., M. A. SANDE, R. AUSTRIAN & O. J. HENDLEY. 1975. Spread of *Streptococcus pneumoniae* in families. II. Relation of transfer of *S. pneumonia* to incidence of colds and serum antibody. J. Infect. Dis. **132:** 62–68.

93. HEIKKINEN, T., O. RUUSKANEN, M. WARIS, T. ZIEGLER, M. AROLA & P. HALONEN. 1991. Influenza vaccination in the prevention of acute otitis media in children. Am. J. Dis. Child. **145:** 445–448.

94. GIEBINK, G. S., I. K. BERZINS, S. C. MARKER, *et al.* 1980. Experimental otitis media after nasal inoculation of *Streptococcus pneumoniae* and influenza A virus in chinchillas. Infect. Immun. **30:** 445–450.

95. GIEBINK, G. S. & P. F. WRIGHT. 1983. Different virulence of influenza A virus strains and susceptibility to pneumococcal otitis media in chinchillas. Infect. Immun. **41:** 913–920.

96. GIEBINK, G. S. 1989. Studies of *Streptococcus pneumoniae* and influenza virus vaccines in the chinchilla otitis media model. Pediatr. Infect. Dis. J. **8:** S42–S44.

97. TOP, F. Y., JR. 1975. Control of adenovirus acute respiratory disease in U.S. Army trainees. Yale J. Biol. Med. **48:** 185–195.

98. SHURIN, P. A., G. S. GIEBINK, D. L. WEGMAN, D. AMBROSINO, J. RHOLL, M. OVERMAN, T. BAUER & G. R. SIBER. 1988. Prevention of pneumococcal otitis media in chinchillas with human bacterial polysaccharide immune globulin. J. Clin. Micro. **26:** 755–759.

99. TOEWS, G. B., D. A. HART & E. J. HANSEN. 1985. Effect of systemic immunization in pulmonary clearance of *Haemophilus influenzae* type b. Infect. Immun. **48:** 343–349.

100. JORGENSON, F., B. ANDERSON, L. A. HANSON, O. NYLÉN & C. SVANBORG-EDÉN. 1990. Gamma globulin treatment of recurrent acute otitis media in children. Pediatr. Infect. Dis. J. **9:** 389–394.

101. KALM, O., K. PRELLNER & P. CHRISTENSEN. 1986. The effect of intravenous immunoglobulin treatment in recurrent acute otitis media. Int. J. Pediatr. Otorhinolaryngol. **11:** 237–246.

102. HAMMILL, R. J., D. M. MUSHER, J. E. GROOVER, P. J. ZAVELL & D. A. WATSON. 1992. IgG antibody reactive with five serotypes of *Streptococcus pneumoniae* in commercial intravenous immunoglobulin preparations. J. Infect. Dis. **166:** 38–42.

103. SHAHID, N. S., M. C. STEINHOFF, S. S. HOQUE, T. BEGUM, C. THOMPSON & G. R. SIBER. 1995. Serum, breast milk, and infant antibody after maternal immunisation with pneumococcal vaccine. Lancet **346**(8985):1252–1257.

104. PUKANDER, J., J. LUOTONEN, M. SIPILA & P. KARMA. 1982. Incidence of acute otitis media. Acta Otolaryngol. (Stockholm) **93:** 447–453.

105. MARCHANT, C. D., P. A. SHURIN, V. A. TURCZYK, *et al.* 1984. Course and outcome of otitis media in early infancy: A prospective study. J. Pediatr. **104:** 826–831.

106. DALY, K. A. 1991. Epidemiology of otitis media. Otolaryngol. Clin. North Am. **24:** 775–786.

107. WISCHNACK, L. L., R. M. JACOBSON, G. A. POLAND, S. L. JACOBSEN, J. M. HARRISION & P. A. MURTAUGH. 1995. The surprisingly high acceptability of low-efficacy vaccines for otitis media: A survey of parents using hypothetical scenarios. Pediatrics **95:** 350–354.

108. GONZALES, F. R., S. LEACHMAN, M. V. NORGARD, J. D. RADOLF, G. H. MCCRACKEN, JR., C. EVANS & E. J. HANSEN. 1987. Cloning and expression in Escherichia coli of the gene encoding the heat-modifiable major outer membrane protein of *Haemophilus influenzae* type b. Infect. Immun. **55:** 2993–3000.

109. NELSON, M. B., R. S. MUNSON, JR., M. A. APICELLA, D. J. SIKKEIMA, J. P. MOLLESTON & T. F. MURPHY. 1991. Molecular conservation of the P6 outer membrane protein among strains of *Haemophilus influenzae*: Analysis of antigenic determinants, gene sequences, and restriction fragment length polymorphisms. Infect. Immunol. **59:** 2658–2663.

110. BARENKAMP, S. J. & E. LEININGER. 1992. Cloning, expression, and DNA sequence analysis of genes encoding nontypeable *Haemophilus influenzae* high-molecular-weight surface-exposed proteins related to fliamentous hemagglutinin of Bordetella pertussis. Infect. Immunol. **60:** 1302–1313.

111. BAKALETZ, L. O., B. M. TALLAN, T. HOEPF, T. F. DEMARIA, H. G. BIRCK & D. J. LIM. 1988. Frequency of fimbriation of nontypable *Haemophilus influenzae* and its ability to adhere to chinchilla and human respiratory epithelium. Infect. Immunol. **56:** 331–335.

112. KAR, S., S. C.-M. TO & C. C. BRINTON, JR. 1990. Cloning and expression in Escherichia coli of LKP pilus genes from a nontypeable *Haemophilus influenzae* strain. Infect. Immunol. **58:** 903–908.

113. OGRA, R. L., S. J. BARENKAMP, G. MOGI, *et al.* 1996. Microbiology, immunology and vac-

cination panel report. *In* Recent Advances in Otitis Media. *Rep. 6th Research Conf.,* D. J. Lim and C. D. Bluestone, Eds. Ann. Otol. Rhinol. Laryngol. In press.

114. KLINGMAN, K. L. & T. F. MURPHY. 1994. Purification and characterization of a high-molecular weight outer membrane protein of Moraxella (Branhamella) catarrhalis. Infect. Immunol. **62:** 1150–1155.

115. HELMINEN, M. E., I. MACIVER, J. L. LATIMER, J. KLESNEY-TAIT, L. D. COPE, M. PARIS, G. H. MCCRACKEN, JR. & E. J. HANSEN. 1994. A large, antigenically conserved protein on the surface of *Moraxella catarrhalis* is a target for protective antibodies. J. Infect. Dis. **170:** 867–872.

116. SETHI, S., S. L. HILL & T. F. MURPHY. 1995. Serum antibodies to outer membrane proteins of Moraxella (Branhamella) catarrhalis in patients with bronchiectasis: Identification of OMP B1 as an important antigen. Infect. Immunol. **63:** 1516–1520.

117. CAMPAGNARI, A. A., K. L. SHANKS & D. W. DYER. 1994. Growth of *Moraxella catarrhalis* with human transferrin and lactoferrin: Expression of iron-repressible proteins without siderophore production. Infect. Immunol. **62:** 4909–4914.

118. SARWAR, J., A. A. CAMPAGNARI, C. KIRKHAM & T. F. MURPHY. 1992. Characterization of an antigenically conserved heat-modifiable major outer membrane protein of Branhamella catarrhalis. Infect. Immunol. **60:** 804–809.

119. MURPHY, T. F., C. KIRKHAM & A. J. LESSE. 1993. The major heat-modifiable outer membrane protein CD is highly conserved among strains of Branhamella catarrhalis. Mol. Microbiol. **10:** 87–98.

120. BHUSHAN, R., R. CRAIGIE & T. F. MURPHY. 1994. Molecular cloning and characterization of outer membrane protein E of *Moraxella (Branhamella) catarrhalis.* J. Bacteriol. **176:** 6636–6643.

121. MURPHY, T. F. & L. C. BARTOS. 1989. Surface-exposed and antigenically conserved determinants of outer membrane proteins of Branhamella catarrhalis. Infect. Immunol. **57:** 2938–2941.

Mechanisms of Recurrent Otitis Media: Importance of the Immune Response to Bacterial Surface Antigens[a]

TIMOTHY F. MURPHY[b] AND KYUNGCHEOL YI

Division of Infectious Diseases
Department of Medicine and Microbiology
State University of New York at Buffalo
Buffalo, New York 14214
and
DVA-WNY Healthcare System
Buffalo, New York 14215

Recurrent otitis media is a common problem that is associated with substantial morbidity and enormous health care costs. A subset of children experiences repeated episodes of otitis media caused by nontypeable *Haemophilus influenzae* (NTHI) in spite of the development of an immune response to the infecting strain.[1] This protective immune response is specific for the infecting strain leaving the host susceptible to infection by other strains of the bacterium. Little is known about the mechanism by which NTHI induces a strain-specific antibody response. The goal of the present study is to analyze that mechanism.

Five rabbits and five mice were challenged with whole bacterial cells of NTHI strain 1479.[2] Analysis of the sera in immunoblot assay with a whole bacterial cell lysate revealed that the most prominent antibody response detected was directed at the P2 protein, which is the major outer membrane protein of NTHI (FIG. 1).

The P2 protein is the most abundant protein in the outer membrane of NTHI, constituting approximately half the protein content of the outer membrane. P2 is an important target of the immune response to *H. influenzae*.[3,4] A topographical model of the protein as it is arranged in the outer membrane has been determined. P2 contains 16 transmembrane regions and 8 potentially surface-exposed loops (FIG. 2).[5–7] The transmembrane regions are relatively conserved among strains, while considerable heterogeneity exists in several of the loop regions of the molecule.[6–8] Many of the monoclonal antibodies that we have developed by immunizing mice with whole bacterial cells of different strains of NTHI recognize abundantly expressed epitopes on loop 5 of the P2 molecule.[9,10] These observations suggest that loop 5 contains an immunodominant epitope. We hypothesized that the expression of an immunodominant epitope by the bacterium induces a strain-specific host immune response.

To analyze the regions of the P2 molecule to which antibodies were directed, the

[a]This work was supported by Research Grant AI19641 from the National Institutes of Health and by the Department of Veterans Affairs.

[b]Address for correspondence: Timothy F. Murphy, DVA-WNY Healthcare System, Medical Research 151, 3495 Bailey Avenue, Buffalo, New York 14215. Phone: 716/862-3303; fax: 716/862-3419; e-mail: murphyt@acsu.buffalo.edu

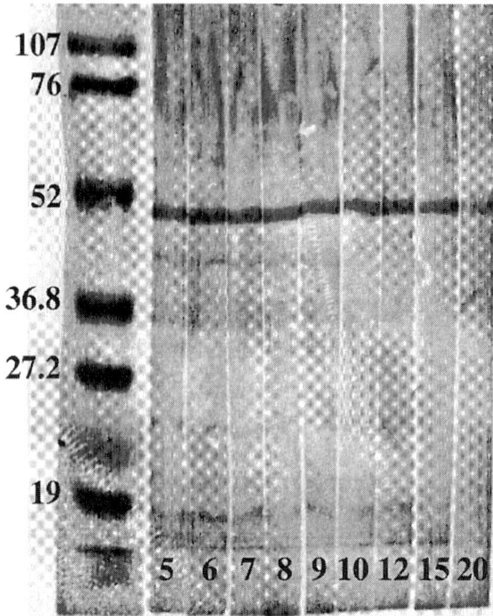

FIGURE 1. Immunoblot assay of rabbit antiserum to a whole bacterial cell lysate of strain 1479. The dilutions ($\times 10^3$) at which the antiserum was tested are noted at the bottom of each lane. Following overnight incubation with antiserum, the immunoblots were incubated with protein A peroxidase and horseradish peroxidase color developer. Molecular mass markers are noted on the left in kilodaltons.

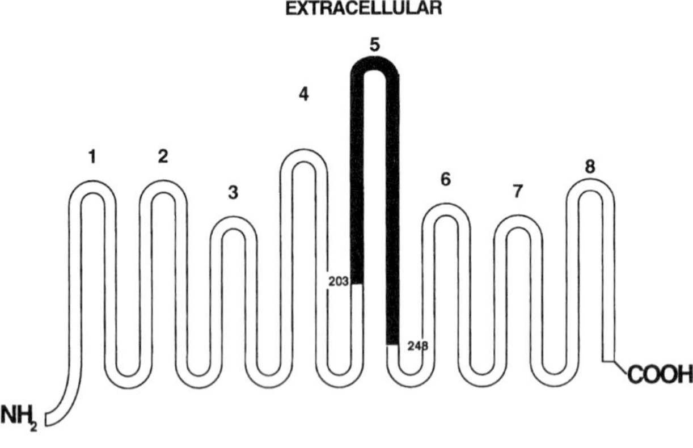

FIGURE 2. Schematic diagram of the P2 molecule of nontypeable *H. influenzae* strain 1479 depicting eight potentially surface-exposed loops. Each loop is numbered at the top. The region of loop 5, which is expressed as a fusion protein, is noted with amino acid numbers corresponding to those in the mature protein.[6] (From Yi and Murphy.[2] Reprinted by permission of the American Society for Microbiology.)

eight potentially surface-exposed loops of P2 of strain 1479 were individually expressed as fusion peptides with glutathione-*S*-transferase using the pGEX2T plasmid vector.[9,11] The purified fusion proteins were subjected to immunoblot assays with antisera. FIGURE 3 shows a prominent antibody response exclusively to the loop-5 peptide. All 10 sera showed an identical result. The results indicate that all of the antibodies detected by immunoblot assay are directed at loop 5.

Both primary structure and three-dimensional structure play important roles in the antigenicity of proteins.[12] The experiments just described are effective in detecting epitopes defined by primary amino acid sequence. However, alternative methods are required to detect antibodies to conformational epitopes that are dependent on the secondary, tertiary, and quaternary structure of the protein. Two additional approaches were used to study the sera from animals immunized with whole bacterial cells for antibodies to conformational epitopes on P2 and other surface antigens.

In previous work, antibodies to conformational epitopes on P2 were detected in ELISA with whole P2, which was purified under nondenaturing conditions.[4,13] This method detects antibodies that are not detectable in immunoblot assay.[4] To determine whether sera from animals immunized with whole bacterial cells contained antibodies to conformational epitopes on P2, aliquots of rabbit serum were individually adsorbed with the loop-5 fusion protein to remove antibodies to epitopes expressed on the loop-5 peptide. The adsorbed serum was tested in ELISA and in immunoblot assay, along with aliquots of unadsorbed serum, serum adsorbed with the GST protein, and serum adsorbed with the loop-8 fusion peptide as controls. FIGURE 4 shows that adsorption with loop 5 specifically removed all reactivity for the loop-5 fusion pep-

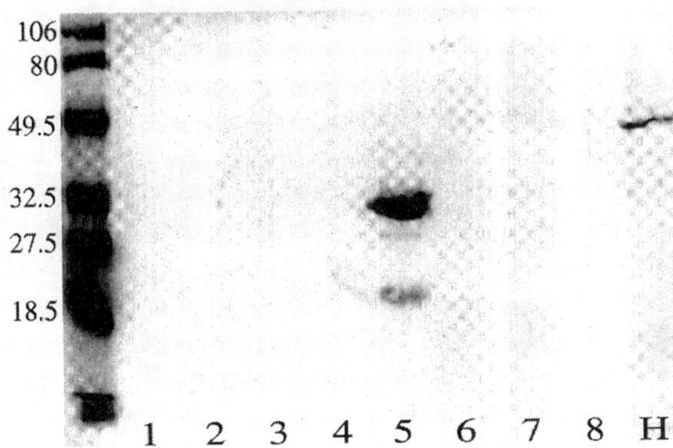

FIGURE 3. Immunoblot assay of mouse antiserum (1:500 dilution). Lanes 1 through 8 contain bacterial cell lysates of clones expressing peptides corresponding to loops 1 through 8 of the P2 protein of strain 1479. The peptides are part of fusion proteins with glutathione-*S*-transferase. Lane H contains a whole bacterial cell lysate of strain 1479. Following overnight incubation with antiserum, the blot was incubated with peroxidase-conjugated antimouse IgG and horseradish peroxidase color developer. This immunoblot was subsequently stained with amido black to verify adequate transfer of protein antigens. Molecular mass markers are noted on the left in kilodaltons. (From Yi and Murphy.[2] Reprinted by permission of the American Society for Microbiology.)

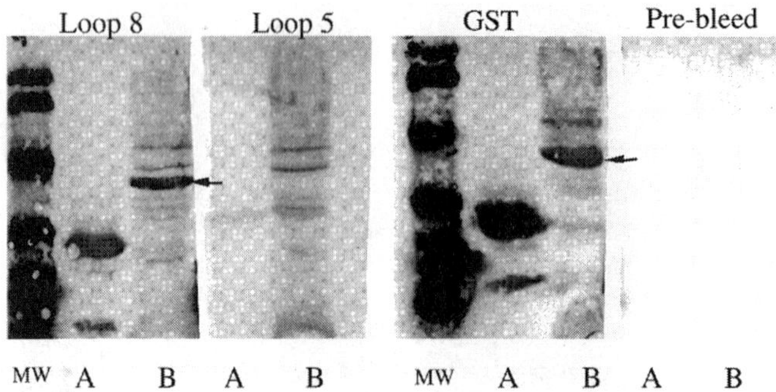

FIGURE 4. Immunoblot assays of rabbit antiserum (1:2000 dilution). Lanes A contain the loop-5 fusion protein of strain 1479 and lanes B contain whole bacterial cell lysates of strain 1479. The four panels were incubated with antiserum as follows: **loop 8:** antiserum adsorbed with loop-8–GST fusion protein; **loop 5:** antiserum adsorbed with loop-5–GST fusion protein; **GST:** antiserum adsorbed with GST; **Prebleed:** serum obtained before immunization with strain 1479. *Arrows* denote P2. After overnight incubation with antiserum, the blots were incubated with protein A-peroxidase, followed by horseradish peroxidase color developer. Molecular mass markers are as noted in FIGURE 3. (From Yi and Murphy.[2] Reprinted by permission of the American Society for Microbiology.)

tide and for the P2 molecule in immunoblot assay. FIGURE 5 shows that adsorption of the sera with the loop-5 fusion peptide completely eliminated reactivity for the P2 protein in ELISA. This experiment indicates that all of the detectable antibodies to P2 bind to epitopes that are present on the loop-5 peptide and that no significant populations of antibodies to conformational determinants on other regions of the P2 molecule are present in the serum.

The second approach used to detect antibodies to conformational epitopes was whole-cell radioimmunoprecipitation (RIP).[2] This method is effective in identifying antibodies to linear and conformational epitopes on molecules that are present on the surface of intact bacterial cells. FIGURE 6 is an autoradiograph that shows that RIP detects a single band corresponding to P2, indicating that antibodies to surface structures were directed exclusively to P2 (by this method of detection) when animals were inoculated with whole bacterial cells. To assess the possibility that RIP was detecting antibodies to conformational epitopes on other parts of the P2 molecule, aliquots of sera were adsorbed with the loop-5 fusion peptide. We reasoned that if the loop-5 peptide adsorbed antibodies that were detected by RIP, one may conclude that the majority of antibodies in the serum were directed at epitopes on the loop-5 peptide. The adsorbed sera were subjected to RIP in parallel with aliquots of unadsorbed serum and serum adsorbed with GST as a control. FIGURE 6 shows that the loop-5 peptide adsorbed almost all antibody detected by RIP. This result indicates that when the animals were challenged with whole bacterial cells, antibodies were made predominantly to epitopes on loop 5 of the P2 molecule.

Polyclonal antisera consist of populations of antibodies to linear and to conformational epitopes. For example, antiserum raised to the globular protein, myoglobin,

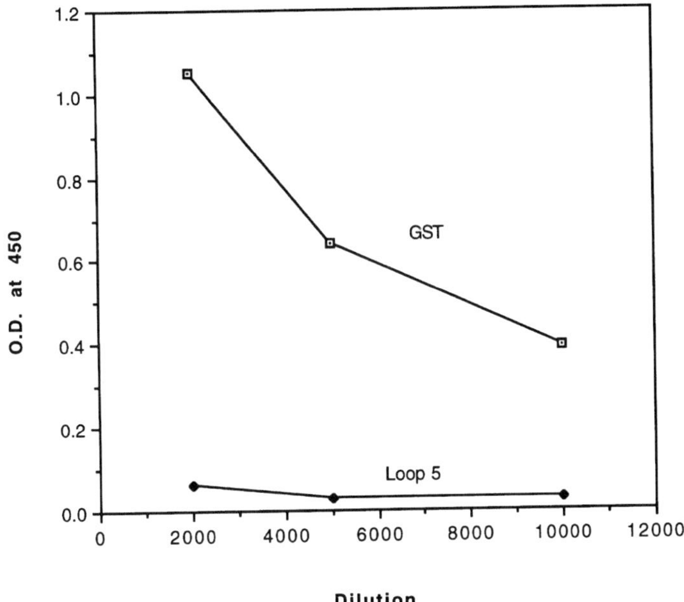

FIGURE 5. Results of ELISA with adsorbed antiserum. The *y*-axis represents optical density at 450 nm, and the *x*-axis represents dilution. P2 purified using nondenaturing conditions was used as coating antigen. The curve marked "GST" depicts the results of serum adsorbed with GST, and the curve marked "loop 5" depicts results of serum adsorbed with loop 5. (From Yi and Murphy.[2] Reprinted by permission of the American Society for Microbiology.)

consists of 60 to 70% antibodies to peptides (linear epitopes) and 30 to 40% antibodies to the native molecule (conformational epitopes).[12] By contrast, the present study shows that immunization with a complex set of antigens (whole bacterial cells) produces an antiserum that contains a defined population of antibodies. Most of the antibody is directed at the P2 molecule, the major outer membrane protein on the bacterial surface. All or most of the antibody to P2 binds a single peptide of 46 amino acids. The high degree of surface accessibility of the loop-5 region of the P2 molecule is likely an important factor in the generation of the restricted population of antibodies following immunization with bacterial cells.[9,14]

These observations have important implications in understanding how children experience recurrent episodes of otitis media. Faden *et al.*[1] demonstrated that children develop serum bactericidal antibody to the infecting strain of NTHI following otitis media. The presence of serum bactericidal antibody to a strain of NTHI is associated with protection from infection by that strain. Children who experience recurrent episodes have persisting serum bactericidal antibody to their original strain, but lack bactericidal antibody to the new strain.[1] A serum bactericidal antibody response then occurs to the new strain following infection. These observations indicate that children develop a protective immune response to NTHI following otitis media.

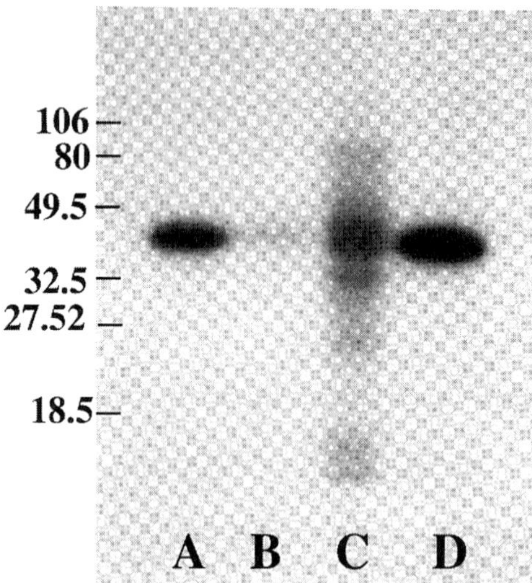

FIGURE 6. Autoradiogram of radioimmunoprecipitation of cells of strain 1479 labeled with [³H] leucine. Cells were incubated with aliquots of rabbit antiserum prepared as follows: **Lane A:** antiserum adsorbed with GST; **Lane B:** antiserum adsorbed with loop-5 fusion protein; **Lane D:** unadsorbed antiserum. **Lane C** contains an aliquot of the [³H] leucine-labeled cells. Molecular mass markers are noted on the left in kilodaltons. (From Yi and Murphy.[2] Reprinted by permission of the American Society for Microbiology.)

However, this protective response is directed exclusively at the infecting strain so the child remains susceptible to infection by other strains of NTHI.

We hypothesize that otitis-prone children develop an antibody response to an immunodominant, strain-specific region of the P2 molecule following otitis media, just as the animals challenged with NTHI in this study did. This would explain how certain children experience recurrent episodes of otitis media in spite of developing a protective immune response to their infecting strain.

Many children are not otitis prone. Such children experience few or no episodes of otitis media throughout childhood. It is tempting to speculate that otitis-prone and non-otitis-prone children develop antibody responses to different antigens on the surface of NTHI, and that this difference accounts in part for susceptibility to recurrent episodes of otitis media. NTHI contains a variety of antigens on its surface. As noted earlier, the P2 protein contains antigenically heterogeneous epitopes among strains. However, other surface proteins are more antigenically conserved among strains. For example, outer membrane protein P6 is a 16-kDa surface protein that is highly conserved among strains of NTHI.[15] An immune response to such a protein would have the potential of protecting against infection by all strains of NTHI. We speculate that non-otitis-prone children generate an immune response to antigenically conserved antigens such as P6, and that these antibodies render the children less susceptible to recurrent otitis media.[16] By contrast, otitis-prone children have antibodies primarily to antigenically heterogeneous, strain-specific epitopes on the P2 molecule. The observation that otitis-prone children have less antibody to P6 compared to non-otitis-prone children would support this idea.[17] However, the hypothesis has yet to be rigorously tested.

A vaccine to prevent otitis media caused by NTHI would result in improved quality of life for millions of children worldwide. In addition, an effective vaccine would have an enormous impact in reducing health care costs. In order to develop effective vaccines, it will be critical to understand the human immune response to NTHI.

SUMMARY

Otitis-prone children experience recurrent episodes of otitis media due to nontypeable *H. influenzae* (NTHI). A protective immune response occurs following infection, but this immune response is specific for the infecting strain, leaving the child susceptible to infection by other strains of NTHI. Little is known about the mechanism by which a strain-specific antibody response occurs to nonencapsulated bacteria. To explore the mechanism by which this strain-specific response occurs, animals were inoculated with whole bacterial cells and the antibody response was studied. The antibody response was predominantly directed to a highly strain-specific, immunodominant surface loop on the major outer membrane protein. This exquisitely restricted immune response leaves the host susceptible to recurrent infections by many strains of NTHI. The ability of the bacterium to direct the host to make a strain-specific antibody response has important implications in understanding the immune response to otitis media due to NTHI and in designing strategies for vaccine development.

ACKNOWLEDGMENT

The authors thank Yasmin Thanavala for helpful advice and discussion.

REFERENCES

1. FADEN, H., J. BERNSTEIN, L. BRODSKY, J. STANIEVICH, D. KRYSTOFIK, C. SHUFF, J. J. HONG & P. L. OGRA. 1989. Otitis media in children. I. The systemic immune response to nontypable *Haemophilus influenzae*. J. Infect. Dis. **160:** 999–1004.
2. YI, K. & T. F. MURPHY. 1997. Importance of an immunodominant surface-exposed loop on outer membrane protein P2 of nontypeable *Haemophilus influenzae*. Infect. Immun. **65:** 150–155.
3. MUNSON, R. S., JR., J. L. SHENEP, S. J. BARENKAMP & D. M. GRANOFF. 1983. Purification and comparison of outer membrane protein P2 from *Haemophilus influenzae* type b isolates. J. Clin. Invest. **72:** 677–684.
4. MURPHY, T. F. & L. C. BARTOS. 1988. Human bactericidal antibody response to outer membrane protein P2 of nontypeable *Haemophilus influenzae*. Infect. Immun. **56:** 2673–2679.
5. SRIKUMAR, R., D. DAHAN, M. F. GRAS, M. J. H. RATCLIFFE, L. VAN ALPHEN & J. W. COUL-

TON. 1992. Antigenic sites on porin of *Haemophilus influenzae* type b: Mapping with synthetic peptides and evaluation of structure predictions. J. Bacteriol. **174:** 4007–4016.

6. SIKKEMA, D. J. & T. F. MURPHY. 1992. Molecular analysis of the P2 porin protein of nontypeable *Haemophilus influenzae*. Infect. Immun. **60:** 5204–5211.

7. DUIM, B., J. DANKERT, H. M. JANSEN & L. VAN ALPHEN. 1993. Genetic analysis of the diversity in outer membrane protein P2 of non-encapsulated *Haemophilus influenzae*. Microb. Pathogen. **14:** 451–462.

8. BELL, J., S. GRASS, D. JEANTEUR & R. S. MUNSON, JR. 1994. Diversity of the P2 protein among nontypeable *Haemophilus influenzae* isolates. Infect. Immun. **62:** 2639–2643.

9. HAASE, E. M., K. YI, G. D. MORSE & T. F. MURPHY. 1994. Mapping of bactericidal epitopes on the P2 porin protein of nontypeable *Haemophilus influenzae*. Infect. Immun. **62:** 3712–3722.

10. YI, K. & T. F. MURPHY. 1994. Mapping of a strain-specific bactericidal epitope to the surface-exposed loop 5 on the P2 porin protein of nontypeable *Haemophilus influenzae*. Microb. Pathogen. **17:** 277–282.

11. SMITH, D. B. & K. S. JOHNSON. 1988. Single-step purification of polypeptides expressed in *Escherichia coli* as fusions with glutathione *S*-transferase. Gene **67:** 31–40.

12. LANDO, G., J. A. BERZOFSKY & M. REICHLIN. 1982. Antigenic structure of sperm whale myoglobin. 1. Partition of specificities between antibodies reactive with peptides and native protein. J. Immunol. **129:** 206–211.

13. MURPHY, T. F. & L. C. BARTOS. 1988. Purification and analysis with monoclonal antibodies of P2, the major outer membrane protein of nontypable *Haemophilus influenzae*. Infect. Immun. **56:** 1084–1089.

14. BERZOFSKY, J. A. 1985. Intrinsic and extrinsic factors in protein antigenic structure. Science **229:** 932–940.

15. NELSON, M. B., R. S. MUNSON, JR., M. A. APICELLA, D. J. SIKKEMA, J. P. MOLLESTON & T. F. MURPHY. 1991. Molecular conservation of the P6 outer membrane protein among strains of *Haemophilus influenzae*: Analysis of antigenic determinants, gene sequences, and restriction fragment length polymorphisms. Infect. Immun. **59:** 2658–2663.

16. MURPHY, T. F., M. B. NELSON & M. A. APICELLA. 1992. The P6 outer membrane protein of nontypeable *Haemophilus influenzae* as a vaccine antigen. J. Infect. Dis. **165**(1): S203–S205.

17. YAMANAKA, N. & H. FADEN. 1993. Antibody response to outer membrane protein of nontypeable *Haemophilus influenzae* in otitis-prone children. J. Pediatr. **122:** 212–218.

An Introduction to the Genetics of Normal and Defective Hearing[a]

ALESSANDRO MARTINI,[b,d] MANUELA MAZZOLI,[b]
AND WILLIAM KIMBERLING[c]

[b]*Servizio di Audiologia*
Clinica ORL dell' Università di Ferrara
Corso Giovecca 203
44100 Ferrara, Italy

[c]*Department of Genetics*
Boystown National Research Hospital
Omaha, Nebraska 68131

INTRODUCTION

Basic research and clinical work do not very often come together, but the recent rapid development of molecular biology techniques applied to the genetics of normal and defective hearing shed new light on old questions. For this reason, the interest of clinicians in the development of this field is particularly lively and intense.

Often in our daily practice we tend to underestimate hereditary factors as a cause of hearing impairment, especially in those cases of late onset and progressive hearing loss. The fundamental processes involved in the mechanism of hearing seem to be controlled by hundreds of genes,[1] and hereditary hearing impairment may be caused by a large variety of genetic mutations in different genes. Genetic hearing impairment may be congenital, but it also may develop at any decade throughout life or deteriorate as part of a preexisting congenital or acquired hearing impairment. To date, 350 different genetic conditions associated with hearing impairment have been described. Over the past five years, hereditary diseases associated with hearing impairment have been mapped, and several genes have already been identified (see TABLES 1–4 from the Hereditary Hearing Loss Homepage[2]). As the causative genes are identified, it is often found that the original syndrome is in fact a mix of several similar syndromes caused by mutations in different genes.

The extensive genetic heterogeneity along with the paucity of clinical criteria and the vagueness of definitions used by the different professionals involved, have been a serious obstacle to progress in understanding hearing losses with genetic cause. Progress in nonsyndromic hearing loss has been particularly difficult, given the extensive genetic heterogeneity and paucity of clinical criteria. It is thus essential that the phenotypes for such monogenic abnormalities be carefully defined. Furthermore,

[a]This work was partly supported by Grant PL950353 from the European Concerted Action Biomed.

[d]Author for correspondence. Phone: 30.532.295341; fax: 39.532.295887; e-mail: mma(dns.unife.it

TABLE 1. Dominant Nonsyndromic Hearing Impairment According to Hereditary Hearing Loss Homepage

Locus Name	Location	Gene	Screening Markers	Most Important Reference	OMIM Entry
DFNA1	5q31	Unknown	D5S640, D5S410, D5S412	Lion *et al.*, 1992	124900
DFNA2	1p32	Unknown	D1S255, MYCL1, D1S193	Coucke *et al.*, 1994	600101
DFNA3	13q12	Unknown	D13S143, D13S175, D13S292	Chaib *et al.*, 1994	
DFNA4	19q13	Unknown	D19S208, D19S224, ApoC2	Chen *et al.*[20]	600652
DFNA5	7p15	Unknown	D7S629, D7S673, D7S529	Van Camp *et al.*, 1995	600994
DFNA6	4p16.3	Unknown	D4S1614, D4S412, D4S432	Lesperance *et al.*, 1995	600965
DFNA7	1q21-q23	Unknown	D1S194, D1S196, D1S210	Fagerheim *et al.*, 1996	601412
DFNA8 (See Note 1)	11q	Unknown	D11S1345, D11S934, D11S1320	Kirschhofer *et al.*, 1996	
DFNA9	14q12-q13	Unknown	D11S1345, D11S934, D111S1320	Manolis *et al.*, 1996	
DFNA10	6q22-q23	Unknown	D6S267, D6S407, D6S472	O'Neill *et al.*, 1996	601316
DFNA11	11q12.3-q21	Unknown		Tamagawa *et al.*, 1996	601317
DFNA12	11q22-q24	Unknown	D11S4111, D11S925, D11S934	University of Antwerp, in press	
DFNA13	6p21	Unknown	D6S299, D6S464, D6S276	University of Iowa, submitted	

identification of probands having a similar phenotype is difficult because many genes are involved and different mutations can cause similar phenotypes. Nevertheless, there is now a strong interest in this area and recently about 30 loci involved in nonsyndromic hearing loss have been identified.

CHROMOSOMES AND GENES

Classically, after Mendel, genes were inferred by studying the pattern of inheritance of a character (phenotype) and most of the properties and behavior of genes were worked out from results of experimental breeding organisms. For each locus

TABLE 2. Recessive Nonsyndromic Hearing Impairment According to Hereditary Hearing Loss Homepage

Locus Name	Location	Gene	Screening Markers	Most Important Reference	OMIM Entry
DFNB1	13q12	Unknown	D13S143, D13S175, D13S292	Guilford *et al.*, 1994	220290
DFNB2	11q13.5	Unknown	D11S911, D11S527, D11S937	Guilford *et al.*[53]	600101
DFNB3	17p11.2-q12	Unknown	D17S122, D17S805, D17S842	Friedman *et al.*, 1995	600316
DFNB4	7q31	Unknown	D7S501, D7S496, D7S523	Baldwin *et al.*, 1995	600791
DFNB5 (See Note 2)	14q12	Unknown	D14S79, D14S253, D14S286	Fukushima *et al.*, 1995a	600972
DFNB6	3p14-p21	Unknown	D3S1767, D3S1289, D3S1582	Fukushima *et al.*, 1995b	600971
DFNB7	9q13-q21	Unknown	D9S50, D9S301, D9S166	Jain *et al.*, 1995	600974
DFNB8	21q22	Unknown	D21S212, D21S1225, D21S1575	Veske *et al.*, 1996	601072
DFNB9 (See Note 3)	2p22-p23	Unknown	D2S144, D2S171, D2S158, D2S174	Chaib *et al.*, 1996a	601071
DFNB10	21q22.3	Unknown		Bonni-Tamir *et al.*, 1996	
DFNB11	9q13-q21	Unknown	See DFNB7	Scott *et al.*, 1996	
DFNB12	10q21-22	Unknown	D11S4111, D11S925, D11S934	Chaib *et al.*, 1996b	601386
DFNB13			Reserved		
DFNB14			Reserved		
DFNB15	3q21-q25 19p13	Unknown	D3S1309, D3S1593, D3S1553 D19S591, D19S592, D19S221	Chen *et al.*, 1996	
DFNB16	15q21-22	Unknown	THBS1, D15S132, D15S123	Campbell *et al.*, in press	
DFNB17			Reserved		
DFNB18	11p14-15.1	Unknown		Jain *et al.* (NIH), presented at the American Society of Human Genetics, 1997	
DFNB19			Reserved		

TABLE 3. X-Linked Nonsyndromic Hearing Impairment According to Hereditary Hearing Loss Homepage

Locus Name	Location	Gene	Screening Markers	Most Important Reference	OMIM Entry
DFN1 (See Note 4)	Xq21	DDP	DXS101	Tanebjaerg *et al.*, 1995	304700
DFN2	Xq22	Unknown	COL4A5	Tyson *et al.*, in press	304500
DFN3	Xq21.1	POU3F4	DXS26, DXS995, DXS232	De Kok *et al.*[23]	300039, 304400
DFN4	Xp21.2	Unknown	DXS997, DXS992	Lalwani *et al.*, 1994	300030
DFN5	Reserved				
DFN2	Xq22	Unknown	DXS8036, DXS8022, DXS8019	del Castillo *et al.*, 1996	300066
DFN7			Reserved		
DFN8			Reserved		

(type of gene), an organism has two alleles (alternative versions of a gene), one inherited from each parent. The two alleles may be the same (homozygous) or different (heterozygous). Across a population, a given gene may have only one allele, two different alleles, or a very large number of different alleles.[3]

Although over 5000 Mendelian human characters are known, the great majority of genetic or part-genetic human characters do not follow the well known typical Mendelian pedigree pattern (autosomal dominant, autosomal recessive, X-linked dominant, and X-linked recessive). Such characters are variously called polygenic, oligogenic, or multifactorial.[3]

Genes are DNA sequences that specify characters, normally by specifying the sequence of aminoacids in a protein. The majority of genes are located in the chromosomes (human chromosomes have perhaps 80,000 pairs of genes). The chromosomes are located in the cell nucleus and each chromosome consists of a single immensely long double helix of DNA (typically 50–150 million base pairs), packed around a scaffold of proteins.[3] In addition there are 37 mithochondrial genes that are inherited only from the mother.

TABLE 4. Mitochondrial Nonsyndromic Hearing Impairment According to Hereditary Hearing Loss Homepage

Gene	Mutation	Most Important Reference
12S rRNA	A1555G	Prezant *et al.*, 1993
tRNA-Ser(UCN)	T7445C	Reid *et al.*, 1994

THE HUMAN GENOME PROJECT

The Human Genome Project has as its goal the determination of the complete sequence of the human genome, and is allied with the localization and determination of all the DNA sequence coding for the full complement of genes. At the same time, a number of genomes of so-called model organisms are the focus of similar programs (e.g., the mouse genome[4]). Most of the genes in the mouse genome are conserved and show homology with their human counterparts, species, including genes between mouse and human.[5] Outside of man, the mouse is the best genetically characterized mammalian organism, and it occupies a unique place as a model organism for studing human genetic disease.[4]

COCHLEAR cDNA LIBRARIES

One method used to identify candidate genes based on their function or pattern of tissue expression involves the construction of cDNA libraries from the target organ or tissue, in this case from the cochlea. The construction and characterization of cochlear cDNA libraries from humans and other species provide an important resource for rapid identification of cochlear genes involved in normal hearing and hearing disorders.[6–9] A cochlear cDNA library will provide copies of the messenger RNA of most genes expressed in the cells of the cochlea. Many of these genes code for proteins that are needed by all cells in the body; these are called *housekeeping genes*. However, other genes code for proteins that give the organ its unique or tissue-specific properties. A cDNA library can be enriched for tissue-specific messages by subtraction hybridization. This approach permits the enrichment of the tissue-specific genes found in the cochlea by the elimination of unwanted housekeeping genes. Selected cDNA clones from a cochlea-subtracted library can be examined individually to confirm that they are expressed only in the cochlea.[8]

Studies of the molecular genetics of the inner ear are hampered by its relative inaccessibility, by the limited numbers of cochlear and vestibular cells, and by our inability to mantain many of these cell types in long-term cultures. The production of cochlear cDNA libraries from single cells or small cell populations is difficult with current conventional methods, even using PCR amplification methods. The so-called "amplification of mRNA (amRNA) technique"[10,11] allows creation of a cDNA library from a single cell, and it is becoming critically important to molecular studies of the inner ear. For example, amRNA should allow the construction of libraries specific to inner hair cells, outer hair cells, stria vascularis cells, and afferent and efferent neurons. The amRNA technique can be combined with the patch microelectrode technique to study gene expression in individual cells important in the hearing mechanism.

Several rodent inner-ear cDNA libraries and a human fetal cochlear cDNA library have already been constructed.[7,8,12–14] Human and rodent cochlea-subtracted cDNA libraries have a great significance for identifying genes controlling the development and maintenance of hearing. cDNA libraries constructed at different stages of development, and subtracted from each other, could be instrumental in identifying genes important at each stage of development of the cochlea. Libraries made from different tissues within an organ (e.g., inner versus outer hair cells) could be compared to identify genes that are needed for the differentiation of the cells into specific types. In addition, these libraries have the potential of fostering the identification of other proteins unique to the cochlea and will contribute to the identification, characterization, and functional analyses of these cochlea-specific proteins.

Another important application of cDNA libraries is in identifying hearing loss genes. Once the candidate gene for a given type of hearing loss is cloned and decoded, the structure of its protein product can be determined. This will provide insights into biochemical function of the gene product in normal cochlear tissue, and will show why the genetic mutation result in hearing loss. The validity of this approach is exemplified by the identification of the alpha-rhodopsin protein in dominant retinitis pigmentosa,[15] the dystrophin protein in Duchenne muscular dystrophy,[16] the cystic fibrosis transmembrane conductance regulator protein in cystic fibrosis,[17] and most recently by the identification of myosin VIIa in Usher type 1B.[14,18] These discoveries have all led to a better understanding of their respective mechanisms of pathogenesis.

cDNA libraries do not necessarily have to be of human origin; a murine gene library is of equal importance. From such a library, the murine equivalent of the human cochlear genes and their gene products can be identified. Alteration of the expression and/or structure of these proteins by site directed mutagenesis of the coding sequences will allow the structure–function relationship to be studied. In addition, through the use of homologous recombination and transgenic technology, *in vivo* mouse models of inner-ear genetic disorders can be created.

RECENT RESEARCH ON THE MOLECULAR BASIS OF INNER-EAR DEVELOPMENT AND FUNCTION

The vertebrate inner ear, and in particular the mammalian inner ear, is a remarkably complex structure both at the gross and cellular levels. The molecular mechanisms that dictate its morphogenesis and differentiation are largely unknown, but the research in this field is very active and new findings are continuously being reported in the scientific literature. There is evidence in the chicken that both hair cells and supporting cells arise from a common progenitor.[19]

In many animals the gene expression of several transcription factors and growth factors in the inner-ear development was characterized. Ocp2 gene encoding OCP-II was recently mapped.[20] OCP-II is localized abundantly in neurosensory cells in the organ of Corti (and not in any other tissue) and at lower concentrations in vestibular sensory organs as well as auditory and vestibular brainstem nuclei; and it seems to be involved in transcription regulation for the development or maintenance of specialized functions of the inner ear. Bone morphogenetic protein (BMP)-4 was shown to be involved in the induction and/or differentiation of the chick inner ear.[21]

Several genes encoding POU-domain proteins are expressed in the developing mammalian inner ear. Recently Ryan and coworkers[22] found that the expression of POU-domain genes remained high in all tissues of the labyrinth, excluding neuroepithelial and neural cells until postnatal day p12 in the rat, and then declined abruptly at day p14. Low-to-moderate levels of expression continued in the spiral ligament, spiral limbus, supralimbal cells, and suprastrial cells into adulthood. Erkman *et al.*[22]

suggest that the Brn-4 gene has a critical role in maintaining the phenotype of the cells in which it occurs. Members of the Brn-3 gene family were expressed only in neurosensory cells; expression was limited to auditory and vestibular ganglion neurons, beginning as soon as the ganglion cells separated from the otocyst at ell and continuing at high levels until around birth.[22] De Kok and coworkers have recently isolated a gene, POU3F4, which is responsible for a specific X-linked form of human hearing impairment, DFN3.[23]

Neurotropic factors are also important for inner-ear development. During development, the mammalian inner ear requires intrinsic and extrinsic regulating factors,[24–26] which include target-derived neurotrophins that are implicated in maturation and maintenance of both central and peripheral nervous system.[27] The inner-ear sensory epithelia and the brainstem nuclei trophically support cochleovestibular neurons.[25] It is suggested that members of the family of neurotrophins play a major role in this process and that they are involved in the development and maintenance of innervation.[28] Five of these neurotrophic factors are nerve growth factor (NGF),[29] brain-derived neurotrophic factor (BDNF),[30] neurotrophin-3 (NT-3),[31,32] neurotrophin-4 (NT-4),[33] also named neurotrophin-5 (NT-5).[34]

In situ hybridization studies suggest that both BDNF and NT-3, but not NGF, function as neurotrophic factors for the sensory neurons of the inner ear.[35,36] Gene knockout studies reveal that both BDNF and NT-3 are critical factors for the survival of both type 1 (NT-3) and type 2 (BDNF) auditory neurons of the spiral ganglion during the developmental process.[37,38] Van De Water and coworkers[39] have shown that both BDNF and NT-3 can act as neural survival factors in dissociated cultures, while NT-3 appears to predominate as the survival factor in organotypic cultures. NGF stimulates the production and repair of injured neuronal processes in cultures of dissociated adult auditory neurons but does not support neuronal survival *in vitro.*

BDNF and NT-3 show a partially overlapping distribution in sensory epithelia of the developing ear of mice[35] and their receptors, trkB and trkC, are somewhat overlapingly expressed in the developing statoacustic ganglion of mice.[40] Mice lacking BDNF expression show a reduced innervation of all vestibular sensory epithelia and a reduced number of vestibular ganglion cells.[41] Fritzsch and coworkers[42,43] demonstrated that the vestibular sensory epithelial innervation is more dependent on trkB, whereas the cochlear sensory epithelial innervation is more dependent on trkC. Ylikoski *et al.*[44] reported that trkB mRNA is expressed in the sensory epithelium of the utriculus and sacculus, whereas trkC mRNA is expressed in the subepithelial mesenchyme of these organs, in the late-embryonic and early-postnatal cochlea. According to these authors,[44] NT-3 is the predominant neurotrophin in the adult organ of Corti and BDNF is that in vestibular organs and these neurotrophins participate in the development of cochleovestibular (CVG) neurons and may be involved in the maintenance and protection of mature CVG neurons.

MOUSE HEARING IMPAIRMENT

Recent catalogues of mouse mutations[45,46] document over 100 genes having effects on the inner ear, either on its development or its function. As in the human, mouse mutations causing hearing impairment can be divided into the following three main classes according to the nature of the underlying pathology.[5,47]

1. Morphogenetic abnormalities represent malformations of the labyrinth arising through defects in its proper development and correspond to Mondini and Michel abnormalities in humans and are usually classified as a syndromal hearing loss.

2. Cochleo-saccular defects arise from disturbances in the stria vascularis and are usually associated with pigmentation defects. Melanocytes are known to populate the stria vascularis and are thought to play a role in its function.[48] The cochleo-saccular abnormalities are classified as syndromal hearing loss because of the association with pigmentation defects.

3. Neuroepithelial defects: a primary defect of the sensory neuroepithelia (including the organ of Corti) will lead to uncomplicated hearing loss or nonsyndromal hearing loss.

A number of mouse mutations have been identified both for morphogenetic and cochleo-saccular defects, and in a number of cases, the underlying genes have been identified. Only recently a number of loci involved in the largest class of mutations (the neuroepithelial defects) has been mapped. The discovery of myosin VII gene as the cause of Human Usher Syndrome has drawn attention on its role in hearing.

Myosin VII Gene

Mice homozygous for the recessive shaker-1 (sh-1) mutation shows typical neuroepithelial-type defects involving dysfunction and degeneration of the organ of Corti.[49] The sh-1 mutation maps to mouse chromosome 7, in the vicinity of the beta-globin and tyrosinase loci. Brown and coworkers[50] were able to demonstrate that the Olfactory marker protein (Omp) was very closed linked to the sh-1 mutation on chromosome 7.[51] Kimberling *et al.* mapped the human homologue of mouse Omp (OMP) to chromosome 1 1q13 and in the vicinity of the Usher type IB locus[52] and of the locus for autosomal recessive nonsyndromal hearing loss (DFNB2)[53]. A number of genes from this region was identified; one gene (ET58) was shown to code for a myosin VII.[14] Analysis of the available coding sequence from the motor head region of the myosin molecule, confirmed that the myosin VII was the sh-1 gene.[14] Weil and coworkers[18] discovered that the myosin VIIa gene was responsible for Usher type IB and probably for DFNB2. According to Brown and Steel,[5] the identification of the first neuroepithelial hearing-loss gene represents an important step toward a better molecular picture of hair-cell function, as it is known that myosin VII expression in the inner ear is confined to the sensory hair cells in the organ of Corti and in the vestibule. Hasson and coworkers[54] have recently shown that an antiserum to human myosin VIIa labels the cell bodies and stereocilia of inner and outer cochlear hair cells, but does not label other cochlear cells. The importance of this finding derives from the fact that adaptation of the mechanoelectrical transduction mechanism in hair cells of the auditory and vestibular systems appears to be mediated by adjustment of the tension on the mechanosensitive transduction channels and there is growing evidence that tension is controlled by molecular "motor" molecules in the tips of hair cells' stereocilia.[55,56] These motor molecules are members of the myosin superfamily. According to Dumont and Gillespie,[57] the tension in each gating spring is controlled by an ensemble of myosin molecules that are coupled together to generate forces exerted during adaptation. Within the retina, myosin VIIa is expressed solely by the retinal pigmented epithelial cell and these results provide compelling evidence that the impairment of hearing and vision phenotype associated with Usher disease are due to the lack of functional myosin VIIa polypeptide within a specific subset of cochlear and retinal cells.[54]

CLINICAL AND MOLECULAR STUDIES ON
GENETIC HUMAN HEARING IMPAIRMENTS

A major difficulty in the coordination of efforts toward resolving problems of genetic heterogeneity, particularly in nonsyndromal hearing loss, has stemmed from vague definitions used by the different professionals concerned. The lack of uniform terminology, descriptions, and definitions is a major obstacle to obtaining more detailed knowledge on these rare genetic disorders and, thus, implementing any preventative measures. The importance of this aspect was stressed, for audiological terms, by a recent editorial in the *Journal of Audiological Medicine.*[58]

Another important problem stems from the variability of certain genetic disorders in terms of the range of abnormalities found and the degree of such abnormalities associated with the same gene alteration. The phenotypic expression of the mutant genes in question may vary considerably, as do definitions of various genetic diseases including hearing impairment.

Furthermore, since the knowledge about the prevalence of the genes, their transmission, and phenotypic expression is limited, more epidemiologic data must be collected. In fact, nonsyndromal recessive hearing impairments are very common disorders, although the prevalence, which is certainly low, of each clinical entity is yet unknown. Considering the involvement of 20 different genes with equal relative frequency, a prevalence of 1:50.000 can be modeled (1/1000×0.5×0.8/20). Some of these disorders will have an even lower prevalence and may be considered as "private disease." Regarding syndromal conditions, data are available for the most frequent disorders: oculo-auricolo-vertebral spectrum (hemifacial microsomia) stime: from 1:3500 to 1:26.500;[59,60] BOR Syndrome 1:40.000;[61] Treacher-Collins Syndrome 1:50.000;[62] Waardenburg Syndrome 2–3:100.000[63] (Type III is rarer); Pendred Syndrome from 1:100.000[64] to 1:130.000; Usher Syndrome 3–4.5:100.000.[65,66] The latter includes at least seven different conditions each with only two subtypes accounting for our 75% of all cases.

Due to the very low prevalence of individual genetic hearing impairments, basic and clinical research within the field is virtually impossible on a national level and requires international collaboration in order to obtain more knowledge.

Identification of genes causing hereditary deafness, as with other genetic diseases, goes through two stages: first mapping, then cloning. Mapping is wholly dependent on the availability of samples from families affected by the condition. For the genetic analysis it is important to study groups of patients whose hearing loss has, as far as possible, the same genetic cause. Genetic heterogeneity among the study group greatly complicates the task of mapping genes by linkage analysis. In any case, it is essential to study families that have been meticulously characterized clinically.

For syndromal hearing loss, the main obstacle to obtaining a homogeneous series of families is the difficulty of finding a sufficient number of cases since these conditions are usually rare. Extensive collaboration is usually necessary and has led in the past to the foundation of study groups (e.g., the International Waardenburg Consortium, The International Usher Consortium). For nonsyndromal hearing loss, the research strategy must be designed to accommodate genetic heterogeneity; careful clinical documentation, using uniform protocols and definitions, is one tool for distinguishing disorder subtypes. To achieve these objectives, extensive collaborations are invaluable.

Following this line of interest, a European Working Group on Genetics of Hearing Impairments was created and financially supported by the European Community. The objectives of the project include the establishment of common terminology and definitions and the coordination of the multidisciplinary approaches: audiologists, otologists, maxillo-facial surgeons, ophthalmologists, clinical geneticists, and genetic laboratories for DNA studies. Homogeneous classification of families based on the characteristics of hearing impairment, vestibular function, inner-ear malformations and other phenotypic criteria, and genetic transmission could be obtained.[67,68]

It is an ambitious project, but the European Community (scientific community and involved families) will benefit from the outcomes of this project, since a European network of experts will be available for reference and counseling on such rare disorders. Data will also be useful in programming medical costs and services for diagnosis, care, and rehabilitation.

The European Concerted Action HEAR and the Hereditary Hearing Impairment Resource Registry (HHIRR) of the National Institute on Deafness and Other Communication Disorders will provide an impetus for future research in this field.

SUMMARY

The recent rapid development of molecular biology techniques applied to the genetics of normal and defective hearing shed a new light on old questions regarding hearing and deafness.

Genes are DNA sequences that determine characteristics, normally by specifying the sequence of aminoacids in a protein. The majority of genes is located in the chromosomes (human chromosomes have perhaps 80,000 pairs of genes). In addition there are 37 mithochondrial genes which are inherited only from the mother.

One method used to identify candidate genes based on their function or pattern of tissue expression involves the construction of cDNA libraries from the target organ or tissue, in this case from the cochlea. The construction and characterization of cochlear cDNA libraries from humans and other species provide an important resource for rapid identification of cochlear genes involved in normal hearing and hearing disorders.

Studies of the molecular genetics of the inner ear are hampered by the relative inaccessibility of the cochlea, by the limited number of cochlear and vestibular cells, and by our inability to maintain many of these cell types in long-term cultures. Several rodent inner-ear cDNA libraries and a human foetal cochlear cDNA library have already been constructed. Human and rodent cochlea-subtracted cDNA libraries are very useful for identifying genes controlling the development and maintenance of hearing. cDNA libraries constructed at different stages of development, and subtracted from each other, could be instrumental in identifying genes important at each stage of cochlear development. In addition, these libraries have the potential of fostering the identification of other proteins unique to the cochlea and will contribute to the identification, characterization, and functional analysis of these cochlea-specific proteins.

Another important application of cDNA libraries is in identifying hearing-loss genes. Once the candidate gene for a given type of hearing loss is cloned and decoded, the structure of its protein product can be determined. This will provide insights into the biochemical function of the gene product in normal cochlear tissue, and will show why the genetic mutation results in hearing loss, that is, the recent identification of the myosin VIIa gene in Usher type IB. In addition, through the use of homologous recombination and transgenic technology, *in vivo* mouse models of inner-ear genetic disorders can be created.

To date, 350 different genetic conditions associated with hearing impairment have been described, and during the past five years several of the genes involved in these forms have already been mapped and identified.

REFERENCES

1. NANCE, W. E. 1980. The genetic analysis of profound prelingual deafness. Birth Defects **16:** 263–269
2. HEREDITARY HEARING LOSS HOMEPAGE. 1997. http://dnalab-www.uia.ac.be/dnalab/hhh.html
3. READ, A. P. 1996. Basic genetic mechanism. *In* Genetics and Hearing Impairment, A. Martini, A. Read, and D. Stephens, Eds.: 18–32. Whurr. London.
4. BROWN, S. D. M. 1994. Integrating maps of the mouse genome. Cur. Opin. Genet. Dev. **4:** 389–394.
5. BROWN, S. D. M. & K. P. STEEL. 1996. Mouse models for human hearing impairment. *In* Genetics and Hearing Impairment, A. Martini, A. P. Read, and D. Stephens, Eds.: 53–63.
6. WILCOX, E. R. 1992. Strategies for constructing a guinea pig organ of Corti cDNA library and its potential use. Otolaryngol. Clin. N. Am. **25:** 1011–1016.
7. RYAN, A. F., S. BATCHER, L. LIN, D. BRUMM, K. O'DRISCOLL & J. P. HARRIS. 1993. Cloning genes from an inner ear cDNA library. Arch. Otolaryngol. Head Neck Surg. **119:** 1217–1220.
8. ROBERTSON, N. G., U. KHETARPAL, G. A. GUTIERREZ-ESPELETA, F. R. BIEBER & C. C. MORTON. 1994. Isolation of novel and known genes from human fetal cochlear cDNA library using subtractive hybridisation and differential screening. Genomics **23:** 42–50.
9. KIMBERLING, W. J. & K. BEISEL. 1996. The use of gene libraries in the study of the molecular genetics of the auditory system. *In* Genetics and Hearing Impairment, A. Martini, A. Read, and D. Stephens, Eds.: 48–52. Whurr. London.
10. VAN GELDER, R. N., M. E. VON ZASTROW, A. YOOL, W. C. DEMENT, J. D. BARCHAS & J. H. EBERWINE. 1990. Amplified RNA synthesized from limited quantities of heterogeneous cDNA. Proc. Natl. Acad. Sci. USA **87:** 1663–1677.

11. EBERWINE, J., H. YEH, K. MIYASHIRO, *et al.* 1992. Analysis of gene expression in single live neurons. Proc. Natl. Acad Sci. USA **89:** 3010–3014.
12. WILCOX, E. R. & J. FEX. 1992. Construction of a cDNA library from microdissected pig organ of Corti. Hear. Res. **62:** 124–126.
13. BEISEL, K. W. & J. E. KENNEDY. 1994. Identification of novel alternatively spliced isoforms of the tropomyosin-encoding gene, Tmnm, in the rat cochlea. Gene **143:** 251–256.
14. GIBSON, F., J. WALSH, P. MBURU, A. VARELA, K. A. BROWN, M. ANTONIO, K. W. BEISEL, *et al.* 1995. A type VII myosin encoded by the mouse deafness gene shaker—1. Nature **374:** 62–64.
15. DRYJA, T. P., T. L. MCGEE, E. REICHEL, *et al.* 1990. A point mutation of the rhodospin gene in one form of retinitis pigmentosa. Nature **343:** 364–366.
16. ROWLAND, L. P. 1988. Dystrophin: A triumph of reverse genetics and the end of the beginning. New Eng. J. Med. **318:** 1392–1394 .
17. ROMMENS, J. M., M. C. IANNUZZI, B. S. KEREM, *et al.* 1989. Identification of the cystic fibrosis gene: Chromosome walking and jumping. Science **245:** 1059–1065.
18. WEIL, D., S. BLANCHARD, J. KAPLAN, *et al.* 1995. Defective myosin VIIa gene responsible for Usher syndrome type IB. Nature **374:** 60–61.
19. FEKETE, D., S. MUTHUKUMAR & D. KARAGOGEOS. 1995. Hair cells and supporting cells share a common progenitor in the chicken basilar papilla. Abstract (1). The Molecular Biology of Hearing and Deafness. Bethesda, Md.
20. CHEN, A. H., I. THALMANN, J. C. ADAMS, K. B. AVRAHAM, N. G. COPELAND, N. A. JENKINS, D. R. BEIER, D. P. COREY, R. THALMANN & G. M. DUYK. 1995. cDNA cloning, tissue distribution, and chromosomal localization of Ocp2, a gene encoding a putative transcription-associated factor predominantly expressed in the auditory organs. Genomics **27:** 389–398.
21. WU, D. & S. H. OH. 1995. Gene expression in the developing chick inner ear. Abstract (2). The molecular biology of hearing and deafness. Bethesda, Md.
22. ERKMAN, L., R. J MCEVILLY, L. LUO, A. K. RYAN, F. HOOSHMAND, S. M. O'CONNELL, E. M. KEITHLEY, D. H. RAPAPORT, A. F. RYAN & M. G. ROSENFELD. 1996. Role of transcription factors Brn-3. 1 and Brn-3. 2 in auditory and visual system development. Nature **381:** 603–606.
23. DE KOK, Y. J. M., S. M. VAN DE MAAREL & M. BITNER-GLINDZIC, *et al.* 1995. Association between X-linked mixed deafness and mutations in the POU domain gene POU3F4. Science **267:** 685–688.
24. VAN DE WATER, T. R. & R. J. RUBEN. 1984. Neurotrophic interactions during in vitro developmental ear. Ann. Otol. Rhinol. Laryngol. **93:** 558–564.
25. ARD, M. D., D. K. MOREST & S. H. HAUGER. 1985. Trophic interactions between the cochleovestibular ganglion of the chick embryo and its synaptic targets in culture. Neuroscience **16:** 151–170.
26. SWANSON, G. J., M. HOWARD & J. LEWIS. 1990. Epithelial autonomy in the development of the inner ear of a bird embryo. Devel. Biol. **137:** 243–257.
27. YLIKOSKI, J., U. PIRVOLA, M. MOSHNYAKOV, J. PALGI, U. ARUMAE & M. SAARMA. 1993. Expression patterns of neurotrophin and their receptor mRNAs in the rat inner ear. Hear. Res. **65**(1–2):69–78.
28. PIRVOLA, U., U. ARUMAE, M. MOSHNYAKOV, J. PALGI, M. SAARMA & J. YLIKOSKI. 1994. Coordinated expression and function of neurotrophins and their receptors in the rat inner ear during target innevation. Hear. Res. **75**(1–2):131–144.
29. LEVI-MONTALCINI, R. 1987. The nerve growth factor 35 years later. Science **237:** 1154–1162 .
30. BARDE, Y. A., D. EDGAR & H. THOENEN. 1982. Purification of a new neurotrophic factor from mammalian brain. EMBO J. **1:** 549–553.

31. ERNFORS, P., C. F. IBANEZ, T. EBENDAL, L. OLSON & H. PERSSON. 1990. Molecular cloning and neurotrophic activities of a protein with structural similarities to nerve growth factor: Developmental and topographical expression in the brain. Proc. Natl. Acad. Sci. USA **87:** 5454–5458.

32. HOHN, A., J. LEIBROCK, K. BAILEY & Y. A. BARDE. 1990. Identification and characterization of a novel member of the nerve growth factor/brain-derived neurotrophic factor family. Nature **344:** 339–341.

33. HALLBÖÖK, F., C. F. IBANEZ & H. PERSSON. 1991. Evolutionary studies of the nerve growth factor family reveal a novel member abundantly expressed in Xenopus ovary. Neuron **6:** 845–858.

34. BERKEMEIER, L. R., J. W. WINSLOW, D. R. KAPLAN, K. NIKOLICS, D. V. GOEDDEL & A. ROSENTHAL. 1991. Neurotrophin-5: A novel neurotrophic factor that activates *trk* and *trk*B. Neuron **7:** 857–866.

35. PIRVOLA, U., J. YLIKOSKI, J. PALGI, E. LEHTONEN & U. ARUMAE. 1992. Brain-derived neurotrophic factor and neurotrophin 3 mRNAs in the peripheral target fields of developing inner ear ganglia. Proc. Natl. Acad. Sci. USA **89:** 9915–9919.

36. ERNFORS, P., J. P. MERLIO & H. PERSSON. 1992. Cells expressing mRNA for neurotrophins and their receptors during embryonic rat development. Eur. J. Neurosci. **4:** 1140–1158.

37. FARINAS, I., K. R. JONES, C. BACKUS, X. Y. WANG & L. F. REICHARDT. 1994. Severe sensory and sympathetic deficits in mice lacking neurotrophin-3. Nature **369:** 658–661.

38. ERNFORS, P., T. VAN DE WATER, J. LORING & R. JAENISCH,. 1995. Complementary roles of BDNF and NT-3 in vestibular and auditory development. Neuron **14(6):** 1153–1164.

39. VAN DE WATER, T. R., H. STAECKER, R. KOPKE, W. LIU, C. HARTNICK, B. MALGRANGE, P. P. LEFEBVRE & G. MOONEN. 1995. Neurotrophic factors: Maintenance and injury-repair of auditory neurons. Abstract (7). The Molecular Biology of Hearing and Deafness. Bethesda, Md.

40. PIRVOLA, U., U. ARUMAE, M. MOSHNYAKOV, J. PALGI, M. SAARMA & J. YLIKOSKI. 1994. Coordinated expression and function of neurotrophins and their receptors in the rat inner ear during target innervation. Hear. Res. **75(1–2):** 131–144.

41. ERNFORS, P., K. F. LEE & R. JAENISCH. 1994. Mice lacking brain derived neurotrophic factor develop with sensory deficits. Nature **368:** 147–150.

42. FRITZSCH, B. & D. H. NICHOLS. 1993. DiI reveals a prenatal arrival of efferents at the differentiating otocyst of mice. Hear. Res. **65:** 51–60.

43. FRITZSCH, B., I. SILOS-SANTIAGO, A. FAGAN & M. BARBACID. 1995. The role of the neurotrophin receptors *trk*B and *trk*C for maintaining the innervation of the developing ear: A study on single and double knockout mice. Abstract (6). The Molecular Biology of Hearing and Deafness. Bethesda, Md.

44. YLIKOSKI, J., U. PIRVOLA & M. SAARMA. 1995. Expression of neurotrophin receptor genes in the inner ear. Abstract (4). The Molecular Biology of Hearing and Deafness. Bethesda, Md.

45. LYON, M. F., S. RASTAN & S. D. M. BROWN. 1995. Genetic Variants and Strains of the Laboratory Mouse. Oxford Univ. Press. Oxford.

46. STEEL, K. P. 1995. Inherited hearing defects in mice. Ann. Rev. Genet. **29:** 675–701.

47. STEEL, K. P. & S. D. M. BROWN. Genes and Deafness. TIG. Vol. 10, No. 12, Elsevier Science. New York.

48. STEEL, K. P., D. R. DAVIDSON & I. J. JACKSON. 1992. TRP-2/DT, a new early melanoblast marker, shows that steel growth factor (*c-kit* ligand) is a survival factor. Development **115:** 1111–1119.

49. STEEL, K. P. & D. HARVEY. 1992. Development of auditory function in mutant mice. *In* Development of Auditory and Vestibular Systems, Vol. 2, R. Romand, Ed: 221–242. Elsevier Press. Amsterdam.

50. BROWN, K. A., M. J. SUTCLIFFE, K. P. STEEL & S. D. M. BROWN. 1992. Close linkage of the olfactory marker protein gene to the mouse deafness mutation *shaker-1*. Genomics **13:** 189–193.

51. EVANS, K. L., J. FANTES, C. SIMPSON, B. ARVEILER, W. MUIR, J. FLETCHER, V. VAN HEYNINGEN, K. P. STEEL, K. A. BROWN, S. D. M. BROWN, D. S. CLAIR & D. J. PORTEOUS. 1992. Human olfactory marker protein maps close to tyrosinase and is a candidate gene for Usher syndrome type 1. Hum. Mol. Genet. **2:** 115–118.

52. KIMBERLING, W. J., C. G. MOLLER, S. DAVENPORT, *et al.* 1992. Linkage of Usher syndrome type 1 gene (USH1B) to the long arm of chromosome 11. Genomics **14:** 988–994.

53. GUILFORD, P., S. BEN ARAB, S. BLANCHARD, J. LEVILLIERS, J. WEISSENBACH, A. BELKAHIA & C. PETIT. 1994. A non-syndrome form of neurosensory, recessive deafness maps to the pericentromeric region of chromosome 13q. Nat. Genet. **6:** 24–28.

54. HASSON, T., M. B. HEINTZELMAN, J. SANTOS-SACCHI & D. P. COREY. 1995. Expression in cochlea and retina of myosin VIIa, the gene product defective in Usher syndrome type 1B. Proc. Natl. Acad. Sci. USA **92:** 9815–9819.

55. COREY, D. P., B. H. DERFLER, T. HASSON & M. MOOSEKER. 1995. Four myosins and a hair cell: Molecular cloning of motor proteins from bullfrog saccular macula. Abstract (74). The Molecular Biology of Hearing and Deafness. Bethesda, Md.

56. HASSON, T. & M. MOOSEKER. 1995. Molecular motors, membrane movements and physiology: Emerging roles for myosins. Curr. Opin. Cell Biol. **7:** 587–594.

57. DUMONT, R. A. & P. G. GILLESBY. 1995. Properties of myosin Iβ'S tale are consistent with its proposed role as hair-cell adaption motor. Abstract (75). The Molecular Biology of Hearing and Deafness. Bethesda, Md.

58. PARVING, A. & V. NEWTON. 1995. Editorial guidelines for descriptions of inherited hearing loss. J. Audiolog. Med. **4:** ii–v.

59. POSWILLO, D. 1973. The pathologies of the first and second brachial arch syndrome. Oral Surg. **35:** 302–329.

60. MELNICK, M. 1980. Hereditary hearing loss and ear dysplasia-renal adysplasia syndromes: Syndrome delineation and possible pathogenesis. Birth Defects **16**(7):59–72.

61. FRASER, F. C., *et al.* 1980. Frequency of brachio-oto-renal (BOR) syndrome in children with profound hearing loss. Am. J. Med. Gen. **7:** 341–349.

62. DIXON, M. J., J. DIXON, T. HOUSEAL, M. BHATT, D. C. WARD, K. KLINGER & G. M. LANDES. 1993. Narrowing the position of the Treacher-Collins Syndrome locus to a small interval between three microsatellite markers at 5q32–33. I. Am. J. Hum. Genet. **52:** 907–914.

63. WAARDENBURG, P. J. 1951. A new syndrome combining developmental anomalies of the eyelids, eyebrows, and nose root with pigmentary defects of the iris and head, hair, and congenital deafness. Am. J. Med. Gen. **3:** 195–253.

64. NILSSON, R. L., N. BORGFORS, I. GAMSTORP, H. E. HOLST & G. LIDEN. 1964. Nonendemic goitre and deafness. Acta Paediatr. Scand. **53:** 117–131.

65. HALLGREN, V. 1959. Retinitis pigmentosa combined with congenital deafness; with vestibulo-cerebellar ataxia and mental abnormality in a proportion of cases. A clinical and genetico-statistical study. Acta Psychiatr. Neurol. Scand. **34** (Suppl. 138): 1–101.

66. BOUGHMAN, J. A., M. VERNON & K. A. SHAVER. 1983. Usher Syndrome: Definition and estimate of prevalence from two high-risk populations. J. Chronic Dis. **36:** 595–603.

67. MARTINI, A. 1996. European Working Group on Genetics of Hearing Impairment. Infoletter, Vol. 1, No. 1.

68. MARTINI, A. & M. MAZZOLI 1996. Organizing a European working group on genetics of hearing impairment. Editorial. J. Audiol. Med. **5**(1): ii–viii.

Index of Contributors